TO HUMANITY

ON PROOF FOR THE EXISTENCE OF GOD, AND OTHER REFLECTIVE INQUIRIES

BY PAUL VJECSNER

PENDEN, NEW YORK

Library of Congress Catalog Card Number: 87-62964
Published by Penden, P.O. Box 464, New York, N.Y. 10101
ISBN: 0-9619519-0-7
Manufactured in the United States of America

First printing 1988
Second printing 1990
Third printing 1992

CONTENTS

INTRODUCTION

Unexpected claims from unexpected quarters usually meet with much resistance and often with resentment if they disregard what is widely or authoritatively believed to be true. Attempted past contributions to knowledge are well known to have been rejected because they conflicted with contemporary stands, and upon eventual acceptance as of merit of what was offered intentions have been to forestall similar adverse responses. Yet the acceptance of new views tends again to harden opposition to subsequent attempted contributions in conflict with them. The previous relinquishment of a then prevailing outlook for what seems a truer one brings about a reluctance to consider that the later of these, too, might be corrected. This is especially true if what is offered, however of value, does not follow current avenues of thought. Men can be overcome by successes, perpetuating searches in those directions to the neglect of what presents itself, in the perhaps most common fallacy, that of undue generalization.

The opposition to the unacknowledged may intensify if what is submitted is not merely presumed wrong, but is, even if supposed right, of determinations regarded as either unlikely or impossible to make, as are ones propounded in this treatise.

Among determinations regarded long as unlikely or impossible to make are the demonstration of axioms or postulates underlying mathematics and logic, and the resolution of paradoxes or other incongruities held to be of the same fields. More recently certain propositions in these fields came to be believed demonstrated unprovable though true, and on a wider philosophical scale statements customarily referred to as metaphysical have been thought impossible to demonstrate as true likewise, if not looked upon as meaningless.

The questions in metaphysics, which has been a major philosophical branch, concern such issues as what sort of fundamental entities, as may be mind contrasted with matter, exist, and various speculative systems were in the past constructed to supply the answers. For some time ancient mathematical accomplishments were of extensive influence. Some thinkers accordingly essayed corresponding methods in philosophy, among them notably Spinoza, who built inferentially on assumed axioms in the manner of the geometry of Euclid. However, not only did the inferences lack sufficient rigor, but the axioms, the initial assumptions supposed true, were far less self-evident than those of geometry. A point taken up in the present treatise is whether science indeed must depend on initial assumptions of fact, or whether all its presumable truths should not alike be ascertained. Aside from that consideration the progress of natural science, repeatedly overturning the results of metaphysical speculation, gained a predominant position for its methods of physical experiment and observation. And truths in metaphysics came to be held not capable of proof because they seem not amenable to these methods. It is for not being subject to similar verification that statements were even declared meaningless, unless of logic or mathematics. The last mentioned exceptions have been, further, regarded as merely tautologies, true by definition.

The tendencies can be viewed as denying the existence in consciousness of conceptions of things not physical, not to speak of denial of consciousness, and accordingly pronouncements like those of ethics or aesthetics, admittedly of meaning, are considered not to be statements allowing of truth or falsity, but expressions of other kinds, such as conveyance of feelings.

To deny consciousness itself is, to be sure, not only to forego finding of any reality at all, since finding it means it is of consciousness, but because all things, real or otherwise, are of recognition only be being of consciousness, without it there is no certainty of any thing.

As regards the meaningless statements contended, the intimation is that a statement can be inferred meaningless on determining it not to be verifiable as proposed. But a statement is understood to be verified in accordance with its meaning, and its meaningfulness is accordingly not pending its verifiability. Irrespectively, one can conceive of not only physical states but what might be termed otherworldly ones, whether they have actuality or not, and these conceptions can likewise be made the understood meanings of statements.

Considering statements of mathematics or logic, they can, regardless of whether of definitions, equally be held to be of conceptual entities, as exemplified by the ideal figures of geometry. And that they should be tautologies, supplying no new information, is refuted by the very dependence on them as major sources of learning.

And in regard to expressions not looked upon as statements of truth or falsity, this position does not prevent the reality again in consciousness of feelings or other ingredients, however expressions asserting the same be designated.

Distinguishing nevertheless between fleeting elements of consciousness and realities of a more tangible kind, more moderate viewpoints than the preceding have for a longer time been that such realities can only be known by means of sense experience, not the aid of deduction. A distinction has been made thus between matters of fact, concerning things of the world, and matters of reason, concerning logic and mathematics, with the latter ones, while highly regarded, not admitted to furnish any truths about the former. In deliberation of the usefulness of logic it was suggested that facts are at best by it substantiated but not discovered. But substantiating a fact can be taken to mean none other than discovering it.

Because of the spoken of reliance on scientific method, the sciences of which it is the province have alone been considered by philosophers to have the competency to determine what exists. Hence metaphysics became either frankly conjectural or was abandoned as a fruitful enterprise. Philosophy in general is for the same reason no longer concerned with determining worldly facts. There appears even a prevalent notion that anything discovered about the world is at once carried to, as it is said, its logical conclusion, although mathematics is evidence that conclusions drawn about things, as in findings in that science, can be virtually limitless. In lieu of the other inquiries and with the prospect of aiding them in other fields, philosophy thus directs its attention largely toward clarification of concepts, the nature of many of which, too, is believed to be, if not indeterminable, indefinable.

The physical character of scientific method, however, incorporates a host of presuppositions, of understandings or knowledge on which the authenticity of the observations depends, and these understandings, possessed by everyman, are not verified by that method. They are of metaphysical entities, of what things have reality, as well as of deductive principles and last brought up concepts, and their oversight, beside preventing insights, gives rise to mentioned paradoxes. The last is remindful that inasmuch as these understandings comprise presupposed knowledge they cannot, in accord with the well known and in a coming chapter discussed law of contradiction, be defensibly denied.

Inasmuch as they comprise knowledge they might also be thought to represent knowledge as an innate attribute of man, as said to be put forward by Socrates. He is storied to argue for it by eliciting a mathematical principle through reasoning from an unschooled boy. The knowledge presently at issue, however, is not necessarily one that has been ever present, but that underlies scientific or other particular knowledge about the natural world. But as knowledge which is presupposed by other findings, it and anything that may be deduced from it, is by strength of implication at least equal in certainty to other findings and susceptible to exploration.

To disclose how such an exploration can be carried out, how in general fundamental or other truths can be reflectively demonstrated and thereby an actual rather than speculative edifice of existence revealed, is together with such demonstrations the object of this writing. It is an investigation that, as made known by the title, includes such subject matter as the existence of God, which, irrespective of the arguments used, may in its exalted objective encounter strongest opposition.

For this reason and those given earlier it is urged that in reading this exposition one set aside preconceptions and rely on one's apprehension regarding the determinations herein made.

The existence of God is uppermost in consideration, because of its momentousness. But as indicated, other realities are in like manner explored, among them, beside realities in a customary sense, truths by which, as by logical principles or even meanings of words, they may be determined, as well as the reflective methods by which, as by deduction, it is possible to determine either of these. In the process, the difficulties associated with the seemingly indemonstrable and insoluble matters spoken of will be found surmountable.

PROCESS OF INQUIRY

The relied on methods of inference, of reflective determinations made on the basis of what is known, have traditionally been those of induction and deduction. Popularly stated, the first, applying to nature, is inference of principles or laws from constancies in it although these are conceivable otherwise, and the second, exemplified in logic and mathematics, is similar inference of one thing from another but with the other not conceivable without the first. This distinction may not coincide with everyone's. What the difference between the two kinds of inference is, or whether there is any, has been debated. It should suffice at this time that the difference here meant by the terms is, more exactly than in the preceding, between, in deduction, inference of what is intrinsic in things, in the sense that it, although not known before, is part of the things as conceived, and, in induction, inference of what is extrinsic to things, of what is not of those parts. The concept of conceivability or not may not be adequately useful, because in for instance lengthy deductions in mathematics it is strange to say that the result is not conceivable otherwise. And it remains later in this book to find that both connections, the intrinsic and extrinsic, exist, how, for the matter of that, they become deductive and inductive knowledge.

The two connections, respective ones also called analytic and synthetic, can as ones that are negations of each other be seen exhaustive, in conformance with the likewise known and in a later chapter discussed law of excluded middle. Further, since both inductive and deductive inferences are based on unfailing connections as to things and what is true of them, they provide complete certainty. These two means of inference are therefore those utilized herein as well.

As apparent in the foregoing, it is not the intention here to conjecture on possible realities, but to base determinations only on criteria not wanting in certainty. The criteria used will in point of fact be seen to exceed in certainty the scientific ones customarily resorted to. The discovery in natural science, in the inductive sciences, of particular laws, of invariabilities, encounters utmost difficulties, and the scientist relies heavily on theory for determination of fact. And, as noted, basic principles in mathematics and logic, in the deductive sciences, have defied their ascertainment as unquestionable, and, while held to be so inconsistently with holding them unprovable, they, too, have been consigned to theory.

The use of theory, beside experiment and observation another prevailing method in natural science, is, again, for that reason respected elsewhere. It should be recognized in this respect that theory unreserved is but a return to speculation.

Still, in sciences of the physical world theory might be of assistance, because the very nature of an extrinsic connection allows for unlimited possibilities, and a reasonable but tentative judgement could be made as to the area in which to look. The same is not the case when the connections are intrinsic. The area is already delimited, and only what is contained in it can be the object of a search. This does not render the search easy, but a theory can becloud a survey of what is already in cognition.

A theory can be a burden in other sciences as well, because of the conviction it can carry by help of accompanying arguments. An accepted principle in reasoning has been reductio ad absurdum, whereby if a hypothesis leads to a false conclusion it is inferred false. It is tempting to think that if it leads to a true conclusion it is true, which is fallacious as to be found. Although the fallaciousness is not unknown to science, there is nonetheless considerable reliance on the hypothetico-deductive method, which follows that reasoning. The point is that a theory can rest partly on cogent arguments, as by use of mathematics, instilling certitude, and in consequence an opportunity for other answers, of which there may be quite many, can be hampered.

A worse yet effect of implanted beliefs is that they can be pursued with too much zeal, as are often doctrines and ideologies and as can be the inexactly or falsely based theses of such as behavioral sciences, so as to be deleterious to humankind. Emphasis is given to these pitfalls of theory since false conclusions may well be responsible for nearly all of man-made ills.

While to surmise the truth in many situations is unavoidable in life, it can frequently be avoided in research. In statistical researches, often of scantest and misleading evidence, theoretical conclusions need be drawn very far from lightly, and in the researches engaged in in this disquisition they need, for the opposite reason, not be drawn at all. As indicated, the inferences in the present researches are of the certainty of, on one hand, inductive criteria which apply to experiences more fundamental than particular physical findings, and of, on the other hand, deductive criteria which apply to factors that can be found already contained in the concepts. Unquestionable knowledge is accordingly possible in both.

In addition to these methods of inference, there is the question of premises, material on which conclusions, the inferences, are based. This material might be simply referred to, as earlier above, as that which is known. But to determine what is initially known is by no means a simple problem, as attested by another major branch of philosophy, epistemology.

Much of what may be considered known is itself the result of inference, to include many of the referred to presuppositions, which will be examined correspondingly. Accordingly, in order to consider the material for earliest inference, it will be required to revert to the entities of interest themselves, as represented by their concepts, before anything, including their existence, is inferred, whether or not the entities be spoken of as objects of knowledge. Thus, to establish what truly may be known, the initial task will be to determine the nature of the entities or concepts considered, a task usually identified with definition. This procedure, the determination of the nature of the things considered, may, in harmony with the procedures of inference, be termed eduction. It is differentiated from definition, because the primary concern will be apprehension of the concept, rather than its formulation in language.

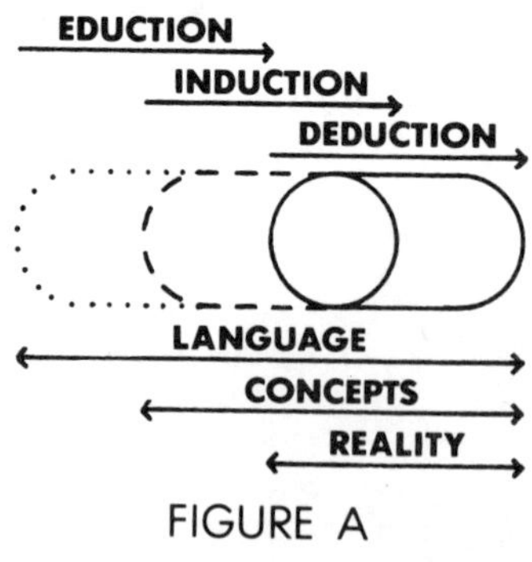

FIGURE A

Figure A here correspondingly delineates this step alongside the two of subsequent inference, as taking place in the present investigations. Inquiry proceeds by educing beyond the language through which they are in this and other discourse conveyed the concepts of concern; by inducing from these concepts realities by which a world is known; and by deducing from these realities further ones. Since realities determined, as are other things, are treated of through both, concepts and language, these two subjects extend beside the third to the end of the diagram. Their reverse extensions, past that of reality (solid line), in addition signify imaginary concepts (dashed line), and language void of meaning (dotted line).

Whereas above the diagram the three procedures are applied to the subjects as noted, they may be used extensively in intermediate searches. Eduction can also be of any concept later acquired; induction is usually from occurrences within a reality already determined; and deduction may concern purely conceptual entities as ground for logical or mathematical principles. It stands to reason that the use herein will be in such a comprehensive manner.

Similarly, the three subjects below the diagram are designated in the titles of the first and second chapters but are likewise concerned in the further of the four. The third chapter deals with principles by which one thing can be deduced from another, the things intended to be of reality, and the chapter is hence a furtherance of what realities may be determined, with language and concepts, mentioned as pervasive, accordingly also involved. And the concluding chapter, similarly proceeding through language and concepts, is of realities that are derived via the other determinations and are outside of what is viewed as worldly experience.

The repleteness and range of this undertaking may appear discouraging as a reading to some. However, while the material may be difficult to construct, it should not present the same difficulty in comprehension. It is, as known, often the case that the more extensive an inquiry the simpler its outcome, and the same proves to be the case at present.

This, too, may be contrary to expectations, for solutions to philosophical problems in particular, because implicitly encompassing, are looked to as exceptionally complex. So dominant is this anticipation that a thesis not elaborate to the point of being unfathomable can be refused outright, unawares that failure of accomplishment may hide behind a veil of inscrutability. Authors are often indeed praised for the depth of their insights, while endless scholarship is expended to estimate what they may be.

There may also, contrariwise, be expectations of lesser multiplicity, frequently in seeking immoderate uniformity. But in accordance with the accustomed view of the issues, the findings made should be seen to be of unawaited simplicity.

The writing itself can furthermore, in the light of the voluminous other writings on its subject matter, be seen to be of substantial brevity. This because of its dependence on conclusive demonstration. The large number of supporting arguments through which a speculative work may gain conviction can be omitted, as can arguments that are irrelevant, which a work often includes.

Approachability of the discussions may be further enhanced by the common ownership of the ideas discussed. They reside at the basis of everybody's conscious existence and require no specialized knowledge. For the same reason there is no need for use of esoteric language, and terminology not of wide currency is avoided.

This accessibility may likewise not be expected, and the reminder may therefore be appropriate that one be guided not by expectations about the nature of the findings or their circumstance, but by one's cognitions concerning them.

It may in addition to the above be mentioned that parts such as chapters or sections can be read individually by individual readers. Although premises on which conclusions there are based may be substantiated elsewhere, they should appear true as a matter of course. Pertinent other parts will nonetheless be referred to, as was done with respect to certain logical laws in this introduction.

The reader may over and above these be attracted by the process of deductive discovery, as readers have been for centuries regarding the geometry demonstrations in Euclid's Elements, or in recent times regarding the detective exploits of Sherlock Holmes and other fictional investigators.

The considerations listed should make acquaintance with much of what follows feasible for every contemplative reader.

Chapter I
LANGUAGE AND CONCEPTS

Section 1
THE SIGNIFICATION OF LANGUAGE

The presence of language in man's pursuit of knowledge is critical, since language is almost the only form in which all known, as well as assumed, is set down and communicated. Accordingly words are often viewed as inherently standing for certain entities, and it is endeavored to discover what the entity represented by a given word is.

What constitutes life, for example, is a matter of appreciable debate; as an illustration, the Encyclopedia Britannica offers five alternative and protracted definitions. As another example, light has been progressively redefined, in the confidence that it is in the course described more accurately; instead of for instance defining it as, initially understood, visual sensation, it would be defined as electromagnetic radiation of wavelengths beginning and ending with, in contradiction of the first meaning, invisible ultraviolet and infrared.

Language as used by man does not presume undiscovered meanings, however, which man is to investigate. Language is by definition, as would be said, and in conformance with the beginning of this chapter a form of conveyance of things in the awareness of man, who thereby assigns the meaning to the words.

The preceding statement, as can any other, may afford the first occasion for disputation in the body of this treatise. What linguistic expressions are about or mean is a matter of extensive theory, known as semantics. Notwithstanding a frequent acknowledgement that the meaning of words is decided by consent of its users, it is maintained that it has a more remote inception. It is likened to government, which likewise may have a more obscure beginning than a sometimes supposed social contract. However, the origin of a meaning is not relevant, as need not be the origin of a government. Men do agree or not to use the meaning, or to abide by the form of government.

As was indicated in the introduction, of account with regard to language herein is that the inquiry centers on entities however worded, not, in a linguistic study, on the words. That is to say, what is herein of account is not the initial meaning of the language used, nor what other meaning it might have, but what is wished to be expressed by it. It is here thus dependent on agreement or decision what the words mean. The same can be taken to be the case in regard to the customary philosophical or comparable search for the meaning of expressions. The search is not for the meaning of words as used by someone else, in which case the issue might be considered a linguistic inquiry into a foreign or obsolete language. The search is for the meaning of words as used by the inquirers themselves, as happens with "life" as used by physiologists, or "light" as used by physicists. In that event, however, the inquirers know the meaning, which is the one intended by them.

The truth of this inference, as of any, would still be challenged, and a frequent query concerns the understanding of language as conveyor of things in man's awareness, in man's consciousness. The contention is that, at one extreme, abstract words like "and" and, at another extreme, concrete words like "chair" do not designate things residing in consciousness, aside from the mentioned view that there is no consciousness. It was also mentioned that all things are of recognition by being of consciousness, which is to say more generally that anything that might be considered, whether something merely contemplated or of a determination like a decision or discovery, is so by manifestation in consciousness. Thus an abstract word like "and", although not designating an independent entity, is represented conceptually by the presence of more than one thing in some circumstance, and a concrete word like "chair", although designating an object viewed as separate from the perception of it, is represented conceptually by that perception. The words are used to designate those entities in accordance with those conceptual representations. The representations in awareness need not even be what are held to be direct perceptions of the objects. The objects one speaks of may only be thought of, and in the case of hypothetical ones they furthermore need not exist although the words used for them, not referring to the thought of them, would refer only to existing ones. What matters is that one has a conception of the thing referred to, perhaps indirectly, rather than using words empty of such content.

This issue is not the present one, however, which is the awareness that certain words stand for certain things, rather than the awareness of those things. It is similarly beside the point to question whether that awareness of what the words mean can be said to be knowledge. That the users of words have knowledge of what they mean was asserted in the above inference, and inasmuch as previous to it only such as consent to the meaning by the users was spoken of, it might be argued that its knowledge is not the consequence. The argument may be advanced because of the alluded to belief that knowledge can only be acquired through sense experience. It concerns the synthetic connections spoken of as contrasted with analytical ones and held alone to comprise facts, compared to the supposed definitional truth of the other. Someone may therefore propose that definitions do not constitute knowledge, and that as a result the above determination does not hold. But as suggested regarding statements supposed meaningless or neither true nor false, a decision over language, as presently whether something may be termed knowledge, does not dispose of underlying matters. The users of a language were said above to know their meaning because the of concern understood awareness of it is normally referred to as knowledge. And it may be specified here correspondingly that by knowledge of a meaning is meant awareness of it, instead of awareness of its assumption, however the awareness be obtained, as by one's own definition. It may be remarked that by awareness and hence knowledge is not meant present consciousness alone of a thing, but its mentioned being sometime considered, in the sense that it may be stored in memory. And the question is whether the users of a language do in this sense not know their meaning, accordingly seeking it, or whether they do.

The affirmative reply should by the foregoing be obvious, the meant knowledge consisting in the very having decided the use, and it should be observed that the inference is made about other persons by induction. The elucidation of how the induction is made can be postponed, however, because the comprehension altogether of this writing, as of the writing or other forms of communication by others, presupposes, is proof, that the induction has been performed. It has been learned that others convey meanings through language in the same manner as oneself does. As a matter of fact, since a form of language is generally not devised by oneself, one uses it in that manner because one learns that that is the usage by others.

This writer thus has likewise induced that language is used in this manner by others, and the induction of understandings held in common extends farther. It concerns also any observations herein made through the language, observations which were noted to be of basic matters in man's life. The observations can be of the mentioned educed entities themselves which man has cognition of, as well as of the inferred facts about them as brought out in this treatise. In all of this is implicit of course that the induction as pertains to language is not only that it is used by men alike for conveyance of their meaning, but that particular meanings are likewise held in common.

All particular meanings, it is clear, need not be understood by every speaker of the language. Language is an inconstant thing, differing not only with communities, but with individuals. Of pertinence at present is that while the hearer of a language need in instances be informed of its meaning, the user need not, but knows it.

The recognition of this knowledge can be of estimable value to thinkers, since corresponding calling forth of what entity is named provides a basis for further knowledge about it. The like took place in inferring that since consciousness is meant to extend to all objects of man's consideration, all meanings man considers for words are of consciousness. The recognition that a meaning is known can also dissuade from supposing a different one, to thereby wrongly infer a fact about, ironically, the originally meant. Such inference takes place in the frequent argument that if the self is held to include the body then the destruction of one's body is the destruction of oneself, although the self first meant with respect to immortality is one dissociated from the body.

The presence of knowledge of the meaning of the words man uses does not imply that a verbal definition, or even a suitable eduction in thought alone, is an easy task if not a prohibitive one. One often thinks of only familiar instances of what is named, and as with other knowledge a taxing of memory may be required. The knowledge does imply, however, that the search for knowledge of various fundamental entities, which has been a concern of philosophy, is misconceived. It has been continually sought to know what entities like virtue are, with volumes sometimes devoted to the questions, without cognizance that, insofar as the concern is not with an unfamiliar language, what the entities named are is known to the seekers in accordance with their sometime deciding.

These mistaken searches for knowledge already possessed are perpetuated among leading schools by phenomenology and analytic philosophy, in their main enterprises of investigating essences or concepts. It is the investigation mentioned in the introduction as having replaced former ones in philosophy, so as to furnish information for others elsewhere. But in concord with observations in the same place and by the above, possession of that information belongs to the understandings presupposed in science as in all human activity making use of language.

Accordingly, as regards linguistic meaning the formulation of theory is not only not required, similarly to the situation in logic, but it is misplaced. In deduction, though conclusive answers may be reflectively available, they may be difficult to attain and theory the only substitute. But what the meaning of words is has been determined, and theory but infringes on it.

Be determinations dependent thus on definition or on other factors, once any have been appropriately made they cannot, lest engaging in contradiction again, be controverted by argument. It has as remarked of Socrates (page 3, fourth paragraph), assuredly, been put forward that man possesses what is sometimes called a priori knowledge, knowledge that precedes any determination. It is contrasted with a posteriori knowledge, knowledge derived from experience, and it should be explained that it is meant here in the sense in which it excludes any finding, physical or reflective. Thus certain logical principles are held to be known without confirmation. But something proposed to be true, as would be a theory in any field, becomes by definition admittedly known to be true only if it is found to be so.

The preceding speaks again of knowledge, but with respect to more than meaning, and its implied definition as including a certainty would be questioned. It would be maintained that the knowledge one has before findings need not have the certainty attached to things afterward. But the issue is exactly the certainty that can be attached to things. By knowledge here is meant, as can be held to be its common meaning, the complete certainty connected with having determined that something is the case. Otherwise a fact would not be held known, but merely perhaps quite certain. In other words, in following through from the definition of knowledge of a meaning (page 11, first paragraph), by knowledge in an inclusive sense is meant awareness of something actual, in whatever the form by which something is meant to be so, instead of awareness of something assumed, however probable the thing. Among the assumptions are meant to be beliefs, which accordingly, howsoever infused with conviction, fall short of knowledge. The definition of knowledge as justified true belief, frequent in philosophy, is accordingly inadequate. Objections to it are of the contention that it is not apparent what makes a belief justified. But the justification can be characterized independently, by again the particular way by which something is meant to be fact. Justification for a belief only, however, is insufficient because of its very limitation by its meaning, even though the belief may be true.

In the light of the foregoing it should upon appropriate demonstration of something not be requisite to address opposing arguments. If therefore such arguments are in this exposition intermittently surveyed it is because they may be well known or their discussion instructive. In the one case the inaccuracy may not be discerned, with men laboring under misapprehension, and in the other case additional observations can be made, supplementing primary ones.

With reference to linguistic meaning, theories dealing with it as a whole tend correspondingly not to investigate the meaning of individual expressions, but what sort of things are meant by them in general. Proposals on individual meanings will in this treatise in the main be considered when they come into question. As to what sort of things are meant by words in general, any attempt to particularize those things, since they are up to the speakers, is as misapplied as are theories about individual meanings. The issue has been moreover confounded with the question of what is sometimes phrased as the meaning of meaning. It is a question concerning an individual word again, rather than words in general.

The phrase "meaning of meaning" is of course begging the question, since, contrary to the intimation, if what "meaning" stands for is not known at the end of the phrase it is not known at its start, the purport of the whole not understood. But the question being, in using here a presumably understood synonym, what "meaning" stands for, the situation is such that, in asserting to try to know what words in general mean, one cannot make up one's mind about what one wishes to say by "mean" or other words used in the process.

Furthermore in the questioning of particular expressions others, less accustomed ones, are often substituted for them, forgetting that since unusual, they are more difficult yet to comprehend. In place of thus asking "What does this word mean?" it is asked "What is it to say this word?", and the second phraseology is evidently the one unclear to the usual hearer. Rather than responding with a definition as customarily desired, one might try to assist in pronunciation. How by replacing in these attempts other words as well beside "meaning" language is, contrary to intention, not clarified but obfuscated, is illustrated with respect to speaking of a person as "one", as done at the end of the preceding paragraph. The notion being that the second and third use of the word in a like sentence can be taken to speak of someone other than the first does, writers would replace them by "his" and "he". But by usage the interpretation is the opposite. The substitutions signify thus a reading into words meanings at odds with those agreed to.

That the word "meaning" itself be in this way held ambiguous is interestingly attributable to a supposed twofold signification of words in general, regardless of whether the signification be called meaning or not. The duality does not concern an expression's two what are generally called senses, but two kinds of things an expression is in, inconsistently, a single sense thought to designate. In further inconsistency as observed, since what expressions designate is arbitrary, they cannot all designate the same particular kind of thing, let alone two.

That they are believed to can be viewed as due to the cognition that while language can designate worldly objects, it is made to do so by reference to conceptual representations of them. Approximately corresponding to these conceptual and worldly interpretations, the respective two signfications supposed of words or composites of them have been variously named intension and extension, connotation and denotation, or sense and reference. The last mentioned and most recent division is argued by adducing the difference in expressions by which a given thing can be referred to. Accordingly it is contended that whereas "the morning star" and "the evening star" both refer to the planet Venus, they cannot have the same meaning. If they did, it is maintained, then by knowing the meaning of both, one would know that they refer to the same thing, when in fact the sameness is an astronomic discovery.

The specific argument can again be seen a matter of definition. "Refer to" and "mean" can be considered synonyms, and by "morning star" and "evening star" is in fact respectively said to be meant a certain star seen at sunrise and one seen at sunset. That is to say, the star itself, not the circumstance of its observation, is said to be meant, and despite thus meaning in both cases the same thing, one may not know that the same star is at issue.

To hold that meaning only concerns a certain character of the thing referred to, not the thing itself, also contradicts the purported dual aspect of meaning spoken of in the same regard, by which one of the aspects concerns the thing itself. This duality further, whether termed one of meaning or not, does not take place in the above designations of the planet. While they concern it as wholes, their parts, those of the composite designations specifically, concern other things, ones connected with it. One and the same unit does not have two kinds of meaning. The different meanings regarding the two phrases do not concern their wholes but their parts, simply because different things are named by them. The duality is for the same reasons not true of complete sentences, to which it was also proposed to apply.

What a sentence, a declarative one in particular, as a unit refers to is, naturally, also subject to debate. The referent is usually said to be a proposition, and it is not always clear what that word refers to either. The issue is again one of consent, and a declarative sentence, herein in short called a statement, is, alike with other linguistic units used in more than one sense. In its widest use a statement can be held to be of a straightforward assertion of fact.

By an assertion, to be clear, is not again meant a statement, but its content, the discussed object of consciousness. That content of a statement is, worded otherwise, the internal ascertainment, the affirmation, of the state described in it. As an object of consciousness the affirmation can be characterized as a taking into cognizance the actuality of that state. The affirmation may have been made at any time past though conveyed by a present statement. A statement, it should be noted, does not, contrary to some contention, stand for the state itself, which is done by a phrase. The state in "Birds fly" is referred to by "the flight of birds", but whereas the first expression, the statement, signifies the affirmation of the state, the second expression, the phrase, signifies the state, as if its affirmation had been granted.

Statements can, certainly, also be falsehoods, in which case they may signify intent to delude that the stated is true, or unwarranted certitude of it. Statements are, further, frequently used to signify suppositions regarding which something is to be demonstrated, furnishing ground for speaking of them as about propositions. A discourse may set out to demonstrate the truth of a proposition, as done in mathematics, or to assume it for the sake of argument, as done in logic. When its substantiation is conclusive, the proposition can in truth be regarded as an above assertion of fact, and when it is not, or the proposition merely serves as a postulate, then the sentence stating it informs in effect tacitly that the supposed fact is a supposed one.

Of interest is that sentences and other word combinations have, as do words, in single senses, redundantly, single meanings. And the word "meaning" can as others also be used in more than one sense, by a sense understood, as suggested by in the last sentence mentioned redundancy, a meaning as in the preceding explicated. What is of pertinence is that when two meanings, e.g. connotation and denotation, are said to be associated with expressions, said is that associated with them are two things, that may happen to be called by the same name. But of interest in the linguistic inquiry is a particular sense of meaning, which word it will be seen can be used in more than two senses, as can more than two things be associated with a word. One can associate with a word its pronunciation, as remarked, its etymology, and so forth. And one can associate with it in connection with the thing named various things known about the thing. The point is that in the case of for instance the planet Venus, one can associate with it things about it such as being the morning or evening star, without those things being what is meant by its designation.

It is in fact because different utterances speak of the same thing that something what is called informative is said about it. This thought was in the arguments for two meanings expressed by saying that whereas "*A* equals *A*" is uninformative, "*A* equals *B*" is not. Hence, it was argued, *A* cannot mean the same thing *B* does. And by the present sense of "mean" it is owing to the very identity that the same thing is meant. What is not the same is the name, the description, or perhaps the unspoken particular attribute considered. Only in the last case, the other cases assumed to name the attributes, can an additional content different from the present sense of the meant be spoken of. To explain, when making a statement about something named by a word, one considers under it, unless the word itself is the subject, some particular attribute known of the thing, of which more is then stated. "Earth is the planet man lives on" may merely be a definition of a word, but in "Earth is the third planet from the sun" some particular attribute other than stated may be considered under the subject. In other words, both the subject and what is said of it speak of the same thing, but under the first less of particular attributes is understood. All this is natural to all learning, in knowing about things talked about only so much and then determining more.

When the particulars known are unspoken, they can be considered understood premises, with demonstrations including them familiar in logic as enthymemes, in which conclusions may be reached from unstated facts. By the preceding it should be clear that the silent understandings under words, inasmuch as things talked about are seldom described, abound, and they can generally be held to coincide with the particular attributes by which the entity first becomes known or defined, whereafter other attributes are determined. They can also be, however, of particular attributes known besides, and in either case one might speak of these understandings as meanings, in another sense of the word than described. But because it is another sense, one would be dealing with something else associated with words, not with their signification as expounded. This other sense of meaning can further unlike presumed differ from occasion to occasion, although the same name is used. When making a statement about the planet Venus, one may think of it as either the morning star or the evening star. In speaking of particular attributes as a meaning, furthermore, meaning can be split into additional two senses. One is of attributes in consciousness when a thing is considered, and the other of attributes by which a thing is fundamentally understood and often defined. Both meanings, it will be seen, can be drawn upon for inference.

When the limited attributes by which a thing is considered, moreover, are intended to be what is meant when using its name, the distinction between this meant and the whole entity referred to is not the assumed one between the conceptual and the worldly. The goddess Venus may be considered by the limited attributes of being either the Roman goddess of beauty or of love, but the possessor of the whole of the attributes need herself not exist; the opposite takes place concerning the planet of that name, the attributes of its morning and evening appearance existing with it.

In contrast to intending meaning to apply to those aspects of what is named that are conceptual, meaning is sometimes regarded as applying only to things of the physical world, as suggested in the introduction in relation to statements held meaningless. Those statements, it was noted, were considered ones whose truth or falsity could not be verified through natural science. It was noted also that some pronouncements were in conjunction acknowledged not to be so verifiable though meaningful. They were accordingly viewed as nondeclarative sentences, neither true nor false. Irrespectively, however, of the often declarative form of those sentences, stating such as that something is beautiful, all sentences can be seen as declarative in content, asserting something that is true or false. As language they, in keeping with what was said, are meant to transmit information about something in awareness, the informing of it a declaring, an asserting, true or false. A question informs of the wish to know something; a request of the wish to receive something.

This sameness of assertion in sentences notwithstanding, it has been maintained that the meaning of the sentences in question has to do with such as the attitude of the speaker or listener, as would be their expression of approval or disapproval. The speaker's wishes referred to in the preceding could indeed be held attitudes meant, explicit or implicit. But to hold the attitude of the listener as the meaning adds but another, nonlinguistic, sense of it, that of the purpose, the use, of the sentence. The use language is put to is another of the things associated with it and not meant to be its content. That content as its meaning is a precondition for its use, as when informing someone about something in order to gain a certain response. It has been also submitted that the meaning of words is the accompanying outward behavior of their users. Overlooking how farfetched, this opinion has only to do with a further nonlinguistic sense of meaning, that of what goes with a thing, what is implied by it. It is another association, now of the user's behavior with the words, to wit with their meaning as content.

What that meaning is by consent of its users, by which it is therefore known to them, was expounded in this section. And because of the pervasiveness of the correspondingly mistaken search for the meaning of linguistic expressions, in discussing various entities herein it will recurrently be stressed that the meaning of the terms used for them will not be determined by an estimation of it, in accordance with an enigmatic origin. Their meaning will instead be determined by choice, in accordance with the entities of concern. If there should be estimation it will be as to the suitability of the terms in the light of usage.

Since the entities dealt with are of common acquaintance, there should for the most part be no trouble correlating an entity with a sense of a word or term in use. The attention is nevertheless on the entity considered, and that it should be that particular entity which is considered will be either expressly or tacitly made apparent. That is to say, it may for instance be at times specified in this writing that an expression used in it has a certain meaning, with the understanding that that is the meaning of concern to the reader as well as to the writer. Not to impoverish language, moreover, the use of words will not be needlessly restricted to a single sense, their particular sense no doubt recognized from their context, and more than one expression may be used for the same entity as well.

The search may then proceed toward what may be known about the entities, the objects in awareness, that are of concern, however named. And since objects in man's awareness take for man the form in which they are presented to it, the knowledge will be sought with respect to those forms, which may inclusively be termed concepts.

Section 2
CONCEPTS AND THEIR CONSTITUENTS

Because it does not seem out of the ordinary that entities that are the contents of man's awareness be called concepts, it should not be important to give reason for, though doing so, the use of the word. As in instances herein where the intended meaning of a term is only given, there is no problem in affixing the word to the entity. The preponderance of the terminology used will evidently not be defined at all. The defining terms may be asked to be defined also, and so on endlessly. Most of the meaning must therefore perforce be grasped from the context, as it is in all discourse and is of course practicable accordingly, as explicated. It may be added that far from giving a reason for use of a word for an entity of a discussion, giving definitions of key terms is in many expositions refused on grounds that it is unworkable, in resemblance to the believed uncertainty of meaning described in the first section. These presumed difficulties were in the introduction mentioned with regard to concepts, by which term, it may be remarked, discussants, though disputing the same, refer to the very things represented by words, in accordance with the present definition.

Despite these considerations, because "concept" in the present sense refers to all things of human apprehension, including those of language itself, it should be favorable to supply ground for the word's use, in order that its signification be comprehended with ease.

Unlike "consciousness", "concept" is less frequently used for all apprehended, this time for anything belonging to that all, rather than for the entirety alone. Accordingly it would be objected that the definition of the word is too sweeping, that there are important differences among objects of human awareness. The domain of an expression, however, can be as wide as desired, without taking away from either inside or outside its boundaries. Any intricacies associated with the subject should therefore not be layed at the door of definition, but investigated separately. The more particular things in consciousness that sometimes would be meant by concepts are usually the ones distinguished from things in the world, and concepts are at times even within that limited range distinguished from else.

As concerns the exclusion of worldly things, one can again be misled into wondering if one knows in any way the nature of for example chairs, contrary to the observed knowledge of what entities one names by words. One identifies a thing, including a worldly one, by the nature by which considered, and should one suppose a nature different from that, it would contradictorily not be of the thing considered.

As pertains to concepts as still more particular things of the part of consciousness not of the world, they are regarded in opposing ways. Concepts are sometimes viewed as ideas of classes of things, while classes of things, in the traditional debate about universals, are sometimes considered to exist in name or in reality rather than as concepts.

The problem of universals offers a prominent example of the pursuit of linguistic meaning already possessed, and of the potential deceptiveness of language side by side with its utility in succinctly denoting multitudinous things.

A universal is, or is what is represented by, a term such as "man", which does not refer to only one individual but to a class, in this instance to all men. But since a universal term does not refer to a class as a unit, man e.g. being two-footed rather than of all the feet of mankind, the question has been outstanding as to what sort of being a universal term designates.

As can be seen all words except proper names can be held to be universals, applying to many instances of something. And if it is taken into account that some dictionaries do not list proper names, all words in a language may be held to be universals. The problem can accordingly be a wide-ranging one. In conformance with the aforesaid, however, the problem is illusory. What the words are about is decided by their users. The users can nevertheless be deceived by the words of their choice, especially since anyone's language is largely received from someone else.

If the intended meaning is obscured, then "man", as an example, could, being a singular noun, be expected to refer to a single entity, as was suggested. What that entity is is accordingly wondered. However, the word is not meant to refer to such an entity, but to all humans individually, despite its concise singularity.

Varied arguments have, regardless, attempted to demonstrate the presence of behind universal terms universal single entities as well, of, as sometimes worded, one over many. The arguments are irrelevant, however, since it is each of the many to which the universal term is intended to refer, whether or not there is a single other one.

A most frequent argument for a single entity is that it is required as a standard by which members of the class can be recognized as alike. It has been sought of late to circumvent the question by asserting a frequent absence of common attributes in those members. Things named by a universal term are thus said to often have only family resemblances, some of the things being similar to some of the others, without any attribute being shared by all. That observation, however, deals with the universal term in differing senses, when the things denoted are not, as otherwise, defined by the same attributes. As dictionaries already inform, the same term often designates through differing senses things differing in the attributes concerned, not the case with single senses. And as noted elsewhere, the interest in what is named by a term has to do with one of its senses at a time. The question as to a standard by which things named by a universal term are found to be alike can accordingly remain. But as implied in the last paragraph, such a standard, thought of as the universal behind the term, is usually not a thing named by it.

Alluded to are named things of the world, and by the time names are used for classes of some found in some respect alike, an attribute by which one of them is determined to be like another is usually thought of apart from actual observation. That is to say, it is in accordance with a thought of the things named that an actual thing is determined to be one of them. But the thought, the standard, is not one of those things. In conformance with an earlier remark, the universal "chair" refers to actual chairs, not to the thought of them by which their being chairs is determined.

It may be noted that the oft debated question of what form a thought of a universal entity takes is likewise irrelevant. Since consciousness, a part of which other than apprehension of the world is meant by thought, is seen as the ultimate arbiter of all that takes place, there is no need to support by argument what takes place in consciousness. The taking place in it is its own confirmation.

With the foregoing in view, it may be added that the ancient argument of "the third man", disputing in fact single universal entities, is erroneous. By the argument if two things are alike through their likeness to a third, then the third is like the others through their combined likeness to a fourth, and so on indefinitely. Not so. The presence of a standard in thought by which real things are judged to be the same in some respect does not mean that they cannot be so judged without the standard.

Its use, as suggested, is due to the passing quickly into memory of things perceived, and it is much apter to compare things to that memory than to seek out past seen instances, which action makes use of memory regardless. Memory indeed serves as indicated (page 11, first paragraph) the function of storing knowledge, on which to draw in the future for comparison, and a sense like hearing can compare alike sounds only through memory.

But a likeness between two things at once perceived is, as the mere fact of consciousness of the resemblance again confirms, observed without a third thing, provided the pertinent attribute is, as in weight, not observed somewhere else only. A worldly thing can respecting some attributes, as in the case of size, indeed not be compared to a memory but only directly to another worldly thing.

With universal terms not referring to at least the standards only, or to other single entities which somehow represent classes, but to the members of the classes themselves, they bear a likeness in meaning to concepts as here considered. These, too, concern in such as classes of worldly things the actual entities as presented in awareness. They can, however, also concern the single as well as objects of thought. In brief, "concept" is here used in the sense in which one would ordinarily query what concept any linguistic expression refers to. One may speak of the concept of the single and real universe, or of the concept of the multiple and ideal geometric figure.

Sometimes objects in human awareness in general are instead spoken of as ideas, as happens in British empiricism or is reflected in references to some philosophical doctrines as instances of idealism. But nowadays "idea" appears to connote mainly a proposition, with the broad application accorded to concept. That application, it should be clear, includes propositions or any assertion as described, in concord with the inclusion of all that is in awareness, as represented by any linguistic expression.

Although all that is considered may accordingly be named concept, it may be added that, in keeping with the varied usefulness of language, there is no abstention herein from speaking of, rather than concepts, entities or things, especially when concerning realities. Similarly, there should be no reluctance to speak of the conceptual in the sense contrasting it with the worldly.

The inclusive meaning of concept being thus specified, the material of which a concept is constituted may, further, be termed perception. Specifically, by perception is meant all that is a distinct ingredient of consciousness, all that, unlike for instance quantity, is conceivable not only in connection with something else. Among perceptions are for example colors, sounds and other qualities associated with the senses. But such as emotions or even intellectual effort likewise belong to them. It should also be noted that no differentiation is made here between perception as the object confronted and as the act of confronting, because the act of perception can be considered to consist in the characteristic that the object is a perception, a certain occurrence to someone.

The term "perception" is in philosophy today mainly confined to sense perception, to conscious occurrences found to be the result of the processes of the senses. In a previous time John Locke for one instead defined perception as the first operation of all intellectual faculties. Such a definition was rejected by others as failing to distinguish between perception and other cognition. The rejection can again be seen itself to fail, by not recognizing that meanings of words are assigned.

Through the debating of what words should mean, as was suggested, it has been attempted to resolve factual problems. Views in opposition to each other have thus been tried to be vindicated by adjustments in language. Behaviorism, eschewing consciousness, would define names for man's perceptions with language for man's overt behavior, thereby thinking to eliminate them. Phenomenalism, uncertain of physical objects, would refer to them with descriptions of their perceived attributes, although the single words for the objects refer to the same phenomena.

As pertains to perception itself, the tying of its meaning to physical occurrences may give rise to the notion that as a result they exist. This was to counter an extreme skepticism about worldly reality, but to have a word concerning it does not imply it.

There may be objection to speaking of perceptions even with respect to worldly reality, insofar as they identify it with something in awareness. It is often argued that worldly things cannot be identified with a content of private consciousness, because of their public reality. But as observed (page 20, fourth paragraph), the objects require no more for their identity than their nature in awareness. If they can be considered public, it is because they coincide in appropriate ways among numbers of persons, in contrast to parts of consciousness such as dreams, which can accordingly be regarded as private.

The word "perception" as used here should rather be an accustomed one, inasmuch as things of which consciousness is composed are in general said to be perceived, while things that like quantity are not distinct entities as described are not said to be perceived independently. The use of the word need as before yet not be restricted to this sense, it being sometimes convenient to call anything in consciousness, distinct or not, perceived.

However, the consideration of the distinct elements of consciousness presently named perceptions is important, because they consist in the qualities by which concepts, perhaps fanciful, are apprehended, and by which accordingly anything factual about them comes to be known.

These perceptual elements may, as in the preceding, also be referred to as qualities, as is the practice in some of science, with the attention less on entities as objects of consciousness. And it may be remarked that these elements are themselves concepts as spoken of, which are meant to, again, include all kinds of entities, from the simplest to the most complex, from perceptions of a moment to objects that, as in the case of material ones, are conceptually constructed out of myriads of perceptions repeated.

And the just mentioned matter of apprehending concepts by those qualities, by perceptual elements, and of accordingly acquiring about the concepts further knowledge can be impeded by their intimate connection with language.

Considering that in interdependence among men a large part of information one obtains is received from others, language plays by its basic communicating function already an important part in acquiring personal knowledge. In additionally serving to preserve knowledge in forms like writing, language functions similarly as a medium. For these purposes languages developed into systems of most economical signs, taking the place of the likes of pictorial representation. For that reason language serves well even in thought, where rather than transmitting information, it codifies the concepts contemplated. But language became simultaneously an obstacle, for by formulating thoughts in language, the concepts behind it can be obscured, and findings about them correspondingly prevented.

In order to observe concepts and what is resultingly true about them, therefore, it is necessary to take special care to separate them from their names. Frequent pronouncements to the contrary, it is required to so to speak think by means of concepts instead of by means of language.

To that end it is requisite to, in the parlance of the introduction, educe the concepts in accordance with what may be termed their perceptual attributes, in accordance with described perceptions by which they may be apprehended. To elucidate, since what is sought in concepts are objects of consciousness apart from the language signifying them, if a concept, such as quantity, is not a distinct object of consciousness, not a perception, it must be educed by some other concept aside from the language. Quantity for example can be educed in relation to things as it applies to them.

In connection with this observation, a still further sense of linguistic meaning, next to those of the last section, can be spoken of. It concerns the question of whether or not an expression has meaning, and it was alluded to before (page 10, last paragraph). In its primary sense the "meant", as noted and used in dictionaries, concerns the actual entity considered, not something regarding it. In that sense by "man" are meant actual men, not the thought in some form of them. But by that sense of "meant" it could be said that nothing is meant by an expression for an assumed entity that happens not to exist. And upon misunderstanding, the expression could be dismissed, as thinkers have tended to. Assumed, looked for, realities are, however, an integral part of man's everyday as well as scientific pursuits. They are put into words not only in parts of but whole sentences, in statements and questions with responses of true or false and yes or no. The positive response signifies the reality of the state in question, the negative response the unreality. But in the last case, too, the sentences, or their concerned parts, will be held of meaning.

This meaning can be said to in lieu of the entity or state be about the thought of them. It can even be about something logically impossible, though expressed in words. What matters is that language for assumed things expresses thoughts of something as connected with something else as the assumed, possibly existence, even if the connection between the two cannot occur conceptually either, each of them conceived only separately. For example a sometimes cited round square can be considered though contradictory, as can any deductive proposition though proving to be false. More generally, to conceive behind expressions certain things, to specifically have perceptions regarding them as explained, is the requirement for meaning in the present sense. Quantity need not have a distinct existence, in reality or in thought, but the term has meaning because of perceptions it represents.

This sense of meaning appears similar to one in which the things named are considered only by particular attributes. Even when so considered, however, the attributes can be ones assumed real, and hence if they are not, there is no thing that is meant. Instead what is meant in the present sense of meaning behind words is merely the described perceptions, so as not to render the words vacuous.

Knowledge of what in particular cases the perceptions, the perceptual attributes of the things named, are is needed for, as indicated, findings to be made about them, findings specifically that are not linguistic only, having to only do with names of the things. That a thing of a name is also of another name could be learned without knowing what the thing is, the saying so by one who uses the words the criterion. But knowledge that something else is true about a thing, the issue being one's own confirmation, requires more. Any truth about something, any fact, becomes one for man, it will be recalled, in the form in which presented to consciousness (e.g. page 24, third paragraph). Put differently, for something to be true about something for man, it must be presented to consciousness in the form concerned. That form was observed to consist of concepts, identified by perceptual attributes. Specifically now, in order to know whether something is true about something, the things are meant apprehended by their perceptual attributes, be they the contents of words or words themselves. Regarding the last this took place in the above example, and the same takes partly place in usual definitions. They speak partly of words and partly of concepts named by them, in which case the concepts must be apprehended by their perceptual attributes, as are the words by theirs. And if what is to be determined, nonlinguistically, is something about something when these things are taken as of attributes behind their names, then it is those attributes which must be of perceptual awareness.

With regard to attributes of things treated of in this writing, the determining, the ascertaining, is, as made clear, by what may be held reflective inference, rather than by, as concerns things of the world, physical observation. Therefore the perceptions relied on, if things of the world are at issue, are of their conceptual representations, whereafter something may be induced or deduced of them. As was remarked (page 22, fifth paragraph), memory is relied upon for knowledge. In the case of induction laws of nature are inferred from memories of constancies already perceived, and in the case of deduction inferences about nature from its conceptual awareness are made in what may be held conformance with logical principles. The conceptual awareness is adequate for application of constancies of this kind, because logical principles hold, as it is said, in all possible worlds. And the awareness is required, in order to know that the particulars conform to the conditions of the logical principles, or in order to, as more common, perceive the inference directly from the particular concepts. That logical, or mathematical, principles themselves hold must of course be perceived likewise, in consonance with the requirement that something is true only if in awareness in the form that makes it true.

Some of the findings may only be made step by step, when a connection is not perceived at once but after a train of reasoning, it being of account presently that for these and other purposes concepts behind words be sufficiently educed by perceptual attributes.

The accurate identification of concepts as a result of their sufficient eduction will as suggested be seen to prevent often found erroneous inferences, as well as to promote revelatory new ones.

This can in symptoms of linguistic deceptiveness be true because, as seen in the case of "meaning" itself, the meaning of one word can be variant, and the meaning of more than one word the same, these characteristics frequently called respectively homonymity and, referred to, synonymity. The fallacies connected with homonyms are well known as equivocations; they will be found nevertheless committed professionally. The unwarranted differentiation to which synonyms are liable is recognized less; the contradictory results will be observable in paradoxes. More contributively, synonyms can through their identification lead to additional knowledge, by enabling recognition that things of attributes known under one of the synonyms have attributes known under another. Likewise the uncovering of ambiguity in homonyms, which virtually all words because of their multiple senses can be said to be, aids in separating the meanings, whereupon what is not true of one may of another be found to hold.

It is worthwhile to add that the harm that can be wrought by language without due attention to the represented concepts exceeds failures in inference. At issue are particularly homonyms or synonyms, in uses like those of metaphor and euphemisms. Euphemisms are known to make the bad sound good, leading to the acceptance of numerous evils, and metaphor makes as often the good sound bad, with words of disparaging senses that bring equal injustice.

Language can conceal other factors beside those from which synonyms and homonyms mislead, factors the eduction of which enables further findings, and therefore if in discourse something about an entity is to be demonstrated, it may be requisite that the term used for it be appropriately defined.

Section 3
DEFINITION

It is said that some entities, called simple or unanalyzable, are undefinable. Among them are held to be the elementary perceptions or qualities spoken of, because they cannot be reduced to other entities. But considered among them are also concepts such as the good, for the very reason that they are thought not to be identifiable with such perceptions or qualities.

That to define an entity should require that it be analyzable can be understood from the usual definition of one term by several others. An explanation of the entity, not furnished by a single term, is often desirable. However, the corresponding reference to things by which an entity is identified is, in what can be held an equivocation of "analyzable", confounded with the reference to things of which the entity is composed.

Not only the many concepts that like "and" are indistinct as described are identified by circumstance. Material objects are likewise often defined by function, as are localities by place, and so forth. Circumstance can similarly identify mentioned qualities, as blue is in dictionaries defined by the color of the clear sky.

The issue as said is that the meaning of the words be so educed as to make known what is talked about, of especial importance for demonstrating what is true about the things named. For that purpose any definition bringing the concept to consciousness will do, even a synonym, whereupon one may assure oneself whether or not something about the concept holds. All sorts of defining attributes made explicit are in fact commonly part of deductive proof, illustrated by the traditional syllogism. In likely the best known it is from definitional "Socrates is a man" and knowledge of "All men are mortal" deduced "Socrates is mortal". It is immaterial to the deduction whether a defining, or other, attribute of the thing in question is about some of its components or about something else connected with it. What matters is that the attribute figure in the inference, and that it be known through identifying its possessor by whatever definition.

As an early proponent of indefinability of simple entities, Locke defended it by noting that a blind man could not comprehend the concept of light however described. But a subsequent reference to the rainbow inadvertently reveals that the problem need not apply to simple entities alone. The rainbow, a complex thing, can, also, not be described to a blind man. The question indeed is not whether something, simple or complex, can be defined for someone who is not acquainted with it or with, at least, things by which it is conceived.

As indicated in this chapter, men in communicating use language to speak about things in possible mutual awareness. If the participants are unable to share the meaning, then the language does not have its communicating function. In the example of the blind man the inability to acquaint him with a concept is not due to the weakness of language, but to the lack of visual meaning for him.

In the present treatise, as in many others, definition of unknown concepts need, as suggested, not even arise. The matters dealt with are predominantly inseparable from everybody's conscious life, and the definitions accordingly are in general of concepts well versed in by the average reader.

As pertains to definability of these or other concepts, the point is, as explained, to bring them to consciousness by perceptual attributes.

Correspondingly, if definition of perceptual elements, the described qualities, itself is the issue, it is doubtless enough to use a synonym, having understood that the term defined is not comprehended, perhaps not in the intended sense. More likely it is comprehended, and no definition is needed. For inasmuch as these qualities are the elemental things perceived, they have an abundance of well known names, the use of which will make the concepts specific.

As to definitions of other than the perceptual elements, definitions of the nondistinct concepts not containing them or of those containing more, they can be performed by way of perceptual elements likewise. The nondistinct concepts, too, must be, as noted (page 25, third paragraph), identified by some perceptual attribute, by way of which circumstance, as noted also (page 28, last paragraph), they would be defined. By circumstance definable were also indicated (page 28, next to last paragraph) to be many that are composites of perceptual elements. In defining either concepts, furthermore, defining words can refer to nondistinct concepts themselves, to ones not perceived alone. While the name for the concept defined is again taken not to be appropriately comprehended, the same is not necessarily true of the words defining it. As in the case of perceptual elements, there is a richness of understood language for all objects of knowledge held by men in common, in particular for basic concepts by which further things are characterized, and including ones not perceived alone, such as motion. As remarked with respect to words in general, these concepts can at the least be grasped from their context, without continued definition.

It is the through shared cognitions avaliable choice of all kinds of words in all kinds of arrangements that makes definition of all concepts that can be shared by men possible. That fundamental concepts and correspondingly the meaning of any language for them are shared was discussed as determined by induction, which as observed will be amplified later, since the sharing is presupposed by comprehension of this writing.

It should be added that there are qualities not of acquaintance to everybody who can perceive them. Whereas one may have no trouble calling forth an image of a color by defining it, perhaps by a synonym, the same may not be true regarding a taste. In those cases it is the difference between actual and possible conception, one said of account, which is in effect. Though the thing defined may not be conceptualized thereupon, it can be conceptualized on finding the defining circumstance. These definitions are of little significance here, however, such as tastes not even bearing names, the concepts of concern enjoying as indicated universal familiarity.

Because there should in either event be by the preceding no concept that, as sometimes said, defies definition, it is justified in discourse to ask for a definition if a term is not understood. It is justified, specifically, to ask for identity by perceptual attribute as expounded, be the identity unspoken in the definition, so long as apprehension does not remain linguistic.

Much of deductive demonstration includes, as observed, such definition, insofar sometimes as recourse is not had to mentioned enthymemes, arguments in which some pertinent factor is not stated but taken to be in consciousness. The omission to state the factor is acceptable in obvious situations, but evidently not when consciousness of it is in doubt. Such can be the case when the to be omitted is a definition, and it is, as was indicated, in fact maintained that all things deductively derived follow by virtue of definition.

Definitions, in spite of their avoidance, are thus accorded a central place in logic. They are regarded as referred to (page 4, last paragraph) analytic statements, as accordingly necessarily true, that status often explained by using as example the statement "No bachelor is married". It is noted that if "bachelor" is replaced by its definitional equivalent "unmarried man" then the resulting statement, "No unmarried man is married", is true logically and accordingly analytically, or necessarily. Since the definitional statement can thus be turned into a logical truth, it is inferred that it is likewise analytic or necessary.

This explanation can be viewed as prompted by the desire to demonstrate that definitions, while not appearing as logical truths, possess the same internal coherence discussed in the introduction as intrinsic or deductive. The interchange of definitional equivalents in getting logical truths has been supported by what is known as Leibniz's law, by which if two expressions refer to the same thing then on replacing in a true statement one of them by the other the statement remains true. By thus complying with that law, however, any statement whatever, even when of an accidental fact, can by that interchange be made logical. In recognition it is attempted to in various ways qualify the statements in which the interchange can be carried out. But the interchanges are irrelevant.

Allowing that on replacing "bachelor" by "unmarried man" in "No bachelor is married" the resulting statement remains true, the statement is not the same one as the first. The process is an instance of deduction by to be treated transitivity, as when from "*A* equals *B*" and "*B* equals *C*" inferring "*A* equals *C*", without the inferred stating the same that either of the inferred from did. "*A* equals *B*" can stand for " 'not unmarried man' equals 'not bachelor' ", "*B* equals *C*" for " 'not bachelor' equals 'married man' ", and "*A* equals *C*" for " 'not unmarried man' equals 'married man' ". Indeed whereas the two premises, or the reversely ordered previous "No bachelor is married" and equivalence of "(no) unmarried man" to "(no) bachelor", may be held to state definitions, the conclusion, or "No unmarried man is married", states something else, a logical truism as it were. That is to say the statement revealed logically true through the interchange is the derived one, not the initial one.

It may be wondered though whether in consequence the initial one is not logically true also. It may in fact also be wondered whether basic logical principles, notoriously resisting proof, cannot in some such manner be proven. But the logical truths derived in the preceding are the consequence of their being already employed in the statements from which derived. For instance " 'not unmarried man' equals 'married man' " is logically true by later examined law of double negation, used in the second of the premises from which the statement is concluded. The first premise, to explain, follows from the definition " 'Bachelor' equals 'unmarried man' " by also later transposition, and the second premise is the equivalent of the first but for the replacement by "married man". But this replacement is itself licensed by the law expressed in the conclusion, which follows as a result. The conclusion expresses the law because it is applied to the definition of bachelor, which merely serves as a premise with the others, none of which results likewise in a logical truth, in an intrinsic one, as to be seen.

A similar situation occurs when oppositely a statement like that premise is through the interchange obtained from a statement like that conclusion. In the dispute as to necessity in a definitional statement like "No bachelor is married" it is contended that that interchange cannot work for facts that lack necessity. A statement like "Necessarily no unmarried man is married" is construed as expressing the one previously inferred, and a statement reversely inferred from it is maintained to likewise have necessity, since the interchangeability means that what is true under one name is true under another. It is thought in other words that if the interchangeability were always to hold then from for instance "Necessarily no toothless feathered creature has teeth" would follow "Necessarily no bird has teeth", taking the interchanged as equivalent. And the inferred statement would be held to falsely assert necessity.

But what can be inferred is here, too, mistaken for something initially posited. The conclusion that no bird has teeth is truly necessary, provided the premise that all birds are toothless is true. In a general explanation, if, or when, "*A* equals *B*" is true, and "*B* equals 'not not *B*' " being by law of double negation necessary, then "*A* equals 'not not *B*' " is necessary as well, without the same required of the first equality. To be more specific, the last necessity, namely logicality, is here one not only because resulting by mentioned transitivity law, but because it, due to the first premise, is an instance of the second, logical, one. Were the second premise a causal law, the conclusion would similarly be an instance of it.

The preceding would suggest that Leibniz's law, by which the equality admits the interchangeability, holds after all. But the law relies too much on language, whose delusiveness was noted in the foregoing. Expressions overtly naming certain things refer covertly often to only particular attributes of them, possibly the names themselves. Thus it was observed in the past that if something true is said about a word, perhaps that it has so many letters while using the word as if the thing meant by it were spoken of, the same may not be truly said about a substitute word of the same meaning. Likewise with other attributes. "Being the city of the Acropolis makes Athens a favorite tourist spot" may not be true if the part describing Athens is replaced by "the capital of Greece".

If the sentence began with the addition "The attribute of" it would be explicit that something is said about the particular attribute, not the city. Things differ if something is said about the city, even if still identified by a particular attribute. Since Athens is both the city of the Acropolis and the capital of Greece, the city of the Acropolis is the capital of Greece. The issue is that if one thing is identical with another then what is true of one is by transitivity in fact true of the other, but that what the things talked about can be obscured by language.

The effort to prove definitions, definitional identities, to be in an indicated sense necessary is thus ill-conceived if only because the reasoning offered as ground for proof, e.g. something like Leibniz's law, applies to all identities, including accidental ones. It can moreover on a much simpler basis be determined that identity by definition is not an intrinsic necessity. Since names are arbitrary, what is named by a word can be identical with a certain thing at one moment and not at another.

A reason that the necessity is held plausible can be found in a confounding of definition with properties that a thing by its nature always has, in likeness to mentioned analyzability. But as likewise indicated, things are not always defined by such properties. The moon is defined as the heavenly body revolving around the earth, but that it always revolve is not required in order to be the same object.

Argument is also advanced that a statement like "All bachelors are unmarried" is somehow necessary because an analogous statement can be found in most any language. But aside from no logical basis, other languages are apt to have a word for unmarried men, as they have words for the many other things of common human acquaintance.

More pertinent than these, a definition has to do with elucidating what is meant by an expression, and that meaning can be changed at will. At the base of instead arguing that that meaning possesses some sort of necessity can be held to lie the proposal that deductive truths are somehow grounded on definitions rather than unchanging facts. Since those truths are nonetheless considered to possess that necessity, so are definitions. In defense of this point of view inconsistency is engaged in.

In presenting truths of logic as ones founded on meaning, their traditional understanding as ones contained in the concepts concerned is discarded. It is customary in logic to not surprisingly view its problems in terms of sentences or statements, in place of states of things. Hence logical containment has been expressed as containment of predicate in the subject. This is objected to as limited to subject-predicate forms and as making containment unclear, as evident from the linguistic separation. However, there is no such limit or unclarity as regards containment in concepts, explained to cover all apprehension, with the containment factual. It is more the notion offered that the logically true is so by virtue of meaning that lacks clarity, and interpreted as following only from definitions it is these truths that become limited, precluding deduction from other conditions. But really of account is that what comprises deductive truth depends as with other entities on what is chosen to be meant by it. Meant by it traditionally and in its present role was noted to be inference of something part of the concept of the inferred from. The inconsistency in the arguments disowning this meaning resides in their attempt to show that the definitional replacement possesses the disowned internal necessity nonetheless.

Thus definitional statements were as discussed endeavored to be reduced to logically necessary ones, or to be explained as describing the necessary nature of the things defined. The last necessity is sometimes called essence, and because it and other conceptions of necessity, together with those of possibility and related ones, all usually named modal, appear, due to their relation to certainty, important to definition as well as to subsequently explored actual and logical truths, an examination of them should be timely.

The question is again what is meant by them, and the definitions here will again be in conformity with what the writer understands to be their generally held meaning and, more pertinently, the concern. With all definitions herein, if a reader's concepts of concern are not the same, it is hoped that the concepts discussed will at least be found of interest.

As regards "necessary", it might as frequent be defined by "indispensable", or "what cannot be otherwise", or similarly. These, however, contain forms of "impossible", itself a modal concept and hence wanting in the desired definition.

The necessary can in a broad sense rather be simply defined as that which is completely certain, in a factual sense rather than the previous one regarding knowledge (p. 13, fourth par.). It is the sense in which what has happened would be called necessary in that it will no longer, for good or for bad, be prevented, whereas the same may not hold for the future. That is to say that if all is not determined beforehand, if there is chance or free will, then some of the future is not of a necessary outcome. Otherwise, should all be predetermined, as by unbroken casual chains or by divine decree, all things would be necessary. In either event, those things are broadly necessary which have been the case or are predetermined to be the case at some future time.

By what reason something may be held predetermined may further be asked. And as indicated (e.g. p. 4, last par.), correct inference, in which ascertainments about the future by having to by what was said be based on previous perceptions consist, is meant based on unfailing finding. Things are certain to at some future time be the case, accordingly, if they always are the case under any condition or a particular condition an instance of which has occurred. To the first of these belong the, inductive or deductive, principles themselves, by which other things to be the case in the future are inferred.

Whichever the situation, in the light of the preceding the necessary in a wide sense may be newly described as that which—as little as by chance—has been the case, or that which—as might be the effectuality of a deity—is always the case, whether independently or in connection with something else.

The necessary so comprehended can be seen as identical with fact in a likewise broad sense of the word, when by fact, also, are meant those things that have been true together with those always true, independently or in connection with something else.

It may be objected that the necessary is meant to be somehow more substantial than fact in this sense, that for something to be necessary it should have a reason other than something with which it is connected however lastingly, not to speak of its merely being the case at any time. The reason for anything is seen to be none other, however, supposing that such other be wished to be called necessary. For let something be the reason, in whatever sense, for the first thing. But then the last thing is none other than something with which the first thing is connected.

That fact as well as the necessary be about what has been true along with principles and what consequently will be true, can be attributed to the regarding as fact or necessary those things that need be taken into account in man's presumed free actions. It is for that reason that the necessary as the completely certain was above described as what will not be prevented. If mentioned chance be possible too, then though it by its present meaning cannot be caused, it still would be pertinent as not necessary if it can be prevented. Of bearing is that the necessary is about no more than the, by man dependent on, certainty of fact.

Although the necessary is accordingly synonymous with fact, its terminology can be useful, as exemplified by "need" in the preceding paragraph. It is simpler to say "This is necessary for that" than to state as a factual principle "Whenever that occurs this had occurred". Consequently forms of "necessary" or acknowledged synonyms, or other terms proving not to stand for supposed additional concepts, are again not avoided in this writing if they facilitate it.

In the last paragraph the mention of forms of "necessary" with regard to principles suggests that the words may in a narrower sense be used for that purpose only. It is indeed the practice to say of a past event that it was not necessary, meaning that there was no compulsion by such as a causal law. It may be remarked that the very speaking of necessity customarily with respect to laws of nature, which are referred to synthetic truths contrasted with the analytic, makes the term as suitable for them as for laws of logic, often argued to be the only applicable ones. What the term is used for is, to repeat, a matter of choice, and it is in logic that in fact, in contrast to above, principles are stated, making the designation of necessity superfluous. It would there be stated that if *A* then *B*, not as in causation that an event, *B*, is necessary due to another, *A*; this likely since in logic the interest is more abstractly principles, and in nature concrete particulars. A stricter sense of necessity can thus herein concern principles in general. The narrow sense of fact instead, it may be added, usually concerns only what has occurred.

Having defined the necessary, by "impossible" are meant indirectly, by denying the possible, facts which are contrary to those meant by the necessary. That is to say, those things are in the wide sense impossible which in fact have not been or never are the case, independently or in connection with something else. The narrow sense is as before confined to what in fact never is the case. In either sense, accordingly, whereas "necessary" asserts affirmative facts, "impossible" asserts negative ones. For the matter of that, the necessity associated under determinism with all things refers to the impossible as well, to absences as to presences.

By "possible", next, is meant the denial of the impossible, of negative fact. It may be wondered if this meaning, taken as common, does not without warrant, by saying that the possible is the not not possible, presume common knowledge of the mentioned law of double negation. Ordinary life is continually, however, guided by, as cases of the discussed presupposed, knowledge conforming to these and other principles, without formal acquaintance with them.

Specifically, then, in denying the broadly impossible the possible refers, by later law of complements, to a thing as having been the case, or to what is sometime, maybe always, the case in itself or with the specified, or would sometime be the case in itself or with the specified if certain things were done or because, as may be an act of will or event of chance, it is merely not precluded by a principle. In denying the narrowly impossible, that something never is the case, the possible refers to the same as in the preceding, but for a thing as having been the case. Viz., that something in the past was possible does, as normal, not mean that it was the case, but that it was not impossible by some principle.

The possible thus includes the necessary, inasmuch as it in the broad sense refers to what has been true and what beside sometime is always true as explicated, and in the narrow sense to what is always true likewise.

It might be proposed that the necessary should not be included in the possible. It can be heard stated that something is not possible but necessary. This can, however, be regarded as an emphasizing figure of speech, there being likely no misunderstanding if after "not" in the preceding sentence is inserted "only". Not to be possible and to be necessary, both asserted in that sentence's figure of speech, are ordinarily viewed as contraries, and the present definitions will be fitting for the purposes.

It may also be noted that as it can be useful to speak of the necessary in place of stating entire principles, so can it be useful to speak of the possible in place of denying them. It is simpler to say "This is possible" than "It is not true that this is never the case".

Corresponding to the possible, by "not necessary" is of course meant the denial of the necessary, of affirmative fact, the things specifically included being the negative counterparts of those included in the possible.

At this point it may be observed that these modal expressions, the necessary, the impossible, and their negations, are often without qualifying used with respect to human knowledge rather than its objects. When it is said that something is not necessarily true it can be meant that it will not necessarily turn out to be so. A future event may thus be held not necessary in accordance with experience, while the event may in fact be necessary as a result of others. For the same reason the necessary would in that usage refer to only facts which are known in accordance with experience, not also to those true independently of it. The possible and impossible are spoken of in the same dual manner, leading to later observed equivocation.

The significance of the above defined concepts is at this time their referred to correspondence to what is considered the essence and any related characteristic of entities.

Designating herein anything that is true about an entity its attribute, by "essential" can regarding an entity be held to be in general meant an attribute without which an entity is not the one considered. But since without any attribute a thing has had it is not the thing considered, any attribute a thing has in fact had is in that sense essential. There appears thus the same factuality that was encountered with regard to the necessary, and the sameness is seen to extend throughout. When considering broadly as necessary what has been true, then since truth concerns a fact regarding something, something has been true of something, which by the preceding is the same as saying that something has had a certain attribute. The necessary, further, concerned principles, constancies, likewise happening to essential attributes. Things necessary by being always true independently are, again, about something always true of something, namely about constant attributes. And things always true in connection with something else are about constant attributes under some condition, e.g. about an effect on a thing under a cause. Only the undetermined future is of things not counted as true, as attribute.

The only distinction between essence and necessity that might be made is that in a narrow sense by essence the referred to as true of a thing, as its attribute, can be that by which the thing is first considered, not what is learned about it later, though perhaps a principle. This strict sense of essence has to do with the interest presently, which is concepts as mainly first considered, of which more is then determined.

Both, the attributes referred to by the broad and the narrow sense of essence, can be seen of importance in the light of earlier observations. The first because a thing can be defined by any attribute applying that distinguishes it, and the second because a thing cannot be redefined by denying a first meant attribute without speaking of something else.

The contradiction in similar denials is also pertinent to the longstanding contention that existence is not an attribute. As regards that contention it should suffice to remind that as elsewhere what is named an attribute, the present meaning of it as anything true of a thing another common one, is arbitrary. More to the point, if a thing considered is an existing one then something not existing is not the thing considered. That is to say, the existence is, along with other things, essential, whether or not called an attribute. To repeat a former example, of a yet more stringent requirement, for something to be a chair, although there may not be any, it has to, beside else, exist. A thought of a chair is not a chair.

It may again be remonstrated that the essence of a thing

should be something deeper than an attribute that in fact applies, even something other than an attribute, as has long been argued in reference to substance.

A distinction made between substance and attribute can be understood as counterpart to the grammatical distinction between subject and predicate. However, in line with the discussed disparity between language and its content, the utility of making a statement in terms of subject and predicate does not imply a like separation in actuality. To suppose the separation amounts to needless differentiation mentioned as to synonyms, which in fact are knowingly used in definitions, which are instances of statements with subject and predicate. Similarly, subject as part of a sentence is as a homonym equivocated with subject as object of consideration. With these misconceptions the impression that attributes differ from subjects has led to varied interpretations of the two, akin to the discussed twofold meaning assumed of words, although both words and attributes can in their respective designating and characterizing way be of any content.

Most often the subject, in relation to the notion of substance, is equated with the concrete individual said to be denoted, and the attribute with the abstract universal said to be connoted. But when the former is indeed a concrete, an existing, entity, then so can be regarded the latter. In "Socrates is a man", the mentioned and oft cited paradigm of a singular proposition, a living Socrates is also a living man. Even in "All men are mortal", the companion universal proposition, living men are living mortals. And the difference between the individual and universal is merely that the second concerns more than one.

Moreover, it can be the subject which is abstract, a conception, without the attribute the same, in reversal of the contention. This happens every time a thing is stated to exist. Since the information is new, the thing is known without its existence before declared. In cases where the thing is a conjectured reality, it may be wondered how it can be referred to without its being. Thus by a quark, as by a chair, is not meant a thought, but a physical object, if not a confirmed one. Here again the flexibility of language can deceive. In "Quarks exist", by quarks are provisionally not meant real things, but the conception of them, in concord with the last discussed sense of meaning (p. 25, last par., through p. 26, second par.). As long as hypothetical, with all entities the referred to, often as subject, is thus their conception.

When it comes instead to substance, it, as could existence, can also, perhaps as material, be called an attribute by fiat. It has been argued besides that there must, based on the assumption of a world independent of the perception of it, be an unknown substratum in objects, one that may be called their substance and the truly essential. But as observed (p. 20, fourth par.), things are identified by the nature by which apprehended, not requiring a further nature to be the things meant. Furthermore whatever unknown things may be true about something, such as the composition of matter, they still would be none other than what in fact is sometime or always connected with it, as explicated of the necessary.

Many entities do in addition, as indicated above, not concern substance, mostly conceived as concrete matter. Apart from sometimes being abstract in the conceptual sense, entities can be so by not having a distinct, an independently perceived, nature as previously described. Size is an example. And in many material things attributes like function, as in tools, are, in place of the substance of which they consist, considered the essential ones.

Designating as the essential in likeness to the necessary thus factual attributes, the same should not be required in likeness to the impossible. The essential should be adequate to designate factual absence of given attributes as well. As to the nonessential, it designates the denial of the essential, in continued likeness. Since the interest now is identification, definition, this means that nonessential attributes, such as those a thing has not had, are those by which a thing would not be described as desired.

In seeking accordingly definitions, of account is that in concord with the aforesaid an entity is fully characterized by its attributes, simply because "attribute" can, and does, designate anything that an entity is, e.g. the entity itself.

This state of the matter notwithstanding, counterargument is advanced. Thus it is maintained that if things that basically identify an entity be, like other things about it, termed attributes, a contradiction arises. The first accordingly termed attributes, identifying the entity, then include the perhaps later discovered others. Namely, it is argued, the number of attributes is both that of the first ones and its combination with the number of the others.

Needless to repeat, anything that identifies a thing can at will be called an attribute, and dependence on language, therefore, does not provide a solution. It is dependence on language, rather, which brings about confusion. A combination of attributes is commonly spoken of as a single one, in seeming contradiction. This is due to the compactness of words, wherein combinations of often a multitude of attributes are given a single name. The generality of this is as a matter of fact manifested in most of definition, where one thing, as represented by a word, is defined in terms of a number of others. It is a process involving classification, when for example man is defined as animal and certain further attributes, animal is defined as living thing and certain yet further attributes, and so forth. It would be awkward then to say that being a man is attributes instead of an attribute, in keeping with the singularity of "man". The same holds for animal and so on, either of which can be said to have numbers of attributes, though spoken of in these contexts as single ones.

Taking into account the foregoing, certain theorems or principles of definition may be formulated. These can be thought of as eductive principles in similarity to deductive principles or laws and inductive laws of nature, because they comprise rules by which the process of eduction or associated definition may be guided. The truth of these principles, as of others, may appear self-evident, but what may be regarded as formal logical proof is for the sake of better assurance furnished.

Instead of, then, speaking of what defines a particular thing as something necessary or essential to it, it can be spoken of as the factual attributes of the following.

THEOREM I.1. *A thing is defined if and only if referred to by attributes all and only those things have.*

As diagramed below in Figure I, a chair (circle) could accordingly be defined as a single seat with a back, which in fact all and only chairs are. It would not be defined as only a single seat (left oval) or a seat with a back (right oval), which in fact not only chairs are, and it would not be defined as also a seat with arms (bottom oval), which in fact not all chairs are.

Proof. (Formal proofs of theorems are in this treatise contained in single paragraphs.) The theorem is an instance of a principle treated in Chapter III, and it can—in at least its "if" half, the "only if" half often not given—be held equivalent to what is known as the axiom of extensionality. In accordance with the principle, if and only if all and only things of one kind

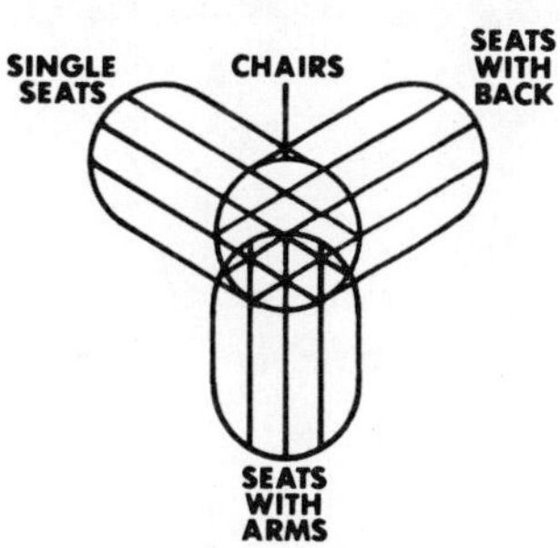

FIGURE I

(those named chairs) are of another kind (those of the attributes listed) then the first and second things are identical.

The principle is disclosed in the diagram, by which all of and only the circle (the first thing) contains the combination of (the second thing) descending and ascending diagonals, while not all of the circle contains also verticals. As the singularity of the circle as a thing may suggest, by all can be meant a single thing alone, the principle applying to also a definition of an individual entity, when the question of not all having an attribute does not enter.

For the above definition of chair the fiqure does not assign to being a seat a separate attribute. Since the attributes are viewed as characterizing things, those a chair is, the listed attributes other than of merely a seat, which are not suited as nouns, would separately be referred to by phrases like "things with a back". Seeing that being a thing can likewise be held an attribute, the attributes listed by separately giving that of being a seat would needlessly multiply. That fewer are listed will be remindful of the practice of regarding as a single attribute a combination of them, often by a single name. The one attribute chair is defined by a few others. An entity, as was indicated, can be defined by sparsest attributes, so long as the above theorem on identity is conformed with.

This is accomplished even in definition by a single term, a synonym, although it may not be as illuminating as required. For that reason, because a concept can require eduction by some other attribute, a further theorem is furnished, for which the preceding concepts of term and synonym will first themselves be defined.

By "term" is meant a word or phrase which, as approximately defined in dictionaries, has a definite meaning, but which, more precisely, refers, through its whole, to only one kind of entity, not, through its parts, to more than one, which combined would identify it. When a term is a phrase it is sometimes called idiom, and "bring about" serves as an example. Its meaning is to be "cause" as a verb, without here an independent meaning of the words within the phrase, whereby it would be explicated. A single word can by this understanding, as a matter of fact, consist of more than one term. "Knowable" refers to both the concept of knowledge and its possible object.

By "synonym" is then meant a single term referring to the same entity a given other term does. It may be remarked that it has been proposed, in particular in connection with the spoken of interchangeability, that no two expressions are exactly synonymous. But as with other meanings, it is merely a matter of choice that one expression refer to the same thing as another.

THEOREM I.2. *An expression, perhaps in part, does not define a term by a synonym if and only if it defines it solely by more than one term.*

Proof. By the above definition of synonym as one term, if an expression, perhaps in part, defines a term by a synonym, it does not define it solely by more than one term. Therefore by later principle of transposition, by which if from *A* follows *B* then from the negation of *B* follows the negation of *A*, the "if" half of the theorem is true. Further, since part of a term has by the above no independent meaning, if an expression does not define a term solely by more than one term, it, perhaps in part, defines it by a synonym. By transposition therefore the "only if" half, equivalent to placing "if" in front, is true.

When accordingly a definition by a synonym is not suitable, as in defining discussed nondistinct things by distinct ones, then by the "only if" half of the theorem more than one term must be used, and by the "if" half none of them can be a synonym of the term defined.

Having set forth these principles of definition or eduction, of identifying concepts of concern, inquiry, in keeping with the process outlined in the introduction, may begin as to what realities can be discovered through concepts so identified.

Chapter II
REALITY

Because the object of this treatise is to determine realities, it appears especially important that reality be comprehensibly defined.

The determination of fundamental realities has been, as noted, the primary interest of metaphysics, which had been called the queen of sciences, and its general omission of a definition of reality, its identification, reveals how a major field of inquiry can fail to decide what the inquiry is about. In conformance with the expounded, when without an established concept behind the word, the query about reality amounts to a linguistic one, about what sort of things would be referred to as real. In contrast once the nature of the concept intended is settled, it is possible to, sometimes immediately, learn with certainty what particular things have reality, obviating much of the speculation and doubt of metaphysical doctrines.

Since by "reality", to accordingly proceed, is not meant a mere quality like color, the concept—in order to indicate with some specificity what qualities, what perceptual attributes, apply to it—must by what was said be defined by language other than for its whole, and consequently a definition by a synonym, such as "existent" or "actuality", falls short. The concept must for that purpose therefore, by above Theorem I.2, be defined by more than one term. But in accordance with Theorem I.1 that definition, too, can be inadequate. Were reality defined as, for instance, the object of sense perception, then sense perception, if itself thought a reality but not its own object, would be excluded.

In consonance with what went before, the question of the meaning of reality should be better answered by asking what the meaning of concern is.

It can then be said that the reality sought in this treatise and, it can doubtless be safely presumed, in most every quest for the real, are those objects of man's possible awareness, possible perception, that are the case and on which, good or bad, the outcome of man's pursuits can depend, which are accordingly consequential in man's purposes. While a mirage of an oasis as nearby may be the case, the oasis would not be considered real without further possible perception such as through touch and, ultimately, fulfillment of a desire such as quenching a thirst.

The real thus bears a resemblance to the necessary and fact again, these having been noted (p.35,. last par.) as of things that need be taken into account in man's actions. The now considered stricter sense of reality, of being, does not concern, however, anything that has been or is the case, nor merely principles, constancies. As indicated, something that is the case, e.g. the oasis of a mirage, may not be considered real, whereas something not a principle, e.g. an actual oasis, may. More specifically, when describing reality as something the case on which the outcome of man's pursuits can depend, by this specific "can", a synonym of a form of "possible", is meant, by what was said about the possible, that this reality, existence, concerns facts on which the outcome of man's pursuits either depends always, or sometime, or if certain not by principle precluded things are done, not to mention dependence simply not precluded. On reaching an oasis and drinking its water, these not precluded in principle, one quenches one's thirst.

There is also a broad sense of existence or synonyms, corresponding to that of fact or the necessary. Any occurrence, even an object of thought, would be said to have being. Forms of the last word are frequently used to connect subject and predicate, when the word is likewise a means for expressing asserted facts, existences of states, in conformance with earlier observation (p.16, first through third pars.). And this use is suggestive of why words like "existence", similarly to "fact" and the like, would be applied in the wide as well as a narrow sense. All that has been the case is in the vast contents of man's consciousness, with many of them found crucial to man's purposes, ascribed a tentative existence like that in propositions, which may be confirmed or disconfirmed.

Reality as described has an affinity with fact and the necessary also by supposing a free will (p.35, last par. again), through which upon knowing realities, things in the above way consequential in one's purposes, one may strive to realize those purposes, rather than be at the mercy of events. The freedom is especially supposed by the things most often looked upon as real, those that occur in the material world. Only a fraction of facts in that world is depended on in one's purposes. It is of indifference whether a larger portion of particular facts in it, e.g. the location of some object, occurs or not, the more so the more removed from one's life. That is to say these occurrences are in the required sense consequential only inasmuch as they would be depended on if through a free will one acted accordingly.

Whereas one may at no time depend on all things in the world, one may at times, as in an act of concentration, virtually depend on all of one's consciousness. This observation further highlights the discussed importance of consciousness in man's endeavors. By these endeavors are meant, in point of fact, efforts made through the employment of consciousness. They do not pertain to the human organism's activities in which one's consciousness is not made use of. Of consciousness to be sure are as said earlier all things under human consideration. What differs regarding the body's activities and all things material is that they are considered to be present also when not perceived. But like things stored in memory they like all else acquire actuality in their form in man's consciousness (p.26, last par.), and for that reason presently discussed reality was described as of man's possible awareness, possible perception. That material realities, or contents of memory, be considered present when not perceived thus signifies that, as in other possibilities, under certain in principle not precluded conditions they would be perceived.

The real was spoken of as perceivable by man, and it cannot be argued that, for instance, animals depend on the same things, things accordingly consequential to them, and that these things are by the aforesaid therefore realities even if man did not exist. The reality of animals might conceivably be only theirs. In other words, in order that something be man's reality, it must be consequential to and by the preceding therefore perceivable by man.

That it be perceivable accords somewhat with the pronouncement of the 18th-century philosopher George Berkeley that to be is to be perceived. A difference is that he did not specify man as perceiver, positing instead that all reality is perceived by God. He correspondingly also speaks of the perceived instead of the perceivable. And what is perceivable is in the present writing, further, not identified with what is real. I.e. unlike the converse, not all perceivable is real, as opposed to how Berkeley's view can be interpreted.

What is real can, however, be identified with what is knowable, knowable by man. In agreement with the definition in the first chapter (p.13, fourth par.), knowledge can be understood as awareness of something actual, compared to awareness of something assumed, and "actual" can, as indicated (p.44, third par.), be replaced by "real". By the real is for the meantime meant, if not all that is, the explained consequential broadly enough to include, as suggested in the introduction (p.4, third par.), things like logical principles or even definitions, things on which one may depend in seeking more proximately consequential facts. They include negative facts as well and represent truths that may be known, in contrast to hypotheses assumed. Transforming then the definition of knowledge, so as to speak of the known as the real meant to be the object of the awareness, something known is something real of awareness. This is the same as saying that something knowable, as what can be an object of the awareness, is something real of possible awareness. This sameness here of the known and the knowable, or of any occurrence and its possibility, is due to the comprehensive meaning of a word like "known". Used as in definitions, the word covers not only the actually known, but anything known possibly. And since the possible was seen to also cover the actual, the known and the knowable are in this use the same. By saying in the preceding thus that something known is something real of awareness, all possible times of the knowledge and awareness are meant. Thence something knowable is something real of possible awareness. But in accordance with the meaning of real (p.44, last par.), all of it is of possible awareness, which qualification of it is therefore superfluous. I.e. what is knowable is what is real.

A few more remarks about reality as perceivable and knowable.

The perceivability may be questioned in the light of accepted realities like the atom, seen as unviewable. The issue may be likened, however, to that of nondistinct entities like quantity. Particles of matter are determined in accordance with what are regarded as their effects, and while invisible, their description accords with attributes of visible things with similar effects. The descriptions are thus conceptual aids, the things referred to being truly the connections between things observed, as between certain experiments and their results. What matters with respect to the realities is that things of possible dependency are in fact perceived. Without the perception the dependency would not be held ascertained.

With regard to knowability it may be added that for something to be known does not imply strictly that it has been perceived. The entire process of correct inference about worldly reality rests on an absense of perception of the inferred. Nevertheless all that is known presupposes its perceivability, its possible presence in consciousness in the form making it actual, instead of an image. For even when something is known by inference, meant is by the very inference that what it conceives in the form of an image is actual, namely perceivable accordingly. It is by the same token that it is the circumstances of such as atoms that are actual, real. In whichever case it is not the image but the real which is the described consequential, correspondingly perceivable.

Doctrines inconsistent with the finding that what is real is humanly perceivable are certain realisms, sometimes including an idealism. The concerned things in the latter can be exemplified by Plato's forms, or universals, associated with attributes, and those in more exclusively the former by Aristotle's assumed underlying substance. Both, abstract archetypes of properties, and concrete substrata as their bearers, have been thought real but unperceivable by man. That what is real is what is knowable controverts, in addition, the skeptical position that no reality, some being provided, is knowable.

On the positive side, the furnished understanding of reality, as was indicated, makes it possible to establish whether and what realities exist, what accordingly, because of their identity with the knowable, is or can be known. In consequence speculation in epistemology, dealing with theory of knowledge and comprising the other major sphere of philosophy, is made likewise unnecessary. What is or can be known is what has been found to be or is real, i.e. consequential as explicated.

In the search for the real, for knowledge, there is between the real, the known or knowable, and knowledge also the issue of means by which knowledge is acquired. What these means are, a question in epistemology, is equally determined by what in that regard is consequential, whereby the means, too, can be held real, as suggested near the beginning of this chapter with respect to the senses (p.44, third par.), and elsewhere with respect to reflective methods and other matters. The reflective methods, distinguished before as eduction, induction, and deduction, and by means of which other realities that include broadly comprehended ones are herein sought, are examined in the course of seeking those realities as treated in various chapters. And the chapters immediately preceding and following the present one treat of further things that are realities by being means to knowledge. They concern reflective generalities, the first as to concepts of awareness, whereof subsequent realities may be discovered, and the second as to findings in logic, bases for discovery of additional realities. It is for the present chapter to for the first time explore realities other than of general reflection, although the reflective means of eduction and deduction used in the other chapters mentioned, and used here abundantly as well, are yet prominently supplemented here with the one of induction. The presently explored realities, represented by nature, are largely no longer means to knowledge, but more exclusively its sought after objects, as often, more directly, means toward human fulfillment which is no longer a means, but is desired for its own sake.

What fundamental entities belong to these realities, including any that might be held to extend beyond nature, has, as previously indicated, been a matter of much metaphysical debate. And the general requirement that the real be of those facts of one's possible awareness on which one can be dependent in one's pursuits was observed in the foregoing. Particular laws of nature as things of that dependence are for example accordingly realities.

It may be further observed that since the concern in realities is in what can be of knowledge, if something is presupposed by that knowledge, something one may find to be dependent on for it, then the presupposed can be held a prior reality. The dependency of one thing on another is a form of implication, and by later law of transitivity, hence, if something is dependent on the first thing, it is on the second. Accordingly since the knowledge at issue is of dependency in man's pursuits, and the presupposed spoken of is of dependency in that knowledge, the presupposed is of dependency in man's pursuits and is therefore by the discussed a prior reality mentioned. It is so insofar as it at least may be found a means to that knowledge, as are the senses found in relation to the outside world. And evidently if such a presupposed reality presupposes something else then that is by repeat transitivity a prior yet reality.

The priorities are still more emphatic if representing, as presuppositions by knowledge of another reality, not only realities but their knowledge. It can correspondingly be found that the common acceptance of particular realities presupposes, as noted in the introduction (p.3, third par.), not only certain realities questioned, but knowledge of them.

It is in accordance with the preceding thus possible to determine an order of priorities of reality, supplying a framework for more extended searches regarding it.

Section 1
THE SELF AND MIND

As observed, all things are known by man through the medium of one's consciousness, past, present, or future. In agreement with the above, hence, since knowledge of all reality accordingly presupposes consciousness, consciousness is a prior reality. This is of interest in view of the traditional opposition between espousals of only a material world and of only a conceptual one, more on which subject later. Since all apprehended is, to proceed, an ingredient of consciousness, however, it remains to be asked which ingredients have reality prior to which others.

Because the justification for things to be considered real was seen their consequentiality in man's pursuits, in man's purposes, these purposes, hence presupposed by knowledge of other realities, have prior reality. Many of the purposes, to continue, have as interest more basic ones. One has certain ends as objective so as to lead to ones of more concern. There are then as was suggested (p.48, third par.) eventual ends aimed at not for the sake of others but for their own sake, fulfilling what can be regarded as a person's fundamental purpose of being satisfied, of attaining one's what is spoken of as happiness. This what can be held a fundamental quality of purpose or concern, whose knowledge as ground in one's conscious pursuits is by the foregoing presupposed by all other knowledge, can be accordingly seen as primary as a reality. Since what is, further, principally meant to identify a person, a self, is, as in hope for surviving the decease of one's body, that quality of purpose, the concern with being satisfied, that quality can be considered to be the self.

This definition of the self may seem unusual. The self is frequently identified instead with the whole of consciousness, or what is called mind, although the soul as the self and subject of consciousness may be heard of. And materialism identifies the self with the body, alone or with consciousness as a component. Whether or not consciousness is accordingly inseparable from the body, it can be separately considered in its manifestations, and these manifestations are often held to represent the self. It is the self conceived of again as possibly disembodied. Consciousness encompasses, however, all of what is called the external world, and the self is not meant to consist of also that world. Nor is it meant to consist of all the internal world, of objects of such as dreams or the imagination. The self is rather thought of as different from these objects, sometimes as somehow unperceivable except for a manner of functioning. Viewed from the outside it might thus in fact be considered vaporous and not discernible, as are all of another person's perceptions. What is accordingly meant to distinguish continued life after the death of the body is indeed the functioning that is meant to distinguish all life, namely the functioning, the presence, of certain purpose. The writer will not at this point address the alluded to arguments (p.9, second par.) on what constitutes life, but for reminding that it is a matter of definition. And by the preceding whereas the purpose found to distinguish living organisms is preservation of them and others, the purpose found to distinguish sentient, conscious, beings is satisfaction in general. This purpose distinguishing the self is while perceived from outside by effects only nevertheless like other purposes an internal perception or quality, which may be named individual sensibility, called at times ego.

The question may be raised again as to how a perception, said to occur to someone, can occur without a subject different from it. The topic is sometimes presented by proposing the self to be a substance like matter, and the argument is irrelevant, the point as in other cases being what is chosen to be meant by the self. In addition the linguistic nature of the issue may by now be evident. Though perception might in subject-predicate fashion be said to occur to someone, the language does not require that a perception, a quality, may not exist as an autonomous subject of other perceptions, and as perception conscious of itself in what is called apperception. It may be asked how that can, in view of the seemingly more palbable processes of such as the body, occur. But it does and, as in the case of e.g. resemblance (p. 22, sixth par.), requires only its own confirmation. As a matter of fact a person of a body, viewed as the subject, is, as all else known, itself made up of perceptions. These perceptions of the person accordingly could themselves be thought to require a subject of them. But since all is perception, there is no subject outside it to which it occurs. Indeed one would be loath to declare that something is perceived by one's body, and not by oneself as the inner sensibility of concern.

The maintenance that the self be an entity distinct from the body is by some thinkers a most vehemently assailed one. The attitude can be understood as recognition of only material reality, and it is irrelevant once again, the meaning of the self being a matter of choice. As presently disclosed, furthermore, the described self, far from subordinate as reality to the body or other material things, is a prerequisite for them.

Other arguments in behalf of a bodily self have been advanced, likewise containing irrelevancies. Upon finding no entity thought to qualify as a mental substance representing the self, former philosophers, adhering to a conceptual one, questioned the presence of a criterion by which many perceptions can be held to belong to one person. Since attempts at an answer were by later thinkers thought to be useless, the body was again proffered as criterion of an individual. But the issue is not relevant to the, once more arbitrary, definition, instead concerning what makes the defined a single entity.

This question can be asked about a sought after substance as well, spiritual or corporeal. And what makes an entity a single one, whether at a moment or through time, is characteristically left out of definitions. The comprehension is normally implicit, and there should be no wonder, since there seems no common criterion, with designation of unit another arbitrary matter. The simplest unit can be the smallest discernible part of a perception, and a single perception, one that may be held to be of a moment, can be one that undergoes no change. Units can become more complex depending on the interest, familiar ones among these being material objects, of a single identity though of, as earlier remarked (p.24, sixth par.), manifold simultaneous perception and subsequent changing ones.

With many of these objects it may be of comparatively small importance whether they remain one and the same. The sameness of the self is of paramount importance, however, because it figures in the very seeking of fulfillment of one's purposes, by which other things become important. The sameness figures as stated inasmuch as one wants to know it is the same oneself whose purposes may be fulfilled. In the long run the interest, as explicated, is that oneself as the sensibility, the fundamental quality of purpose or concern, is satisfied. It is in the form of this sensibility, perhaps lastingly satisfied, that one wishes to survive. This sameness of the self is also the interest of persons outside it, in what is known as the question of responsibility. Others wish to know that an action is performed by the same person that, depending on the action, is treated correspondingly, so that the person's purpose in the actions be in harmony with the purposes of others. The sameness of the self accordingly hinges on self-awareness as of the same purpose, concern, since the interest both of the self and others is whether perceptions, pleasing or displeasing, of different times are regarded by the self as its own, and its unity is related to that sameness. A self is chosen to be called a single one because it identifies itself with the selfsame purpose concerned. In similarity to the above singleness of a least perception of a moment, it identifies itself with a purpose by its whole, not separately by any part, and it continues to do so through time, not undergoing change, any different part as the purpose, or any through change different purpose, not being by that difference, as self-determined, the selfsame. How the identification is accomplished is again immaterial, it mattering to self and others that it is.

Thinkers who identified the self with an internal entity described its unity through time by, while seeing only consciousness in general, its memory of awarenesses of things. Consciousness as a whole—made up of varied things, including phenomena of the material world—cannot of course be held the subject of past awarenesses, nor is it clear what makes any a unit at a time. But as factor in defining unity of an individual, memory was irrelevantly criticized as leaning on something unreliable. An entity, including unity through time, can, again, be defined by any attribute of interest.

The objection to the memory was as before intended to support the concept of a bodily self. It is contended that one's memory of having perceived things cannot, in view of failures of memory, be a criterion for one's past existence, that it is therefore the sameness of the body which identifies the individual. It can be noted that even if the body were better suited for that purpose, it would not thereby have to be a part or the whole of the self, not to repeat dependence on definition. Things can be signs of something, e.g. of the same individual, without being its constituents. What is more, memory is relied upon for all that is past, including acquaintance with someone's body. Still more, the body can change to a point of losing any individual resemblance to its previous state.

Regarding failure of a memory in general, it has to do mainly with the very particulars of the external world, including individuals. An amnesiac will even fail within a short span to recognize his immediate family. But he will remember general things such causal connections. Similarly men at large remember to considerable detail fundamental things required in their lives. Since they remember these as of account in their purposes, they remember themselves as of those purposes. Or simply, since their remembrances are of perceptions by themselves, they remember themselves as of the perceptions.

As last of the arguments put forward, the contention may be mentioned that since by person is often meant the outer appearance of someone, that aspect be held to be constituent of oneself. But in this case merely a choice of definition takes place. Reference to persons was in what went before here made sparingly, because the self as discussed can apply to animals as well. Apart from this, bodies are known to be accoutrements of sentient beings, and it makes sense to give a name to the combined attributes. But the question is what entity is wished to be talked about, and presently it is the discussed individual sensibility, referred to customarily as soul or the self.

By the foregoing the knowledge or reality of this entity, as the concern in seeking other realities, is presupposed by all other knowledge while not presupposing any of it since not requisite, and it can therefore be stated that

THEOREM II.1. *The self is the primary reality.*

Proof of theorems in this chapter is contained in the discussions preceding them, instead of being formally given after them. Since the chapter functions as a digressive whole in establishing these theorems, an informal style is preferable.

It will next be suitable to return to the concept of consciousness, noted at the start of this section to be presupposed by knowledge of all other realities. Among these is the self, and the reason it can be considered the primary reality nonetheless is that its knowledge presupposes consciousness by being an instance of it, and thus does therein not presuppose knowledge of another thing. The self knows all further realities by consciousness of them, however, and hence consciousness can be placed after the self as a presupposed reality, as can its knowledge, by reason of one's very knowledge of things as phenomena of consciousness.

The consciousness under discussion might also, and in a way less confusingly, be called mind. Consciousness often connotes apprehension of the physical world, in contrast to, for example, dreams; the consciousness of this writing, as should be evident, is of all human, or animal, apprehension. Consciousness also connotes apprehension in the present, not in the past, or perhaps the future; in the now written about, consciousness is meant to include, as in the case of knowledge, apprehensions committed to memory, from which they might be recalled. The consciousness meant here is in brief the sum of all perceptions that have been those of an individual and to a large degree preserved in memory. This totality may in accordance with usage more suitably be termed mind.

This naming is reminiscent of mind as spoken of in psychology and including the unconscious. With the unconscious to mean things that were never in consciousness, however, it is not included in the present concept of mind. Things that were never in one's consciousness though part of the individual are simply by definition part of other than mind in the organism. This as dictionaries attest is manifested as the common understanding of mind, and efforts to prove it false can again not accomplish more than give the word another meaning. That meaning is also unable to delimit what part of the organism is the unconscious, which since all is known through consciousness nothing can be. In response to frequent further objection it may also again be noted that, as observed in relation to the self, mind need not be described in terms of substance, perhaps as receptacle for perceptions, but can be comprehended by the attribute of perception alone.

With mind accordingly naming consciousness as the known reality determined above, it may be stated that

THEOREM II.2. *Mind, including the self, is a reality prior to every other.*

It should be added that by the mental, as by the conceptual or the like, can as common be herein also meant only the inner, nonworldly, objects of awareness, as normally understood from the context, or occasionally referred to as purely mental. In compliance with what was said this narrower sense of mind was seen likewise not to be identical with the self, and taken strictly it does not include it, but is of things in its cognition that are not of the external world, examined in the next section.

The conclusions stated by the preceding two theorems are in certain agreement with the one in the famous "I think, therefore I am" of Descartes of the 17th century, asserted in his search for indubitable reality. His conclusion that he exists was not well substantiated, however. He did not furnish, primarily, a concept of being, of reality, and, to a lesser extent, of the I, the self, from which the inference within the statement could be drawn. He made the assumption that the world is as unreal as are dreams, and since even this form of doubt consists in his thought, he inferred that at least he and his thought are real. The contents of even dreams and the world assumed imagined, however, could in their occurrence be regarded as having as much being as he and his thought does, and explanation is wanting as to why the latter entities should have more being than the former. Further, the use of "I" in "I think" does not imply the existence of an I distinct from the doubted physical matter. The phrase can be a succinct way of saying "Inside this bodily shape occurs thought". Or, the "I" can be merely the discussed subject of a sentence, not implying an entity distinct from the predicated thought. Descartes nevertheless recognized that a thing can be identified by its attributes, in this case mind by thinking.

The much debated dualism of mind and body, or mind and matter, propelled by his views is further of interest. Man, reality, and other things can in truth be arbitrarily and correctly seen as twofold, threefold, or more by repeated dichotomy. By considering any particular feature as distinguished from the rest of a thing, a twofold division is made; by continuing the same in regard to either of these parts, a threefold division is made; and the procedure can go on. Thus in accordance with above, man as known might be divided into the self and other attributes, which attributes might similarly be divided into mind, in the restricted sense, and body. But the insistent questions regarding the dualism have been whether either mind, in a wide sense and as often equated with the self, or matter is not part of the other, or whether one or the other exists at all.

In the case of whether matter is the inclusive entity, as proposed by materialism, the questions can be understood by considering that matter and its events can seem to, compared to for instance the imaginary, be the only objects of cognition that are effectual with regard to man's interests. This explanation illustrates as basis for a reality the possible dependence on it in man's pursuits. By holding then matter and its behavior to be the only reality, mental occurrences are accounted for by regarding them as part of it or by denying them altogether, in what can be viewed as needless equivocation of worldly reality with any form of being.

In the case of whether only mind is real, a proposition of idealism, the questions can be understood in the light of the same cognition, the manifestation in mind of all, the world of matter as well as other things, as aided by finding all perceptions to converge in the brain. Matter can be considered to nevertheless exist in that manifestation, and not as part of a self not synonymous with mind.

These remarks notwithstanding, since presently mind and the self are at issue, the bearing of these questions on their status, namely whether they are forms of matter, if not nonexistents, may be considered.

That mind or the self be part of matter, specifically the brain, can be seen to be impossible. Whatever the brain portion assumed to be indentical with mind, with consciousness, might be, inasmuch as it would be manifested in particular perceptions characterizing matter, it cannot be identical with other or all perceptions, i.e. mind. And inasmuch as the self was observed to be of a quality distinguished by no more than the sensibility spoken of, it cannot be identical with certain matter, distinguished otherwise.

At the basis of this impossibility lie as well the mentioned diverse ways in which things are identified as selfsame. Beside the character distinguishing individual perceptions of material objects from the other perceptions, those objects were indicated to admit of different perceptions of them through time while held to retain their identity and even be unchanging. The self and states of consciousness, however, do, as noted alongside (p.51, last par., through p.52, second par.), not allow that variety of perception, whereby a version of them could be found identical with some perceived matter. A state of consciousness, a perception of a given time, is not the same as another perception, e.g. of some matter. And a perception that differs from one of a sensibility which is a self is not of the same sensibility, if any.

As to the existence at all of mind or a self, it, their reality before others in fact, was determined precedingly herein.

Doubts about it have extended from the denial of discernment of oneself in consciousness to the mentioned denial of consciousness itself. The first of the denials is associated with the 18th-century philosopher David Hume, who on introspection averred to find nothing but a bundle of perceptions. His views differed from materialism, by giving no more credence to matter than to a self. But he fell short of recognizing that either of them need be manifested by nothing more than certain of the perceptions he spoke of, ranging from touch, signifying the material, to concern, signifying the self. The second of the above disavowals is as indicated associated with behaviorism, which seeks to understand men through observations of their overt actions. Its refusal to recognize consciousness, as readily apparent and suggested before, belies the nature of its own observations, the form in which the behavior of others is known.

The last doctrine is an example of the influence of observational science, with a related scientific determinism, the belief that there is no freedom of action, that all events are determined by physical or chemical laws. If they are then men's behavior might indeed be studied from their physical response to stimulus, without paying to their conscious at least attention. That men's behavior be studied would then not seem of interest, however, with the actions of those who study it predetermined likewise, whatever they may learn of others.

Whether or not man's mind is thus subject to physical or chemical laws may be seen presently, in its further exploration.

While the self and mind were found to be prior as realities to any other, it has not yet been determined what further entities, entities apprehended through the mind, may be regarded as realities, as objects of knowledge. Traditionally the major dispute in epistemology, in theory of knowledge, has been between rationalism and empiricism. The two doctrines contend that the source of knowledge is, respectively, reason and experience. The distinction between the two, though, is not entirely clear. There is little question that the rational is meant to be of mind contrasted with a physical world, and the empirical had been referred to in terms of sense perception. But the classical empiricists tend to discount a reality of senses and other physical entities, relying only on mental impressions. It may be asked in that case, which of the mental occurrences, before acknowledgement of a physical world, consist in experience, and which consist in reason.

An answer suggesting itself is that the first are the involuntary and the second the voluntary. The division should reveal itself to be a useful one, but it can now be asked whether such a division exists if there is no free will, if volition is not free. For by voluntary things are meant here, as appears customary, things resulting from volition independent of external compulsion. If they were compelled by something else, they should be considered involuntary.

It might be suggested that by voluntary mental occurrences those be meant that emanate from the mind distinguished from the physical world, without being free from compulsion. The distinction of a physical world is assumed not to have yet been made, however, preventing knowledge of whether something emanates from it or otherwise. And should such a world, of the all-pervading physical and chemical laws argued, be assumed, then no mental events could be free of them.

It may thus be of benefit to see whether a valuable difference cannot be established in accordance with the initial meaning of the voluntary and involuntary, whether some occurrences, purely mental or other, arise from a free will, and whether some do not.

It should be understood that the freedom at issue is not one completely unrestrained. Supposing an initiating free will, even the imagination may be hampered by conditions like fatigue, and bodily action is always constrained to function in accord with material laws of nature. At issue is whether one's will, one's effort directed at an intellectual or physical end, is wholly determined by factors external to it, such as divine or natural laws, or even logical ones in the sense that one could not deduce a false conclusion from given premises. The question of complete jurisdiction of man-made laws is understandably not often raised. The question of their futility in absence of free will, however, is raised frequently, since in that absence man-made laws are seen as not influencing men's actions, and it may be noted that in absence of free will, again, legislation would be likewise not a matter of choice.

In order then to find if free will exists, it will be well to recall, from the discussion of necessity, that a universal law, an invariable fact about something, depends for its truth on no more than that invariability. The mentioned laws of nature are of course accepted as preponderous realities. Questioned is that man's will is to any degree exempt from them or perhaps otherwise not compelled to take a certain course. But in conformance with the preceding, if some other fact about something is determined equally invariable, then that connection is equally a principle. It is a principle, a corresponding reality, even more emphatically if the connection can always and fully be observed, and if, in keeping with the order of priorities spoken of, knowledge of the other realities depends on it.

And the finding is not merely that circumstances do sometimes but perhaps not always not impose one's will. If that were the case, it could be presumed that when an act of will seems to have no cause, it is because none has yet been found. Such presumptions are made about physical states, because all of them are taken to have a cause, due to the constancy regarding them in observable cases. The constancy, however, applies to will in the opposite way, an absence of connection. One's will is always found unimposed by any circumstance. One is free to choose or not any object of volition, even if the object, as may be a recollecting or a physical action, cannot be realized. That one can do so can in addition be found at every try and without a lapse in particulars, in contrast to such as physical causation, not always observable of an event, while inferred as indicated above, and intractable in particulars, as remarked in the introduction (p.5, second par.). The knowledge by principle that one is free to will any object, that one can in fact thereby realize many of them and their desired consequences, is furthermore presupposed by regarding, as suggested (p.45, last par.), as realities any of those results and their world, including the corresponding laws. One is cognizant that one is free to make choices regarding one's fate, accordingly considering the entire world that enables the same consequential, real.

It has been argued that volition does have a cause in its purpose or reason, in the objects of one's will. As one is not compelled by any other circumstance to will something, however, one is not compelled by the objects of one's will, by given prospects, but can will any other thing or none. The belief that the reason for a volition may be its cause can be attributed to equivocation regarding senses of reason and cause. The cause of an event is sometimes called its reason, and a reason for an action is sometimes called a cause for it. The first case can be taken as reflecting mental explanation of the event, and the second as of reasons as preceding volitions, as causes precede effects. But the issue concerning free will being that a volition is not required by something else, cause and reason in this context are of opposites. In concord with former observations, one thing requires another by being always accompanied by it. This can apply to cause and effect as well as to logical implication. Accordingly the cause requires the effect. But a volition instead requires, by its meaning, a purpose, the reason, not the reason the volition, contrary to the supposed causation.

The purpose contained by meaning in volition has in some arguments for will as predetermined been omitted. Presumedly thinking a purpose a cause, it is maintained that if a will is undetermined it is tantamount to chance, having then no reason, by which persons are expected to act. It is in this vein put forward by some that widely accepted free will exists though predetermined, its freedom residing in an absence of impediment to carrying it out. But such an absence was observed missing. One can indeed be prevented from carrying out one's will, whether by physical factors or lack of knowledge. Furthermore, the contended freedom from impediment is not the one meant, which is just that one's will is not predetermined, that one is free to seek required knowledge and to accordingly choose one's actions, so that one may correspondingly pursue one's ends, not otherwise ensured.

The will can as a matter of fact be regarded as free by, in consequence of its, definition, if understood as the power of commencing purposive activity. This meaning is the one herein adopted in a precise sense and can be viewed as the general one considered above, when volition is regarded as a starting force directed toward some end, as in the frequent definition of will as the power of self-direction, contrasted with direction by something else. And, as noted to also apply to organisms at large (p.50, second par.), by purposive activities or events, by ones directed toward some end, are more specifically meant those that by appropriate adjustment accomodate whatever circumstance toward what does, or appears to, attain, or is likely to attain, the end at issue.

The qualifications of appearance and likelihood should be elucidated. The appearance has to do with man's supposition that the object of the will can be attained, and the likelihood concerns actual probability of the attainment. The difference is analoqous to that between possibility of something insofar as man knows and insofar as not precluded by a law, in accord with observations in the last chapter. But purposiveness also has a more solid base. After the initial force now identified with the act of will, assuming it to have at least the most immediately aimed at result, comes what is accordingly already a purpose fulfilled although most often only a possible means to a further end. Ends that are purposive outcomes, toward which circumstances are adapted and which may be called purposive events in a restricted sense, are consequently much more frequent than the above qualifications make it seem. For instance man's acts of will result more often than not in the intended bodily motions, toward which intermediate processes also function, and which normally succeed in, in what can be held purposive events in a nonrestricted sense, some further material purposes, like taking care of mundane needs.

With purposive events so understood, and the will the power giving rise to them, it may be asked if some other condition does not compel the unqualified will to do so. But if it did then since the will's behavior would be decided by it, that behavior would not adjust to whatever circumstance to fulfill the purpose, but would be the same irrespectively. Hence the will would not be the force initiating purposive activities, contrary to its meaning, and therefore it is not compelled by something else, but is free.

By this determination the previous finding that one has a free will is equivalent to one that men, and animals, possess the power of will, the otherwise redundant ascription of freedom usable in making it explicit. The finding takes the form of a principle in that one can if not at all times then when of a minimal alertness exercise one's will, exert, purposive, effort.

The by the foregoing established free will should be of much pertinence to behavioral or social sciences, when on the order of natural science endeavoring systematic studies of men's actions. The tendency has been to look for hidden causes, to the dismissal of men's conscious grounds. Men, not to mention animals, are often thus degraded to the rank of objects, if somewhat complex ones. For the solution of problems professionals may try to influence or gain information from men regarding their actions not by addressing their reason, but by eliciting unreasoned replies, as in psychoanalysis, though even animals have reasons for their actions. Similarly, history is thought to be moved by inexorable laws, and in thinking to know what they are, governments impose them on populations. To boot, in the well known notion that responses to stimuli can be conditioned is implicit a presumption that the experimenters can create natural laws of their own, in conformity to which mankind is expected to eventually acquire attributes according to plan. The conditioning is based on reward or punishment of its subjects according to their behavior, in the familiar method of coercion, made worse by the detachment of assumed science. The assumption is additionally that men can be stupefied into holding the connections between their actions and the requital to be laws of nature, in denial of an intelligence even animals, fleeing a cruel master, possess. The denial is in tandem with the belief that one's will is but subject to forces imposed on it. The general error of behavioral sciences is indeed their thinking to be ones, neglecting that one's behavior is guided by one's free will.

That one has a free will can be regarded as, in view of the constancy by which it is determined a principle, the first induction about now discussed reality. The finding of the continued existence of something, as would be the case regarding the world of matter, could likewise be called an induction, and since the reality of that world is not known without the reality of selves, their continued existence might be considered an induction also. Whereas there is little argument about the continuance of the physical universe, however, there is much argument about the continuance of individual selves. The induction of a free will concerns instead, similarly to customary causal inductions, a power, a capability, namely that of exerting effort, perhaps a minute one of refraining. The induction, it is again notable, is a prescientific one, found to be present in the very holding of knowledge in science as elsewhere worthwhile, by understanding that one has corresponding choices of action.

Speaking of knowledge and action, there are other prescientific inductions having to do with the will and requisite in one's pursuits. The action is brought about by the will, as is for that purpose the recalling of remembered, known, things. The inductions are that, in conjuction with other enabling conditions, willing of the recollections and actions will produce them.

It has been questioned what the willing consists in, and

things suggested in that regard, such as a thought of the aimed for, were determined not to have the desired effect. This question, too, is, however, irrelevant. Men and animals have knowledge of the nature of a volition, be it only referred to by such a general word or none, of account being that whatever the willing consists in, one learns of it as a cause of certain events regarding oneself.

Insofar as this finding of causation is about bodily action, it has been called interactionism, which also refers to causation of mental events by bodily ones. The existence of the interactions has been beside free volition denied, by holding it incomprehensible that an immaterial mind be causally connected with a material body. The connection is of course comprehensible and fact in the very finding of it, and causal interaction among material things rests on scarcely as firm a ground. Its legitimacy is secured by being through physical causation, as through light rays and the sense of sight, conveyed to consciousness, where it is as a mental effect manifested. Should this causality between matter and mind terminate, the cessation would be physical at all events, since if mental then the physical by being dependent on its perception for its reality would likewise lose it.

Whereas the perception of physical reality is involuntary, not the direct result of volition, the before spoken of actions, at least their beginnings, and the rememberings were seen as voluntary. These, too, are in a sense involuntary, by being results of volition in accordance with spoken of causal laws. What is truly voluntary are the volitions themselves, rather than their results. The existence of these voluntary mental contents, of those of free will, was determined above. And it is possible to determine with no lesser ease the existence of involuntary ones. As it is discernible that one can produce voluntary thoughts, so it is discernible that one has involuntary experiences, as suggested at the beginning of this paragraph. Among these experiences are those of physical realities, which since dependent on the involuntary perceptions render them also realities. The common awareness of both the voluntary and involuntary is sometimes expressed by the distinction between active and passive mental contents, referring to the use or not of volition, both contents otherwise involving mental activity, change, unlike connoted.

There should be thus no trouble to examining the contents of mind with respect to the distinction between the voluntary and involuntary, another division exhaustive by dichotomy. Specifically, the division can serve as a stepping stone for exploration as to what ingredients of any of the two parts may be further realities.

Having determined the real to be what is of possible dependency in man's pursuits, it follows that all reality must be subject to universal law, to explicated constancy. As indicated before (e.g. p.4, last par.), the reason that something is found of possible dependency in some regard is that it, perhaps as existence itself, always accompanies a certain other thing of account. This lawfulness is exemplified by the implication by which the self or mind are real because other realities depend on them.

As a result those mental ingredients, those concepts, that are solely voluntary, that are not confirmable by involuntary perception, are not realities. Since voluntary concepts are free from compulsion, they are free from constancies by which they would be of dependency. Concerning either intrinsic, logical, truths, or extrinsic, natural, ones, one can if relying on volition make any, e.g. a false, determination, even if contradicting the concept in view.

This conclusion invalidates the contentions of rationalism if understood as upholding that, intrinsic or extrinsic, knowledge is acquired through the mere use of thought or reason as a voluntary exercise of mind. The understanding is in accordance with (p.57, fourth and fifth pars.) distinguishing between the rational and empirical as between knowledge through the voluntary and involuntary, and it was adumbrated when distinguishing between the a priori and a posteriori (p.13, third par.). As remarked there, some of logic is thought to be known true without proof, and the same was proposed of such as causality. The latter finds less support today, but the former is likewise excluded by the foregoing. This negation of rationalism does not apply to knowledge by way of deduction. That method will be seen securely grounded in involuntary perception, and as purely mental might be called a rational means to knowledge.

The preceding does not of course deprive voluntary mental activities of value. They were already a few times referred to as source of man's actions, in the interest of which knowledge, dependent on the involuntary, is required. And they equally assume an extensive role as pertains to that knowledge. Relative to their likewise referred to use for recollecting, the will is used for calling forth the concepts, the premises, from which above mentioned deduction can proceed, as well as for recalling experiences leading to induction. As observed, further, anything learned is equally summoned from memory, to apply it to subsequent purposes. In addition to these uses of volition for actions and for evoking for their sake such as past determinations, volition is also used for making to that end the determinations, as when affirming what is perceived, the act distinguished before from perceived states alone (p.16, second par.), or when deciding a definition. These determinations serve to fix situations in memory, and they are for like reasons made into linguistic statements, to represent forms of knowledge.

The voluntary mind thus also has a direct part in acquiring knowledge, along with the involuntary as conveyor of that which is to be known. It should be noted that although awareness of a definition was earlier viewed as loosely a form of knowledge, definitions naturally are not of the dependability accorded other objects of knowledge, those comprising stricter realities and observed to in their law-based dependability require involuntary perception. There is a degree of man-made lawfulness in definitions too, insofar as it is for utility agreed upon to abide by them, and when that consent by others is learned, it is so in an involuntary way. But when a definition is specified by oneself, it can be quite arbitrary, and though still useful to adhere to, it rests the less on established and to that degree dependable meaning. The upshot is that above voluntary determinations need not be assertions of, dependable, realities, involuntarily perceived, but may be, changeable, choices made where desirable. Voluntary mind nevertheless partakes in the acquisition of knowledge by ascertaining what is supplied by the involuntary.

Volition participates in that acquisition also more indirectly than observed before. Recollecting for and acting is done also to gain knowledge, not only to put it to use for other purposes. Whichever the purposes, both the voluntary and involuntary mind are by the preceding indispensable to knowledge of any of the mind's content as reality.

While both are thus indispensable to knowledge and hence are realities, they understandably do as before not assume therein priority over the self, which after all is the possessor of these capacities. More in keeping with the aforesaid the prior reality of the self may in the following again be explained by the presupposition by other realities of not only the self, but the knowledge of it.

The introduction above of affirmation as, in acquiring knowledge, another voluntary act brings more subtlety into the discussion of mind, as befits its all-encompassing nature. But the discussion should be distinguished from those which propose theories of mind as comprising what is labelled man's psychology, somehow distinct from man's conscious and freely purposeful life. It was already noted that by the usual meaning of mind any such subconscious life would be consigned to other parts of the organism, not to mention the impossibility of an unconscious as a real entity. More critical is that this psychological structure, rather than chosen conscious purposes, is purported to supply the drive behind man's actions. As indicated, such conceptions of mind find their basis in holding the behavior of matter as foundation by which to know all reality, the grounds for human actions sought accordingly in physical causation. But to seek the grounds one need only resort to introspection, it being origin in purposeful consciousness which belongs to the meaning of action, as compared to other bodily activities. And what truly matters is that it is the mind of consciousness, presently the free volition responsible for action and omitted by psychology, that is now explored.

It might be as well to dispense with the discussion of finer points in mind's volitional part. The discourse could proceed by simply observing that the self is part of conscious reality as soon as anything else is, and then seeing what subsequent priorities can be found. But volition as mere affirmation or the like is of interest both in making determinations as wholes and in considering subjects of which determinations are to be made. These become issues in logic. Something is often said to follow from propositions, whereas it actually follows from the things proposed. It is not from acts of proposing, but from the conditions, that Socrates is a man and that all men are mortal that it follows that Socrates is mortal. Instead the propositions function in mentally setting down the conditions, from which to deduce results. Similarly one may mentally regard a subject, e.g. a triangle, from which to deduce an attribute, e.g. three sides. The like referred to before as a calling forth, these preparatory mental acts of bringing conditions or subjects to awareness then are volitions, designed here to lead to what may be deduced. Notable is that the things deduced, as earlier explained, are contained in the initial conceptions, though not likewise brought to awareness.

The significance is that these things can hence be viewed as dormant ingredients of consciousness, of perceptions, and the bringing them to awareness in deduction a volitional taking into cognizance, an affirmation, of them. These and other ingredients of consciousness become in this manner objects of awareness or knowledge, which may thereafter be committed to memory. Counting now is that there are many things in perception that, though often implicit as in the preceding, are not brought to awareness, which bringing may be done in varying degrees, as one exerts varying amounts of effort regarding things. This lack of awareness is sometimes voiced by saying that someone is looking at something but does not see it. One may see it as a result of slight attention alone, as in ascertaining particulars of a natural scene, or through lengthy inference, as in mathematical chains of equations. Volition thus serves many functions, from slight attention to thorough determinations—these figuring mainly in gaining knowledge—to more active employment.

Returning to the self and other parts of consciousness at issue, they were seen to be, as deductive facts, implicit in the knowledge of all other reality. They were in fact indicated to be of awareness, known, and can be so regarded even with the addition of the act of affirmation to the gaining of knowledge by man or animal. Unlike when something is contained in a conception but is not in awareness and must be deduced, and as when bringing to awareness conditions or subjects to find what can be inferred, the present entities belong to those of awareness, those known, with respect to which other things are or become known. One again has in awareness, is knowing of, oneself as the subject of concern in one's purposes, one's pursuits that render other things realities, and one is knowing of one's voluntary and involuntary mind as means required for those pursuits. That the knowledge of the self should as said have priority over the other two is decided on the basis that knowledge of these mental powers is only required for those pursuits, while knowledge of the self as the concerned is required for knowledge of those powers.

In detailed scrutiny common to philosophy, it may be asked how if knowledge requires a volitional act of affirmation can the self be an object of knowledge prior to volition being one. However, as can other things be part of perception without being affirmed, so can volition. One can by help of volition affirm oneself, without having so affirmed the volition. As a matter of fact each volitional act cannot be affirmed, since the attempt leads to a so-called infinite regress. An affirmation requires volition, whose affirmation requires another volition, and so forth. What is more, for affirmation of oneself to be as a volition likewise affirmed, the volition must have been performed, namely the self affirmed first.

There is little need in this matter, however, for further reasoning so intricate. That one possesses or not knowledge of things is made certain without the preceding consideration of volition in gaining it, and it will be apparent from what went before that knowledge, or the reality, of one's voluntary and involuntary mind presumes the knowledge or reality of oneself as the described sensibility possessing those powers, that the knowledge or reality of all else presumes the knowledge or reality of those powers, and that therefore

THEOREM II.3. *Voluntary and involuntary mind, including the self, are realities prior to every other.*

The certainty of the reality of objects of voluntary and involuntary mind seen supplied by the second of the two, the succeeding task is to find which of its objects may be considered realities beyond the already determined.

Section 2
EXTERNAL REALITY

The further realities presently sought concern a world and its inherent laws, through which that world is consequential in man's active pursuits, by linking one's purposes with their fulfillment. In conformance with what was said, this world as compared to other objects of consciousness, such as dreams, is a reality because it is thus consequential, and since it functions as the mentioned link, extents of knowledge of it by man are requisite.

This knowledge, as observed, is obtained in involuntary perception, and it may then be asked what, apart from that consequentiality, distinguishes that world from other objects of involuntary perception, to which such as dreams also belong. The question is rightfully asked, because the interest is in what things the consequentiality applies to, so that they may be heeded for that reason.

EXTENSION

The things in question are normally designated as matter, and its identification cannot be made in accordance with the most recent findings on submicroscopic particles. As mentioned previously (p.47, third par.), such particles are known by their effects, and by the preceding the question remains what the things of those effects are. More pertinently, these and other realities detected in some regard through instruments concern in those instruments objects of the macroscopic world, the familiar world found to be perceived through the unaided senses. That is to say it is the objects of this larger world, e.g. the instruments, which are found in this and other ways consequential, and it is these objects that are initially designated as material. If the meaning of matter is accordingly to remain the same then, although it might also be defined by later findings, it must be definable by attributes of the above objects first considered.

More important, since what is meant by a word is a matter of choice, of concern are the above worldly objects in general as consequential as found. And the question is what characterizes these suitably called material objects, whereby they may be distinguished from others.

It could be proposed that material objects are those that occupy space, since space as a three-dimensional expanse is considered the container of physical objects. Objects of dreams and the like, however, seem to occupy space also. Space can in point of fact be seen not to be the presumed entity distinct from the objects in it. A distinct concept referred to by a term, it will be remembered, must be independently perceivable. Any worldly entity independently perceivable, however, is regarded at most as occupant of space, space itself meaning to designate a void. The word is applied to quantitative attributes of these entities or objects, to their volume and location, chiefly to any absence of them in some part of reality, the part being determined by some dimensional relation of further of the objects. In either case space is distinguished in accordance with material objects, rather than material objects being distinguished in accordance with space.

Physical reality need therefore be distinguished by some other characteristic, and the three dimensions mentioned can furnish the answer. It is those objects encountered in perception that are regarded as of three dimensions, of extension, which are found subject to the laws at issue and are accordingly real. Other objects encountered, those that are purely mental, are only accorded an existence that is two-dimensional. The definition of the objects of the physical world as those of extension is fitting because in conformance with Theorem I.1 of the first chapter all and only objects of that world are of extension.

An understandable reply to the definition may be that the contents of a dream or hallucination can have as much a semblance of extension as they can of spatiality. They can, and a distinction between a real and an illusory world is not necessarily easy to make. One frequently believes to be awake while dreaming, and an argument from the objective, or public, experience versus the subjective, or private, will not do. The assurance by someone else that one is not dreaming is, as all experience, perceived by oneself and can be part of a dream. It is left to one's own judgement to make the discernment.

The discernment, if accomplished, is through the constancy justifying other inferences of reality. Real objects manifest themselves as extended things of continuing existence, perhaps changing in form, compared to the evanescence of the illusory. This constancy of the material world of extension is implicit in finding it a reality, expounded to be of dependency through its constancy.

Whether that world is truly extended or, more particularly, external to mind has been debated. In both cases the question revolves around the meaning of the terms. By the extension can be understood the above explicated continued perception itself of volume, and it is accordingly and by the expounded an object of knowledge, viz a reality. As to externality, if mind is understood in the broad sense delineated, then physical reality, determined in perception, is not external. But if mind is understood in the also viewed narrow sense, as what is purely conceptual, then physical reality is external to it by meaning alone. It is external at all events to the self, which was seen as a sensibility separate from other objects, those of its perception and including extended physical reality.

This reality of physical objects is one because, as explicated, corresponding knowledge of them and of what happens to them can be of dependency to man. The knowledge involves identifying these objects, distinguishing one from another, at a single moment and through time, as considered before in connection with the self (p.51, last par.). What the identities consist in has, as indicated there, been a subject of philosophical inquiry, and the determination of them, as likewise indicated, is one of choice, though decided by suitability in accordance with experience. The issue is also confused with the one of identity of a thing when contemplated by different attributes, perhaps names, as treated in the first chapter. The present issue is any one attribute that would define a thing as it may last through possible changes.

Changes of one kind or another are indeed profuse as regards a physical object viewed as remaining the same one. They are so not merely in a living thing, drastically changing during development, and most often the subject of discourse about them. Inanimate objects as well as the animate are continually perceived from different angles, under different lighting, or by other phenomena not held to signify changes in the objects though of changing perceptions, as before suggested. Particular material things are thus identified through a changing complexity of characteristics.

The description of the things, as in a definition, may be simple, because attributes named concern already understood material entities. But even the most general character of individual material things consists of accumulations of many perceptions all of which are of the same objects. Their three-dimensionality, their extension, may sometimes be perceived through the combination of perspective, light and shade, and touch. Perception through both eyes, and hence from different mentioned angles, is a further means. The angles together with lighting were also indicated to change in time, while still signifying the same unchanging objects. The lighting can also change their degree of lightness or darkness or their color, and distance or foreshortening can change their size, the objects regarded as all the while not changing. They remain the same ones by equally elaborate associations, by which an object of certain like perceptions is seen to have a, perhaps moving, continuity, although the continuity is not always observed. The continuity applies to other, changing, material things that remain the same things, as well as to ones that do not remain the things. Among the first of these, the now discussed ones, lifeless objects are considered to remain the same ones if retaining some principal feature though changing otherwise. Living organisms, further, seem often, as indicated, not to retain any individual physical feature at all, their identity viewed as remaining by their function to preserve a form of themselves, if not by, unlike in the case of plants, being of a sentient self described.

Despite this multifariousness of perceptions by which material entities may be recognized, men do know what they mean by words for them, as they do by other expressions. Not only men, but animals, recognize material things as of repeated daily experience, knowing that they behave according to certain laws, constancies, by which the perceivers regulate their own lives.

Knowledge, the reality, of the material, extended, world is accordingly presupposed by the knowledge or reality of those laws by which men live, and therefore

THEOREM II.4. *The world of extended matter is a reality prior to laws applying to it.*

It can hereupon be inquired what kind of laws, laws that make it consequential and therein real, this world is subject to.

CAUSALITY

In consonance with what has been said, the answer immediately suggesting itself is that it is causal laws. It is causation of events, leading to the satisfaction or dissatisfaction of man's concerns, which makes the world the reality of interest. Similarly to the case of that world, it may then be asked what distinguishes causal laws from any others.

It could be proposed that causal laws are of occurrences in time, wherein the cause is followed by the effect, since by the foregoing the issue is what event that has not occurred would if some other did. Sometimes cause and effect appear simultaneous, however, as when one object is pushing another. Time can as a matter of fact like space be seen not to be the presumed entity distinct from the occurrences in it. It is not meant to refer to something independently perceivable. The word is applied to quantitative attributes of occurrences or events, to their duration and occasion or absence, each determined in relation to further events as characterized by change. In analogy with space, time is distinguished in accordance with occurrences, rather than occurrences being distinguished in accordance with time.

Causal laws, the constantly connected events called cause and effect, need therefore be distinguished otherwise, and the answer can be supplied by the preceding characterization of events as changes. A causal law can be characterized as a constant connection of certain changes.

What distinguishes, what defines, causal laws is of course again a matter of deciding what laws are to be called causal. The interest herein is in, as said above, what event that has not occurred would if some other did. In other words, the causation of the effect means its coming about as a change from one state into another, a change that by knowledge of causal laws may be brought about if desired, or prevented if undesired; and since the cause implies by its meaning the effect, and the effect is a change from its absence, that absence implies by transposition the like former absence of the cause, namely that it also consists in change. The common comprehension of this meaning of causality is exhibited in regarding occurrences not preceded or succeeded by a change as having respectively no cause or effect.

The just mentioned concepts of preceding and succeeding were made use of somewhat freely. The causally connected changes, as noted, appear sometimes simultaneous. But many do not, and, in accord with their usual sequence, in a simultaneity the event considered the cause is customarily the one known to be independently of the other caused by an event occurring earlier. The reference to this sequence as customary is made because the ends of purposive events are, reversely, sometimes called final causes. But even then it is the aim rather than the outcome which is of account, and the ordinarily meant sequence of cause and effect can be adopted here without confusion.

The difference between cause and effect clarified accordingly, it can be stated with exactness that a causal law designates the constant accompaniment of one event as change by another, the first of which would be the cause and the second the effect. The cause and effect, it should be understood, can be combinations of things, each of which things can be regarded as a cause or effect, though not the only one.

It should be worth repeating here that the accompaniment of one thing by another is the only criterion by which a connection can be established, as brought out in the last chapter's discussion of necessity.

That no causal connection but only a constant conjunction can be found between events is known as the observation of Hume. But that only a constant conjunction is possible does not repudiate a causal connection. Whatever is meant by it, taken as constant, the meaning cannot be of other than a constant conjunction, and therefore the connection is not denied by it. Hume thus did not refute causal connections, but he saw correctly that there are none other than conjunctions. However, the same applies to logic, with which he contrasted causation, or to any other relation between things.

And on examination it can be seen that the oft heard distinction noted in the introduction, that inability to otherwise conceive something inferred applies to logical, deductive, laws but not to natural, inductive, ones cannot on more serious grounds than before be maintained.

It was before observed that in difficult deductions it is odd to say that the result is not conceivable otherwise. But in view of the involuntary perception found in the preceding section requisite for determining a principle, it is indeed not possible to so perceive a false deductive result, although the true one may also not be perceived. The conceivability really means this perceivability, extending in deduction to so-called all possible worlds, including the actual one. The reason for that inclusiveness is that the conditions to which deductive laws apply are extremely general. The laws nonetheless apply to certain conditions, such as combinations of numbers. Laws of nature, however, likewise apply to conditions, though much more particular ones. They are conditions regarding nature itself, not conceptual ones, and under them results opposed to its laws can equally not be perceived, while their confirmation may not either. That is to say, what above is thought to distinguish deduction is true of induction as well.

It has also been thought that compared to deductive laws inductive laws concern only the possible, in an equivocation alluded to earlier (p.37, sixth par.). Because laws of nature are difficult to observe with precision, many of its manifestations are inferred only probable, and hence the belief that the laws are exceptionable. The possible has in this case to do with man's knowledge, however. A law, a principle, is by definition true of all instances, and should a connection turn out not to be invariable, it is for that reason not a principle. It may in this regard also be recalled that deductive principles, sometimes called demonstrative, have in their fundamental cases been equally unsubstantiated.

Despite these similarities between the deductive and inductive, there remains the difference that in one the inferred is found to be part of the inferred from as conceived, it is intrinsic, and in the other it is not, it is extrinsic.

It may yet be wondered whether the observation of an extrinsic constant connection between two events is truly sufficient for the connection usually called causal, whether perhaps a causal connection is not an intrinsic one. Night always follows day, but it will not be alleged that the occurrence of day causes the occurrence of night. Like acquaintance with an external world of complex persisting objects despite their ever changing appearance, however, acquaintance, in man and animal, with persisting causal connections is much more profound than isolated observations admit. The occurrence of day and night is comprehended by a child as depending on illumination by the sun, and even an animal will discriminate in its attributions of causation. That causal connections are not intrinsic ones can furthermore be simply confirmed, by seeing that perceptions of familiar causes do not contain as part of them the familiar effects, which can moreover be largely found to occur subsequently.

Regardless of the type of connection in causal laws, the material world is found subject to them. This is the case even if, as noted earlier, the connections are not always observed, and the exact nature of the laws is not known. The physical world has as indicated the peculiarity that, unlike the contents of consciousness, things in it are taken to occur even when not perceived. Correspondingly laws in it will be considered to hold even if not precisely recognized, provided there is good reason for the inference. It could be mentioned that even the above probability can sometimes be regarded as a law, as apprehended in statistics. If the probability is based on a constancy within a range, then that constancy can be viewed as a law. If for every hundred occurrences of *A* there are from forty to sixty occurrences of *B*, then this proportion of the connection, though not a constant connection between *A* and *B*, can be held to be a law. But the presence of causal laws in the external world can be inferred on more substantial ground.

The experience of particular causations is more overwhelming than the preceding proportion. A blowing wind is expected to bend the grass; a stone released in air is expected to drop; a pot of water placed over the fire is expected to boil. One's entire life is regulated by such particular reliabilities. One's understandings go deeper. One learns of more assured general connections behind particular ones. Not only does the wind move the grass, but objects of many sorts move many others, and they do so more efficiently in some ways than in others. If an animal does not secure a fruit from a tree by a certain motion, it will try other motions, till hopefully succeeding. Its lessons were that while there is some reliability that certain kinds of actions bring certain results, there is an accuracy of the actions yet more fruitful. One finds that underneath the likelihood of a certain connection there is a more dependable one, on which the first one rests. This experience generalized means that one induces from progressive findings of fairly well working first connections, then better working ones on which based, etc., that all deficient connections are based on more exact ones, with an unvarying one, in which exceptions are reduced to zero, at the basis. It is so to speak induction of induction, of inductive laws of nature. The experience that all that occurs in this world is thus causally connected, whereby that world is as expounded consequential and hence real, is so thoroughgoing that the occurrence of things in that world is considered the criterion of their reality, if only in a general, material, sense and not a particular one exemplified by the artificial, which may not be a real specific thing, but is real by being of the world. And since the reality of things in that world is established by its conformity to causal laws,

THEOREM II.5. *That the material world is subject to causality is a reality prior to other realities in that world.*

This theorem and what went before can be seen to entail certain familiar principles of nature. They are that every, extrinsic, material state, every condition of matter aside from its existence, has a cause and at least a possible effect, and that elemental constituents of the world persist or are conserved.

In agreement with the previously established nature of reality, the material world is found real or consequential because its states can be caused by and of effect on man. In consequence, since the states of the world of matter, future ones that are not determined, can be caused by man, they cannot be uncaused. If they could, if a future state could occur by chance, then man could not effect it, could not be responsible for it. In other words, with the future requirement learned as a principle from the past, every material state has a cause. And since the states of this world can be of effect on man, every material state can have an effect.

As regards the permanence or conservation of elemental entities, it has to do with what is known as conservation of matter and energy, or of mass-energy. By their conservation is meant that the total quantity of the entities is constant, and the constancy of the world of matter, which does not appear and disappear, was already observed as distinguishing it from illusory ones, i.e. as true by definition, and as in that dependability presupposed by its reality. As to energy, it is defined as the capacity for doing work, and it is hence a causal property. It can at once be noted that energy cannot therefore be an independent entity, let alone the constituent of material reality, as proposed in physics. A causal property is meant to hold of something other than itself, in this case the very material objects. Regarding energy's conservation, it is often explained through concepts of potential and kinetic energy. A weight suspended above ground is considered to have potential energy, in being able to do work on being released and falling to the ground. After release the energy is considered to in fall become kinetic, energy of motion, for the same reasons. The magnitude of the two energies, the capacity for doing work they signify, is determined unchanging, conserved. This determination is, however, not a matter of ascertaining conservation, but a redundancy. Both names for the energy stand for the same capacity of doing the work due to the combination of factors, e.g. the height of suspension and the amount of weight, the different names merely used to speak of that energy with regard to stages before and after release respectively. The energy is in fact an expression of forces like gravity, and energy is thus a reified fictitious entity, unduly added to those forces. The forces, having to do with what occurs under what conditions, comprise nature's causal laws, and it is they that are conserved. This conservation, this constancy, is implicit in the laws, proclaiming constancy. Like that of matter, it is required by their consequentiality, also presupposed by their reality.

As in other matters here observed to be presupposed by acknowledged realities, the principles of the last two paragraphs have in some of their form been disputed.

In particle physics, the exact sequence of events has been found indeterminable, and thinkers have inferred that causality must be abandoned as a scientific concept. This is formulated in the dictum that science should not explain, only describe. But the two procedures can be seen to be here synonymous. With an individual occurrence, a description differs from an explanation, which amounts to giving a cause. But in now concerned observation of generalities, the observation is its own explanation. Reasons in the present sense, not in the earlier sense of motives, are generalities, accounting for instances and not required for generalities themselves, unless they can be found to be based on broader ones. The interest is in principles, and, as noted several times, there cannot be any other than constant conjunctions. Moreover, the observations that in particle physics are thought to dismiss causality themselves contain causal conjunctions. The physicist makes the observations about particles under certain conditions, which constitute causes, resulting in the observations as effects. Particles were mentioned before as known by effects, and there exist series of causal ties producing them. The researcher knows that his will causes his actions, his actions the managing of implements, and so forth till the observations.

In relativity, the famous equation of Albert Einstein,

$$E = mc^2,$$

enunciating the equivalence of mass and energy, led to the denial of certain laws of conservation, in particular of matter. Matter is regarded as synonymous with mass, and since mass and energy are found to be mutually convertible, conservation of mass-energy is instead upheld. Matter, as mentioned (p.74, last par.), cannot be formed of energy, and therefore if energy is convertible into it, not remaining energy, its conservation should likewise have to be rejected. The notions find their basis in a conceptual confusion, however, traceable to the inception of classical mechanics. Isaac Newton spoke of the principle of inertia, the property of bodies to as regards their motion resist forces impressed upon them. Inertia has thus been treated as a body's property separate from those forces. It is, however, merely a manifestation of them. To hold that a body has a certain resistance to a force is to hold that the force has a certain magnitude, because the magnitude of the force is measured by the effect on the body. Formulated either way, inertia is, by concerning effect, a causal property. But conceived as separate from force, it is today the property by which mass, namely matter, is measured, rather than by such as bulk and density, which concerns matter as here considered but may be difficult to gauge. The concept of matter was accordingly misconstrued to be a causal one, and its maintained equivalence with likewise causal energy does not assert a lack of matter's conservation, but a causal relation.

In point of fact, the energy of the above equation was originally a kinetic one and can correspondingly be found identical with the mass, viewed as above resistance. The energy can be held to be the force of a moving body on another, and that force can in accord with the above be translated into the moving body's resistance, to wit mass.

Apart from the mistaken differentiation of the force on a body from its mass as resistance, there is a similarly false differentiation of mass as either inertial or gravitational, but not in conformance with a like tenet of relativity. By "inertial mass" is meant the amount of the said resistance of a body to a force, as when pushing the body, and by "gravitational mass" the amount of attraction of a body by gravity, as when weighing the body. The two measures seem opposed, because in one case the motion of the more massive body under the respective force is smaller, and in the other case larger. That the two measures are proportional is thought to be evidenced as follows. It has long been observed that all bodies falling side by side toward earth, supposing no obstruction such as air, do so at the same speed. The reason is believed to have been supplied by Newton, who argued that since resistance to a force, e.g. to gravity, differs according to the body's mass, the pull of gravity, in order that all bodies fall at the same speed, must be proportional to that resistance. As explained, however, the amount of resistance is the very manifestation of the force, the pull of gravity, making the resistance of all bodies and hence presumably their mass during fall in fact the same. That the motion of the more massive body be larger during its weighing and smaller in the other cases is accordingly not due to opposite measures of mass. It is due instead to the same resistance, inertia, by which these objects, resisting motion in other cases, resist hindrance of their motion during weighing. Of present account is that since the inertia here has to do with the pull of gravity, inertial and gravitational mass are indentical by definition, to which the uniform fall is irrelevant.

The uniform fall of objects can be explained by way of Newton's law of gravitation itself. In accordance with it equal particles of matter are attracted with equal force. This is to say that a more massive object does not, so as to actually fall slower, resist gravity more, which reaches every part of the object to result in equal fall. In contrast in normal pushing or pulling of one object by another, the force is acting on only those particles of the first that are held to be in contact with the second. Hence in order to affect through these parts the others, the force must surmount the combined resistance, mass, of all, which increases accordingly with more massive objects.

An interpretation of the uniform fall and with it, as indicated, a contention of the identity of inertial and gravitational mass was put forward in relativity. This identity is instead, as observed, unrelated to that fall, but holds by the understanding of mass in terms of force. Relativity's explanation of the uniform fall of objects, further, commits a rudimental fallacy, known as affirmation of the consequent and alluded to in the introduction (p.5, fifth par.). By it from true premises "If something is a bird it is an animal" and "This is an animal" it would falsely be concluded "This is a bird". In the present case in place of the second premise is relied on a recognized relativity of motion, specifically motion as change in position. In a vehicle travelling on earth, a reposing passenger appears at rest in relation to the vehicle, but in motion in relation to the earth. This relativity is a logical matter, to be substantiated in the next chapter, and it does not mean that in actuality a further attribute may not distinguish what may be viewed as a moving object from one at rest. The other premise is, further, that if bodies fall equally toward earth then, as in all motion, the motion is relative, the earth for instance viewable as moving toward those bodies. To simplify, by this premise if bodies fall equally then their motion is relative, and by the preceding premise their motion is relative. It is concluded that they fall equally, i.e. that this reasoning explains the equal fall. But the relativity of motion is irrelevant, true no matter how bodies fall.

The contended equivalence of falling of bodies and motion of the earth or like frame of reference toward stationary ones, the contention a staple of theory of relativity, does in fact not hold. Differences have been noted by science. Since falling objects tend toward the center of the earth, those equally distant from it approach each other; and since the speed of falling objects gradually increases, those of unequal distance from the earth recede from each other. In other words when those objects are held in motion, the distance between them changes, and when the earth would be held in motion, that distance remains. To maintain equivalence of the falling of bodies and the opposite motion of the earth is hence in effect to maintain that there is an equivalence insofar as there is one.

The more general thesis of relativity pertains to the above question as to whether, apart from relative change in position, a moving material object can be distinguished from one at rest, and the thesis of the theory is that it cannot. The question is of longstanding interest, and of interest is here motion in general, because it appears as the physical world's principal form of change and therefore of causal events. Additional attention may therefore be paid to it.

It may be noted that Newton's famed laws of motion constitute a partial announcement of the discussed prevailance of causal laws in the material world. The laws of motion are

1. *Every body continues in its state of rest, or of uniform motion in a straight line, unless it is compelled to change that state by some force impressed upon it,*

2. *The change of motion is proportional to the force impressed, and is made in the direction in which that force is impressed,*

and

3. *To every action there is an equal and opposite reaction; or, the mutual actions of two bodies upon each other are always equal and in opposite directions.*

The first of these is sometimes interpreted as a definition of force. Force would accordingly be that which acts on a body when it changes from a state of rest or the described motion. But then it is assumed that something always acts on a body when it undergoes these changes, and this assumption should be considered a principle, in the fashion of the principle that every physical state has a cause. It is evidently a principle of this kind that Newton declared, that a body will not undergo these changes without a cause, although he did not necessarily equate force with cause. He spoke of the force of gravity, for instance, while owning to ignorance of its cause. He thus did not perceive the mentioned synonymity here of explanation and description. To look for a cause of something is to look for some event resulting in it by some principle. At present it would mean to find events that along with e.g. the freeing of distanced bodies result in their gravitation toward each other. But the freeing has already that result, and the force of gravity needs no causal description beyond its own.

Because a force is determined by the effect, to speak of force in the first law above can also be misleading, as it has been in regard to inertia and is in regard to the second law.

The second law could by the meaning of force be understood to redundantly say that if a force is such that it causes a certain motion in a certain direction, then it causes that motion in that direction. Regarding direction there is no escape from this interpretation. Force can be understood in the law to refer to the causing event, and its direction is not always the same as the effected one, as exemplified by billiard balls. Regarding the rest of the law it can by its author's comments be held to state that if a certain event causes a certain motion then double the event causes double the motion, and so forth. That is, the connection between the causing event and the motion is constant. But this is a form of causality itself, which is of constant connections. The law accordingly asserts that there are causal connections between certain events and certain motions, magnitudes included.

An added interpretation is accepted, however, which can be seen not to state a presumed law of nature but a definition, one, unlike the first law, of force, this time by effect and quantitatively. The law is held to state that the force on a body equals the body's mass multiplied by its acceleration, its change of speed or direction, the equality symbolized as

$$F = ma.$$

What is in practice asserted by the equation is that if some action has the force of accelerating by a certain amount a certain mass then it will accelerate another mass in inverse proportion. I.e. the mass and acceleration, though varied, when multiplied by each other equal the same. But in concord with previous observations, this is a result of the definition of mass as resistance to acceleration, beside numerical choice. To clarify, when at first the same action, as by a moving body, is considered in relation to different masses, it is practical to assign it the same numerical force, attained mathematically by multiplying whichever acceleration by its reciprocal, the number

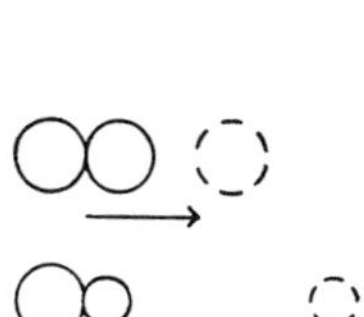

which if multiplied by it yields 1, and which is assigned hence to the mass. Accordingly a certain force is numbered 1 by numbering the same a certain affected mass and its corresponding acceleration, and if another acceleration is 2, its mass is numbered ½. Of account is merely that these multiplied result in 1, signifying the force as cause, with either mass or acceleration signifying the effect. When a mass is measured by volume, to be sure, there indeed apears the experience of an inverse proportion, the changes of size and acceleration of two masses the reverse. But with mass measured by acceleration, the proportion is a mathematical convenience, defining in the above equation quantity of force. The definition is useful because when for instance knowing the mass of an object and a certain acceleration is required, the needed force can be computed.

The third law of motion can be viewed as but an indication of whatever causal law applies in the pertinent event. As an effect need not be in the direction of the cause, so need a reaction not be in the direction opposite the action, or be equal to it. That these should be thought otherwise is understandable in view of the notion that resistance, rather than being a measure of the force, is a separate and commensurate opposition to it. Thus Newton cites a horse which by drawing a stone is drawn by it, although its progress signifies merely the horse's power. What the law suggests, if flawed in particulars, is that in an event among things should be considered effects in not only some but all of them.

Although the three laws are about motion, they do not say when motion of an object occurs. Whether no distinction can be made in material objects between their relative motion and rest was noted to have been a persistent issue, and it has involved the concepts of space and time.

Newton argued absolute, independent, space, in relation to which the motion of objects is determined. He alleged besides similarly absolute time, which would determine the speed of objects. Einstein asserted relativity of motion and acordingly of speed, as well as of the measures of space and time. He nonetheless described a separate though dependent universe of space-time, with a curvature placed apart from material objects and determining their course.

It will regarding space and time be recalled (p.68, second par., and p.70, last par.) that they by their meaning are not independently perceivable entities, but are delineated by material objects and their events. As expounded in the first chapter, in consequence, by speaking of space and time as independent, absolute, entities though not perceivable, no entities can be referred to. For the same reasons a universe of space-time as a dependent, relative, entity cannot be characterized by a curvature separate from material objects.

Newton acknowledged that space and time are commonly conceived in relation to sensible objects. Yet he posited a truer, mathematical, meaning of them by which motion and duration is determined. These are determined in relation to physical things, however, such as the earth in the one case, and the phases of the moon in the other, not to say that a true meaning is one in use. Einstein proposed similarly a geometry of space and time, the mentioned curvature held to be the cause of corresponding motions of objects near massive bodies like planets. These motions, associated with gravity and whatever their nature, are again, however, found connected with the nearness itself to those bodies, and as before need no other explanation, especially the impossible curvature as cause.

Despite the discussion in relativity of, as in the case of the moon's orbit around the earth, the path of one object near another, in a geometry of all such paths as associated with space-time, the theory does not establish that any of the objects describes those paths, because it holds motion to be relative.

That it is was asserted first with regard to rest and constant velocity, constant speed and direction. These are the two states of Newton's first law, and inasmuch as they remain unless acted upon, objects in those states are called inertial frames of reference. It is then maintained that no distinction can be made between an inertial frame at rest and in motion. Compared to these later were reference frames that are accelerated, as was indicated when speaking of objects falling under gravity. These frames are additionally then said not to be distinguishable from inertial ones. It should be remarked that this can be true in spite of the noted changing distance between falling objects, as it can be true if they did not fall equally otherwise. The issue is whether there is a difference due to their states of motion alone. The contention thus is that there is no difference between rest and motion in general, since the alternatives of constant velocity and acceleration, the last the negation of that constancy, exhaust all motion.

To support this main contention of relativity it is argued that the speed of light, if not affected by other particulars, is in all frames of reference, regardless of any of their motion, always measured to be the same. If it were not, if the speed of light, assumed constant if not affected by other particulars, were found to differ in the frames, motion would not be relative, to be gaugeable with respect to that speed.

The thus argued invariance of the measurement clashes with common sense, for if, for example, relative to one thing another is in motion in a straight line, and in the same direction relative to the second thing a third, then the speed of the third thing, which may be a ray of light, is taken to be greater in relation to the first than in relation to the second. In order to therefore justify asserting the invariance of the speed of light, relativity offers a definition of particular time, of when an event, as is the onset or finish of a motion, can be said to occur.

It should be of value to remark that in various areas, as earlier suggested, attempts are made at demonstrations by way of offering corresponding definitions, and that if the definitions do not denote the entities at issue than the demonstrations are not achieved. The definition presently discussed is among these.

It is taken into consideration that the time of an occurrence is associated with simultaneity. For an event to occur at a certain time is for it to be in some way simultaneous with another, for instance with a designation on a clock. It is accordingly queried how simultaneity is determined, and the definition by relativity is as follows. It is taken into account that since the transmission of light is not instantaneous, e.g. it takes years for the light of distant stars to reach the earth, two events cannot be judged simultaneous because they appear to be so to the observer. Hence to decide that two events occur at the same time, a synchronization of clocks placed at the events is considered. The two clocks are held synchronized if when a light signal is sent from one to the other and reflected back, the time on the second clock when it reflects the signal is midway between the times on the first clock when it emits and receives the light.

It may be noted that to speak of when these events occur is question-begging. It can be asked what makes a time on a clock and an adjacent stage of the light signal simultaneous. But the present point is that this definition of synchronization, of sameness of time, is meant appropriate regardless of any motion of the clocks relative to something else. The clocks are viewed as fixed in the same reference frame, but a little thought will reveal that ordinarily if the frame is held to be in motion parallel to the signal the definition does not apply. If the unit is seen as moving in the direction of the second clock, both of the clocks moving accordingly, the light is held to travel proportionately farther to reach that clock then to return to the first one. The second clock recedes from the light, and the first clock approaches it. The times on the clocks would hence not be synchronized as above, the light taking proportionately longer on its first trip between the clocks than on its return trip. What the above definition does correspondingly is to individualize time for every reference frame, deciding by fiat that in each of them the time of the trip is the same for the same distance in the frame. In other words, the conclusion that the speed of light is measured the same in all frames of reference is circularly inferred from the premise that the measure is decided to be the same.

By the foregoing it should become evident that to thus define particular time separately for each reference frame is not in accord with the meaning by which the time in question is considered. By the individualized definition it was determined that simultaneity, or measures of time, and measures of space are relative, and it will be suitable to explain these contentions before seeing the untenability of the concerned definitions and of what is inferred from them.

As regards measures of time, if when one frame moving in a straight line relatively to another passes it a light is flashed nearby, then by the above different measures a ray parallel to the motion reaches a place next to a given place in the one frame at a different time according to it than according to the other frame. For by then the place corresponding in the other frame in distance from the light source has passed that place in the initial frame, and since the same time is assigned to both of these places in their frames, the times are not the same where the frames are next to that stage of the ray. That is to say, the same events would occur according to different frames at different times.

It may again be noted that there is a question-begging in speaking of when things pass or are next to each other, viz when aligned perpendicularly to the motion. If time in the two frames varied as supposed, the time when parts of them pass each other could as above not be always the same for both, although it is at a time as a single one when the ray is held to be next to such passing parts. Thus relativity presupposes by the instant of passing or adjacency a common supertime it denies.

As regards measures of space, or length, an additional definition is offered. By it in two frames moving in a straight line relative to each other the length of an object in one is measured in the other by finding where with respect to it the corresponding ends of the object lie at one time. If then the length is parallel to the motion, the same time for the ends is measured by clocks passing them, and the length by the distance between the clocks. And by the different measures of time, when one of those clocks passes one end, a clock passing the other does not read the same time. Consequently when a clock there does read that time, the first clock is not passing the first end, and hence the distance between those clocks differs from the length in question as measured in its own frame. That is to say, the same objects would according to different frames be of different sizes.

Neither time nor space are meant to be measured according to points of view, however, wherefrom different quantities of each follow depending on the frame of reference.

In relativity it is often said that the differences depend on what is seen by the observers. But as in the case of light from distant stars, informing of long past events as brought forward by science itself, men continually make allowances as to what situations in the world obtain, rather than judging by subjective appearances. As was observed regarding identity of physical entities, judgements made about them differ from individual perceptions on which founded, with the perceptions of for instance size or tonality not necessarily representing what is attributed to the objects (p.69, last par.). The actual attributes are meant to be perceived under certain conditions only, and it is these perceptions that are comprehended as potential through the others. All creatures have the capacity for objective appraisal, inferring facts from merely signs of them, an animal knowing that the small perception of a distant prey represents a full-fledged meal.

While the sign can differ in its nature, perhaps owing to the standpoint, the fact cannot, lest it be contradicted. Accordingly in measures of space, i.e. size in some respect, there may as mentioned be varied appearances of it according to e.g. the object's distance, but only one size is meant to apply, one that at least ideally is perceived if the object is appropriately placed alongside the chosen standard. All other judgements of size are inferences. Similarly in measures of time a certain one only is meant to apply to an event, namely the occasion when by discounting representative perceptions through such as distance the event would ideally be perceived simultaneously with the chosen standard. Simultaneous perception, it may be remarked, need not be substantiated, because, as all perception, it is not an inferred, but a known, state. One has a capacity to distinguish between present and past perceptions. As in the case of space, accordingly, other assessments of time of an event than by that direct perception of its occurrence are made by inference. To these belong inferences allowing time for the travel of light, or for other production of signs of past events, as in archaeology, these allowances made in relativity inconsistently for the speed of light but not the speed of relatively moving reference frames, by which speed the arrival time of light perceived may be shortened or lengthened. Through these and other faulty premises more than one conclusion of such as a time or a size may be reached, but only one of them can be correct, the one corresponding to the mentioned ideal perception. Differing designations of measures, as for time zones, are of course a convenience of language only, in time zones enabling similar hours for day and night.

It may be added that it has been questioned that ideal perceptions are appropriate in considering reality. It has been objected that Newton's first law of motion does not apply to reality, because no straight motion can be said to occur in it. It could also be objected that if it did occur it could not be precisely measured, as cannot be other worldly things despite methods like magnification and slow-motion photography, by which concurrence in size and time may be more exactly observed. This exactness may also raise questions about defining these concurrences by their perceptions, though ideal ones. But straight motions or deviations from them, as well as other measures in reality, are as through instruments determined just in accordance with ideal perceptions of them, which it is regarding reality the aim to more and more approximate in accuracy. Laws of nature that concern these measures, as any of motion, can be expressed in ideal form to facilitate their use, and for the same reason ideal measurements, sometimes expressed in mathematics as limits, are conceived as if perceived in full precision, which real measurements are held to approach.

It may also be wondered whether the measurements one person finds worldly things to have or approach are the same ones other persons find. The answer lies in the referred to sharing of the experience of the same world by all, the induction of which enlarged on later. One shares the experience of the same laws of nature, from which the same consequences are deduced, by likewise shared laws of logic. From the former laws, from any known fact, can by the latter laws not be deduced contradictory results. By being deduced the results are likewise facts, which cannot be contradictory. That is why the correctly inferred time or size of something cannot differ with different observers. It may be added that should someone's perception of a worldly particular be abnormal, allowance is likewise made for physical misdirection.

On the basis of its mistaken belief that time and space differ in different frames of reference relativity holds in more mistaken reasoning that these extents differ in an exactly reverse manner with respect to two frames moving relative to each other. It is argued that from either frame time in the other appears equally slower, and space shorter in the direction of the relative motion, the appearances called time dilation and space contraction.

The unsuitability here of the concept of appearance was spoken of above, and at the speed of light, of account now, the concept becomes figurative. What is actually meant by time dilation is that when relative to one frame another is considered in motion then the clocks in the other are slower than the clocks in the first. It may at once be noted to be ludicrous that the pace of clocks should change merely by considering one of the frames instead of the other as relatively moving. If this relativity were to hold then certain clocks would impossibly be slower than others while speedier.

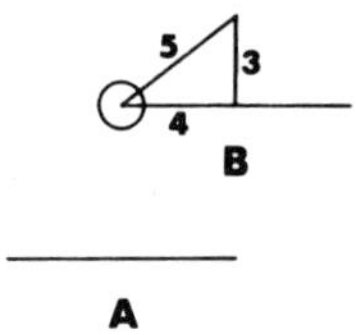

How the dilemma is encountered should be evinced by giving an instance of the argument used for this relativity. In the diagram the horizontal lines depict reference frames *A* and *B*, with *B*, having passed *A*, moving horizontally relative to it at 4/5 the speed of light. When *B* was passing *A* the clocks in both of them read zero, and a flash of light, pictured by the circle, occurred in the center of *B*. In the diagram, *B* has moved 4 units since, and with it the source of light, now the right bottom corner of the triangle. At this stage a light ray, forming the right side of the triangle, reached a place vertically above in *B*. But relative to *A* the ray travelled diagonally, forming the left side of the triangle. Hence since by postulate light travels relative to *A* 5 units for each 4 of *B*, the diagonal is 5 units long. And by the renowned Pythagorean theorem the square on the diagonal equals the sum of the squares on the triangle's other sides. In consequence the right side is 3 units long. Then in accord with the supposed sameness of speed of light for all frames, if units on clocks are chosen to match units of length travelled by light relative to the frames, *A*'s clock reads 5, and *B*'s clock 3. Accordingly the clock in *B* is slower than the clock in *A*, and it is argued that the reverse would be true if the light had in like manner occurred in *A*. There is more than one flaw.

By what was said the argument of another light is irrelevant; it is enough that with the first light the clock in *B* is slower than the clock in *A*, whence the opposite cannot be true of those very clocks, contrary to the contention that all clocks of *A* would be somehow slower from the viewpoint of *B*. Further, since light travels relative to *A* at 5/4 the speed of *B*, when the base of a like triangle in *A* is 4, signifying 4 units of relative motion by *B*, then the vertical, depicting the corresponding ray relative to *A*, is 5; consequently the triangle is of different proportions than the other, contrary again to contention. Furthermore even with the flash as first conceived in *B*, the time on *B*'s clock need by the theory itself not be less than on *A*'s, and for that matter if a horizontal ray to the left is considered, the time is three times the previous one; since as before relative to *A* the source of light moved 4 units to the right while the rays travelled 5 units, the ray in the left direction travelled 9 units relative to *B*, whose clock accordingly reads 9.

It is also maintained that by the argued measurement of time Pythagorean relations as discussed, well known as of Lorentz transformations, always hold. That this is not the case is evidenced by the last described example. The horizontal ray of

9 units in *B* is in the same line with the 4 units of relative motion of *B*, as well as with the 5 units of the ray relative to *A*. These lengths form no triangle, nor do they have Pythagorean proportions. The error of thinking all the lengths to have them can in accord with the supposed measurement of time be ascribed to the belief that light travels in either frame the same distance in all directions. In the example diagramed, since the verticle ray in *B* travels 3 units, it is supposed the other rays do too, and since the other distances marked, those travelled by *B* and light relative to *A*, remain by postulate, the proportions would always obtain. That the vertical distance be the one attended to first can be held due to experiments gauging speeds of light perpendicular to the motion of its source.

It may be additionally noticed that in the diagram, as depicted by the vertical and base of the triangle, light travels relative to *B* at 3/4 the speed of *A*, in negation of the contention that from these believed relativities it follows that nothing travels faster than light relative to any, at least nonaccelerating, frame of reference.

In preceding paragraphs it was merely disclosed that things thought to be the consequence of the measuring of time proposed in relativity do not follow, the measuring itself seen inappropriate, and there should be no need to make similar observations on space. Some likewise undue derivations may further nevertheless be surveyed, because they touch more closely on whether or not motion is relative.

Certain of the derivations are that there are objective differences of duration and other measure in objects in accordance with their motion. Principally, events are said to slow down in an object as it gains speed. The conclusions are firstly uncalled for because the premises offered state that the differences are subjective. They are posited true from a point of view of one reference frame and not another, and to then hold them true from the point of view of each frame is contradictory. In addition, to infer from a lesser time on a clock, as done, the slowing of other events in the frame is likewise without foundation. The time on the clock is by the theory less not because it is so affected by the putative motion, but because it is so set by men. Should motion have the effect on things, it should have it on the clock apart from that setting.

The initially intended inference that light behaves the same in relation to all frames of reference does, lastly, also not follow. Returning to the diagram this becomes clear by merely considering that the rays travel different lengths relative to *A* than to *B*. The clocks, that would also read different times, are irrelevant, it sufficing that during the relative motion of the frames the light travelled different distances relative to them.

Under the presumed constancy of the speed of light, its noncapriciousness, motion is, accordingly, not relative, in the sense that due to it there would be no distinction between relatively moving frames, a distinction e.g. between the distances light travels relatively to them.

That the speed of light is thus constant, not capricious, presupposes moreover, since speed is measured relative to something, a, also perhaps ideal, reference frame relative to which the constancy takes place. In the diagram such a frame is *A*, in relation to which light is postulated to travel 5 units in all directions, to have a constant speed. That frame can hence be held to be at rest, by the customarily meant equilibrium, with the other frame, relative to which the light was seen to travel varying distances, in motion. More generally, under that constancy, assumed in the theory not to be otherwise affected, there is a distinction between motion and rest.

There need be no such distinction merely because light travels different distances for different frames, however. Should the distance travelled be e.g. dependent on the one of the source of the light, then the light might relative to the source travel equal distances in all directions, as do due to inertial law other things in moving frames when propelled with equal force. In that case the same light can travel different distances relative to other frames, but its source need not be at rest relative to for instance another source of light, the light travelling relative to that source equal distances for the same reason.

Contrastingly, if though impossible it were true after all that the speed of light, the distance it travels, be the same with respect to all relatively moving reference frames, the sought after relativity of motion would not follow either. There may be some other factor by which motion of an object can be distinguished.

The assertion in relativity that events in an object slow factually down with its motion (last p., fourth par.) has been found ill-supported by some, not because falsely derived from settings of clocks, but because it is in the same breath maintained that motion is relative. The inherent contradiction had been illustrated by the so-called twin paradox. In it it is by the theory found that a twin space-traveler at high speed, upon leaving the earth and returning after years, has as a result of the speed aged much less than the other twin, who remained on earth. But since by relativity the earth can be held in motion and the traveler at rest, there should be no difference in age. That there is a paradox is persistently denied, with many arguments advanced against it. But as observed in the first chapter, if something is demonstrated then argument cannot confute it. To say both, that there is nothing by which things can be considered to be in motion, and that there is something, the speed of events in them, is a contradiction, which cannot be explained away.

In effort to counter the paradox it is often adduced that experiments amply demonstrate that physical processes slow down in objects at high speeds. But aside from the argument's denied supposition that the motion is distinguished before that difference is observed, if that difference among relatively moving objects is detected, then the contended relativity of motion is false. It will not do to ignore a contradiction in order to by procrustean means save a theory.

Newtonian mechanics already contained a principle of relativity, by which motion could not be distinguished in either of two bodies in relative motion to each other at constant velocity. The principle has been thought incomplete, and modern relativity holds to extend it to other, accelerated, motion, as observed. But classical mechanics was, instead, deficient in the opposite way.

According to Newton an attribute distinguishing motion is in rotating objects centrifugal force, the force by which things in circular motion recede from its axis. That rotation can be thought relative is illustrated by the one-time view that, as everyday experience still has it, the earth, rather than rotating, is unmoving and the heavens, e.g. the sun, revolve around it. But the centrifugal force, of receding from the axis of circular motion, applies to certain only of things in that relative motion. It applies to a centrifuge or its contents, receding from its axis, but it does not for the same axis apply to the surroundings, though relatively rotating about it. It is accordingly justified to among two relatively rotating objects regard one as in actual motion.

This inference of Newton, that there is an absolute motion of rotation, has been, together with the like in other motion, denied under the influence of his corresponding claim of an absolute space. It being noted that space is about no observable object, and that what are considered rotating ones appear so relative to the fixed stars, it was proposed that centrifugal force is causally connected with those stars. There is no need, however, to postulate an absolute space for the motion to hold. It suffices that the difference occurs to one object moving relatively to another. And for this reason it is also irrelevant what the cause of the difference may be, or what else may be connected, in another needlessness of explanation (p.79, first par.). It remains that the centrifugal force occurs to one of the objects in relative motion, the motion itself nameable the cause without groundlessly the stars, and it is convenient to refer to that object as in motion and to an object without the force as at rest, in comparison to which absence of the force, in keeping with said equilibrium, the force in other objects occurs in varying degrees and directions.

The centrifugal motion of objects was observed by Newton to be due to their property of moving in a straight line if not prevented by some force, in conformance with his discussed first law. The rotating elements if able recede by that law from the axis, to continue in a straight line at a tangent instead. He overlooked an underlying situation, however, extending to other motion beside rotation.

It has to do with what can be said to be resistance to deflection from a straight course in things that may be held in motion, the resistance increasing with speed. Resistance in things was observed before to be a manifestation of force on them (p.76, second par.), and the usual naming of the above law as of inertia is correspondingly misleading. Inertia was mentioned to refer to the resistance (same paragraph), whereas the law speaks merely of absence of force. A state of rest or uniform velocity is thus not a state of resistance, and when presently observing that things held in motion have a resistance, it is meant that a force affects them to a lesser degree than it does things at rest. That this difference exists is easily evidenced through those circular motions, which signify restraining forces exerted on objects moving otherwise in a straight line. The mentioned centrifuge, as exemplified by the domestic washing machine, can provide an illustration. Outside the machine if clothing is pressed against an obstacle and released, elasticity will push it back to some of its former state. The same will not happen during a spinning cycle in the machine. Because of the speed of the items, they, unlike those at rest, will resist the elastic forces that would deflect them from outward motion in a straight line. A more ordinary example is provided by a whirling around of an object on a string. Should the string while lying still be stretched by means of the object thereafter released, elasticity would pull the object back. Not so when the string is stretched by the object in whirling. The speeding object will resist its deflection from a straight course. To further disclose the widespread observability of this difference between motion and rest, gravity can be considered. An object suspended what would be held motionless above ground and then released will fall to earth quickly. But when hurtling parallel to the ground an object resists falling, to the point that at high speed, as in the case of the moon, it does not fall to earth at all.

There is then a quite evident difference between what would be regarded as motion and rest, although the difference escapes notice as a clearly formulated phenomenon. This phenomenon could side by side with other forces of nature be termed motive force, inasmuch as more resistance in an object usually translates into more impact on the object resisted, and it should not be confounded with energy of motion, the kinetic energy mentioned (e.g. p. 75, first par.). Without the present motive force that energy is merely of the law of inertia, that a moving body will as much keep its velocity as a still one its station, without offering more resistance to the change of its state. Since by the law of inertia a moving object tends to continue in a straight line, it will upon meeting in that direction another object exert on it a corresponding force, ascribed to kinetic energy. But by that law the effect need be no different if the other object is regarded as instead moving toward the first one. There still would be no difference between the powers of motion and rest. This was seen not to be the case in the above examples, where the forces of the moving object were, in the spoken of form of resistance, perpendicular to their motion. The same resistance was seen not to occur when the objects are what is normally viewed as stationary while the same, perpendicular, action is taking place. The perpendicularly depressed clothing, similar to the above meeting objects, will normally push apart, but not when speeding in a washing machine. It should be remembered that the rotation, motion, can be viewed as relative, and hence the difference in resistance between it and what is viewed as rest.

With motion thus possessing added force, it should be no wonder if clocks and other physical processes slow down within objects at high speed. The parts of the clocks and other elements, partaking in the motion of the whole, likewise resist deflection from that motion. Their actions not of that motion are retarded.

The retardation of action in moving objects does as made apparent moreover not require in order to be discernible the high speed supposed in relativity. As a matter of fact, as known of centrifugal force but not known as hence true of all motion, the motive force, the retardation of action, increases as the square of the motion's speed. A tenfold increase in speed, for instance, means a hundredfold increase in the force. And the force, the retardation, can accordingly be easily confirmed to act in all directions. Clocks and other objects are found to function at a constant rate in all directions while partaking in the speeding of the earth through the universe at over 100 miles per second, by which the solar system stays aloft. It could be asked if e.g. a clock's constant speed in all directions can be illusory, in that one what seems an equal period on a clock may not truly last as long as another. But if another clock is positioned at other angles than the first, a sameness of time is still observed. The motive force accordingly all-directional, it should be likewise no wonder that it is found that the higher a particle's speed the more difficult its increase. The particle gains in resistance, and it is in this regard falsely inferred that the object's mass, its size, becomes larger as well. Mass as resistance to force is again mistaken for mass as quantity of matter.

An effect similarly resulting from resistance was by likewise erroneous argument determined about gravity. As spoken of before (p.77, last par., through p.78, second par.), there is contended a relativity between bodies falling due to gravity toward the earth and the earth moving instead toward them, each viewpoint held correct about the same event. The relativity is further considered extended to a more general one between gravitation and accelerated systems. What is viewed as happening by gravitational force is thought to be viewable as happening by corresponding acceleration of what is otherwise the object of the force, and vice versa. Hence since in accelerated systems time is determined to slow down, it is argued that time slows down under gravity.

That matters are not the same regarding what are found to be gravitational forces and what are found to be corresponding accelerations was noted with respect to falling bodies (p.78, second par.). By the supposed relativity, in addition, time in those bodies when considered at rest and free of gravity, with the earth falling toward them, is unlike in falling ones not held to slow down, in further negation of the equivalence.

Things do in fact slow down under gravitation, but simply because as in the case of motive force, or any other, gravitational force counters opposing ones, and consequently their action is impeded. This interaction of forces takes place in the very examples of the operation of motive force listed. That force impedes the action of others, e.g. the falling down due to gravity, while the others prevent motion in a straight line.

Whereas action slows down in things under the gravitational force of reference frames like the earth, the same was seen above not requisite in things with regard to which a reference frame is accelerating instead, the general equivalence claimed on the basis of certain instances. Among them are those where things seated on, or hanging from objects seated on, earth are respectively compared to things pressed against, or stretched from, a reference frame due to its respective acceleration toward, or away from, them. But in the later things action slows down progressively more, due to the acceleration, not the case in those on earth. Also compared are to things falling toward earth ones that inside a rotating reference frame fall toward its peripheral wall due to centrifugal force. But in these things, in uniform motion by the law of inertia, action is slow at a constant rate, not the case in those falling to earth and hence accelerating, not to mention the referred to changes of distance between objects falling toward the earth, and the compounding of slowing in them due to increasing force of gravity.

The believed relativity of gravitation and accelerating systems is thus persistently wrong as were others, specifically the relativities of time or simultaneity and space or distance, and most notably the main thesis, relativity of motion. The mistaken theories, by way of which a number of correct conclusions was argued, illustrate the pitfall of consequently holding the premises, the theories, right. Conclusions in relativity, as often happens elsewhere, were seen also not to follow from premises given, to as much as contradict them. Inasmuch as these errors occur in the most exact sciences, they remind that theory in general be treated with great caution, that knowledge be not presumed lightly.

Upon having determined the existence of motive force as a correlate of other forces, all of them the expression of causal connections, a more general inquiry can proceed as to whether there exist other invariable connections in nature, whether, as sometimes supposed, other laws of nature exist beside causal ones.

The reason that the laws or principles treated are discussed as connections was referred to previously. These laws declare in the quest of what may be held true of things that something is the case about some things, and thereby establish a connection between these things and what is the case about them, be it their existence alone. The continued existence of nature at large can thus be considered a constant connection, and it could be considered a law of nature. So could the fact that all of nature is subject besides to laws peculiar to it. In seeking laws of nature, however, it is these laws themselves to which nature is subject that are the connections meant.

In endeavoring accordingly to find what other such laws or constant connections beside causal ones, broadly ones of causation, might exist, the interest is by the preceding not in merely whether the existence of some matter, of the described stuff which happenings in the external world concern, altogether is always accompanied by the existence of some other. That connection would only be of an instance of the continuance of all matter. The one existence would be known as always accompanied by the other simply because the other, as well as the first, is already known as constant and thus accompanying everything.

The connection sought in a law of nature must consequently be about some condition of matter beside its existence, it must be about some material state, as earlier referred to (p.74, second par.). And since the connection would concern a thing and something the case regarding it, i.e. it would concern the accompaniment of the first thing by the second, at least one of them should by the preceding be about some material state, beside the existence of some matter, since the mere coexistence of matter was excluded.

If then it were the first thing which is a state and not the second, the situation would be of no interest as before. The first thing would be known as always accompanied by the second —still only of the existence of some matter—simply because the second is already known as constant, accompanying everything.

And if the second thing and not the first were a material state, perhaps a vicinity, it, as observed (same p.74), would have a cause, and hence it would be of a change, not constant. But then as before observed differently (p.71, third par.) it could not always accompany the first thing—which is constant—and could in consequence not be of a law of nature.

Consequently not only one of the two things connected, but each of them, must be a state and therefore the connection a causal one, since both states connected, having causes, would be of changes (e.g. p.71, fifth par.). It may be added that the connection can be the reverse of the causation, by which one event might be always preceded, rather than succeeded, by another. In that case, since nothing can bring about the later event without the prior one, the prior one is at least a contributing cause of the later. The law would accordingly be that a certain event always has a certain other as a cause.

As a result of the foregoing, causal laws are the only laws of nature, further searches into which laws need therefore be conducted among them. At present the search can be directed at any type of causal law presupposed by knowledge of more particular ones.

It can initially be noted that all facts about nature are found to be conveyed by means of one's body as a living organism.

The issue of what defines life was mentioned at the beginning of the first chapter, and later with regard to the self (p.50, second par.), and it was observed that the definition, as elsewhere, is a matter of choice. In the later mention it was indicated that what is of concern when speaking of life is that it is characterized by certain purpose, one, more specifically, not in the sense in which purpose characterizes a what is regarded as lifeless tool, but in the sense that purposive behavior in the living is considered to stem from within.

It was indicated also (p.60, first par.) that by purposive behavior is meant one that by appropriate adjustment accomodates whatever circumstance toward attainment of a particular end. This has to do with living organisms inasmuch as they are entities which whatever the circumstance are found to utilize it toward the same ends.

These meanings of life and purposiveness may be thought to be by some not appropriate. It may be proposed that to speak of purposiveness in living organisms unjustifiably connotes design. Or it may contrariwise be put forward that some man-made machines function purposively but would not be said to be alive. Life should thus signify less than purpose in the first case and more in the second. The important question, rather than being what names to assign, is, however, what sort of differences can be discerned between organisms and other material entities.

And there is discernible a fundamental causal difference. It is that other material entities do not function purposively as described. They do not utilize circumstances toward the same ends, but respond in different directions according to different circumstances. This is the case also with man-made machines built to respond to different circumstances in a way resulting in the same end, for instance the same temperature in an enclosure. There are in general of course varied circumstances resulting should they occur in the same ends, and that is a very factor made use of by organisms, in adjusting their behavior in order to through varied means obtain the same results. The machine, however, will lead to constant results only insofar as its user supplies conditions required. It will not do so under all conditions even if unimpaired, and should it it may well be called alive.

The causal laws by which machines and other lifeless objects exclusively function are customarily called physical and chemical ones, and it is, to be sure, very often proclaimed that organisms, too, are subject only to these laws. The outlook is termed mechanism, and it is so widespread that to contest it should meet with especial opposition.

But the refutation is contained in the above, and it is similar to the earlier demonstration of free will. The invariable finding that unlike things solely subject to those laws organisms, availing themselves of them, function in accordance with ends as described, with what may be called final cause, cannot be overturned by another finding, which can be no more then likewise invariable and cannot contradict fact.

This presupposes that things acting only in conformity with mechanical cause do not also act in conformity with final cause. That this presupposition is pertinent is attested by the frequent contention that the components of organisms have as part of physical and chemical forces a built-in property to act in accordance with ends. What is meant by these forces could thus be all sorts of things, without distinguishing them from the vital or life force that is spoken of by some and that mechanism argues against. The point is that if the behavior of organisms be wholly explainable by physical and chemical laws as purported, it must be decided what is meant by these laws. If they are meant to include activity occurring in accordance with ends, and with it perhaps the gamut of laws of nature, then the behavior of organisms is in fact explainable by them. But this would not nullify the purposive activity. It would embrace it as part of the laws. Neither is the activity nullified by calling it functional instead, as has become the practice.

Without considering volition of sentient beings, there exists in nature a distinction thus between things that act in accordance with ends and those that do not, and in concord with accustomed designations they may respectively be termed animate and inanimate, or of, as said, final cause and only mechanical cause. These two kinds of cause represent then different laws of nature, in that the laws usually regarded as physical and chemical are of forces not leading to described purposive ends, whereas organic laws are of forces that do. The last mentioned laws are in their general aspects known as principles of preservation of self and the species, and in particulars organisms strive to preserve diverse functions, each in behalf of the, largely cyclic, goals of the entire unit.

In the body of a sentient being those functions include transmitting of information to the mind, as well as ability for subsequent action. The information transmitted is of course one depended on for knowledge of the external world, and consequently that knowledge presupposes the purposive function of the body, with other physical processes part. To wit, in conformance with what has been said any reality learned of the material world, e.g. its particular causal laws, presupposes the reality in it of the purposive organism, namely of final, together with utilized mechanical, cause.

With these types of cause presupposed by the body as informant of material realities,

THEOREM II.6. *Final and mechanical cause in the physical world are realities prior to other realities in it.*

The presence in organisms of final cause, of purpose, has been thought refuted in the last century by Darwin's theory of natural selection. It should be remarked that a theory, not being proof, cannot refute. The one in question ascribes the adaptation of organisms so as to cope with their environment to nature's through evolution nonpurposive elimination of organisms not adapted. The minority thought to adapt is held to do so by accident, by random mutation.

As seen, however, the disclosure of purpose in organisms, with their acknowledged life itself distinguished by purpose, does not require evidence extending over generations of numerous members of a kind. Evidence of a single organism's behavior while alive was sufficient. The life and purpose revealed themselves as action toward self-preservation, consisting in, beside development to maturity and retainment of that state, adjustment to new environments, as in acquiring resistance to the harmful. Such acquired characters are irrelevantly argued not inheritable, the purposiveness occurring notwithstanding. Furthermore heredity itself, by which the kind continues, was seen as manifestation of purpose, that of preservation of the species.

Even if these discrepancies are neglected, moreover, natural selection is in itself statistically untenable, as some have argued, if without success. When here discussing the everyday purposive behavior of organisms, it was observed that the behavior of other things differs by not leading toward the same ends under all conditions. Their resulting in disparate ends is as a matter of fact so extensive that results are statistically determined to be progressively less specific to eventually have an equal chance at innumerable possibilities. This diffusion is sometimes referred to as entropy, and compared to an organism's preservative adjustment to the environment it is signified by erosion. Since the diffusion increases with time, a nonpurposive entity's chance of preservative change decreases, and its long-term accidental adaptation, by which it would survive natural selection, is therefore uncountably less probable than, as in the individual behaviors discussed, a short-term act of self-preservation by a likewise supposed unpurposeful object.

The accidental adaptation of one surviving lineage of an organism, ignoring the single organism's constant adaptation, can alone by what was said be seen unlikely at the least. That the same accidental adaptation in addition happen to the many lineages of a species is yet the more unreasonably unlikely, with the topmost unlikelihood the accidental adaptation in the very many species of organisms extant.

While the preceding has to do with how untenable accidental adaptation is in kinds of organisms that have survived, the same is the case regarding the kinds that have become extinct and hence held to fall victim to natural selection. The very fact that they once were alive, not to mention survival through generations, signifies again that they were purposive beings, and they were adapted to function correspondingly. Their past existence lacks as much conformity with mechanical probability as does the present existence of the others.

It has been proposed that probability depends on points of view, in a contradictory relativity similar to those discussed. It is posited as highly unlikely that a man have male descendents in an uninterrupted line for very many generations. Yet every living man is a descendent from such a long line. Ironically the birth of any offspring was seen purposive preservation of the kind and cannot serve to demonstrate lack of purpose. Presuming the improbability true, further, it is not contradicted. Keeping in mind that only fathers of fathers are counted, the more ancestral the fathers the fewer they are, since men have many common ancestors. The few are accordingly the statistically rare ones of their contemporaries. But this sort of justification is not necessary. If something almost never occurs then it is by definition improbable, and if not then not. If mechanical survival of progeny is statistically untenable then it cannot continually occur. In other words a statistic cannot be both true and false if to avoid contradiction.

The contended chance adaptations, meaning here by chance not absence of cause but of purpose, are accordingly not merely improbable but impossible. Statistical probability is as indicated based on fact, and if the fact regarding certain entities, now organisms, is that something is never true of them, now that they not be adaptive, then there is no probability, i.e. no possibility, of it. And the constancy of the adaptiveness, present even when inadequate for survival, renders the adaptiveness of generations, in likeness to the behavior of single organisms, of final cause, purposive.

It is of concern to add that the destructive potential of the theory of natural selection, also known as survival of the fittest, was noted by others, it asserting a hereditary inequality among men, leading to haughtiness in some and hopelessness in others, with many a tragic result in recent history.

Observing in the foregoing the purposefulness of organisms, it can be further observed that specific purposive laws are far more evident than are physical and chemical ones. Whereas laws of an organism, especially where concerning its whole, are comparatively easy to determine, other laws of nature, as indicated in the introduction and elsewhere, are elusive. The most primitive man soon learns of the general action of organisms toward fruition or preservation, and knowledge of the function of particular organs is not far behind. But other causal principles by which events ordinarily observed occur have to do largely with interactions of minutest particles, and their detection hence requires sophisticated instruments and may, if quantum theory is right, meet insurmountable obstacles. The interactions, the causal principles, are spoken of in terms of forces, and the remaining force of acquaintance beside the ones just referred to is gravitation, which waited millennia to be found a principle. The motive force herein described (ca. pp.90-91) was seen yet to be recognized.

The detection of realities by means of instruments, used to ascertain larger phenomena about the universe as well as smaller ones about its particles, is, as was suggested (p.67, fourth par.), in addition subordinate to the detection of realities by means of unaided senses, because the instruments themselves are relied on by being perceived through those senses. There is accordingly subsequent to the previous cases, also an order in priority regarding these two mediums and the realities perceived by way of them.

The combined discussed order in reality is depicted in Figure II. At the end of it knowledge of reality perceived through the aid of instruments presupposes knowledge of the instruments as reality (the two realities circles in dotted line, the horizontal line in one circle signifying means of transmitting knowledge); the knowledge of instruments in turn presupposes knowledge of reality known through sense perception, which knowledge presupposes knowledge of the reality of the body as conveyor of the perceptions (the last two realities circles in dashed line, with again a horizontal line for transmission of knowledge); in accordance further with the theorems of this chapter and as made reference to in its headings, the body as conveyor of realities presupposes the reality of final and mechanical cause, this and in the preceding mentioned realities and their knowledge presupposing the reality and knowledge of the world, which presuppose the reality and knowledge of voluntary and involuntary mind as determiner, by which are presupposed the reality and knowledge of the self as ultimate concern (these realities circles in solid line, with vertical lines for appropriate divisions).

The solid lines thus represent the principal determinations in this chapter, the other lines representing, in the form of the body and instruments, successive extensions of the self as receiver of knowledge, together with knowledge received through them. Should the self be postulated of possible disembodied existence, that knowledge, perception of external reality, might also come about without those intermediaries, as hinted by the subject matter of the first half of the diagram.

Returning to that subject matter, it may again be observed that both processes in accordance with ends, the one of the

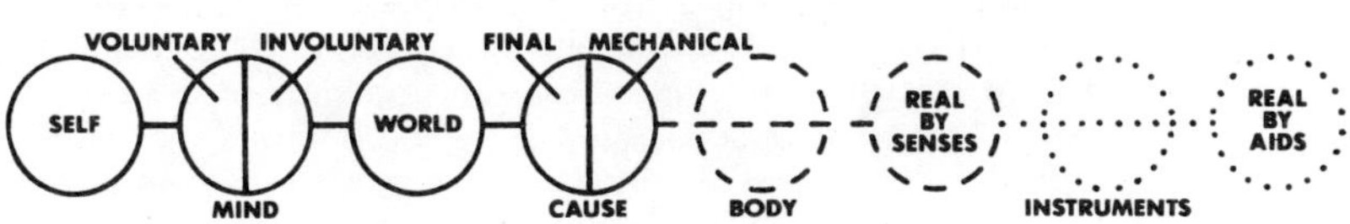

FIGURE II

final cause of unconscious organisms and the one of voluntary mind, represent additional forces beside the mechanical ones dealt with, because they are not results of mechanical forces alone. That an organism like one's body should have its own force of final cause and in sentient beings the added force of voluntary mind is specifically of value in one's purposes. In one's body the force was observed to strive for preservation of one's functions, including transmission of knowledge to the mind and ability to act accordingly, to act in accordance with, that is to say, one's purposes, that action an expression of the other, mental, force. Even in plants the force by which they grow and propagate serves to replenish man's sustenance to therewith have a function in man's purposes, toward which other forces of nature are likewise applied.

Man's purposes were highlighted at the beginning of this chapter as ground for determining what is real, and for identifying the self as primary reality. In the process the self has been taken to apply to others beside this writer. That it does has for the matter of that, as indicated largely in the last chapter, been taken to be true from the beginning of this writing, in supposing a readership for it. Similarly the existence of selves other than oneself, of other conscious individuals, is presumed in all ordinary human transaction and is thus taken for granted. It is nevertheless the subject of debate, in what is called the question of other minds, and its examination here should bring out an instance of inference of entities not perceived, not at least by each individual. As a matter of fact inferred entities, because of the need for their inference, are unperceived as a rule, at least temporarily, but because the act of inferring is an everyday recourse in coordinating one's manifold perceptions, its foundation can be overlooked, and disputes on the order of the present one arise.

It can first be noted that in raising the question of other minds in discourse, as done in these queries, the words used, including "mind", are for the most part received from other men. The question could accordingly be accurately whether what other men mean by their mind corresponds to the entity of one's own one learned to associate with the word. The underlying question would be whether they, too, possess that entity. But since however the issue is put in language, understanding of the meaning by such other minds is here presumed, minds and the like may as well be spoken of, and the task is to explicate why the presumption of that understanding consists in knowledge, because of which the explication should be comprehended by the reader.

Arguments denying such knowledge start from the justified contention that inductive knowledge, to which the questioned knowledge belongs, can be obtained only from the experience of numbers of instances, on the basis of which a generalization can be made, in this case that other human forms beside one's own are imbued with minds. It is maintained that the requirement of the repeated instances is in this case not met. One only has the experience of one's own mind, and it is proposed that one cannot accordingly infer the others. The numerosity experienced, however, is here not of beings with minds, but of attributes of oneself that have counterparts in other beings. From the constant known accompaniment of one's attributes by counterparts in other beings, counterparts of other of one's attributes, e.g. consciousness, can be inferred.

The constant known accompaniment does not, of course, hold for all of one's attributes without exception. The color of one's eyes may not be repeated in someone else. What does correspond are fundamental functions of even the most primitive animal, functions in regard to which animals can in fact be said to be distinguished from plants by having minds, by perceiving, as in the form of feeling. Animals are often said to in contrast to plants feel pleasure or pain, and should these attributes be held not to distinguish the first of these beings from the second, one need only be reminded that the matter has to do with definition, with what is wished to be meant by an animal compared to a plant. What is of account is that even at the simplest level creatures usually called animals display behavior sufficiently parallel to one's own and, in continuing induction from the more to the less complex, to that of other animals to warrant the inference that they also perceive. From the great multiplicity of shared functions in other men one can induce their mind in corresponding function, as one can in multitudes of progressively less complex but still very similar animals, and from these many correspondences one can induce the same of the simplest creatures that display the appropriate behavior. They in the main react to injurious or seemingly so events by through motion at once trying to avoid them, thus instantly seeking their well-being, from which behavior like that of other animals their corresponding feelings of pain and pleasure is inferred. Should entities regarded as plants be consistently so responsive, they may be considered to have like feelings.

That also certain other living beings beside oneself perceive can be determined by more than induction, furthermore. In practice it is really other beings' actions that determines their consciousness. Their attitude like one's own toward the world is equivalent to their like consciousness of it as by demanding treatment like that desired for oneself. These functions accordingly not only signify in other beings consciousness, but selves as possesors of it, in keeping with former observations (e.g. p.50, second par.) on the self as characterized by a basic purpose of satisfaction. The import is that other beings' attitudes as analogous to one's own cannot be ignored, whatever the exact nature of others' perceptions.

The nature of the perceptions even in beings otherwise most alike need not be precisely the same, as illustrated by colorblindness. Nonetheless the more similar to one's own an animal's overt characteristics, the more justified one is to induce that its mind likewise corresponds. As animals gain the ability to communicate, furthermore, they disclose added similar consciousness of, beside their environment, purely mental contents. In man these mental contents are of course especially abounding. They are communicated in the course of history in recorded form through highly wrought languages and find realization in the development of civilization. Beside their actuality other minds in men can accordingly be induced to be like one's own to the utmost.

That they are can, as suggested before (p.100, second par.), be held for the most part taken for granted, as can be the associated induction of which mental content is communicated by which linguistic expression. Words and languages pertaining to given things are known to be variable, and it is accordingly not particular usages that lie at the basis of why communications are comprehended. It is rather the understanding that communication is taking place to begin with. This understanding occurs before individual meanings may be comprehended, as when not knowing the meaning of what someone says though knowing that something is meant to be conveyed, and accordingly one can induce it through not merely one kind of sign but any variety of signs the speaker wishes to make, nonlinguistic ones called ostensive. The gist is that induction of linguistic or related meaning goes beyond signs alone, to have a more thorough underpinning. It is based on the deeper learning of other selves as of, alongside other attributes, perceptions like those of oneself, and one learns, in furtherance of this process, by use of the means of communication more of the sameness of the inner lives of others.

The reality of, as also consequential as described, many alike selves, of within their purview their voluntary and involuntary mental contents, the external world, and its final and mechanical causalities, all explored herein in relation to any one person, should suffice as the worldly realities principally determined in this chapter. To determine more particular realities in nature, aside from occasional exceptions, is not the intention of this disquisition; such determinations are the province of specialized searches, not necessarily proceeding from common observations, mentioned as the material for the present inquiries. And the determination of any reality transcending nature as customarily understood will be considered separately; to that end and for other possible inquiries what has preceded should provide a foundation, supplemented by the following investigation of matters of deduction.

Chapter III LOGIC AND MATHEMATICS

The difference between what is meant by logic and what by mathematics is not well established. Logic is ordinarily regarded as having to do with rules of correct inference, and the kind of inference in question, as indicated, is here deduction. As observed previously, however (e.g. p.13, third par.), the only way in which something, including an inferred thing, is known to be true is by finding it to be so, and that by whatever nature it is meant manifested, presently by being intrinsic. For that reason logical principles are not about how, but what, things can be deduced from given ones. But mathematical principles, too, are about this, and the question remains how do the two disciplines differ.

The generality of the above frequent description of logic may suggest that it in the comparison somehow treats of all things irrespective of quantity, whereas mathematics treats of them with respect to quantity. But logic, too, treats of quantities, as in the concepts of "all" and "some", applied to things unless fully negated, in which case their quantity is zero, a concept part of mathematics likewise.

The concept of "all" in logic can in kinship to discussed necessity be taken to represent the universality of a principle, by which something is true of all of a kind. It is thereby inherent in logical, mathematical, or other principles themselves, which concern all instances of the conditions considered, or of the things considered in them, as a causal law would be of all of certain events regarding all of certain things. The observation is in concord with the allusion in the preceding chapter (p. 67, third par.) that principles, e.g. laws of nature, are expected to be true of certain things, e.g. matter, without exception. "Some" and negation can similarly be taken to concern principles. To assert some can in kinship to possibility be viewed as denying an opposing principle, a necessity if not an impossibility, the last of which can be viewed as signified by negation.

In all, these quantitative concepts take part by that universality in mathematical principles as well, apart from the quantities those principles particularly speak of. Accordingly a distinction between logic and mathematics may be easier to make.

Considering in accord with the preceding paragraph that principles are about what holds or does not of certain things under certain conditions, or perhaps unconditionally, these things—which may be referred to in terms of conditions, states, themselves, as in propositional logic, or in terms of attributes, as in predicate logic—can in logic be anything, whereas in mathematics they are limited to various quantitative concepts. How in diverse logics these things are not limited in concept shall be elucidated later, and the distinction here made between them and ones in mathematics will be appropriate for the investigations ahead.

While considering that logic and mathematics as deductive fields differ by the nature of their principles, it should be noted that principles are not the only things determined deductively. Most of deduction is for that matter of individual instances from principles already determined, and these principles, serving that purpose, can be of all sorts, from causal ones to merely definitions by convention. The deductions are nonetheless regarded as of logic, because performed in conformance with it. However, since, as noted again at the start of this chapter, something can be known to be true only if found to be so, it must also be found that an instance results from a principle, be the principle a logical one prescribing that result.

More about that requirement later, now it being of interest that while questions have often been raised as to the validity of logical or mathematical axioms, basic laws, there has been little question of the validity of inference of instances from them. Furthermore since by the foregoing these axioms must likewise be found true to enter the sphere of knowledge, and they are considered to be indemonstrable, it is in logic and mathematics neither substantiated that their basic laws are true, nor that the inferred instances, which may be further laws, follow.

The belief that initial principles cannot be proven can be explained through the very notion that once these are accepted other principles and single cases follow without need of more confirmation, with deduction thus held to be inference of the particular from the general. Similarly to the belief that certain basic terms cannot be defined, it is argued that since a deductive proof must follow from some principle, proof of which must follow from some other and so on, initial principles must be accepted without proof.

Some terms, as noted in the first chapter (p. 28, fourth par.), are thought undefinable because what they name is regarded as unanalyzable into components, and thus upon defining things by their components, and these by theirs and so on, undefinability would likewise be reached. Accordingly key terms assigned no meaning, ones by which others are defined, are indeed used alongside unproven axioms in logic and mathematics, although these terms may not be unanalyzable.

It can be observed again that in matters of worldly reality such omissions are, with justification, for science usually not accepted. As spoken of in the introduction, existencies believed not to admit of demonstration, as might be ones of metaphysical entities, are repudiated, as are factual statements that are held meaningless, among them ones believed unverifiable likewise. Yet such failures, extending throughout due to the dependence on them of deductions and definitions, are commended in logic and mathetmatics, sciences accorded greater certainty than are others.

That all language can be defined was expounded previously, and, as indicated by what was said, deductive truths can likewise be substantiated. The inference of fundamental deductive principles from the material considered is at least as simple a procedure as is inference of further things through them, and to demonstrate these procedures and what some of the inferences are is the object of this chapter, similarly to objects in others.

In speaking in the preceding sentence of the material considered, the reference is to the content of any language or symbolism used. That content has in much of mathematics and logic been set aside as not pertinent, the concentration being on form, on linguistic symbols and their combination. This inattention to meaning is in accord with the above, as connected with presumed undefinabilities. But the supposing of possible deduction on the basis of language without content, content to which the results are said to apply by accordingly interpreting the language, may be ascribed to added reasons. Such a one can be considered the extreme universality of logic and mathematics, leading to the conception of them as of truths separate from anything they may be applied to. A more contemporary ground can be held to be the disposition not to allow for reflectively acquired knowledge, with reliance on the physicality of language instead. Whatever the reason, the attempt to seek in language solutions to problems outside it is as misdirected here as it was seen to be elsewhere (e.g. p. 23, last par., through p. 24, second par.). It need only be repeated that in order to know whether something, e.g. a logical principle as pertaining to the things it speaks about, is true, it must be found, observed, to be so, in whatever manner what is in question is meant observed, as by reflection. To instead contemplate the corresponding language will not do, unless it takes the form of its content (p. 26, last par.).

The dismissal of the meaning of language in logic or mathematics is thus a hindrance in the search for appropriate knowledge, as well as in the resolution of the paradoxes or other incongruities that have perplexed men in that endeavor.

These incongruities, introduced through the centuries and by and large known as paradoxes, falsely affect these sciences, by motivating elaborate restrictive theories, in effort to avoid concerned contradictions. They display contradictions partly because of faulty postulates, but they can all be found to arise from concealment by language. The language fails to disclose contradictory premises, resulting in contradictory conclusions.

A seemingly consistent statement of the form "*A* is *B*" will accordingly turn out contradictory when it is recognized that *B* designates a negation of *A*. In paradoxes their very disclosure moreover constitutes ironically disclosure of the underlying inconsistency, since the paradoxical parts noticed are thereby determined to have been hidden under the language in the first place. Those parts are nevertheless sufficiently removed from that language to obscure the reason for their notice.

The following section is about how the incongruities fail to inform of the inconsistencies, how they can furthermore fail to impart information altogether. The subsequent section will include the substantiation that factual contradiction is not possible, as a result of which language that harbors contradictions can be disallowed as designating fact, as can be disallowed language that lacks informing content.

Section 1
PARADOXES

"Paradox" is often intended to refer to an utterance which though reasonable on the surface appears to call for both affirmation and denial of the same thing. But some incongruities call for neither affirmation nor denial, in opposition to what appears required, and they may with some liberality also be called paradoxes.

In the paradox perhaps most discoursed about, the ancient "liar", both of these situations take place. It may be phrased as

1. This statement is false.

As appears evident by its content, if the statement is true then it is false, and if false as it says then it is true. This is the situation of indicating both affirmation and denial, which situation is in this instance mainly acknowledged. Less acknowledged is that the statement may allow of neither affirmation nor denial. These two presently examined interpretations combine in illuminating the vagaries of language, as it can pretend to say either less or more than is the case.

The solution to the first and usual interpretation, that the statement is both true and false, may be found surprisingly simple when it is considered that it has for so long been elusive. It has in the past been prefigured and rests on the hidden premise

1.i. By the truth of a statement is meant what it declares.

This premise, in agreement with the aforesaid, is disclosed in disclosing the paradox, by finding statement 1 false if true and true if false, because of the very associating of its truth with, as in other statements, what it declares, namely its falsity.

The conclusion is

1.ii. Statement 1 contradicts definition 1.i

and is accordingly illegitimate, as would be any that overtly declares both the truth and falsity of something.

It may be noteworthy that statement 1, the liar paradox, has been contended false, in keeping with certain presumed logical principles, as based on to be looked into truth tables. By these principles if a statement or proposition implies a contradiction, possibly its own negation, it is false.

It should be mentioned again that (p. 65, second par.) when it is said that a proposition or statement implies something, it is not really they that are meant, but their truth. It is not the statement "This object is a tree", but its truth, which implies that the object is a plant. And the truth, or falsity, meant to apply to a statement, to a declarative sentence in accord with the discussion on its meaning (p.15 last par. through p.16 third par.), is the same one meant to apply to the, mental, proposition it stands for. For it is the same supposed facts that are in question.

And speaking of supposed facts, that a statement or proposition, in accordance with the above, imply a contradiction can be true only if they represent such suppositions, since actualities cannot, by to be seen law, imply contradictions. In statement 1, in the paradox (last p.), that supposition can be said to be that the statement implies it is false, or by the preceding correctly that the truth of the statement implies the statement is false. But it does not follow that the statement is false. From the supposition that the truth of "Paris is in France" implies "Paris is in France" is false it does not follow it is false.

Interestingly by the same belief that a statement or proposition implying a contradiction is false the paradox is again true as well as false. Since it was also determined that its falsity implies its truth, a contradiction, it should not be false, it should be true. This presumes that it is either true or false, as held to be under the believed principles above, which, however, were seen to ensure neither.

That a proposition leading to a contradiction need not be false invalidates as a method of proof the reductio ad absurdum mentioned in the introduction (p.5 fifth par.). The method is used for propositions leading not only to false ones, that disagree with some reality, but to contradictory ones, in the sense that disagreement follows from the first proposition itself, or from it as a result of some other assumed proposition. In this manner the method is perhaps most notably used in Euclid's geometry, and the invalidity does not mean that the conclusions are incorrect. The same inferences can as a rule be reached in accordance with transposition later herein explored. By it again if *A* implies *B* then *not-B* implies *not-A*, with either of the letters and their negations interchangeable, and an affinity with reductio inferences is readily seen. When both *A* and *not-A* are on the basis of assumptions true then since actualities, including conceptual ones, cannot result in contradiction, there is likely a conflicting assumption *B* which implies one of the contradictories, say *not-A*, unless the last is as in the liar paradox assumed independently. Accordingly *A* would be held true first, and by transposition of the preceding it implies *not-B*, which represents the denial of the assumption of the reductio.

As an example can serve Euclid's Proposition 6. It states that if angles *a* and *b* in the large triangle at right, the entire figure representing above *A*, are equal then so are its sides. For proof it is assumed, *B* above, that instead the right side of the small bottom triangle, or of an otherwise like one whose right side extends above the large triangle, equals the left side of the large one. It is then argued that the two triangles thus having those sides equal, as well as the base and the angles contained by these lines, the triangles, too, are, by Euclid's Proposition 4, equal, *not-A* above; but they are by initial construction contradictorily unequal. It is via reductio inferred through deriving by it the inequality, *not-B*, of the pertaining sides of the two triangles that the right side of the large triangle is not unequal to the left side, that it is equal. The inference rests on the further to be considered principle that a quantity (the right side of the large triangle) is either smaller than, equal to, or larger than a given one (the left side).

The inference by transposition follows a simpler route, not needing a false assumption, *B*, and its result, *not-A*. Said Proposition 4 transposed states that if two triangles are unequal then they do not have an equal angle with equal lines containing it. Hence the small triangle or any unequal, *A*, to the other but with an equal angle and base containing it cannot, *not-B*, have the other containing line equal. Therefore as before, the right side of the large triangle equals its left side.

Not only is either the falsity or the truth of paradox 1 (p.107) thus not ensured by reductio ad absurdum, but neither truth nor falsity can be seen to, as mentioned, apply. Because, in improvement of definition 1.i (p.108),

> 1.iii. By the truth and falsity of a statement are meant, respectively, what distinct from its truth or falsity it declares, and the negation of that.

Definition 1.i was relied on on the assumption that every statement is either true or false, whereas in conformance with the last definition it should be clear that if a statement is not about something distinct from its truth or falsity then, like an incomplete or nondeclarative sentence, it cannot lay claim to either. Like other nondistinct entities discussed, the truth or falsity of a statement is meant to concern a content outside themselves, and without such a content, with nothing said that would be true or false, a statement is vacuous and may be termed uniforming.

As with other words, it may be remarked, there exist diverse theories of truth, and the present definition may be questioned. It may therefore aid to be reminded that the meaning of words is a matter of choice, and the present one is the one of interest and presumed to be so commonly.

Accordingly,

> 1.iv. Statement 1 contradicts definition 1.iii

and is neither true nor false but, for that reason as well, illegitimate. Since calling for neither affirmation nor denial it might also not be considered a paradox in its first interpretation (p.108 second par.), unless because of the conditionality by which the truth and falsity result from each other.

Solutions to the liar paradox and similar incongruities have been attempted by rejecting the reflexivity in these utterances, and by replacing it by some form of hierarchy. For instance the use of a metalanguage, a language not the one in which the utterances are made, is thought requried for stating their truth or falsity. The problem is again, however, not solved by means of language. No matter what the words used for concepts or what language they are said to belong to, contradiction in those concepts is not therewith eliminated. As long as the same concepts are at issue, they, redundantly, retain their, perhaps contradictory, identity. E.g. as long as any words of any language, however applied, have the above meaning of "true" and "false", or of other words concerned, statement 1 remains a paradox.

The use of a metalanguage, of an additional deductive formal system phrased in it, is believed requisite for deciding that certain logical or mathematical statements are true. The statements are considered unprovable in the language or system in which they are presented, and they bear a close resemblance to the liar paradox. They can be exemplified by

2. This statement is unprovable.

It is irrelevant again in the system of what language the statement is tried to be proven, what it speaks of and what hence is to be proven remaining whatever its language, which can arbitrarily be meant to be that of the system, whose difference in language namely does not count and whose correctness is rather at issue. The statement is in fact thought demonstrated true by using standard language in reasoning, and it can be found illegitimate on more grounds than is the first paradox.

It should at this point be seen without difficulty that the statement is uninforming in the sense explained. Like a statement's truth or falsity, its provability or unprovability is of something it declares that is distinct from these, and therefore statement 2, saying nothing that would be provable or unprovable, is neither one nor the other and, with these concerned in it, hence neither true nor false.

The recongition that such a statement is none of these should be of pertinence to the foundations of mathematics, allied with logic, to both of which the statement, since presumed true and correspondingly unprovable, brought an above alluded to indeterminacy, with protracted elaborations on whether truths in varied formal systems are decidable. Since these statements are furthermore uninforming, there is, as suggested before the start of this section, no need to fear their insidious appearance in calculations.

Despite the introductive observation here that statement 2 is neither provable nor unprovable, it may be of interest that were it one or the other, and with the additional premises in arguments contending its truth, it would not be simply true, but would, on the basis of a premise unnoted, become a paradox similar to the starting one of statement 1. The argument that 2 is true or unprovable has proceeded thusly.

It is first supposed that

2.i. If a statement or proposition is provable it is true.

By this and 2 it is inferred that

2.ii. If 2 is provable it is unprovable,

and from this and the referred to (p.108 fifth par.) presumed principle that

2.iii. If a statement or proposition implies its negation

the negation is true
it is concluded that

2.iv. 2 is unprovable and hence by its content true.

Some remarks on the justification of these propositions.

The supposing that certain propositions, like 2.i or mathematical axioms, hold is often submitted to be correct intuitively. Perhaps needless to say, the recourse to intuition again belies in deductive sciences the confidence in their unquestionable certainty. The approach does not even participate in inductive generalization from worldly experience, preferable if all else fails. As regards 2.i, it is correct by definition. In analogy with an earlier noted meaning of the knowable (p.47 first par.), by something provable is meant something true that can be ascertained to be so.

The inference, further, of 2.ii from 2.i and 2 presupposes by moving from true in 2.i to unprovable in 2.ii, from the truth of 2 to what it states, the meaning of truth in 1.i, or 1.iii, a meaning, as indicated, often disputed by those concerned.

That 2.iii is not an acceptable principle was explicated.

And conclusion 2.iv twice more acknowledges that meaning of truth, by moving from true in 2.iii to unprovable through 2.ii, and from unprovable in its own statement to true.

Providing nonetheless that premises 2.i through 2.iii are all correct, along with the assumption that 2 is either true or false, by deriving conclusion 2.iv it is believed that further matters that cannot be ascertained were found beside such as logical axioms, to which by the foregoing incidentally statement 2 might have been added without ado about metalanguage. In contrast to the other supposed impossibilities, unprovability and corresponding truth of 2 is thought by the above reasoning to be ascertained. And therein lurks the paradox. In that reasoning the premise is omitted that, as observed with regard to 2.i (this p. third par.),

2.v. If the truth of a statement or proposition can be ascertained it is provable.

Hence since in conclusion 2.iv the truth of 2 is by the premises provided ascertained,

2.vi. 2 is provable, and false.

Therefore and by 2.iv

2.vii. 2 is both provable and unprovable, and true and false,

and correspondingly a paradox.

As in other cases it results from violating underlying premises. By 2.iii and 2.v

2.viii. If a statement or proposition implies its negation the negation is provable.

By this and 2.i

2.ix. The provability and hence truth of a statement cannot be made to be its unprovability.

In consequence

2.x. 2 contradicts 2.ix

and is accordingly illegitimate.

Statement 2 can lastly if assumed either provable or unprovable seen illegitimate on a deeper ground. As suggested when comparing the provable to the knowable (facing p. third par.), the provable can be regarded as identical with the true, as could the knowable with the real. For as indicated when considering that last identity (p. 46 last par.), what is true, not merely hypothetical, can be held synonymous with what is real, similarly to earlier synonymities with it of fact and the necessary. And what is provable, as indicated throughout likewise (e.g. p.3 first par.), can be held synonymous with what is knowable. With what is provable correspondingly identical with what is true, statement 2, meant like 1 and others to be true, should accordingly be provable and is contradictory for that reason as well.

But statements 1 and 2 were both found neither true nor false, since not meeting the described requirement of informing. There are statements furthermore that can be held neither true nor false although they inform. Such incongruities have been exemplified by

3. The present king of France is wise,

or the familiar

4. The husband stopped beating his wife,

it being understood that he never beat her.

Two versions are given, because thinkers have inclined to advance theories that intend to explain a particular incongruity, but are unrelated to other puzzles of the kind.

Statements 3 and 4 can be held neither true nor false, since by the meaning of the attributes the present king of France, who does not exist, is neither wise nor unwise, and the husband neither stopped nor did not stop beating his wife. It could in accordance with all these examples be thought enough to reject the belief that a statement or proposition must be either true or false.

Yet a conviction may linger that the principle must be somehow sound—otherwise a myriad of apparently obvious conclusions, in everyday life or in sciences as exact as those discussed, could not be drawn. Indeed a statement or proposition requires truth or falsity when, as set forth in the next section, matters are in accord with what is conversely required by the truth and falsity. Matters concerning 3 and 4, as in the case of uniforming statements, should have to hence be in accord with those requirements by the truth and falsity, which requirements are as usual unspoken though, as evidenced above, disclosed in the disclosing of the inharmonies.

With respect to 3 the pertinent tacit premise is

3.i. For the present king of France to be wise or unwise he must exist.

But it is a matter of fact that

3.ii. The present king of France does not exist.

Therefore and by 3.i

3.iii. The present king of France is neither wise nor unwise,

and 3 contradicts 3.iii.

With respect to 4 the premise is

4.i. For the husband to stop or not stop beating his wife he must have beaten her.

But it was postulated that

4.ii. The husband never beat his wife.

Therefore and by 4.i

4.iii. The husband neither stopped nor did not stop beating his wife,

and 4 contradicts 4.iii.

It may be noted that the deductions take a form again like reductio ad absurdum, but utilizing instead transposition in a manner known as modus tollens, by which if *A* implies *B* (3.i or 4.i), and *not-B* is true (3.ii or 4.ii), *not-A* is (3.iii or 4.iii).

It can also be observed that the same unmet requirement for truth or falsity underlies many statements alleged meaningless. They may be exemplified by "The sound is blue", in the literal sense of the color. Such statements are not meaningless—having concepts behind them—nor uninforming in the discussed sense—since being blue can be true. They merely give an attribute meant with its negation to apply to something else, here the visual.

That the principle that a proposition is either true or false may not universally apply has been suspected since antiquity. Aristotle's discussion on whether it can be rightly said that there either will or will not be a sea battle tomorrow proposes that the principle may apply to the past and present but not the future. The problem hinges on holding a proposition to be true or false when considered, it being said that it is, rather than will be, true or false regarding a future event. It is argued that since accordingly propositions that anything will or will not occur would respectively be now true and false, all that will and will not occur would be predetermined, with no room for contingency. Since the determinism appears unacceptable, it is concluded that propositions about the future may be neither true nor false.

It is again the deceptiveness of language, however, which

gives credence to the argument. The present tense of "is" when speaking of whether a proposition is true or false does not concern the state at issue—which can be of the past as well—but the present time of the proposition regarding that state. When it is accordingly said, in the present tense, that a proposition about an undetermined future may be true, it is merely meant that it is presently supposed that the future in question will occur. This meaning in general is certainly the one herein when saying that a proposition about the future or any time is either true or false. It is meant that at that time the state has been or will be present or not, though neither may be determined, the principle applying in this sense when the spoken of qualification is met.

That the principle may not apply in all cases has in a vein similar to the one of the present tense of statements been more recently ascribed to problems of existence. As illustrated by statement 3, the proposal is that those propositions are true or false whose subject exists or, in an extended sense as may concern infinities, would sometime be encountered. But as attested by statement 4, propositions can be neither true nor false despite conformance to such requirement. And that Don Quixote is the hero of a romance is true or false without that conformance.

The appropriateness of the principle, as suggested in the preceding, is in fact determined by the intended meaning itself of the particular affirmation and denial, to dissolve the uncertainty. By "even" and "odd" in the mathematical sense are meant affirmation and denial regarding a property of whole numbers. Of other things neither of the two can be predicated. While it will in the next section be substantiated that either affirmation or denial is required within their intended range, it should at present be enough to say that inasmuch as their range is determined by their users, there should be no difficulty knowing where the principle applies.

As regards incongruities which are subject to—instead of neither—both, affirmation and denial, and which might accordingly be called true paradoxes, the next may be cited.

The recently perhaps most discussed is Russell's paradox, named after Betrand Russell, its enunciator and a chief expositor of paradoxes. It may be given in two known versions, the second one closer to everyday life.

5. There is a class which has as its members every class which is not a member of itself, and none which is a member of itself.

6. There is a barber in a village who shaves every man living there who does not shave himself, and none who shaves himself.

As before, two examples are furnished because of attempted solutions of one of them that are not suited for the other.

What is paradoxical is that in 5 if the initial class is a member of itself then—by the second clause—it is not, and if it is not then—by the first clause—it is, and in 6 if the barber shaves himself then he does not, and if he does not then he does.

The neglected premise explaining the paradox in 5 is

5.i. A class is a member of itself if and only if it is a member of that very class.

This, it will be noted, is an application of the meaning of "itself" and the like.

But since in 5 being a member or not in the initial class is considered of all classes, including that initial class, and those that are members of themselves are not members of it, and those that are not members of themselves are members of it,

5.ii. Statement 5 contradicts premise 5.i.

Similarly, the neglected premise in 6 is

6.i. A barber shaves himself if and only if he shaves that very barber.

But since in 6 being shaved or not by the barber is considered of all men of the village, including that barber, and those that shave themselves are not shaved by him, and those that do not shave themselves are shaved by him,

6.ii. Statement 6 contradicts premise 6.i.

The concealed premises can again be seen disclosed in the paradoxical findings about 5 and 6. E.g. the inital class is found to be a member of itself if it is not because of the association of "itself" with that class.

The positing of that class in statement 5 is thought justifiable, because both, classes that are members of themselves and that are not, can be held to exist. The first and stranger ones have been illustrated by the class of nonmen, itself a nonman, and the second by the class of men, itself not a man. Accordingly the class of all the last mentioned classes, of those not members of themselves, might be said to likewise exist, in seeming agreement with 5. The class of these classes, their totality, can indeed be said to exist, but not to the full exclusion of the other classes. The second relation given in 5, or 6, cannot hold if the first does, or the first if the second does, if contradiction is to be avoided. With either relation, e.g. shaving the nonshavers, there is at least one exception to the other, by shaving a shaver, himself.

The attempts at previously solving these two paradoxes were, as in the case of 3 and 4, primarily directed at the first of them. Answers were sought in hierarchies mentioned with 1 and 2, more specifically in restricting the meaning of membership in a class to things other than the class. While this can be done by linguistic fiat, however, it does again not prevent the underlying situation, which, however worded, can be used for the paradox. That the class, the totality, of all things not men is also not a man is a fact, whether or not the totality be called a member or other of itself. And if the totality of all and only totalities not the kind of thing they are totalities of is considered, the paradox remains. If the initial totality is the kind it is a totality of, then, since those kinds are not the kind they are totalities of, it is not, and so forth.

The needless through hierarchies prohibiting of the reflexivities, as of self-reference of a language and self-membership of a class, should for 6 result in no one's shaving oneself. This elucidates that the last paradoxes do not, as theory presumes, depend on the relation between a class and things that are members or not of it. In 6 the relation is instead between a barber and those who are shaved or not by, not members or not of, him.

That the last paradox is in fact one was in avoiding equating it with 5 attempted to be denied, by again recourse to language. It was suggested that the barber is a woman or not a resident of the village, and the language herein in 6 is to accommodate this question. There is no obstacle to expressly postulating that the barber is a man and resident, however, and the paradox is in effect.

Other paradoxes leading to both affirmation and denial have been put forward, and it should suffice here to adequately resolve ones of a wide interest. As with the other incongruities, since actuality admits of no contradiction, there should be no problem with these in practice. The rather laborious debated antinomies of the 18th-century philosopher Immanuel Kant will accordingly not also be discussed here. They cannot, furthermore, be regarded as paradoxes, since the contradictory results alleged do not obtain.

Analogous to the preceding two is the paradox known as Grelling's. It concerns the word "heterological", intended to refer to all and only those words not referring to themselves. "English", for instance, does not qualify. Accordingly if "heterological" refers to itself then, since it refers only to words not referring to themselves, it does not, and if it does not then, since it refers to all words not referring to themselves, it does. The premise that makes the condition contradictory is again that a word refers to itself if and only if it refers to that very word. Hence since being referred to or not by the word heterological is considered of all words, including that word, it cannot be defined to refer to words not referring to themselves, and not to words referring to themselves.

Analogous reflexive paradoxes can evidently continue to be

constructed. Reflexivity is conducive to incongruities, because normally when something has to do with something it is not expected to have to do with itself. Thus when regarding shaving by a barber one may not think of him as shaving himself, or when regarding assertions of truth one may not think of it with respect to the assertions. Accordingly another such paradox may be considered, differing by being viewed mistakenly as concerning number. Known as Berry's paradox, it can be paraphrased as

7. The smallest thing not nameable in fewer than twelve words.

"Smallest thing" replaces a phrase such as "least natural number", which number is groundlessly thought to exist, because nameable thus by description 7. The thing need not be the smallest either, but anything specified, and it appears both nameable and not in fewer than twelve words. The first since description 7 in fact names it in only ten words, and the second since the description says so. The clue to the solution is in the first of these, corresponding to which the tacit premise is

7.i. All things are nameable in fewer than twelve words.

This is the case simply because anything can be arbitrarily named by a single word.

Consequently

7.ii. Description 7 contradicts premise 7.i.

The notion that the numerical form of the description refers to an existing number can be explained by the role played by numerals. Numbers are most often named in terms of numerals, even if put into words, as they can be held if spoken. And in accordance there can indeed be a least natural number not nameable in fewer than a given amount of words—or syllables, as 7 is often presented. The least not nameable in less than two syllables is seven, and in less than two words, compounded, twenty-one. But the issue is naming numbers by other than numerals. And any number can be assigned as short a name as desired, as is "pi" in comparing a circle to its diameter.

The mistaking of the varied nature of other language for that of numerals enters also into what is known as Richard's paradox and consists in, rather than a paradox, a misunderstanding. The postulation is of

8. The list of all finite natural-language descriptions naming a real number,

a number expressible in decimals. It is then observed that in accordance with set theory a description can be added naming a real number not on the list. The description may for present purposes by phrased as

8.i. The next real number not listed.

It is concluded that by 8 and 8.i

8.ii. The list both does and does not include all those descriptions of real numbers.

The conclusion does not follow, however, even with pertinent set theory accepted. While description 8.i may name an unlisted number, it need not be an unlisted description. Once listed, it can be used repeatedly, each time naming a new number.

The assertions of set theory on which the preceding is founded, however, are likewise erroneous. It is argued that the set of real numbers is larger than the set of natural numbers. In support it is assumed that the sets are of equal size, and on believing to derive a contradiction, it is by reductio ad absurdum inferred that they are not. With reductio seen not reliable or necessary, the presumed proof can be as follows.

$$1 \leftrightarrow .1\cdots$$
$$2 \leftrightarrow .2\cdots$$
$$3 \leftrightarrow .3\cdots$$
$$\cdots\cdots\cdots\cdots$$

As pictured, with every natural number is paired a real number in decimals, the mutual pairing assumed with reductio in addition possible throughout. It suffices that it is argued that after a real number is paired with every natural one, another real number can be added by the method known as diagonal.

$.123\cdots$	
$.234\cdots$	$.246\cdots$
$.345\cdots$	

If the decimals were as in the left arrangement, then in accordance with the diagonal there, the number on the right could be produced by changing the first digit of the first number, the second digit of the second number, and the like in the third case. That is to say, there should always be a number differing from previous ones by at least the one digit under the diagonal.

As should be evident, if the digits were limited to three they would soon be exhausted, and the point is that a new number can be produced indefinitely since a new digit can always be added at the end. The same is true of natural numbers, however, in the opposite direction. An opposite diagonal could be used, and in fact when previous digits are exhausted, the next number is produced by adding a digit in front.

The reasoning flaw in set theory lay in supposing completion of these sets, so that by asssuming completion of one of them the other can be continued since infinite. Neither can be complete, for their infinity allows continuance by definition.

As a result it is also not required that the list referred to in preceding 8 (p.118), and held to be the size of the set of natural numbers, be exhausted, although no paradox was seen regardless. The list has to merely by digits name those natural numbers, themselves real, to be endless, giving no occasion for 8.i, much less 8.ii, there being no list reaching all those numbers.

The notion that certain infinite sets are, as in the preceding, of the same size stems from a concept of countability, by which a set in question is paired with the set of natural numbers in a manner like the above. The set of rational numbers, numbers expressible in fractions, is held countable, i.e. the same size as the set of natural numbers, by arranging it for example as pictured, pairing the fractions with natural numbers in for instance the sequence designated by the arrows.

```
1/1→1/2   1/3···
      ↓     ↑
2/1←2/2   2/3···
 ↓          ↑
3/1→3/2→3/3···

················
```

By such a sequence any given fraction, any given combination of the digits, is seen reachable. But this is not true of every fraction there is, it should be noted, since there is an infinity of them. By a fraction to be given is meant that it had been conceived, not that it is reached via that sequence. And this suggests that there is no reason to because of that sequential listing decide that the sizes of the set of rational numbers and the set of natural numbers are equal. Given fractions may as well be listed haphazardly so as to be reached, without in either case implying the equality.

As a matter of fact the same sort of enumeration last displayed is, though denied, possible with every infinite set of numbers. The above set of real numbers, held larger, can serve as example, revealing in fact a mirror image with respect to natural numbers, as did the spoken of diagonal.

.1	1.0	0.01	10.00
.9	9.9	9.99	99.99

Depicted are merely samples in the process, which consistently returns to every former column with every further one. In the first one depicted the digits will be listed from 1 through 9; by the second depiction thereupon the same but starting with zero since considered is repeated in that column with 1 before the decimal point, then with 2, through 9; after by the third depiction likewise listing all used digits in the second column after the decimal point, the same is repeated there with 1 in the first decimal column, then with 2 etc., to repeat the whole process with 1 before the decimal point, and so forth; thereafter by the fourth depiction all the preceding is repeated with 10, with 11, through 99, to continue the same with the third column after and then before the decimal point, and so on with more columns. Accordingly any given real number, any given combination of the digits, is by this sequence again reached.

It might be objected that real numbers such as pi, only expressed in infinite decimals, are never reached. These numbers can by above, however, not be regarded as given. Because of that infinity they are not conceived in their entirety, and to the extent that they are given they are indeed reached by that sequence. More pertinent is that that infinity compared to its lack in rational numbers, so as to distinguish real ones from them, is known without resorting to these counting methods, and still more pertinent, this difference does not imply a difference in the size of the sets, but merely in the way specific numbers can be written. There still is an infinity of them in each set.

Similarly are the counting methods irrelevant to the size of any other infinite set of numbers, aside from the countability of each of them by a method like the last. As can be subsets of sets in set theory, which are likewise held uncountable, any of the sets can be counted by, as in the last case, repeatedly exhausting, with all required additions, all digits from 0 through 9 where they occur.

The faultily thought sizes of inifinite sets gave rise to paradoxes in set theory itself. For their survey it will suffice that the paradoxes, known as Burali-Forti's and Cantor's, assert

> 9. The size of certain infinite sets is both largest and not largest of a kind.

However, by the size of something, by how large it is, is meant the measure of its complete extent in question, and since the infinite is meant not to reach completion,

> 9.i. An infinite set has no size.

Therefore, in another case in which neither affirmation nor denial holds,

> 9.ii. The size of an infinite set is neither larger nor not larger than another,

and 9 and the theses leading to it contradict 9.ii, as well as 9.i.

Although the infinite is never complete—so as to constitute a whole, all of an extent—language need not be so inflexible as not to permit reference to, for example, simply all numbers instead of all numbers that may be dealt with by man in the course of time. But the lack of completeness, of size, should nevertheless be kept in mind, for avoidance of more error than the preceding. With the preceding it is also argued that the whole is not necessarily greater than the part, contrary to longstanding acceptance. As reason it is stated that, for instance, the set of even and odd numbers combined is equal in size to the set of either of the two alone. The claim is based on shared infinity, despite the differences seen argued regarding its size. As infinities, however, cannot be unequal in size, possessing none, so can they not be equal. And when any portion of them, any size, is taken, becoming a whole, it is indeed greater than its part. It is so in fact by the meaning of part, as less than all, the reciprocal confirmed later.

A contradiction like the one between the infinite and the complete is also the cause of ancient paradoxes regarding infinitesimals, as set forth by Zeno of Elea. The most popular of them, the "Achilles", recounts

> 10. In a race between Achilles and a tortoise the tortoise has an early start. As a result Achilles, although much swifter, cannot overtake the tortoise, for when he reaches the place it held at the time of his start the tortoise will be at a farther place, and when he reaches that place the tortoise will be farther yet, and so forth.

In other words, supposing the distance covered by the tortoise discounted for both runners after Achilles starts, in order to reach the tortoise he must first cover an intermediate distance, then an intermediate distance of what is left, to continue the same without end. He accordingly would as suggested by another paradox of Zeno, the "race course", remain stationary altogether, since to reach any place he must reach an intermediate one, to be reached through an intermediate one etc., none of which would by the preceding be hence reached. The contentions were to sustain the thesis of Eleatic philosophers that there is no motion. "Motion" is a name for an experience, however, and therefore cannot be refuted.

In explaining the paradoxes it should be brought out that the distances spoken of are finite. It is not expected that the tortoise be overtaken by Achilles if it is infinitely far from him. No place can for that matter be at infinity, because by it is meant that it reaches beyond any place. The incongruities thus of course reside in inconsistency with experience, by which finite distances are traversed. Yet the assumption of infinite divisibility, or reducibility, of a finite extent, leading to the contradictions, is commonplace. That assumption, however, is not only inconsistent with experience, but with finitude itself.

As the opposite of the above meaning of infinity as never

complete, by the finitude of something is meant that it reaches completion. And by the infinite divisibility or reducibility of the finite is meant that beyond any part of it reached there is an infinity of other parts, that, in contradiction of the last sentence, completion is never reached.

Accordingly,

10.i. A finite distance is not infinitely reducible,

and in consequence

10.ii. Paradox 10 contradicts determination 10.i.

The virtually universal belief that a finite extent can diminish indefinitely can be once more attributed to the capacities of language. A fraction can in notation be continually decreased by increasing its denominator, as is ½ to ⅓. The availability of always enlarging a denominator or other number is a linguistic convention, but, despite the usefulness of setting no limit to the minimum or maximum sizes of quantities in mathematics, the language, as always, does not establish fact, and can contradict it.

The observation that there can be no endlessness to a finite extent nor an end to an infinite one has bearing on geometry, including the much disputed 5th postulate of Euclid, which resembles the Achilles paradox. Before proceeding to it and to those preceding it it will be well to consider certain basic concepts initially defined by him, some of which belong to entities held indefinable.

He has been held not to make use of his definitions of the last mentioned kind, but this will be seen not quite the case, even if the use was not explicit. What matters especially is that such definitions, as indicated, can be factors in deducing propositions in question.

Among the concepts presently at issue are point, line and surface. Euclid suggested that they can be extremities, and the words are indeed used for that, for limits, as connoted by surface. They are defined by him and generally understood as in effect lacking some customary dimension, some quantity by which they would be perceived independently, if only as concepts. It is hence no wonder that they are thought indefinable, and if without perceptual attributes in some connection, they would by the in the first chapter observed criteria not be concepts at all. But they are held to lack some dimension for good reason. They are used to mark the end of one thing and the beginning of another, often by choice without preexisting difference between the things, or with either thing possibly a void. They can thus be regarded not as independent entities, but as limits of things as determined by the adjoining of further things, either a possible void again.

The situation is peculiar as regards surface, however.

Although as surface it is not independent of the volume which it concerns, as perception it is independent, and in fact objects in the world are perceived by surfaces. For that reason, and because of the parts played in defining these three concepts, the usual order of defining them will be reversed, to begin with surface.

It is defined by Euclid as that which has length and breadth only. These attributes, however, imply the vertical and horizontal lines at right angles to each other by which something is held to be of two dimensions, and lines at these angles had not yet been defined. The like could be said if volume, a solid, were now defined by three dimensions. However, volume, depth in things, is detected without geometric knowledge of dimensions, as indicated when discussing matter in the last chapter (e.g. pp. 68, 69, last pars.). Acquaintance with things of volume is by such as diminishment of their parts through distance, and they can correspondingly be used in defining surface. In keeping with the above informal definition of limit, then,

a surface is a limit of a volume,

which, though considered only of the external world, can be conceptual. To proceed, in place of Euclid's definition of a line as breadthless length, i.e. as what has one dimension, it can be said that

a line is a limit of a surface.

And in place of his definition of a point as that which has no part it can be said that

a point is a limit of a line.

It can be seen that as used it is an error to regard points as constituents of lines, lines as constituents of surfaces, and surfaces as constitutents of space, as has become the practice. None of these presumed constituents have the required extent possessed by the things of which they are limits and of which they would be constituents. It may be added that, as an instance, the concept of line has been used to represent single extents such as of time. In that case, likewise, a point, as when marking on a clock the beginning or end of a period, is a limit of it and thus is not its component.

In continuing definitions in accord with what can be held understood meanings,

an angle is a shape formed by two lines meeting at a point and of a distance at next points.

Distance from a point is normally conceived as measured by the length of a straight line, so that if the line starting at that point is rotated all around it, the path described by the other end marks all those distances from the point. But should the straight line, not yet defined and perhaps bending, if prolonged describe a path inside the first, the new path would be held to be nearer the starting point, not farther. Hence distance from a point, a center, can more generally be defined by the circular or spherical path described by a point on any ideally constant shape, as might be a compass, rotated at another point of it around that center. Since any constant shape can describe those paths, it will also be more fitting to soon define a circle and sphere themselves by way of that general shape rather than, as done by Euclid, a straight line.

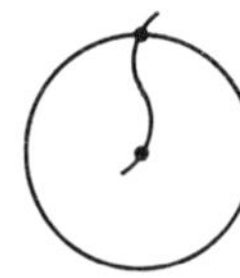

But particular angles above are distinguished by more than accordingly determined distances between points on the meeting lines. Most angles have a reflex angle, a certain larger space on one side of the angle than on the opposite side. The difference is measured by the sum of uniform smaller angles, degrees, between the two lines on a side. It is similar to the rotation above and thought of again in terms of straight lines, as well as planes. The last entity also not yet defined, a more general conception than usual is again suitable.

A plane, as a surface that may not be seen frontally, is part of the concept of three dimensions, although it is regarded as of two dimensions technically. That it is so regarded is understood by considering that an individual perception, as through one eye at one moment, does not determine depth. It only has the semblance of what is held to be a flat picture, although like it it may display such as perspective. A single perception, viewpoint, is thus the basis of area relationships assigned to flat surfaces, to planes, in space. A circle on a plane, as often noted, is seen at best as an ellipse if not frontally viewed. Accordingly those relationships stricly hold in accordance with a viewpoint, not a plane. To go farther, most standard geometric concepts, as suggested when speaking of motion in a straight line (p.84 last par.), are ideal, it being unlikely to find in nature a true circle, square, or the plane in which these are to lie. These concepts are thus authentically conceptual, and the described viewpoint for those in a plane concerns the mere form of their conception. In asserting things that would take place in a plane, it is hence, as frequent, not required to speak of it, the assertions alone of those things informing of conceptions more precise than seen in an actual plane, assuming it possible. In this vein and in accord with the preceding it can be stated that

a circle is a closed line with every part equidistant from a point within,

the definition informing of the conceptual relations without reference to a plane. On what would be held an actual flat surface a figure would be a circle if by suitable measures it compared with that conception.

In consonance with these observations, when speaking of degrees as marking the size of angles, the conception does likewise not require a plane. Nor does it here require straight lines. Similarly to distance, degrees can be conceived through rotation of any constant line about a point on it, and they become uniform by conceiving equal distances between stages of a next point on the line. The distances or degrees are by a later equality principle the same at all other points as well, since there is by postulate no differentiation.

The next definition can be accordingly that

a straight line is a line with angles at every point equal on all sides.

By all sides is meant, conceiving the line to be in a world of depth, the sides of the line from each viewpoint as explained.

This meaning of straight line, in concord with its common understanding as not deviating on any side, has vaguely been shared by science. When the horizon, as demarcated by the ocean for example, was found to represent the curvature of the earth, it was inferred not to be straight, rather than holding a straight line to be curved. Yet there has been an inclination to redefine a straight line in view of physical phenomena, such as the path of light. A straight line is sometimes thought of as the shortest distance between two points, and an interpretation offered of this distance is that it is the shortest route by which two points in nature can in some manner be connected. The path of light in a vacuum would accordingly be regarded as straight although due to gravitation it should curve near a massive body like the earth. Or travel on a globe like the earth would be seen as straight if along a great circle, around the center of the globe. But these curvatures vary, and it can be asked what amount of curvature should serve as standard of straightness. A more general flaw is the attempt to make a deductive science dependent on physical observation. Such a science is, as was indicated, built on what follows from general concepts of so-called all possible worlds, independently of the things in nature to which the results are applied, and therefore to seek in nature answers to the questions is misdirected.

Doing so can be viewed as a form of spoken of bypassing the mental and focusing on the material (e.g. p.2 second par.), as can be the opposite tendency by which a straight line, called only a line, is alongside other words left undefined, seeing the word only as a physical utterance. In continued physicality and conformity with a previous comment straight lines, together with points and planes, are also though invisible held to in infinite number be components of actual space, and straight lines, planes, as well as space to stretch into infinity all around.

The unserviceability of meaningless words was pointed out, and so was the nonexistence, conceptual or real, of invisible things, things without perceptual attributes. As regards the infinite number of those points, lines and planes, it is partly meant present in the infinitesimal direction, in which it was seen impossible even if the entities existed as proposed. Regarding the infinite extent of the lines, planes and space, i.e. volume, these entities are usually in concept, let alone in reality, considered as of finite extent, and therefore they and others are as common meant here to be of some particular size.

Concerning any meaning the question can be raised whether the entity defined is possible, and as made clear in the foregoing the issue here is conceivability, not actual existence. With regard to the first four italicized definitions (p.124), of point, any line, surface, and angle by not necessarily straight lines, the referents can be discerned in nature. But straight lines in nature, as seen, are queried, and circles were likewise noted as ideal (defs. pp.125,126). However, as to the conceivable, although like the physically possible likewise not required if it serves the deductive purposes, the field is much more open. Aside from the logically required, mentioned unconceivable otherwise, it admits of the numberless products of fancy man is capable of. More specifically and to the point, one can by whichever perceiving faculty conceive next to any of its elemental objects any other. It is the conceptually extrinsic compared to the intrinsic, the latter governed by logical requirements, but the former not even by the restrictions imposed in the world by laws of nature. The visual or tactile faculties, not referring now to the senses but their mental counterparts, in addition allow these conceptions all around the elemental objects, in what are known as two and three dimensions.

Accordingly, a circle is possible, because one can conceive a constant shape continuously turned all around a point.

And considering that

a sphere is a closed surface with every part equidistant from a point within,

it is possible on the same ground.

Correspondingly a straight line is possible, because one can conceive an element of a line at equal angles to a next one on all sides. The possibility is more fully elucidated through the meaning of equal angles as their coinciding if appropriately superposed. Accordingly when from a viewpoint the opposing angles of a line are unequal then if superposed at one arm of each, both angles on the same side, the other arms part. But since they can rotate continuously, they can close that distance. Namely the angles can be equal. And they can be so from each viewpoint, because each is distinct. The angles of a line can further be equal on all sides at each point, since one can by the preceding conceive at each the same.

Considering further that

a plane is a surface with angles at every point equal on each side,

the viewpoints meant to be ones seeing the surface as a line dividing two sides, a plane is possible because one can conceive an element of a surface at equal angles to a next one on both sides and from all viewpoints, and one can conceive the same at any point.

The angle of a straight line or plane is called a straight angle, and by definition

a right angle is half a straight angle.

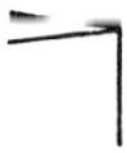

Its possibility should in the light of the preceding be manifest and not necessary to substantiate here, the present depiction of superposed vertical arms of unequal angles, the angles combined equaling a straight angle, viewable if wished like the previous one as closing the other arms.

But Euclid's first three postulates likewise have to do with possibility, in effect asserting it of certain things, and hence warrant examination. They state

1. *To draw a straight line from any point to any point,*
2. *To prolong a finite straight line continuously,*

and

3. *To describe a circle with any center and distance.*

Beginning with postulate 3, the distance can be taken to be any separation, however determined, of the center from the point from which the circle is to be described, and by the above the point can be conceived to rotate all around the center. Therefore the circle is possible.

The postulate may also be understood to say that a circle, or a sphere, can expand indefinitely, viz that the line or surface describing them will upon going beyond previous ones not somehow return to them. This is questioned with regard to a cosmological model of the universe as spherical, by which it has no boundary not exceedable, but by which there is an eventual return to a former one.

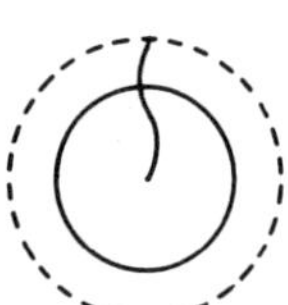

That one can conceive outside a circle or sphere a further point, and thence describe another circle or sphere around the center by a constant shape, was decided by what went before. And as before, because all stages of the rotation are undifferentiated by postulate, the new circle or sphere extends past the old one throughout, i.e. it does not return.

It may be remarked that the return has been held possible for such as a circle on a sphere or cylinder. But these surfaces are not planes, represented by viewpoints as described. An expanding circle on a transparent cylinder may from a viewpoint appear as pictured at right, to eventually in parts return to itself. The expansion in those parts does not signify extension past the previous circle, however, those parts not lying outside the circle. It is conceivability—and accordingly absence of a contradictory return—of extension outside a circle, and correspondingly a sphere, that was noted in the preceding.

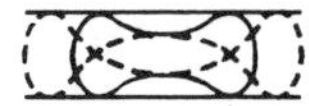

That the continued straight line of postulate 2 is possible should be likewise evident from what was said on the possibility of a straight line and before. But the postulate is similarly to the third one sometimes understood to say that a straight line can extend indefinitely without returning to a previous part, as is likewise questioned.

In answer it will help to conceive an initial part of a straight line to rotate around its starting point, describing a sphere by the other end. Let some initial extension of the line fall on or inside the sphere. This can be conceived from a viewpoint by which the extension is on one side of the starting line. It cannot lie on that line, by the meaning of extension, and it cannot also be on the other side. The two sides are by the foregoing different meant areas, places, divided by the starting line, with difference of things in perception synonymous with difference of place. Accordingly if an extension were also on the other side, not being of the same place it would not be the same one. But with the first extension on one side and not the other, there is a differentiation. Should an extension continue in a straight line, however, there would be no differentiation between the sides. Hence the extension, not falling on or inside the sphere, must by mentioned principle (p.109, end of third par.) continue outside the sphere. Further, upon describing there another sphere, an extension will continue outside it as well. Therefore since by the last postulate expanded spheres do not return to former ones, a straight line extended will neither and will not return to a previous part.

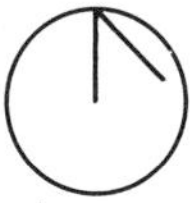

It is by the preceding not surprising that straight lines can measure distance. And if postulate 1 is right then the measure can be applied anywhere.

By the reasoning for the second and third postulates a straight line, beside its rotation all around any starting point, allows extension to the next distance beyond the sphere described, with like rotation there, and so on. Therefore, filling all volume concurrently with the spheres, it can reach any point, and the line of the first postulate is possible.

The postulate succeeding those listed is

4. *All right angles are equal,*

and it follows quickly from the definition of straight line (p.126). Inasmuch as a straight line has at any point equal angles on all sides, and there is no differentiation among parts of the same or different straight lines, all their angles are equal, i.e. all have the same number of degrees. And since right angles are half those angles, they all have half that number of degrees and therefore are equal.

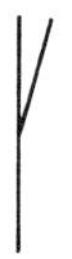

The lack of differentiation in angles of different straight lines can again be illustrated by superposition. If upon a straight line is placed a line of some angle with one arm coinciding with one of the straight angle, and the other arms part, then the second line is not straight, since on the parting side its angle is by that amount larger and on the other side smaller than the straight angle. Therefore another straight line must coincide with the first, their angles equal. The equality of right angles can evidently be illustrated similarly. If on assuming a line dividing a straight angle into two right angles another line starting at the same point of the straight angle extends on the same side of it as the dividing line while not coinciding with it, it will again make different angles with the straight angle. To make equal ones as right angles it must hence coincide with that dividing line, making all right angles equal.

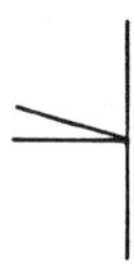

Such equalities are in geometry today often called congruences, and they evidently do not concern selfsameness, but a sameness of things as compared to each other. Both concepts, of selfsameness and of sameness by comparison, apply also to the nondifferentiation spoken of, as, in the first case, to sameness of a line rotating about a point, and, in the second case, to sameness of the angles of straight lines. Selfsameness should need little say here, since simply characterized by the postulated entity. But the other sameness, congruence, requires an added criterion mentioned, by which forms not only have a resemblance, but are held identical. The identity is known to be decided by upon placing one thing appropriately onto another the concerned things coincide.

Notwithstanding that congruence is meant to be in geometry decided by such superposition, it is inconsistently objected that Euclid cannot make certain of it for proving a proposition. It is maintained that in the process of applying one shape to another it may change. The shapes, however, are meant to stay constant by postulate, the process of superposition again ideal. In nature it is no more likely that shapes may not stay the same than that their coinciding may not be made certain. Similar comments are made on propositions in Euclid that speak of ways of construction. They are taken to involve the use of tools, although they can like other proofs be understood as of what follows from given assumptions.

Proposition 2 thus informs how given a certain straight line, separate point, and other geometric assumptions, a straight line equal to the first and starting from that point will follow. It has been argued that a tool like a compass, presumed to be used in other parts of the construction, could be used instead of the geometric reasoning to transfer the line. But it is not tools that are at issue, but what is deductively implied by what. However, the transfer of that line from one place to another could well be merely assumed, as was its rotation to describe a circle in the same demonstration.

And Proposition 4 asserts what will result if two straight lines forming an angle are superposed on an equal, congruent, shape. The objection was that the shapes may change during the procedure, and, as observed, they would by postulate remain the same. There is no need, furthermore, for superposition, since they, as noted, would by definition of the equality or congruence coincide, which is in question. Merely results of the coincidence are needed.

A result stated in the proposition is that since the end points of the two angles would coincide, so would respective straight lines joining those points. In support it is argued that if these lines do not coincide then, impossibly, two straight lines enclose a space.

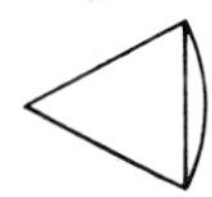

It should be observed that the two lines, as well as the resulting triangles and their angles as also stated, will coincide merely because the shapes are as before undifferentiated. Could two straight lines enclose a space, they might do it with each of the angles. That they cannot is with the proposition informally supposed, and it will now briefly be proven for present purposes.

Let two lines at least one of which is straight enclose a space, and let with one of the meeting points as center be with the other described an arc of a circle. Then the straight line forms equal angles with the arc on both sides, because there is again no difference between them. But the other line does not form equal angles with the arc there, because the enclosed space is added on one side and subtracted on the other. Therefore it cannot be straight, and two straight lines cannot enclose a space.

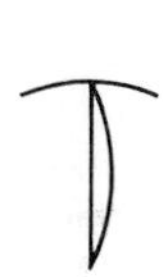

Coming to the mentioned fifth postulate, the last, it in correspondence with the diagram at right states

5. *If a straight line* (horizontal) *crossing two straight lines* (slopes) *makes the interior angles* (a, b) *on its one side less than two right angles, then the two lines, if prolonged indefinitely, meet on that side.*

A recent modification also asserts, as does a Euclid proposition, that if the sum of those angles equals two right angles, then the two lines do not meet on either side, they are parallel. It may be added that the lines lie on the same plane or, in accord with what was said, are seen from a single viewpoint. The original postulate will be proved at present.

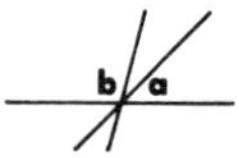

If the distance between the slopes is reduced to zero on the horizontal, they interchange above it their left and right placements. For since *a* and *b* equal less than two right angles, and either, since on the horizontal, equals with the, exterior, angle on the other side of its slope two right angles, *a* e.g. is smaller than that exterior angle of the other slope. Hence that slope, both these angles being on the right side of their slopes, extends now on the left side of the slope of *a*, the side opposite the previous one, and the slopes do not meet again if not to enclose a space. Let the slopes gradually return, to again be distanced at the horizontal, interchanging placements in conformance with the postulate. They cannot pass each other all at once, namely coincide at one stage, since contradicting the less than two right angles; since the angles concerned are on opposing sides of the slopes, they would through the coinciding equal two right angles. And should the slopes pass each other not all at once but still at multiple points, they could not both be straight; either because, if coinciding between those points, they part elsewhere to differ in angles at the point of parting, or because, if not coinciding, they enclose a space. Hence the slopes pass each other at only one point at a time. But since they can be prolonged indefinitely on the side previous to passing, there always remain points not passed. In consequence wherever on the horizontal, the slopes cross each other and therefore meet.

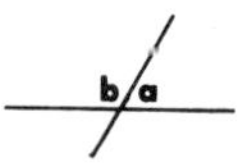

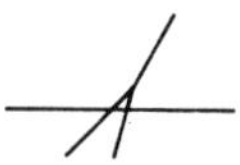

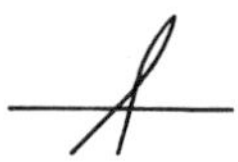

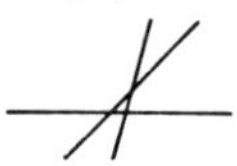

The postulate resembles the Achilles paradox (p.122) by the through the prolongation approaching of one slope by the other, indicating that a finite distance does not take infinity to be traversed, as do the points beyond any one passed indicate that an infinite line cannot come to a finish. These issues do not come into account in the mentioned addition to the postulate, when *a* and *b* equal two right angles. That here the slopes do not meet is proved as follows.

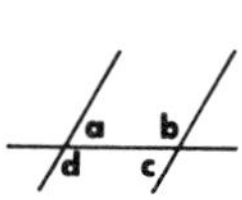

By a method of Euclid angles *c* and *d* in the diagram at left are found to equal *a* and *b* respectively. Since *a* and *d*, like *a* and *b*, equal two right angles, *b* and *d* are, on subtracting *a* from each pair, found equal. The same holds for *a* and *c*, on subtracting *b*, and hence the lower slopes are but the upper slopes turned about. If two such once more undifferentiated lines meet in one direction they meet in the other, enclosing a space. Since the present lines are straight, they cannot enclose a space and therefore do not meet.

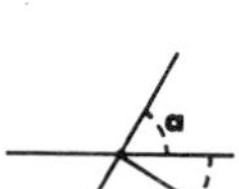

To find e.g. *a* and *d* to equal two right angles Euclid assumed a further line, at right angles to the slope and dividing *d* into two angles. He then observed those two angles combined to equal *d*, and the one of them next to *a* to equal with it a right angle, drawing via additional steps the conclusion, that *a* and *d* equal two right angles. But the premises of the lengthy proof use the sort of evidence that can be used directly. Instead of finding that a right and other angle total *d*, or that a right angle is totaled by the other and *a*, one can find at once that *a* and *d* total the straight angle of the slope, its two right angles, it being exactly that straight angle which *a* and *d* were meant to fill. Also of note is that to know that an angle divided by a line into two angles equals their sum makes alluded to tacit use of defining a line as without breadth, and the like applies to other meanings.

Meanings play instead a misleading part in non-Euclidean geometry, founded on the rejection of the just proven fifth postulate or its companion. These are replaced by postulates on which are built new geometries, which correspondingly, while thought to be consistent, engage in contradiction.

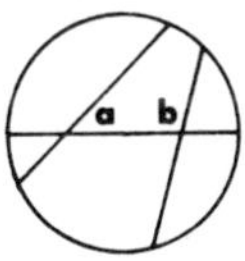

In the geometry known as hyperbolic is posited together with the lines of the fifth postulate (p. 131) a line or circle at infinity. If *a* and *b*, though less than two right angles, are sufficiently large, it is then maintained, the two lines in question, the present slopes, do not meet. As expounded, however, no limiting line can be imposed on an infinite extent without contradiction.

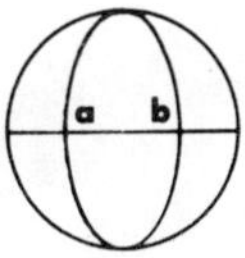

In the geometry known as elliptic a spherical surface is assumed for the proposition in which *a* and *b* are right angles, if not merely equaling two (facing p.). If the horizontal line is conceived as the equator and the intersecting lines as meridians, then the last two meet at the poles. However, the surface is not a plane and the lines accordingly not straight, contradicting preconditions.

It is argued in defense that certain terms must be suitably redefined. It should be reiterated, however, that different definitions do not escape problems of the content behind. The infinite or the straight may be given other definitions, but it can still be asked whether a proposition holds under the previous ones.

The last two geometries are held to be as consistent as the first, because if the original meaning of their terms is retained, e.g. if a curved line is after all not considered straight, then non-Euclidean theorems are found part of Euclidean ones. In that case the assumed conditions considered in the older geometry are not contradicted, but neither are its in the new ones intended to be denied postulates, for the very reason that the new geometries become part of the older. There appears indeed another paradox, wherein, through again conflicting use of language, non-Euclidean geometry is at once in discord and concord with Euclidean.

A more general error is to suppose that if upon appropriately interpreting the language of a deductive system its propositions are consistent then so is the system. As observed, initial terms are often left undefined, and the validity of the system is tested by thus defining them. The terms could be defined in contradictory ways, however. The validity would hence be guaranteed only for a qualifying interpretation, not for the system.

That the validity of a deductive science be held dependent on its consistency can be attributed to the longstanding notion that those statements are deductively true whose denial is a contradiction. But a denial of any fact, including worldly ones, is merely false, not a contradiction, which has to do with opposition in statements, and a fact, e.g. a logical one, still must be established to determine its denial false. The supposed contradiction in the denial of a deduction is further confounded with its consistency whereby no, internal, contradiction is derived through it. Contradiction is of course one of the things barred by logical law, but there are other requisites. A conclusion may not follow for other reasons than that it harbors a contradiction. For instance in mentioned affirmation of the consequent (p.77 third par.) it does not follow that if *A* implies *B* then *B* implies *A*, but although such an inference would be invalid, it would not be a contradiction. I.e. mere consistency, noncontradiction, is not the test of validity. Contradictory results were in paradoxes in fact seen possible through correct inference, their cause lying in some premise. Accordingly consistency rather than being the test of validity of a deductive science, is a test of, possibly nondeductive, consistent premises from which conclusions are through the science derived.

Furthermore emphasis on the, rightly or wrongly found, validity of a system of e.g. geometry, to the dismissal of its particular content and accordingly the truth or falsity of its postulates, merely upholds deductive ways, logical principles, not geometric or other more particular truths. Since the last are in those cases the interest, the postulates should be known true, so that what is inferred be also, and to make the postulates and the rest certain, knowledge of the meaning of the language was observed required. It was also pointed out that both, defining the words and ascertaining the basic theorems is possible. Some of this was done in the preceding regarding geometry, and more general, logical, factors admitting of the same were part.

Section 2
LAWS OF THOUGHT OR OF COMPLEMENTS

The three so-called laws of thought, taken into account severally in what has preceded, are traditionally regarded as fundamental to all logic. They have in recent times been often criticized, sometimes justifiably, but have nonetheless been adhered to, since inseparable from reasoning.

They have been believed indemonstrable, and in accordance with what was said, they are to be here demonstrated, insofar as valid principles. Their formulation is frequent in terms of propositions, such as

LAW OF CONTRADICTION. *A proposition is not both true and false.*

LAW OF EXCLUDED MIDDLE. *A proposition is either true or false.*

LAW OF IDENTITY. *A proposition implies itself.*

Propositions, especially as associated with statements, were observed herein as doubtful objects of logical investigation. A statement may not inform of anything, contrary to the expected. Or, by speaking of a proposition as true or false, no distinction is made between it as a whole and what is predicated of the subject, a distinction that will matter. But even if what is referred to is clarified, by speaking of propositions or statements the inquiry is distracted from its object. Since it is their truth or falsity that is of interest, that is to say broadly facts or realities, realities in question can be referred to directly.

Standard logic does make a distinction between whole propositions and what is predicated of things in them, there being a distinction made between propositional and predicate logics. A similar distinction will be made at present, but in conformance with the preceding it will be about fact or reality, or the absence of the same. As regards predicates, it correspondingly will be about facts of particular attributes or lack of them of things, and as regards propositions, of pertinent existence or nonexistence of things altogether. The truth or falsity of a proposition as a whole, concerning a state, is thus an instance of the existence or non-existence altogether of a thing, the state, as adumbrated earlier (p.45 third par.). The appropriate study about existence can accordingly be named *existential logic,* and the like study about attributes *attributive logic.*

This division can begin with the laws of thought, and related mathematical principles can be adjoined. The adjoining is fitting here because these principles are equally about basic complements, and there are comparable analogies later.

The complemental character is not present in the law of identity, which, however, need not be considered a law, because it consists in obvious redundancy. It is given also, more in keeping with the emphasis herein on things instead of propositions, in a form like

A *equals* A,

noted early (p. 17 second par.) to be found uninformative, while held on to as a law. Whether expressed through implication, when the inferred may be anything associated within given bounds with the inferred from, or through a form in which the inferred is something the inferred from is, the contended law repeats that, granted that what is considered is a certain thing, it is the thing.

It has been maintained that the same takes place in all of logic and mathematics, that all of it consists of tautologies, as mentioned in the Introduction (p. 2 first par.). That it does not was explicated there (p. 2 fifth par.) and is recognized in finding "*A* equals *B*," where things though logically equal are not spoken of alike, informative, as, with the opposite on above displayed "*A* equals *A*", likewise noted early. As mentioned also, it has been argued that deductive principles are true by virtue of definition, and that they are tautologies for that reason. The view is aided by the almost sole reliance for proof of logical theorems on mentioned truth tables. The tables do in fact depend on definitions and can be said to for the most part repeat them. As indicated, however (p. 108 fifth through seventh pars.), they will be seen not to be relied on. Of relevance in point of fact is not whether a principle is true by virtue of definition, but whether it is an inference, deriving, perhaps merely as a name, something not posited before, unlike done in the law of identity, which circularly repeats the premised in the concluded.

In discourse all things are substantiated by virtue of, beside else, definition, meaning, because the things are substantiated of whatever is meant by the words used, hence relying on the definitions. But once it is known what is meant, how it is defined, anything else known or established about it is not of that definition. Furthermore, even if the premises, things known, are true as a matter of definition, conclusions can be drawn not previously recognized. Mathematical learning in general can, in fact, be said to result from definitions.

As an example can serve a proof that 2 + 2 equals 4. Proof of such basic equalities—ones involving single digits and that are, as in the process of addition, assumed true—has been evading detection, in further instance of how hidden premises, here definitions again, can prevent solutions. At present the first definition is

i. 2 equals 1 + 1.

Hence

ii. 2 + 2 equals 2 + 1 + 1.

The next definition is

iii. 3 equals 2 + 1.

Hence and by ii

iv. 2 + 2 equals 3 + 1.

And the last definition is

v. 4 equals 3 + 1.

Therefore and by iv

vi. 2 + 2 equals 4.

The proof also conforms to later equality principles, and what matters now is that although the basic premises here are definitions, the conclusion, with the other inferences, supplies new information. In this case the information was likely acquired already, although one may be hard pressed to say how, but the same does not, of course, hold for more complex equations. What happens is that when considering something, one may not be conscious of all that one, perhaps by definition, knows about it. When considering 2 + 2, one may not be conscious of definition i, only after recalling it to infer ii, and when considering ii, one may not be conscious of definition iii, to infer iv, and so forth. This act of inference illustrates mentioned (p. 18 first par.) drawing upon two senses of meaning, one as attributes in consciousness, and one as attributes that define. And while in this process what is known and deduced seem, as in mathematics, to be mainly diverse wordings for the same things, other things known to be true under those names can be connected. By the above example two children can divide four pieces of sweets equally. That the mathematical deductions only inform of other wordings is accordingly likewise not the case. That 2 + 2 equals 4 informs that one amount of 2, however named, added to another of the same equals an amount of differently known 4, however named.

Ironically, while it is maintained that logical and mathematical principles are true by definition, they are at times unduly proclaimed not to be. Whereas above definitions of particular numbers might not be disputed, it is denied that certain axioms accepted about in general, natural, numbers define them. The axioms state

1. *0 is a number,*
2. *The successor of any number is a number,*
3. *No two numbers have the same successor,*

and

4. *0 is not the successor of any number.*

All numbers but 0 are also, it was failed to be stated, meant to be successors.

Granting that 0 is a number, a definition in consonance with common understanding can, however, be that

a number is, on starting with 0, any quantity counted by successively adding a new unit.

Should 0 not be conceded, the starting number can be 1. Conjointly with the definition numbers are thus said by axiom 1 to include 0, by 2 to include any added unit, by 3 to be new in counting, and by 4 to start with 0. The forgotten axiom, that all numbers but 0 are successors, is in the definition, since definitions are identities.

The axioms are thought not to implicitly define number because, in likeness to non-Euclidean geometry (ca. p. 133), they are held to admit of other interpretation. They can by changing meanings of words in them, it is found, apply to other things. To repeat, however, by redefining words one does not speak of the same things, even if the changed meanings, as in the present case, are merely broader ones. Then spoken of are the things thus referred to, not specifically the others, as in the above definition, which holds of all and only what is here meant by numbers.

In additional irony, a last axiom, though unknown to most who think with numbers, has been held to define them. Known as the axiom of mathematical induction, it states

5. *If 0 has a property, and the successor of any number that has it also has it, then all numbers have it.*

The axiom can as a matter of fact be simply deduced from the others, viz from a usual meaning of number. By it and the if clauses of the axiom, since 0 has the property, 1 has it, hence 2 has it, and so forth for all numbers.

As expounded early herein, something can be technically defined by anything true of, and only of, it. For instance the last above axiom might define number if it meets those conditions. However, aside from the axiom having to be confirmed, that is it could not be used as definition until proven, of interest in general is, rather than all that may define something, how it is initially conceived. This initial character of the concept is normally meant to define the thing, with other attributes findings. And the question at this time is how are the findings made when intrinsic, deductive.

And as indicated at the beginning of this chapter, deductive findings to be made, if certainty be attained, are requisite in places unsuspected. To wit, whenever one thing is said to follow from another, one is justified to ask for the reason. This does not obtain, naturally, if the same thing is in consciousness in each case, even though put in different language. Then the same thing is, circularly, expressed, rather than something yet to become of awareness. But otherwise, even if the deduced, the new in awareness, is a name, the question is why the deduction.

A bit more on the meaning of consciousness and awareness. The words are presently used somewhat freely, their intended sense doubtless evident from the context. Earlier in a strict sense things were meant to be sometimes of consciousness but not awareness. They are the things that though part of conceptions, need be inferred. When now speaking of things already in consciousness, meant are evidently things in conscious awareness, in thought and not needing to be deduced.

What matters at this point is that when it is said that one thing follows from another, there should be a reason why the other, differing from the first, can be inferred, in agreement with the need for finding that something is the case (e.g. p. 26 last par.). And it will not do to state a further, likewise differing, ground. There should be a reason why the conclusion follows from this premise, and if a further one is offered, there should be a reason for the inference from it, and so on. A like need was recognized by the 19th-century author Lewis Carroll, and it is in accordance with it believed that any statement that, as may a logical principle, licenses a conclusion cannot be considered a premise. But what a premise is is again of choice of definition, and if the principle have another name, the need to see why the conclusion follows remains.

This need appears as mentioned strange as regards the very inference of instances from logical or other principles. In accord with the above, at issue are principles regarding which, as loosely the definition "3 + 1 equals 4", instances of the subject, e.g. broadly "2 + 2", are not in consciousness, and therefore a reason is wanting for the deduction, e.g. "2 + 2 equals 4". And the situation in practice always applies, because the instances, far from merely not in thought as part of the principles, appeal to them for the answers.

Accordingly in seeing what deduction consists in, it is not enough to determine the basic principles, all else decided by complying with them. There might be forms of deduction holding only for things more particular than the general ones of logic, or mathematics, but, especially, the principles do not take care of, as seen, the preponderant deductions from the general, including those principles, to the particular, the procedure by which deduction was noted distinguished often from induction, inference from the particular to the general.

To in keeping with previous observations accordingly say that all things deduced must be appropriately perceived to follow is to oddly equally assert a principle. A reason can still be required why as a result a deduction must be so perceived to follow in a particular case. Fortunately or not, ascertained deductions of cases from principles are constantly made regardlessly, and they are founded on the same kind of to be demonstrated conceptualization as are deductive principles.

The demonstration would be awkward if the reader were asked to envision the concepts concerned, so as to mentally observe the results. It is advisable therefore to put the concepts in physical form, in which as diagrams similar substantiations were submitted by men in the past.

Largely known as Euler diagrams, after the fecund 18th-century mathematician, the forms were used to verify Aristotle's syllogisms, but, misapplied and seemingly confined in use, they gave little assurance. They are as much as looked upon with disdain, for which both rationalism and empiricism may offer cause. The one because the use of diagrams seems to diminish the prowess of reason, somehow thought to function without conceptualization, and the other because they are at odds with the conviction that the only principles not tautologies are laws of nature. They are thus used at best for confirming some theorems in a schoolboy environment, without recognition that confirmation is tantamount to proof, as noted in the introduction. In consequence of these, deductive truths remain undemonstrated.

In keeping with the expounded, in order to demonstrate them they must be observed with regard to the concepts concerned, and in physical proof the simplest form, as offered by diagrams, is welcome. They are hence made use of here to that end, and it may only be added that they are representations, with the rest supplied by the imagination.

How an instance is deduced from a principle, a process explained to require the same perceptual validation as do principles, is represented in Figure III. In it all things *B* (small circle) belong to things C (large circle). Thus, being a C can be viewed as a principle regarding every *B*, since a principle is meant to be about all of something (*B*) as a thing (C) of which something is true. And *A* (dot) is a *B*. Therefore, as disclosed by the figure, *A*, also, is a C, a thing of which what is at issue is

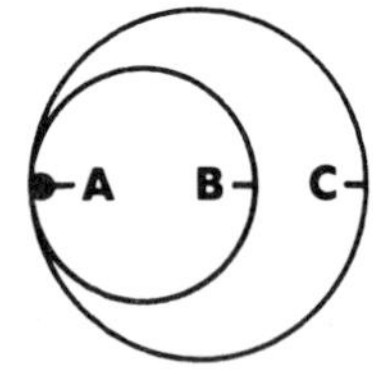

FIGURE III

true. It is easily visualized that the like obtains in the case of identities of *A* with *B*, or *B* with *C*, as exemplified by the earlier numerical equations.

The peculiarity that deduction from a rule calls for the same ascertainment the rule does has bearing on the mentioned syllogism "All men are mortal; Socrates is a man; therefore Socrates is mortal". This inference of an instance, the conclusion, from a rule, the first premise, is in its entirety often furnished as an instance of a syllogistic rule prescribing the inference. And as should be clear now, applying the syllogistic rule calls for the same kind of mental act as applying the rule stated by the first premise.

The former is in fact much more complex. Instead of the "*B* is C" that can symbolize that premise as a principle, the general syllogism as a principle is symbolized by "If *A* is *B*, and *B* is C, then *A* is C". In the simpler case, in accord with Figure III, Socrates (*A*) need by being a man (*B*) merely be perceived as mortal (C) without more specifics. But as to the logical principle, parts of the two Socrates premises (the two now the figure's *A*) must first be perceived as cases of the principle's *A*, *B* and C in the two assumed relations (the two the figure's *B*), thereafter perceiving that another such relation is implied of certain of these cases (the implied belonging to the figure's C), whereupon that relation is concluded to hold. The added conclusion, saying that Socrates is mortal, is needed because, unlike before, it is separate from in the figure the connection of *A* with C. If it is yet considered that the logical law yielding an instance by such complication is a rather ordinary one, it will be appreciated that, as indicated, proof of basic logical laws can be simpler than proof of instances from them.

With these observations the two laws of thought, those not of discussed redundancy, can again be turned to. But their from the onset misleading titles as of contradiction and excluded middle are still less suitable presently.

The first law is regarded with some justification as misnamed, because it, rather than requiring contradiction, excludes it. The second law is also known as of excluded third and contrariwise requires, instead of what it says, inclusion. Its generalized meaning is that

At least one, A *or* not-A.

It does not exclude the third possibility that both be the case, done by the other law by asserting that

Not both, A *and* not-A.

In addition, because the two laws, mentioned as of basic complements, will be formulated here for, beside the described existential and attributive logics, mathematics, they will be about more than two alternatives and their contradiction. But they retain the concepts of inclusion and exclusion and can in their several versions therefore be called *laws of inclusion* and *laws of exclusion*.

Taking the traditional laws of thought for existential logic then, the law of exclusion is

THEOREM III.1.i. *A thing does not both exist and not exist at the same time.*

Proof. In Figure III.1 the circle stands for the times a thing *A* exists, the existence signified by the letter alone. All other area stands for other times, not those when *A* exists, signified by *'(A)*. The meaning of "other area" and correspondingly "other times" and "not those" can be held ostensive (p.102 third par.) in the figure. And by times when *A* does as straight negation of existence not exist, signified by *'A*, are meant not those when it exists. As disclosed by the figure, therefore, not both *A* and *'A* are the case at the same time, proving the theorem.

The distinction between *'A* and *'(A)*, which may be read *"non-A"* and *"not A"*, is made because, as was suggested (p.135 third par.), what is denied of something directly, as in "when *A* does not exist", need not be what is denied indirectly, as in "not when *A* exists". Parentheses are familiar as demarcators, and the apostrophy, often used for omission, offers a compact negation sign placed, as in speech, before its object. It should also be observed that "when" and "time", as well as "existence", are used here extremely broadly. The when or time need not be temporal only, but can also pertain to a particular place; in that case the theorem means that a thing cannot occur and not occur at the same time and place in usually nature, the figure then depicting places at one time. Differently and more generally, the meaning of place can be extended from part of a momentary perception to one of a continuity of them, as understood to occur in time and expressed when saying that something takes place; the theorem means accordingly that a thing cannot be and not be of the same place in perception, be the place part of a momentary perception or a continuity of them, the figure then depicting places thus extended into

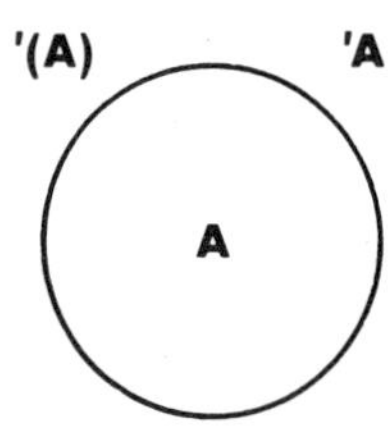

FIGURE III.1

perceptions through time. Existence can consequently likewise be either about presence in the world sometime perceived, or presence anywhere in consciousness, in which case *A* can for instance mean the existence of a logical principle, its place everywhere, and *'A* the nonexistence, its place nowhere, or the opposite. In short, concerned is any sort of being, in any territory.

It has been said that the dividing line between affirmation and denial is not as definite, that sometimes both may apply, that there may be an intermediate area where they overlap. Considering not only existence but anything that may be true about a thing, it might be said that a zebra is both white and not white. What delimits a given thing is, however, again a matter of definition, meaning. For instance something may be meant to be white if more than 50% of its surface is, otherwise not, and it cannot then be both. A meaning of yes and no by which no is not the complete absence of yes, as would black stripes not be absent on a zebra, is not one here considered. By the present meaning if it is too difficult to know that e.g. a zebra is over 50% white, then whether it accordingly is white or not is unknown, but only one alternative is true.

The law of inclusion which is companion to the preceding is

THEOREM III.1.ii. *A thing either exists or does not exist at any time.*

Proof. As disclosed in Figure III.1, either *A* or *'A* is the case at any time, proving the theorem.

It should apart from again the preceding broad application of the diagram be noted that, in keeping with the remark (p.140 fourth par.) that the diagrams only represent, the line describing the circle is of course meant to lack breadth, one that might be taken as a place of neither *A* nor *'A*. Any place, even a limit if wished, other than of *A* is, to repeat, meant to be of *'A*.

The preceding two theorems can also be expressed as certain implications between the states of *A*. As will be seen, for logical purposes all propositions can be put in a comparable form, as indicated by past observations that all states concern something associated with something else.

The general forms, not necessarily speaking of *A* with *'A*, used above for the theorems would be "Not both, *A* and *B*" and "At least one, *A* or *B*", similarly to the laws as displayed generalized before (p.141). These forms are held to be respectively equivalent to "*A* implies *not-B*, and *B* implies *not-A*" and "*Not-A* implies *B*, and *not-B* implies *A*", and they can be seen to be so by their meaning. For the concept behind "not both" can be held to be "To find one is not to find the other", and the concept behind "or" "Not to find one is to find the other". Correspondingly the theorems can have the form

'A *is equivalent to* '(A)

and

A *is equivalent to* '('A).

Equivalence is regarded as the same as mutual implication, which sameness will by a certain meaning be found an inference.

The implications from left to right represent above Theorem III.1.i, and those from right to left Theorem III.1.ii. The first formula was, further, seen as a definition, with only the second an inference, obtained, as suggested in the preceeding, by upon viewing, finding, *A*, not finding *'A*, and upon not finding *'A*, finding *A*. That this formula is not somehow likewise a conscious part of the definition, a part of it at all in fact, is, more than in previous absence of some part from consciousness (p.137 second par.), evidenced by the mere lack of reference in the definition to an area other than of *'A* and *'(A)*. Seeing the place of *'A* to be that of *'(A)*, it is not seen, obvious though it may be, that the place of *A* is that of *'('A)*.

The second formula is known as the law of double negation mentioned (p.32), without the distinction here made by parentheses. Since the two kinds of negation are at present equivalent, the parentheses could indeed be omitted without change in validity. In consonance with former observation (e.g. p.142 last par.), however, the same is not the case in the other, attributive, logic.

Adapting the laws of thought to it, the law of exclusion is

THEOREM III.2.i. *A thing does not both have and not have a given attribute at the same time.*

Proof. In Figure III.2 of a given time the small circle stands for the things that are *A*, or simply every *A*; all other area of the large circle stands for every *non-A*, symbolized *'A*; all area outside *A* stands for things other than *A*, for everything *not A*, symbolized *'(A)*; and the large circle stands for every *B*, thus comprising, whether of a further attribute or not, every *A* and *'A*. An attribute *A* can accordingly be meant to apply to only certain things *B*, and its negation, *'A*, to only the rest of those

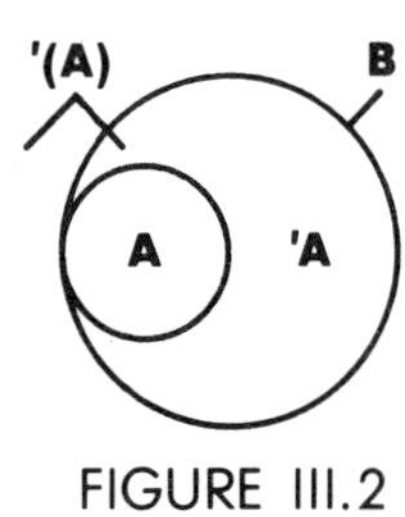

FIGURE III.2

things. This was noted of, among other things, even and odd, applying only to numbers. By 'A is nonetheless meant a thing other than A. By the figure, therefore, a thing is not both A and 'A at the same time.

The letters used for attributes or their absence are the same as those used for things existing or not because, as was suggested (p.105 second par.), the concepts will in the two logics be found easily merged. Since a thing of attribute A can be spoken of as an A, the existence of the same A can be spoken of as well. That it or its negation is spoken of is likely understood by the context, indicated to (p.143 sixth par.) mainly involve association of one thing with another, and specifically implication in one logic and attribution in the other. It ought to be further said that, similarly to the existential case, "thing" and "attribute" are used extremely broadly here, so as to make time again diversely depicted in the figure. The theorem was given as about a time of a thing since, like existence, most things are thought of as worldly, with a discussed continued identity through time. But some things can again merely belong to consciousness, and as perceptions of only a certain time, they need not be specified as of a time by the theorem; whenever a perception occurs, that and only that will be its time, and the figure can correspondingly depict all perceptions regardless of time, with B perhaps visual qualities, and A blue ones. What is more, a thing can be a certain time, or length of it, itself, making the mention of time in the theorem once more unneeded; in that case the figure again depicts all perceptions, along with those of, as on a clock, times, perhaps as durations signified by B, and seconds by A. Concerned are things of any attribute at any of their time.

To the last theorem the, qualified, companion law of inclusion is

THEOREM III.2.ii. *A thing either has or does not have a given attribute at any time if and only if it belongs to things comprising what has and does not have the attribute.*

Proof. As confirmed by Figure III.2, a thing is either A or 'A at any time if and only if it belongs to things B comprising A and 'A.

As seen in the figure, the principle applies, together with the one preceding, without the qualification if 'A is replaced by *'(A)*. In ordinary language, the '(A) counterpart of Theorem III.2.i can then state that *A thing is not both one that has and not one that has a given attribute at the same time*, and the counterpart of Theorem III.2.ii that *A thing is either one that has or not one that has a given attribute at any time.*

As before the two theorems can be expressed in a form like implication, specifically so that a thing can be held to imply an attribute. The simple forms used previously (p.144 displays), however, are now one-directional, suited only for the first theorem.

'A *is* '(A)

and

A *is* '('A).

The attributions do because of the qualifications evidently not hold in the opposite direction, for the other theorem.

As with the previous theorems, the first formula is true as a matter of, partial, definition, only the second inferred. That formula, as indicated, would change in validity without the parentheses, to in that event in truth apply in both directions. The negation would be the limited one, which indeed implies *A* as the alternative. It would seem that the full form can hence be used for both theorems after all, with the first formula redundant without the parentheses. But as suggested by the redundancy and the discussed controversy regarding the law of excluded middle, the usual interest is in whether if either, a certain attribute or its negation, in a limited sense, does not, in a limitless sense, hold, the other does.

Appropriate formulas combined would be

'A *equals* ('(A) & B)

and

A *equals* ('('A) & B)

if and only if

(A & 'A) *equals* B,

with division, as before, into definition and inference. Equality, or identity, will be seen to be the same as attribute in both directions, as in the first chapter observed regarding definition (p. 41 last par.).

For the above counterparts of the two theorems, with *'(A)* in place of 'A, the formulas, no longer qualified, return to simple form. Here, too, the first one, that '(A) *equals* '(A), is redundant, and the second would state that A *equals* '('(A)).

Adapting the two laws to mathematics, the one of exclusion is

THEOREM III.3.i. *A quantity is not more than one of the following, a given one, a smaller one, or a larger one.*

Proof. In Figure III.3 circle Q stands for a given quantity; circle *S* and all other area less than Q stand for smaller quantities; and circle *L* and all other area more than Q stand for larger quantities. The asymmetry indicates that quantities apply to specific things, extending from a (left) point in a certain (right) direction. The theorem is at all events seen in the figure to hold.

The law of inclusion is for mathematics

THEOREM III.3.ii. *A quantity is either a given one, a smaller one, or a larger one.*

Proof. The theorem is substantiated by same Figure III.3.

It should not be required to list the implicational forms of these theorems. It may merely be remarked that they take the form "If one then not another, and if not any of two then the third."

More notably, the theorems can, on the basis anew of underlying meaning, be deduced by logical principle.

That one quantity is less or smaller than another can be held to mean that while all of it belongs to the other, some amount outside it also does. And that one quantity is more or larger than another can be held to mean that not all of it belongs to the other, nor does some outside it. That in the meaning of "less", further, some amount not of that quantity belongs to the other is logically equivalent to not all of the other belonging to the first. And in the meaning of "more" the denial that some amount not of that quantity belongs to the other is equivalent to all of the other belonging to the first. Thus with quantity *A* less than quantity *B*, and quantity *C* more, all *A* is *B*, not all *B* is *A*, all *B* is *C*, and not all *C* is *B*. And if two quantities are equal then by the above alluded to (facing p. third par.) equality principle all of either is of the other, or, by transposition, if not all of either is of the other then the two are not equal. Hence *A* does not equal *B*, *B* does not equal *C*, and since all *A* but not all *C* is *B*, *A*, for fear of contradiction, does not equal *C*. If something *A* equals *C* then by referred to (p. 33 second par.) later principle not all of it is *B* either. With none equaling another, therefore, if a quantity equals either one, it does not, by same noncontradiction, equal another, in compliance with above Theorem III.3.i.

To proceed in correlation with the preceding, if one quantity does not equal another, that is if it is not true that all of each is of the other, then by logical law not all of at least one quantity is of the other. This can in fact be true of one of the quantities only, because by "not all" is here meant an amount additional to the other, meaning at once that the other, all of it, is part of the first. Then if a quantity does not equal a given one then either, all of it is of the other and not all of the other is of it, or

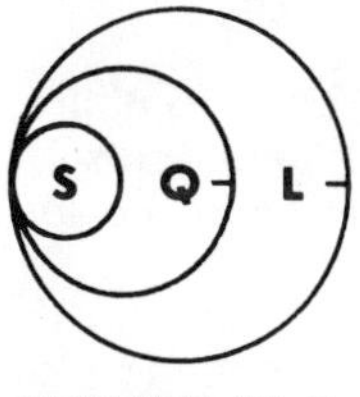

FIGURE III.3

the opposite. But these alternatives were seen to make the quantity either less or more than the other. That is to say, in compliance with Theorem III. 3.ii, a quantity is either equal to a given one, or less, or more.

The last two theorems are manifestly easier to establish by means of a diagram, should even that much be needed, rather than by in the preceding manner inferring them via others. That they and others are logically deducible should nonetheless prove of interest.

Among other theorems are further ones that can be regarded as of complements, this time concerning states usually expressed by means of two variables, e.g. *A* and *B*, signifying things identified by different attributes. The theorems are akin to the familiar square of opposition in syllogistic, which deals with logic here called attributive. But they also have an existential form and can apply to mathematics, although having to do with attribute for the most part. In its connection there is dispute over the meaning of the designations "all" and "some" regarding a subject, the validity of the principles accordingly questioned, and a related issue extends into the other logic. It should at this moment suffice to repeat that what is meant by words is a matter of choice. Addressing the meanings at issue afterward, the principles will now be indicated as pertains to attribute. For exclusion there is, when there is only one *A*,

THEOREM III.4.i. *Not both,* A *is* B, *and* A *is* '(B),

and with more *A*

THEOREM III.4.ii. *Not more than one of the following, all* A *is* B, *some* A *is* B *and some is* '(B), *and all* A *is* '(B).

Both theorems also apply to *'B* (*"non-B"*), as previously (p.144 last par.) distinguished from *'(B)* (*"not B"*). The same is not the case with inclusion, in, treating separately the single and multiple *A* again,

THEOREM III.4.iii. *Either* A *is* B, *or* A *is* '(B),

and

THEOREM III.4.iv. *Either all* A *is* B, *some* A *is* B *and some is* '(B), *or all* A *is* '(B).

As elsewhere, these two theorems apply to *'B* if and only if *A* belongs to things comprising *B* and *'B*. The simpler version is chosen because in this form the theorems represent the other logic as well, the qualified version easily enough supplied mentally. It should nevertheless be noted that, here and subsequently, principles often thought valid may again not be because of the limited range of a negation.

Postponing proof of the preceding theorems, it may first be noted that they, too, are of truths commonly apprehended, as in an awareness of the trichotomy of "all", "some", and "none".

Instead of the trichotomy, however, logic usually states that, for exclusion,

Not both, all A *is* B, *and some* A *is* 'B,

and

Not both, all A *is* 'B, *and some* A *is* B,

and for inclusion,

Either all A *is* B, *or some* A *is* 'B,

and

Either all A *is* 'B, *or some* A *is* B.

In conformance with the aforesaid, the last two formulas must really be qualified, applying instead to *'(B)*. Above Theorem III.4.ii, analogous to the present other two formulas, is ironically at the same time rejected.

It is specifically proposed that all *A* can be both *B* and *'B*. In support is cited the like of the referred to (p.143 last par.) meaning of "Not both, *A* and *B*" as "To find *A* is not to find *B*" and the opposite. In the present case the partial meaning, of similar "A thing is not both *A* and *B*" and expressed in the last above displayed line as the negation of "Some *A* is *B*", would be "All *A* is *'B*". It is then argued that if nothing is *A* then each "A thing is not both *A* and *B*" and "A thing is not both *A* and *'B*" is true, and that hence by the preceding meaning all *A* is respectively both *'B* and *B*.

It may be remarked that here, too, the limited range of *'B* is not taken account of. The denial of "A thing is not both *A* and *B*" would by that interpretation not mean that all *A* is *'B*, but only *'(B)*. Likewise for changing from denial of "A thing is not both *A* and *'B*" to *B*. But more pertinent is that "All *A* is *B* " is commonly not meant to be true if nothing is *A*. If if nothing is *A* then "A thing is not both *A* and *not-B*" is meant true, then the last does not mean the same as "All *A* is *B*". Neither does "A thing is either *not-A* or *B*" if, as maintained also, true if nothing is *A*.

The present meanings of "not both" and "either . . . or" are, as to be elucidated, ones dependent on a connection between the two things at issue, not on the existential status of either, the meanings otherwise not now of concern. A like situation obtains with "Some *A* is *B*". In contrast to the other case, it is said to mean that something is both *A* and *B*, and hence that something is *A*. As a result it is also held false that either some *A* is *B* or some is *not-B*, alternatives likewise ordinarily acknowledged and here implicit in Theorem III.4.iv (facing p.). If nothing is *A*, it is considered, then by that meaning neither is true. But as before, the meaning at issue of "Some *A* is *B*" has to do with a connection between *A* and *B*, irrespectively of their existential status.

As did the laws of thought pertain to any imaginable thing or existence, so do in logical principles here statements about all, some or other of their subjects pertain in them to the same unlimited spectrum. The truth of the statements, as in the variety of them in everyday life, is not dependent on some form of existence or nonexistence of their subjects, in what is called existential import, but has to do with whatever may be known of something of whatever nature. A statement can also declare that a certain thing has worldly existence, or that another has not even a conceptual one. In the first instance the subject, as observed earlier (p. 39 fourth par.), is of a still only conceptual status, and in the second instance of none at all, represented only linguistically. Mentioned argument advanced that existence is not an attribute (p. 38 fifth par.), or that its assertion is a tautology, with a subject held at least in singular propositions to exist by its mention alone, are of no avail. What an attribute is is, again, a matter of definition, and it remains that existence is affirmed or denied of things, with understanding of what is said, and without previous knowledge of the facts.

In the light of these remarks the contention that universal propositions, with "all", are true if the subjects do not exist can run into contradiction. A statement like "All these assumed situations exist" would be true if they did not. To assert that singular propositions, with a single subject, presume its existence is likewise inconsistent with the arguments on universal ones. When there is no more than one *A* it can by "*A* is *B*" be equally meant "A thing is not both *A* and *not-B*" and that this is true if *A* does not exist. Both that existence is not a predicate and that single subjects of statements are assumed to exist are, by holding that to speak of an individual's existence is somehow senseless, propounded in defense of, as to be brought forth in the last chapter, arguments against particular existences, serving to illustrate how premises can be strained to accommodate an aimed at conclusion, not rather seeing what findings can be made. As observed earlier (p. 25 last par.), existences, particular or general, are concerned in all searches for fact, statements made accordingly. Of interest here is what latitudes indeed can be present in statements, or states, as logic applies to them.

In the recourse to the form "A thing is not both *A* and *not-B*" for "All *A* is *B*" its truth is clearly thought also decided if nothing is *not-B*, namely if everything is *B*. That all *A* is *B* does sound more reasonable if everything is *B* than if nothing is *A*. But if the translation of that form is the referred to opposite (last p. third par.) which now is "All *not-B* is *not-A*", then its truth if everything is *B* seems odd again. With less attention to that form, it may be observed that as "All *A* is *B*" is here and ordinarily not meant to follow if nothing is *A*, it is also meant unrevealing if everything is *B*. And this is indicative of the alluded to connection intended between *A*, the subject, and *B*, the thing connected with it, in any statement.

The intent is to assert about the subject something not the case with regard to everything else as well, within whichever area concerned. An example was furnished when seeking to find laws of nature beside causal ones, in seeing it of no interest that something in nature is accompanied by the existence of matter, which accompanies all things (p.93 fifth par. through p.94 second par.). Such an absence of a revealing connection is in current logic part of, beside above predication, implication.

The now treated principles were mentioned adaptable to existential logic, and the connections regarding *A* and *B* in it would as before be of implications. As suggested (p.136 second par.) when discussing the law of identity, implication is herein distinguished from attribution by concerning something, *B*, associated with the subject, *A*, within given bounds, whereas in attribution *B* is something *A* itself is. Attribution can thus be considered a case of implication, when *A* is one with the associated *B*. And implication, in likeness to attribution, is held present if *A* is false or if *B* is true.

Truth and falsity is spoken of in place of existence or nonexistence because, as explained, such as implication has been viewed as holding between propositions, although, while really holding between their truth, they therein hold between actual states, which are but some of the things that can be associated. "*A* implies *B*" was in any event noted (p.143 last par.) equivalent to "Not both *A* and *not-B*", regarded as true in the absence of *A* or presence of *B*. This is, however, not the customary understanding of implication, which, as held in logic also, frequently connotes deducibility of *B* from *A*. There is no need to go so far, since the principles about the connections pertain not only to logical and even causal ones, but to any within any chosen area. Nevertheless the connections are meant to be revealing as observed, *B* to be associated with *A* but not with all other things in that area also. How common this meaning is is disclosed by considering that if one thing, e.g. in nature, does relative to another merely coexist, which all things in nature do, then there is held to be no connection between the two.

With these observations in view, Figure III.4 (next p.) can serve to validate the present theorems (p.148) with regard to either logic, and with as full a versatility as before. Whereas in attribution the diagram, as in previous Figures III and III.2 (pp.140, 144), depicts an *A* as being a *B*, in implication instead the time or place of *A* can be looked upon as a time or place of *B*. Since a thing would be regarded as identical with another if occurring at the very same time and place, though not if only occurring at the same time or the same place, the large circle can represent times or places of certain wider limits within which *B* occurs, the small circle, the times or places of *A*, falling within those limits. In a causal connection accordingly *A*, the cause, is accompanied by *B*, the effect, within a proximate place or time. These proximities make the connections revealing as explicated, since accompaniment anywhere and anytime applies to everything and makes for no connection. Should the connection depicted by the diagram be viewed as causal, then the area for the figure would thus all represent nature, with negations of events *A* and *B* as before outside their respective circles. In that case the discoursed existence, in the world, is indeed presumed of *A* and *B*, or *'(B)* as alternative in the theorems, causality concerning the discussed very coming into existence of the effect upon the cause. This can be viewed as justification here for the title existential logic, since in it dominantly treated implication, much applying to causal connections, is accordingly conspicuously of existence. But the connections can, as observed, be of anything else, deductive ones examples in having one concept entail another, and that is why attribution can be considered to belong to them. The whole area in the figure can hence represent again any specific area of consciousness, from a particular place and time in the world to perception in general. The question then is whether in the limited or unlimited area when, for instance, all *A* in it is *B*, can some not be.

Without the dependance thus on existential factors, particularly worldly ones, with only the question whether *B* is associated with *A* in its area, which can be of the world as well, Theorems III.4.i through III.4.iv can be seen true by means of Figure III.4. For the first one of the theorems compared to the second it will be recalled (p.143 second par.) that by the negation of something, *B*, of a, single, thing, *A*, is meant complete absence of its affirmation. The reader will also find

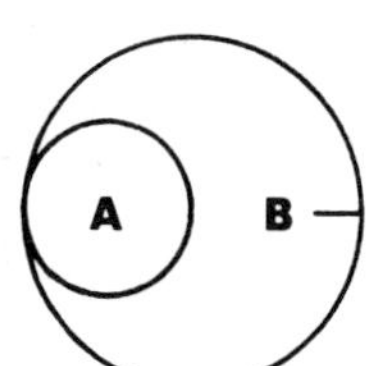

FIGURE III.4

it easy to confirm that the last two theorems hold for *'B* if and only if *A* (e.g. a prime number) belongs to things (e.g. whole numbers) that, perhaps given by a third circle C, comprise *B* and *'B* (e.g. even and odd numbers).

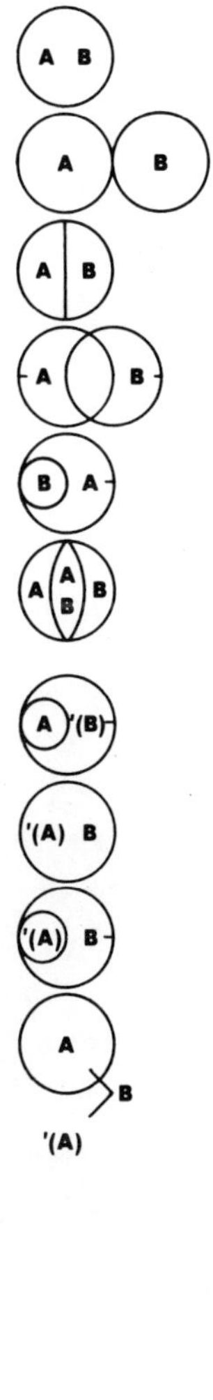

It may be observed that in syllogistic the three alternatives for all *A* in relation to *B* or *'(B)* are viewed by way of as many as seven diagrams. "All *A* is *B*" is, along with the diagram of figure III.4, depicted by a single circle with *A* equaling *B*; "All *A* is *'(B)*" is depicted by discrete circles for *A* and *B*, and, when *A* and *B* exhaust the universe of discourse, by a circle for it of two parts, one for *A*, and one for *B*; and "Some *A* is *B* and some is *'(B)*" is depicted by two circles for *A* and *B* partly overlapping each other, by a small circle for *B* in a large one for *A*, and, when *A* and *B* exhaust the universe, by a circle for it of three parts, one for *A*, one for *B*, and one for both. The exhausting of the universe is added to provide for all connections of "all" and "some" between *A* and *B*, including their negations, the connection "All *'(A)* is *B*" being thus pictured. Even if so many diagrams are used to verify a theorem, however, there is no hindrance to having circles stand for negations, so that three kinds of diagrams will suffice, without the complication of containing the universe in some cases within a shape.

The discrete circles for "All *A* is *'(B)*" can be replaced by a small one in a large one, the succeeding divided circle, for the additional "All *'(A)* is *B*", by a circle alone, and the last, twice divided, circle by also a small one in a large one. There could yet be a circle picturing, as an instance, *B* as exhausting the universe, as would be thing, although the connections would not be revealing as explained.

But regardless of these, not only do the multiple diagrams fail to aid a principle's perception, to rather obstruct it, but that they represent all the alternatives itself requires proof. These alternatives, as is not too difficult to ascertain, are in their various forms in fact established by the theorems presently at issue. That these theorems hold does, further, not require more than, with the aid of Figure III.4, viewing under "(All) *A* is *B*" *A* as confined to *B*, whether to a part or whole of it; under "(All) *A* is *'(B)*" comparably; and under "Some *A* is *B* and some is *'(B)*" *A* as extending over both, *B*, whether part or whole of it, and *'(B)* comparably. These choices become in the added diagrams perplexing to see, and they no doubt need moreover not be enunciated to enable perception of the theorems from the single diagram.

It should be equally simple to perceive from the same diagram the similar displayed principles following them (p.149), as applying to *'(B)* and qualifiedly to *'B*, it being understood that "some" can extend to "all", as "possible" was understood to extend to "necessary" (p.37 second par.). These principles can be of utility in logic, since by them when "all" applies, "some" can at once be denied of the opposite, and when "some" applies, the like can be denied of "all"; and when "not all" applies, "some" can of the opposite at once be affirmed, and when "not some" applies, "all" can be affirmed likewise.

While viewing of all of these principles by means of diagram offers no problem, they can in a lengthier manner be deduced from others in more than one way.

Theorems III.4.i and III.4.iii (p.148), when there is a single *A*, can be deduced straightforwardly from laws of thought. Since *A* is a thing, and by those laws a thing is not both *B* and *'(B)* and is one of the two, the same is by transitivity true of *A*.

For another proof it may be considered that by denying that *A* is *B* is meant that *A* is something *not B*, that it is *'(B)*. For, the conception in the denial is something regarding *A* as a thing, namely that it is a thing other than *B*. One could go even so far as to cover by alternatives such as *B* and *'(B)* also mentioned things not existing even conceptually, but only by name (p.150 first par.). In that case *A* may be just such a thing, and by denying that it is *B* it would be hence likewise meant that it is something *not B*, *'(B)*. What counts is that *B* and *'(B)* are meant to be inclusive in any sense, and by the preceding thus half of each, Theorems III.4.i and III.4.iii, can as in laws of thought be held true by definition, put in, again, implicational form as

*(*A *is '(*B*)) is equivalent to '(*A *is* B*).*

From left to right the implication is half of "Not both . . .", and from right to left half of "Either . . . or . . .". The other halves are stated by

*(*A *is* B*) is equivalent to '(*A *is '(*B*)).*

And by the first displayed preceding formula the second of the equivalent units of the second formula is equivalent to "A is *'('(B))*" and hence, by laws of thought and transitivity, to "A is *B*", the first unit of that formula, the formula therefore likewise true.

From the first formula the second can, in a third proof, be in fact deduced directly by transposition, by which if one thing is equivalent to the negation of another, then the affirmation of the other is equivalent to the negation of the first.

For Theorems III.4.ii and III.4.iv (p.148), and the similar four displayed principles succeeding them (p.149), all on more than one *A*, proof in a manner like the preceding second kind should suffice. It can here, too, first be considered that by denying that all *A* is *B* is meant that some *A* is *'(B)*, and by denying that some *A* is *B* is meant that all *A* is *'(B)*. For, the conception in the first denial, unlike in "All *A* are things other than *B*", is only that some *A* is a thing other than *B*, and the conception in the second denial, unlike in only "Some *A* is a thing other than *B*", is that all *A* are things other than *B*.

Half of the last mentioned four principles can thus, with *'(B)* in place of *'B*, again be held true by definition, put in implicational form as

(All A *is* '(B)*) is equivalent to '(Some* A *is* B*)*,

and

(Some A *is* '(B)*) is equivalent to '(All* A *is* B*)*.

In the same form, Theorems III.4.ii and III.4.iv can be put as

(All A *is* '(B)*) is equivalent to ('(Some* A *is* B *and some* A *is* '(B)*) and '(All* A *is* B*))*,

(Some A *is* B *and some* A *is* '(B)*) is equivalent to ('(All* A *is* '(B)*) and '(All* A *is* B*))*,

and

(All A *is* B*) is equivalent to ('(Some* A *is* B *and some* A *is* '(B)*) and '(All* A *is* '(B)*))*.

Proving in the first of these three formulas the implication from left to right, the first half of the "some" unit, ignoring the negation of the whole, is false by the first above displayed definition, and hence the unit, with its negation, is true. The last inference holds because here, unlike earlier (p.151 fourth par.), "Not both *A* and *B*" is true if and only if either *A* or *B* is false, since meant to be the denial of "*A* and *B*", meant true if and only if both *A* and *B* are true. And the last unit in the formula is true because the first unit implies by aforesaid meaning of "some" (p.153 last par.) that some *A* is *'(B)*, which by the second above definition implies the last unit.

Proving the implication from right to left, the last unit implies by that definition the second half of the "some" unit, and hence to make that unit a negation its first half is false. The last inference holds once more because here "not both" is true if and only if either is false. And because that first half is made false the first unit is by the first above definition true.

In the second formula the second halves of the two large units are equivalent by the second of those definitions. And by that definition the first half of the second unit is equivalent to "Some *A* is *'('(B))*" and therefore to "Some *A* is *B*", the first half of the first unit.

The proof of the third formula is the same as that of the first, but for a reverse treatment of the "some" unit and deriving the equivalencies as in the last proof.

The same method can be used for, regarding *'(B)*, the four principles succeeding Theorems III.4.i-III.4.iv and half of which were seen to comprise those definitions (this p. second par.). The other half can be stated as

(All A *is* B*) is equivalent to '(Some* A *is* '(B)*)*,

and

(Some A *is* B*) is equivalent to '(All* A *is* '(B)*),*
and it actually comprises the last mentioned equivalencies in the third above formula. Hence to prove it the second halves of the present formulas will be found through the definitional ones equivalent to the first halves with *'('(B)* and therefore with *B*.

To see how any of the eight principles can be deduced from others for *'B* it may be recalled that half of them, those that by former remarks may be termed of inclusion, were by diagram seen qualified (p.153 first and last pars.), namely true if and only if *A* belongs to things C comprising *B* and *'B*.

If it does, for the first half of "if and only if," then by Theorem III.2.ii (p.145) and transitivity any one *A*, since a C which thus is either *B* or *'B*, is either *B* or *'B*, confirming for *'B* the counterpart of Theorem III.4.iii (p.148). In consequence follows also the second half of the displayed principles (p.149) succeeding the last theorems. If " '(All *A* is *B*)" or " '(Some *A* is *B*)" is true then, since these were noted (p.154 last par.) to respectively mean some and each *A* is a thing other than *B*, and here as a C an *A* other than *B* is *'B*, respectively "Some *A* is *'B*" and "All *A* is *'B*" is true; by transposition if either of the latter two is true negated then the respective one of the former two is true unnegated. These four implications are counterparts, as forms of last mentioned principles, of displayed ones with *'(B)* (last p. second and last pars., and this p. above), viewed from right to left. From these counterparts follows in addition the counterpart of Theorem III.4.iv (p.148), the last principle now concerned, as, also, displayed as implications (last p. third par.), viewed from right to left. The counterpart can from the preceding ones be derived in the same manner as were those implications.

That only if *A*, for the second half of "if and only if", belongs to things C comprising *B* and *'B* do the concerned principles hold, to signify that if they hold then *A* belongs to C, follows more simply because all these principles assert either *B* or *'B* of the *A*. Hence if the principles apply, if the *A* are either *B* or *'B*, then since both *B* and *'B* are C, the *A* are by transitivity C. This of course is hardly of interest, the question being under what condition the principles hold, not that if they hold then the condition does.

The other principles in the last pages discussed, those that may be termed of exclusion, were to be seen by diagram to hold for *'B* without qualification, because *'B* is an instance of *'(B)*.

To prove via others that they do, it must be true that by the counterpart for *'B* of Theorem III.4.i (p.148) if *A* is *'B* then it is not true that it is *B*. Since by the preceding it is by transitivity *'(B)*, the inference holds by that theorem; by transposition if *A* is *B* then it is not true that it is *'B*, confirming that counterpart. Similarly for the first half of the principles succeeding the last theorems (p.149). If "All *A* is *'B*" or "Some *A* is *'B*" is true then, since hence respectively all and some *A* is *'(B)*, by partial counterparts of those principles (p.155 second par.) respectively " '(Some *A* is *B*)" and " '(All *A* is *B*)" is true; by transposition if either of the latter two is true unnegated then the respective one of the former two is true negated, confirming the principles. From them follows the counterpart for *'B* of Theorem III.4.ii (p.148), the last principle concerned, displayed as implications (p.155 third par.) viewed from left to right. The counterpart can be derived from the preceding in the manner they were.

The difference between *'B* and *'(B)* was seen not to enter existential logic and accordingly implication. The recent principles would hence apply to implication with standard negations, should there not be some problem with linguistic usage. Implication between *A* and *B* is customarily confined to principles, to exclude the single *A* as well as some *A* only. Since principles were seen to consist of no other than, revealingly, constant accompaniment of one kind of thing by another, however, the difference between them, i.e. that all *A* is joined by *B*, and that some *A* or the single *A* are is merely in those quantities. With some liberality and serviceability, therefore, all the accompaniments, as suggested (e.g. p.151 fourth par.), may be spoken of as implications, restricting, as in necessity, the narrower meaning to the constancy. The theorems can for implication accordingly say, for example, "Not more than one of the following, (all) *A* implies *B*, some *A* implies *B* and some implies *'B*, and (all) *A* implies *'B*".

That "some" be less associated with implication is understandable in view of the word's mentioned (p.104 last par.) denial of a principle. With attributes the word has often value, because, although an attribute may not be possessed by all of a kind, it can characterize some for a substantial period, as may a color some animals of a kind. There is hence a degree of certainty that the attribute will repeatedly be observed, if only in some cases, in consonance with earlier observations on worldly things as retaining their identity through time. Correspondingly it can also be of more account that a single thing has a certain attribute than that a single event is accompanied by a certain other. To speak of "some" in regard to implication thus has mainly the significance of denying a principle, normally done by simply denying an implication. Similarly the accompaniment of single things by others is customarily only spoken of as implication when the connections are instances of constant ones.

The usage notwithstanding, accompaniments of some or the single *A* by *B* are of logical consequence and therefore can together with constant ones be considered as outlined. That the preceding principles can be applied to these connections can beside diagrammatically be ascertained in the same ways as above. And being very general, they concern connections between quantities as well, as in the referred to ones between prime numbers and their attributes of even or odd.

Application of the principles to numbers as well as to other things was indicated a matter of course, and the principles of this section can as others indeed be regarded as presupposed in all walks of life. When something is discovered to be fact it is disallowed that it is fiction, one's very pursuits being guided by these fundamental distinctions. It is for the present sections to demonstrate that these presuppositions, though not any, are well founded.

Section 3
OTHER THEOREMS AND OBSERVATIONS

The principles investigated in the last section had much to do with what is called external negation, alluded to at the start of that section when mentioning affirmation or denial of whole propositions, rather than of what is predicated of their subjects. The negation was symbolized by an apostrophy before the parenthesized proposition, e.g. as '(*A* is *B*), with a similar notation, '(*A*), for a similar indirect negation of an attribute. Externally denied propositions were found equivalent to certain, externally, affirmed ones, which may in general be regarded as of more interest, as one would feel closer to one's goals knowing which propositions are true instead of which are false. As was observed in relation to the liar paradox, propositions are in fact meant to be true, even when asserting falsity, and external negations are mainly denials of, affirmative, propositions.

The emphasis on affirmative propositions, which may or may not include internal negations, should prove of special value in deriving conclusions from premises, as already illustrated when seeing how instances are derived from principles. These propositions will also correspondingly be concerned in subsequent further principles.

Beside the laws of complements there are other fundamental

principles in logic, and they are largely accepted as undemonstrated. For that reason and because demonstrations may be faulty the principles may be false. Therefore since, as expounded, substantiation of any truth is made by perceptual finding, basic theorems will continue here to be proven through diagrams. This is not to contend that every deductive theorem must be apprehensible through a diagram, or that any truth whatsoever is determined solely by perceiving it in accordance with the criterion by which the occurrence in question is meant perceived.

As indicated before (e.g. p.4 fourth par.), fine distinctions are not always at once perceived, and many other things beyond immediate reach are ascertained by inference. As brought to attention in the discussion on deduction of instances, however, inference is itself a form of mental perception. While conclusions may thus not be perceived in the subject matter considered, they may be perceived as consequences of premises.

The present theorems are ones that represent the last mentioned sort of perception, and they can hence be simply viewed by diagrams, even if in part themselves deducible from others. In the next two they are in their varied forms known as the law of transposition, contraposition, and modus tollens, these referred to variously before (e.g. p.114 fourth par.). The first is of existential logic.

THEOREM III.5. *If when* A *exists* B *exists then when* B *does not exist* A *does not exist.*

Proof. In Figure III.5 the small circle stands for the times *A* exists, and the large circle for the times *B* exists; when *A* exists, accordingly, *B* exists. As disclosed by the figure, therefore, when *B* does not exist *A* does not.

As previously, that the times of *A* are times of *B* would be thought to require another diagram, a single circle when both times are identical. But as in other cases, it is enough to conceive *A* as confined to *B* to see the theorem hold. The converse of the theorem is usually also given, to say that "When *A* then *B*" and "When 'B then 'A" are equivalent. By *A* and *B* is,

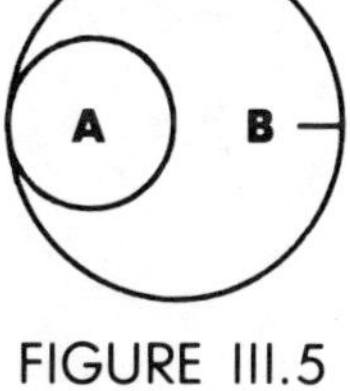

FIGURE III.5

however, meant anything, including negation in one of the things or both, all of which, as said, can be represented by the circles. Hence the converse is true as an instance of the theorem. The theorem, it may be remarked, incorporates by that comprehensiveness laws of thought, since denials of denials in it are by those laws equivalent to the asserted affirmations. These results can be discerned, however, in the present figure as well.

It may be evident that the relations here between *A* and *B*, or their negations, are of the spoken of implications, and as elsewhere they are about any revealing accompaniment except that every *A*, including a solitary one, is involved. "When" can accordingly in this case, too, refer to a place as much as to a time, and perhaps to a conception, as when the connection is a logical principle. The revealingness of interest was also seen (p.152 first par.) to in "when" require a certain limit within which *A* is accompanied by *B*, and that limit can ironically, in further extensiveness of application, encompass in a conception of such as a logical principle all that may be apprehended. The present theorem as a whole itself is an example. If the condition in it, "*A* implies *B*", is a logical principle also, then what it implies, " *'B* implies *'A*", can take effect everywhere the condition does not. In other words the limit within which the condition is accompanied by what it implies could be said to be anywhere. The limit here is the conception itself, however, as represented by the figure. What is conceived to accompany the assumed in the theorem is not conceived to accompany everything.

In the like theorem for attributive logic the accompaniment is conceived as more limited.

THEOREM III.6. *When* A *is* B *then* 'B *is* 'A *if and only if it belongs to things* C *comprising* A *and* 'A.

Proof. In Figure III.6 the small circle stands for every *A* and some of C; the medium circle stands for every *B*; and the area outside it and of the large circle stands for every *'A* and the rest of C. The figure accordingly complies with the conditions of the theorem and demonstrates it.

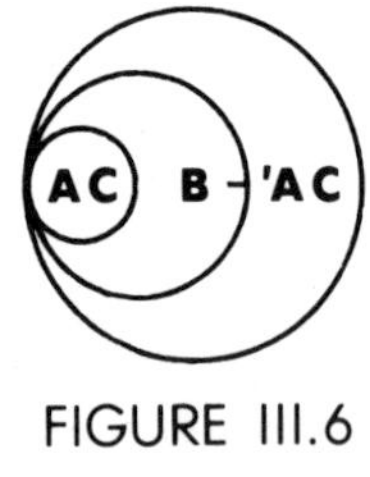

FIGURE III.6

As in other diagrams, *A* might also extend to the rest of *B*, as may instead *'A*, and *C* accordingly. It is only needed to conceive *A* as confined to *B*, *'A* to other than *A*, and *C* as comprising *A* and *'A*.

The situation may appear somewhat involved, but is less so in practice. As elsewhere, one usually knows what sort of things *A* and *'A* concern, viz *C*, as well as whether something, viz some *B* or *'B*, belongs to them. Therefrom one easily infers whether *'B* is *'A* knowing that *A* is *B*. Facts about referred to even, odd, and prime numbers, suited for the restricted coverage of *A* and *'A* in the figure, can serve as example.

For it *A* in the diagram is the number 2, divisible only by 1 and itself and hence named a prime number, *C*; *'A* is every other number divisible only by 1 and itself and hence a prime number *C*; and *B* is every even number. Accordingly since the number 2, *A*, is *B*, even, an odd number, *'B*, is *'A*, another number divisible only by one and itself, if and only if it is prime, *C*.

The example also illustrates how the theorem, like the one preceding it, applies when a connection has only a single subject, *A*. There can in point of fact also be a single *B*, identical with the *A*. That of what is predicated, *B*, of the subject, *A*, there may only be one has been denied in logic. Suffice it to say at this time that, as with affirming a subject's existence (ca. p.150), single things are indeed found with unique attributes, e.g. as, beside what distinguishes them otherwise, the ones of their placement, and those attributes are asserted of them accordingly. Aside from these arguments the last theorem is accepted without the qualification as to *C*, although it is without it that the theorem does not hold.

It does hold without it if applied to *'(A)*, however, as in former theorems. I.e. *when* A *is* B *then* '(B) *is* '(A), as pictorially easily confirmed. *'B* will also do, since included as subject, but *'A* will not, since not assured as attribute of either *'B* or *'(B)*.

Associable with these principles, in particular when about causality, can be a mathematical one of similar form.

If quantity A *is by an amount less than quantity* B *then a quantity by that amount less than a quantity* not B *is* not A.

The same may be said with "more" in place of "less". The by now familiar diagram at right provides confirmation, with letters interchangeable.

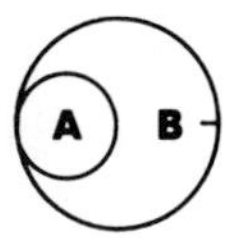

The principle can again also be deduced by means of logic. The condition in the principle can be stated as, equating quantities, *A = B – C*, which implies by transposition, with equality to be seen as mutual attribution, that *'(B – C) = '(A)*. The implied can be seen to be the same as that of the principle, since – C remains by postulate, and hence " *'(B – C)*" is identical with, as in a previous case (p.155 fifth par.), " '(*B*) – *C*". With "more" in place of "less" the inference is obviously analogous. "*A* = *B* + *C*" implies " '(*B* + *C*) = '(*A*)" or " '(*B*) + *C* = '(*A*)".

An example of transposition incorporating the mathematical one, as well as displaying the common comprehension of either, is furnished by the derivation that if for a food to be cooked at a given time one must begin at a certain other then if cooking is not begun at the required time the food will not be done when desired. Notwithstanding the everyday decisions made in accordance with these principles, they, too, are subject to uncertainties. This is not surprising in the light of the qualified nature of Theorem III.6, and Theorem III.5 is likewise a participant object of misunderstanding.

Along with the names "transposition", mainly used for the latter of these theorems, and "contraposition", used for the former, was mentioned "modus tollens". The formula so named is viewed as a separate principle and may be stated as

If when A *exists* B *exists, and* B *does not exist, then* A *does not exist.*

What is asserted by it, however, is the same as what is asserted by Theorem III.5. Each has as conditions that when *A* exists *B* exists and that *B* does at some time not exist, with the consequence that *A* does at that time not exist.

It can certainly be stated that by certain two expressions are meant the same thing, for possible inferences as a result, because, as noted earlier (p.137), something may be known true under the one expression and not the other. A similar likening of two statements is done in the accepted equivalence of "*A* implies that *B* implies *C*" and "*A* and *B* implies *C*", of which statements in fact Theorem III.5 and the last italicized formula are respective instances. Even this equivalence neglects that the contents of the two statements not merely imply each other but are the same. But while these statements are at least in some manner identified with each other, transposition and modus tollens are stated as independent facts, as if to contend different things. Even if two facts merely imply each other, as any under the two sides of transposition itself, is it awry to state them independently.

As companion to modus tollens is known modus ponens, which is of a parallel identity more treacherous and may be stated as

If when A *exists* B *exists, and* A *exists, then* B *exists.*

In accordance with the preceding this is the same as saying that *If when* A *exists* B *exists then when* A *exists* B *exists.*

There is revealed thus a redundancy within modus ponens alone. Indeed it is superfluous to say that if *A* implies *B*, and *A*, then *B*, since for *A* to imply *B* already means that if merely *A* then *B*. The presumed principle has in the capacity of a rule of inference been adapted to formal logic, logic whose symbolism is intended not to require interpretation, meaning. Part of that symbolism is a sign for what would ordinarily be "implies" and which can here take the shape of an arrow. The preceding modus ponens would then be put in a form such as

If A → B, *and* A, *then* B.

The rule, however, only results in allotting the arrow or like symbol a meaning after all, stating it regarding the connection of *A* with *B*.

With this rule is often paired one of substitution regarding variables like *A* and *B*, by stating such as

If a variable in a theorem is uniformly replaced by any other designation then the resulting proposition is true.

This rule equally supplies, however, a meaning to variables, one in conformity with the standard one.

Instead of being rules of inference these statements thus manage to define generalities that, expressed with symbols, characterize logical principles. Because utmost generalities, they contribute, as said, to the notion that they need not be about anything at all. But they concern the characteristic that in logical principles something is generally said to at all times—signified by the implication sign—of all things—signified by the variable—be true.

The adequacy of knowledge of a principle in order to apply it in inference, without the redundancy of the preceding rules, arises also in some of the following, in concord with earlier observations on deduction of instances.

The next theorem is a transitive one, known as the law of syllogism, and it has to do with conclusions from two premises rather than from, in what is called immediate inference, former single ones.

THEOREM III.7. *If when* A *exists* B *exists, and when* B *exists* C *exists, then when* A *exists* C *exists.*

Proof. In Figure III.7 the circles stand as before for the times the lettered entities exist, substantiating the theorem.

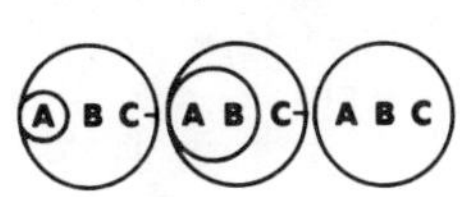

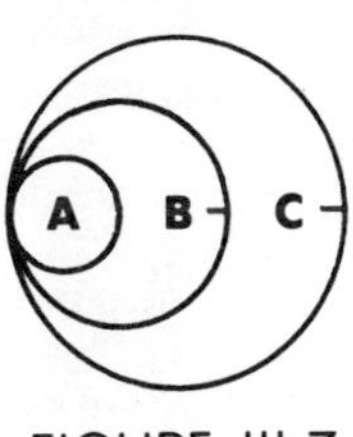

FIGURE III.7

Similarly to other cases, in transitivity the circles, mostly used for attributes rather than present implications, are thought to require the three additional diagrams shown. It suffices again, however, to conceive *A* as confined to *B*, and *B* to *C*. The implications can, further, again be comprehended in the broad sense described, with possible single entities. The comparable is the case with attribute.

When A *is* B, *and* B *is* C, *then* A *is* C.

Same Figure III.7 serves to substantiate, the circles now standing for the things named by the letters, and it serves as well for a transitivity in mathematics, the circles accordingly standing for quantities.

If quantity A *is less than quantity* B, *and* B *less than quantity* C, *then* A *is less than* C.

The place of "less" can be taken by "more", and the principle can once again be deduced by logical means.

As was observed (p.147 fourth par.), that quantity *A* is less than quantity *B* can be said to mean that while all *A* is *B*, some *'A* is *B* also. Hence the principle holds for "less" if all *A* is C and some *'A* is C. The first of these conditions is true directly by preceding transitivity, since all *B* is C by the same meaning. And the second condition is true since those *'A* that are *B* are by same transitivity C.

Concerning "more", it was likewise observed that for quantity *A* to be more than quantity *B* means that not all *A* is *B*, nor is some *'A* as well *B*. These were in the last section seen respectively equivalent to some *A* being *'B*, and all *'A* being *'B*. Hence the above principle holds for "more" if some *A* is *'C* and all *'A* is *'C*. Both of these conditions follow from the preceding ones by transitivity, since all *'B* is *'C* for the reasons just given.

The principle can combine with other transitivity law in causation, similarly to transposition. If *A* is, counting time as quantity, followed by *B*, and *B* by *C*, then *A* is by *C*, the successions viewable as implications, the time, within a latitude, of one thing being a time of another.

That implication can be spoken of in terms of the time of *A* as a time of *B* brings to view that transitivity has to do with inference of instances, a procedure seen (e.g. pp.139-141) to like other inference require justification beyond any principle. With the time of *B* a time of C, the time of *A* is inferred to be a time of C as an instance of a time of *B*. But to follow this principle, or any other prescribing an inference, it must itself be ascertained that an instance of them applies. Transitivity laws, instructing that from a joining of a thing of *B* by one of C follows the same joining of a thing of *A* as an instance of the first, would accordingly seem pointless. That an instance is at issue is, however, not always obvious. It is in implication obscured as about a time or place, since these are not explicit, and in the above mathematical case the connections as about such logical ones are still less evident. The same is not true with attributes, although there, too, arise uncertainties. There is no problem in deducing that one shall die because everyone does, as in the example about Socrates (p.141), but there may be a pause in inferring that the sun is a star because every glowing heavenly body is. When a premise is unfamiliar or the conclusion implausible it may be more difficult to discern the connection directly than through the transitive principle.

The transitivity of implication and progressive quantitative inequality, or equality, is of course as inadvertently applied in life as is the one last spoken of. One knows that if one thing is followed by another, and the second by yet another, then the first is followed by the last.

As a matter of fact one knows that this result ensues however many the connections between the first thing and the last. The general confirmation can easily, if wished, be made by adding circles in Figure III.7, or by regular deduction. Since the principles establish the connection between *A* and *C*, if it also exists between *C* and *D* then by repeat transitivity it exists between *A* and *D*, and so forth. Such prolonged transitivity is well known regarding mathematical equations, in which it functions alike in both directions. The equalities concerned are not, however, customarily treated in logic as of the connections here discussed, as should be apparent from the spoken of (ca. p.39) undue differentiation between subject and attribute. How equality or identity does belong to these connections, and how it results in dual consequences is indicated by the next theorem.

It is one mentioned (p.41· last par.) to be in some form known as the axiom of extensionality, and it speaks of a reciprocity between *A* and *B*.

THEOREM III.8. *When* A *is* B, *and* B *is* A, *then* A *is identical with* B, *and conversely.*

Proof. Figure III.8, the circle standing for *A* and *B*, demonstrates the theorem.

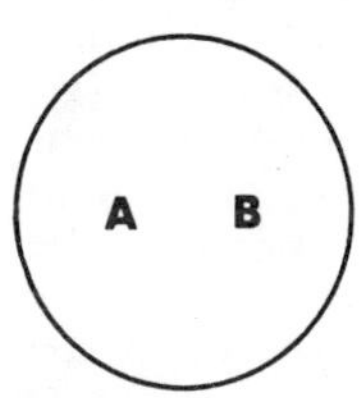

FIGURE III.8

The theorem can be demonstrated through others as well. Similarly to the meaning of "less" or "more" (e.g. p.164 sixth and seventh pars.), the conception that *A* is the same as, identical with, *B* can be held to be that one sees all *A* to be *B* and not some *'A* to be *B* as well. The first of these relations thus makes half of the last theorem true by definition, and since the second relation is by complement law equivalent to all *'A* being *'B* and hence by transposition to all *B* being *A*, it makes the rest of the theorem true.

A note may be added regarding the use of "if and only if" or "all and only" in the earlier formulation of the theorem (p.41 last par. again) and elsewhere. As indicated (e.g. p.156 fourth par.), the "only" part is taken to signify an opposite direction, as in "If *B* then *A*" or "All *B* is *A*" instead of "If *A* then *B*" or "All *A* is *B*". That it does can once more be held the result of meaning, by which "only" is understood as "not some other". By the last, as presently in "Not some *'A* is *B*", was in turn understood "All *'A* is *'B*", found equivalent to "All *B* is *A*". Therefore the opposite direction. The same happens for "if", in compliance with the like laws for implication. The frequent use herein of "when" instead of "if", as in the theorems, should be clear from its explained universality.

The last theorem also holds if the first two relations in it between *A* and *B* are implications and the third is an equivalence. This can be considered to be so in consequence of the theorem, since, as explicated, implication can be taken to speak of the time or place of one thing as a time or place of the other, with equivalence denoting the identity of these times or places.

Mathematics does not of course have a corresponding principle relating to the previous postulation of *A* or *B* as smaller or larger than the other. Each of *A* and *B* cannot at once be smaller than the other, or larger, let alone also identical. Theorem III.8 has bearing, however, on well known mathematical principles.

Anything true of *B* in the theorem can be viewed as attribute *C*, *B* thus being a thing *C* of that attribute. Then since *A* is *B*, by transitivity it is *C*, which is to say that if *A* is identical with *B*, then anything true of *B* is true of *A*. And anything true of *A* is true of *B*. This, seen inaccurately interpreted by Leibniz's law (p.32 last par. through p.33 second par.), applies accordingly equally to mathematics, specifically to selfsame quantities, as when considered in numerical equations independently of things which they concern. Hence the transitivity in the equations, since what is true of one of the numerical forms is true of another, and for the same reason when an operation, such as addition, is performed on one of them, the result is the same as when performed on another.

Equality often has two senses, however, in mathematics, as noted (p.130 third par.), as elsewhere. Beside the one of selfsameness there is one of certain alikeness, as in equating sizes in geometry. In those cases it can likewise be asked whether something true of one of the equal things is true of the other. Everything clearly cannot be the same for each, for instance their location. The question presently is rather whether in substantially mathematics, in analogy with the equality in the last paragraph, if things are equal in the second, nonidentity, sense, anything entailed by one of the things is entailed by the other. By something entailed is meant, as common in logic, something deducible, something intrinsic as explicated.

These equal things, things distinct but regarded by equal, quantitative, attributes, it should be considered, are, as noted about some geometric entities (e.g. p.126 first par.), undifferentiated, in being conceived without individual characteristics that, as may be location, would distinguish one from another. As in superposition of those geometric entities, they are upon their comparison, whatever its manner, postulated indistinguishable. And as in that superposition, if upon the comparison things in question differ in some part, they are contradictorily not equal. Consequently since anything entailed by a thing is, as something intrinsic, part of it, anything entailed by one of the equal things is, as an indistinguishable part, entailed by the other.

Therefore whether quantitative things are equal because the selfsame or because the same by comparison, it can be stated as a general principle that

If quantitative things are equal then what is entailed by one of them is entailed by the other.

This determination furnishes proof for further of Euclid's axioms, known as common notions. The concerned are

1. *Things which are equal to the same thing are equal,*
2. *If equals be added to equals, the sums are equal,*

and

3. *If equals be subtracted from equals, the remainders are equal.*

The equals and equal things can be understood to be quantitative ones, and matters tantamount to these axioms were indicated above with regard to identity (facing p. last par.). While identity allows the likes of these axioms to apply to all things regarding anything, however, the above displayed principle assures that they apply to quantitative ones even if the equality is not selfsameness.

Before specific confirmation, a word on some entailment. As

noted earlier (p.33 fourth par.), definitions are sometimes thought to be logically true, of entailment, because held to speak of properties a thing by its nature always has. But things were seen not always so defined, and the more general issue instead is that properties can be entailed by things by postulate, through definition or otherwise, rather than by inference. One example was the definition that 4 equals 3 + 1, intrinsically true as long as the digits stand for the numbers in question. Another, nondefinitional, example was that one geometric figure, e.g. an angle, equal another.

How these remarks pertain can be seen regarding the first above axiom. The axiom is true by the before italicized principle since by it, if both *A* and *C* are equal to *B*, what is entailed by *B* is entailed by equal *A*, namely being equal to C. If "A = B = C" represents "2 + 2 = 3 + 1 = 4" then "B = C" is a definition. Yet in accord with the preceding it can be regarded as entailment, although since concerning selfsameness, it is not an issue here. But a more pertaining situation occurs if "A = B = C" refers to angles assumed in that order equal.

In the other two axioms the additions or subtractions can be viewed as parts of equal assumptions, from which by the above principle follow the equal sums or remainders.

The remaining axioms of Euclid can be regarded as definitions.

4. *Things which coincide are equal,*

and

5. *The whole is greater than the part.*

The equality in the first of these has to do with geometric shapes, noted to be meant equal by their appropriate coinciding (p.130 third par.). As to the last axiom, it was likewise indicated that a part is meant to be less than a whole (p.122 first par.). There is likely no dispute that correspondingly the whole is more, greater, than the part, although it can be justifiably asked whether "less" and "more" are reciprocal.

This because the thoughts behind the use of the words may differ, and, as in other inferences, it is to be determined whether the things thought of imply each other. With respect to "less" and "more" such a difference was already indicated (e.g. p.164 sixth and seventh pars.). For "Amount *A* is less then amount *B*" one can be held to view *A* first, to find it to be contained in *B*, and some amount outside it to be contained in *B* as well; and for "Amount *B* is more than amount *A*" one can be held to first view *B*, to find not all of it to be contained in *A*, but not some amount outside it to be contained in *B* either. The equivalence of the two relations is without saying quite evident, as made by the already found very serviceable diagram at left, but it can nevertheless be regarded as a

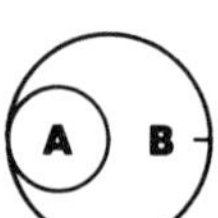

deductive principle.

If amount A *is less than amount* B *then* B *is more than* A, *and conversely.*

As is clear from all said about these relations, the principle can also be deduced by usual logic. "All *A* is *B*", half of "less", is by transposition equivalent to "All *'B* is *'A*" and hence by complement to " '(Some *'B* is *A*)", half of "more"; and "Some *'A* is *B*", the other half of "less", is by complement equivalent to " '(All *'A* is *'B*)" and hence by transposition, since "All *B* is *A*" is by it equivalent to "All *'A* is *'B*", to " '(All *B* is *A*)", the other half of "more".

The reciprocity between "less" and "more" is only one of those that can be seen as deductive. These are best known when the relation is the same in both directions, the mutuality called symmetry or commutativity. That of addition and multiplication in mathematics is the most familiar.

$$a + b = b + a,$$

and

$$a \times b = b \times a.$$

By addition being commutative is more particularly meant that whichever of two numbers is counted first, the total will be the same. This is a consequence of the more general principle that a given number of things, perhaps that total, will be the same whatever the order of counting them. This in turn holds because of the very postulating of a given number of things. The amount of units is postulated to remain during the counting, in whichever order. It is not meant that during the counting some unit is added or subtracted, to result in a different count.

Any quantity is more generally determined in accordance with some standard, which in counting is the number sequence. To count things, they are considered in what is called one-to-one correspondence with the numbers, and to postulate the things to remain of an amount, in whatever order counted, means just that they so correspond. While the number sequence as a standard enjoys quite an unchanging status since a mental entity, other standards, such as measuring tapes, may undergo change, if only in direction used, similar to the order in things counted. Nonetheless any standard as well as the quantity it is used for stay conceptually the same if postulated to, in whatever manner the first determines the second. If in reality a quantity determined should differ according to that manner, then a change occurred in the standard or quantity.

The preceding is germane to the in the last chapter investigated relativity of motion, when considered only as change in position (p.77 last par.). The position means the placement of one thing relative to another, this determined by distances in usually three dimensions. If then there is a change in those distances for one object relative to another, the question is whether the same change occurred for the other object relative to the first. The distances are regarded as measured from one of the objects in one case, and from the other object in the other case. But by the above the same distances as well as measuring means are assumed in question, the sameness decided by the very correspondence of one to the other. Therefore the same change in distances, to wit motion, is measured relative to either object.

Whereas it may be held self-evident that addition or measurement is commutative, that the same is true of multiplication is in textbooks sometimes supported by diagrams. Thus if a horizontal row of three things is multiplied vertically twice, the depicted reveals that a vertical column of two things is multiplied horizontally thrice.

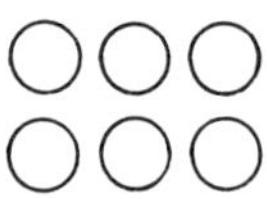

The requirement of proof is in this regard, too, attempted to be skirted by redefinition. Multiplication has been defined in terms of the product of two, or more, numbers. But it is not answered whether the product is the same for *a* × *b* and *b* × *a*. And as in other cases, the proof can also be obtained logically, on the basis of, rather than a numerical diagram, meaning behind language. By "2 times 3" it is not meant that, perhaps, only the third of three things is counted twice, but that each of three things is. Generally, by *a* times *b* is meant *a* of each unit of *b*. That is to say *a* is counted as many times as units of *b*, namely *a* is counted *b* times, or, there is counted *b* times *a*.

Symmetries like these are in logic also held deductive for what are called conjunction and disjunction, "*A* and *B*" and "*A* or *B*", as equivalent respectively to "*B* and *A*" and "*B* or *A*". The latter equivalence can in accord with earlier observations indeed be viewed as deductive. "*A* or *B*" can be taken to mean " '*A* implies *B*", equivalent by transposition to " '*B* implies *A*" and hence "*B* or *A*". By "*A* and *B*" is, however, normally meant no implicational connection, it being merely stated regardless of sequence that both things signified by the letters are the case. "*B* and *A*" is thought to be equivalent deductively in accordance with truth tables, which, as will be seen concerning other principles as well, only restate, however, that both expressions are meant true when both *A* and *B*, in either sequence, apply.

A lack of implicational connection does not pertain, however, to the identity in the last theorem (p.165), with identity, mutual attribution, a form of implication. Whether

If A *is identical with* B *then* B *is identical with* A

could correspondingly be questioned. Indeed by what was observed (e.g. p.166 first par.) the two halves of the symmetry represent different thoughts. The first is that upon viewing *A*, by the attribute concerned, one finds it to be *B*, and not some '*A* to be *B* also; and the second thought is the reverse. It can hence be asked whether one implies the other, and the affirmative answer is of course manifest without such analysis, or even a diagram like that of Figure III.8 (p.165). If desired the implication is available by usual deduction, through complements and transposition.

The symmetry thus applies to equivalence as well, seen as an instance of identity (p.166 third par.), and it does to mathematical equality likewise. For when that equality is not of identity but of comparison, it is still conceived in the described manner, by which e.g. in angles through superposition all of the one amount and not some of another is seen as concurring with the second, and so forth, as would a corresponding inequality be conceived similarly to described "less" and "more".

About symmetry or, as called in this case, conversion, is also the last theorem to be in this chapter featured. It is principally of attributive logic and does not speak of previous "all", including the unitary, but of "some" alone.

THEOREM III.9. *When some* A *is* B *then some* B *is* A.

Proof. Figure III.9.

The circles are believed again to require four more diagrams, depicted, the last one here adjusted as previously (p.153). But it is enough to consider that at least one *A*, among any number, is a *B*, among any number, to see the theorem hold.

Once more, the theorem can be deduced by way of others. "Some *A* is *B*" is by complement equivalent to " '(All *A* is '*B*)", which by transposition, since "All *B* is '*A*" is by it equivalent to "All *A* is '*B*", is equivalent to "'(All *B* is '*A*)", which by complement is equivalent to "Some *B* is *A*".

The theorem is likely not to need a counterpart in existential logic, in which "Some *A* is joined by *B*" would be expressed by "*A* does not imply '*B*". The comparable, as expounded, is not strictly the case in attributive logic, where the denial of "All *A* is '*B*" need not lead to "Some *A* is *B*" (e.g. p.153 last par.). If this seems ignored here in recent notations, it is because either the needed qualification was met, or because '*A* or '*B* was used

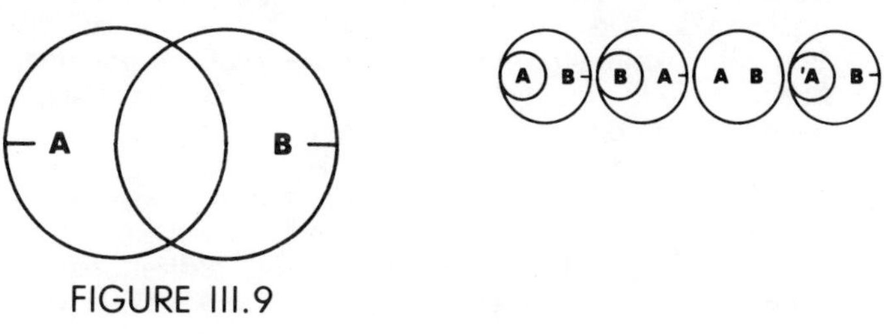

FIGURE III.9

for the exhaustive *'(A)* or *'(B)*. "Some" as explained (p.157 last par.) has besides a more independent significance in attribution than in implication, the present theorem having utility accordingly.

The theorem has been argued to, aside from mentioned like arguments on "some" altogether, require the existence of its subjects. It was rightly maintained that from "Should any *A* exist then some is *B*" does not follow "Should any *B* exist then some is *A*". If no *A* exists but *B* does, the premise can be true, as when *A* is always *B*, but the conclusion cannot. But it was wrongly maintained that the meaning of the theorem cannot be on the order of "When *A* can be *B* then *B* can be *A*". To say that *A* can be *B*, it is contended, is not to say that some *A* is actually *B*. The issue is again, however, not the meaning that expressions may in certain usage have, but what sort of meaning is of concern. And as already indicated regarding propositions used in logical principles, "some" is meant to have, like "all" and other things concerned, an extremely wide application, for all of which the principles hold.

The crux of that meaning of "some" is its herein oft mentioned denial of an "all". "All" was meant, further, to apply to, from all conceivable things of logical principles, to worldly things in causal laws, to particular things of a place or time of any limit. "Some *A* is *B* need accordingly not refer to the denial of "All *A* is *'B*" in an existing situation, although it may. It can refer to the denial of a supposed timeless law of nature. In that event there may be no *A* which is *B*, and it is as appropriate to say "*A* can be *B*" as "Some *A* is *B*".

This broad equating of "some" with "can", with possibility, is in accord with the earlier description of possibility in terms of "some" or "sometime" (p.36 last par.), alongside the description of necessity in terms of "all" or "always" (p.35 third par.). The respective identifying of these meanings with each other, alluded to later also (e.g. p.104 third par.), is indeed suitable for logical purposes.

The second of these identities, one between "all" and the necessary, has likewise been argued against by adducing existential import. An example offered of the necessary has ironically to do with causal rather than supposed logical law. It is that all brakeless trains are unsafe, which, although none exists, can be held true, with the denial false. It is proposed that the same cannot be said of an ordinary "all" proposition. As one reason is cited the mentioned (p.149 third par.) interpretation of propositions as true if the subject does not exist. In that case anything asserted of it is alleged true, and hence a breakless train would be both unsafe and safe. It is further asserted that should propositions be true only if the subject exists (p.115

second par.), the train would be neither safe nor unsafe. It may be remarked again that the alternative meanings of truth or falsity thus submitted seem quite remote from the ordinary meaning, the more so since they are multiple, and hence each meaning cannot be the accepted one. Most of all, what is meant by "all" depends on the intent, and the present one appears much like the customary one.

"All" is commonly used as broadly as found feasible herein, frequently relating to timeless laws without regard to the existence of instances, as in the case of the brakeless train. Correspondingly there is no need to differentiate in logic between such, universal, propositions and necessary ones. As a matter of fact universal ones, as exemplified by causal laws, are customarily about timeless connections, above associated with the necessary. Even singular ones can be regarded as belonging to the necessary, which was observed in the first chapter to be spoken of with reference to any fact.

Likewise observed was that the possible refers to the negation of the negative forms of these, of the impossible, or, as the unnecessary, to their own negation. This is the identity with "some" in the preceding, applying even to limited negation discussed, since "Some *A* is *'B*" like "Some *A* is *'(B)*" denies mostly timeless principles, confined to certain things C. For example some numbers (*A*) are odd (*'B*) rather than even (*B*), all confined to whole numbers (C). "Some" understood thus as the denial of also timeless principles, the last theorem (p.171) refers in the relation between *A* and *B*, as in previous ones, not only to actual states, past or present, but to potential future ones as well. When the relation concerns actuality then "some" indeed speaks of existing things, not merely possible ones, since denying the opposite actual "all", but when denying a constant principle then the relation need be possible only.

This broad understanding of "some" along with "all" of course also enters the laws of complements (pp.148, 149), which is why the possible itself was explicated (p.36 last par.) through those laws. In its wide sense it had to do among them with both, Theorems III.4.iii and III.4.iv. The first by equating the possible, if something is not impossible, with its having been the case; and the second and more pertinent by equating the possible, if something is not impossible, with its sometime, including always, being the case, or with its simply not being precluded in the inclusive sense here of "some".

In this sense "Some *A* is *B*" as depicted in now concerned Figure III.9 (p.171) may merely state something not precluded by a principle in the future, and the figure discloses that should the stated become true, then as in other cases "Some *B* is *A*" is true likewise.

The figure can also serve for elucidating a matter in the first proposition of Euclid. In it two circles are so constructed that the circumference of each passes through the center of the other. It has been put forward that the proposition assumes without support that the circles intersect. That they in fact do is confirmed by the diagram, and it need only be repeated that all deduction is confirmed perceptually. The intersecting can also, as was the case with other principles in mathematics, be deduced by logical means.

Each of the circles extends inside the other, since passing through its center. And each circle extends outside, since its diameter as a straight line does from that center (p.129 third par.). Since both circles are by definition, further, closed figures, of closed circumference with the inside meant to be on one side and the outside on the other, each circumference, being continuous, passes the other somewhere, to therefore intersect it.

In view of the deducibility by logical means of the preceding and earlier mathematical propositions it can be asked, as it has been in the past, whether all of mathematics is so deducible.

In efforts to prove that it is, it has been tried to define numbers in logical terms. It is not necessary, however, that something be a logical concept in order that inferences about it be logical. Logical inferences are made about anything. In this light it should not come as a surprise to find those definitional attempts unsuccessful. For example it is thought that to state, through a connection herein discussed, that every *A* implies one and the same *B*, i.e. that there is exactly one *B* concerned, is accomplished by saying "*A* implies *B*, and if *A* implies also something C then C is identical with *B*". The *B* need not be a single one, however, the statement amounting to saying that *A* implies only *B*. Another effort to subsume mathematics under logic is depending on the omission of definitions, rather than on unavailing ones. Algebraic notations for addition and multiplication, for instance, are left open to other interpretations, e.g. disjunction and conjunction in logic (p.170 fourth par.). Finding that the different contents share properties such as commutativity, it is felt that they consequently consist in the same logic. The shared properties like commutativity, however, need themselves be substantiated, and the question is whether they can logically.

Indeed all mathematical, and other, deduction is performable in accordance with principles of logic. The fact is suggested by apprehensions that appear more common than ones of those principles. They are that certain inferences, as determined by single and often amusing counterexamples (p.77 last par.), are fallacious, in awareness that conclusions that do not follow from premises logically do not otherwise. To examine the matter it will be well to first see better what comprises logical deduction.

In this treatise as in other works a distinction has been made between a logic based fundamentally on implication and one based on attribution. Having noted, however, that attribution is an instance of implication (p.151 third par.), it may also be observed that insofar as the attributional principles parallel the implicational ones, they are likewise true as instances of them.

This is not obvious, for because one kind of thing implies some other it need not be as in attribution one of them. But since implication can be so broad as to be about association of one kind of thing with another within any boundary, including the boundary of the other kind by being one of them, its principles can be read as applying to the boundary at issue. For instance the transitivity of implication can be read as applying to attribution, provided the boundaries within which things are associated are identically their own.

Such a procedure is not the most practicable, with attribution viewed so distinctly as to be favorable stated separately. There were seen other characteristics peculiar to it. Reference to only some of things in statements of it, or a limited meaning of negation, due to the same lasting attachment of many attributes. But what matters is that the two logics deal with any association of one thing with another, with the negation of any of these parts or wholes, and with what in like form follows or does not from any of these parts or wholes.

Accordingly returning to the question whether all deduction can be logical, it can be considered that most things deduced from and deduced can be viewed as associations of one thing with another, rather than as independent units. They are customarily called premises and conclusions. As observed in the introduction and afterward, in seeking knowledge one wishes to find not only what can be known regarding things known, what facts are connected with other facts, but what can be known regarding any concept. In order that findings of facts be made, as in induction or deduction, the concepts were seen to require eduction, usually expressed by definitions. The definitions, seen as fully statements in inferences, thus reflect how almost everything is regarded not independently, but as an association of one thing—here a thing considered, perhaps by a name—with another—here defining attributes, perhaps recalled.

The explanation for these connections may be found in, for the discussed sake of one's pursuits, one's interest in things true in connection with things, even if only identifying attributes are at issue. Subsequent connections may typically be that a thing of given attributes exists, and that it is causally accompanied by some other thing. But the connections, the accompaniments, can be of limitless variety, and of present interest is that they all fall under the equally unlimited accompaniments referred to in logical principles, and which generalized are about whether or not one thing is associated with another.

The associations occur, as expounded, within certain limits, in accordance with which it might be revealingly said that the time or place of one thing is a time or place of the other. Inasmuch as the associations thus concern the same placement of the things, possibly their selfsameness, logical principles regarding them are about whether or not these placements entail certain others.

Logical principles were seen for that matter, in the laws of thought as represented by the law of double negation, not only about what is entailed by placements of one thing with another, but also about what is entailed by individual things as wholes. The things can be viewed as above concepts of which something is yet to be asserted, but they can also be any fact as a unit, without regard to its parts. What is of account is, however, that logical principles about them are likewise about whether their placements entail others.

As observed regarding transposition, an entailment is itself an association, by which the place of what entails is a place of what is entailed, e.g. the place of *A* is the place of ''*A*. When the entailment is not by one thing but by combined things, of presumably things likewise combined, then the difference between those combinations and the entire one is likely that the former are of things within narrower limits. Thus if transposition is applied to causal laws, the entire principle is of nature as place of the association stated, whereas the premise and conclusion are of the, spatial or temporal, vicinity in which the cause and effect, or their absence, occur, as place of these associations. Of significance is that beside the placements with one thing of another respectively represented by premises and conclusions of deductions, when the premises or conclusions do not set down undivided, but combinations of, things as of those places then those combinations are likewise placements of one thing with another.

Those combinations as well as the deductions are, as indicated, the stuff of statements, of concerned assertions of facts, whereby one thing is connected with another, in contrast to concepts as denoted by individual words. Accordingly all deductions are about determinations of placements or their absences, whether again of undivided things or of combined things placed with each other. But such determinations were seen the province of logic, as displayed graphically by the diagrams. They disclose whether or not one thing is placed with another, be the placement only the larger one, of the deduced from with the deduced, or also the smaller one, of something else in addition.

The pertinent factor in the last sentence is that logic informs of, about what is posited, beside what follows, what does not. By saying that it informs of the last it is meant, as indicated, that logic reveals that what does not follow in accordance with it does not follow at all. That logic indeed performs this function may in accord with the preceding be further elucidated.

The disclosure by diagrams of spoken of placements were seen to result from placements posited. When placements in question are not disclosed, it is because the placements posited, known, are not adequate. Thus from knowing only that all *A* is *B* one cannot detect that all *B* is *A*, because the placements can vary as pictured. It may then be asked whether in specific cases one cannot deduce placements in question without knowing more placements than posited. The point is that if one knows added placements required in logic then the deduction can be logical, but that it cannot be if made without that knowledge.

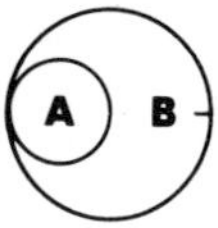

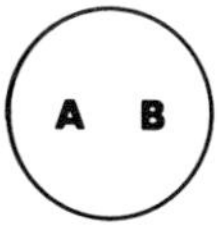

But the sufficiency of the logical information has the same grounding whether it is about what follows from something or what does not. As it can be ascertained through diagrams that if certain placements are known then certain others follow regardless of what the things so placed, so it can be ascertained that if only certain placements are known then certain others do not follow regardless of what the things. The certainty rests on the referred to impossibility to conceive the matter otherwise, in one case than that an inference follows, and in the other case than that it does not, whatever the things concerned.

With knowledge of premises from which conclusions can be logically deduced thus required, therefore, anything deducible from something is so in accordance with logical principle.

The significance is that anything that follows from what is known is by logical steps discoverable, the placements known needing only to be appropriately assembled to perceive resulting ones. The assembly of pertinent premises can nonetheless be quite difficult and the desired conclusions not reached. The task is simplified, however, by the explained reducibility of logic to associations of one thing with another. For this reason there is no need to construct further systems of logic, as is done with regard to spoken of modality, relations, and more. All the concerned particulars of things, their presence at issue in researches, can be treated as just mentioned associations with those things, deriving consequences as expounded.

The dispensability of additional logics does not mean that for clarity a particular application cannot be formulated. This happened when attribution was singled out as a case of implication, it being unlikely that when attribution is meant it will be understood from speaking implication. A distinction between the two connections was noted also made in what are known as propositional and predicate logics. Because much of them is accepted and they suffer from fundamental weaknesses indicated, added attention to them is warranted.

Beginning with the first of these and the concept of implication central to it, it can again be noted that, known as material, an implication, "*A* implies *B*", is held true if *A* is false or *B* true, i.e. under all conditions other than if *A* is true and *B* false (p.151 third and fourth pars.). The spoken of inconsistency of that meaning with the general one is magnified by its usually understood reference to the present as the time *A* or *B* is true or false. Most implications have to do with connections holding at all times, as would be expressed by "When . . . then", and they are hence the less determined by a situation of the present, related to their frequent designation by "If . . . then".

As also alluded to, there has been dissatisfaction in logic with that definition, and another, for what is termed strict implication, has been proposed. It states that "*A* implies *B*" holds not if it is merely false that *A* is true and *B* false, but if it is impossible that *A* be true and *B* false. The definition appears to take care of the above deficiency as to permanence, although the meaning of impossibility and related terms is not made clear. The sought after connection between *A* and *B*, however, was found to still be lacking. If *A* is independently impossible or *B* necessary then the definition applies.

Both definitions in the last two paragraphs also contain the discrepancy that while by them either of "If *A* . . . then" or "When *A* . . . then" are true if *A* is not or cannot be true, either of the expressions assumes *A* as condition. In other words, the purport is that supposing *A* is false, then supposing it is true, such and such follows. Such contradictory suppositions were seen illegitimate, leading to paradoxes and not representing reality.

A paradoxical nature, though not in the same sense, is of these definitions asserted in logic, because of their omission of a tie normally expected between two things when one implies the other. Attempts have been accordingly made for a further definition of implication, one that, as suggested earlier, is thought to require an inner, logical, tie in order to possess any. But what the logical tie, called spoken of entailment and by which one thing is deducible from another, is is itself debated, and as to be seen in truth tables, by which deducibility is held determined, the meaning employed belongs to none other than those found unsatisfactory.

It is also advanced that any essayed definition of entailment, or of other implication involving the tie looked for, faces difficulties similar to the others. The argument in simple form is that for such a definition of implication it is reasonable to state that

1. A *implies (*A *or* B*),*

with *B* standing for anything, and

2. *(*A *or* B*) implies (*'A *implies* B*).*

Taken is then for example the law of contradiction, *Not both* A *and* 'A, which implies by statement 1 that *(Not both* A *and* 'A*) or* B, and hence by statement 2 *(Both* A *and* 'A*) implies* B. The last inferred signifies that something false would imply anything, since any fact in place of the law of contradiction as sample would be denied there. The error can be detected without recourse to a sample.

The undesired result follows by transitivity from statements 1 and 2 directly, by which *A* implies (*'A* implies *B*). Statement 2 was in fact seen true by definition of "or" as "Not to find one is to find the other" (p.143 last par.), and hence statement 1 can be held to in effect say that *A* implies (*'A* implies *B*), giving a very meaning of implication not intended.

The intention indeed when equating "*A* implies *B*", or "*A* is *B*", with "*'A* or *B*", and "Not both *A* and *'B*", was noted to be a certain connection between *A* and *B*, rather than a concern with their independent status (ca. p.149). The connection was observed to be that *B* accompanies within certain bounds *A* but not all things (e.g. p.152 first par.). Accordingly the accompaniment cannot occur if *A* implies everything under *'A*, or, the equivalent, if everything implies *B* under *B*. Should *A* imply everything then there is no restriction to the boundary, and all things would imply the same things; the like result is explicit should everything imply *B*. The gist of this reasoning is that by contradiction the intended connection cannot become true because *'A* or *B* is true. Generally, if implication is defined by a connection between things, the connection cannot contradictorily be deduced absent.

The attention in logic to material implication, meant decided by an independent truth value of *A* or *B*, is, alongside a comparable meaning of "or" and "not both", owing to its use in truth tables, for believed validation of logical theorems. For present illustration of truth tables, as well as for other purposes, implication in general,

A implies *B*,

can be symbolized by means of the earlier arrow (p.163), as

i. $A \rightarrow B.$

The truth table of Table 1 would accordingly be held to demonstrate Theorem III.5 (p.159).

A	B	(A	→	B)	→	('B	→	'A)
+	+	+	+	+	+	−	+	−
−	−	−	+	−	+	+	+	+
−	+	−	+	+	+	−	+	+
+	−	+	−	−	+	+	−	−

TABLE 1

The variables, as indicated, are regarded as standing for propositions though more accurately they would stand for their truth, or falsity, since it is these which are in question. More generally these affirmations or negations were seen extendable to anything in a given domain, not only to propositions. It should hence be fitting to in the tables symbolize them by plus and minus signs for general presence or absence, instead of by frequent ones for truth and falsity only.

In the arrangement then the theorem, as seen, is above the horizontal line, to the right of the vertical line. To its left, *A* and *B* are assigned beneath them all their combined truth values in corresponding rows. Across them the corresponding truth value is then first marked for each occurrence of *A* and *B* in the theorem; for instance with the first assignment for *A* and *B*, true and true, the truth values under *'B* and *'A* are marked false. After, the truth values of the next larger units of the theorem are marked, namely of the first and last implications; these truth values are what is determined in accordance with material implication, true in all cases other than when the premise is true and the conclusion false. Last, by the same criterion, the truth values of the central implication, the theorem, are marked; since true in each row, the theorem is concluded true.

It may be noted first that the truth tables avail themselves of the laws of thought without proving them. They do so in the first two columns, by assuming them exhaustive. Were it not for the laws of thought, there could be combinations in which a proposition is both true and false or neither. The laws are more conspicuously assumed under *'B* and *'A*, by holding them false when *A* and *B* are true, and true when they are false. The issue has been tried to be bypassed by recourse to definition, as observed to happen elsewhere (e.g. p.170 third par.). *"Not-A"* has been defined as true when *A* is false, and false when *A* is true. It is not answered, however, whether, provided when *A* is false it is designated *"not-A"*, *not-A* is in fact false when *A* is true.

It may also be repeated that since the premise of the theorem assumes *A*, its later denials are inconsistent, and likewise for the other assumed conditions in the theorem. But the principal error lies in the conclusion that the theorem is true because it, the central implication, is true under each condition listed.

To begin, although in the theorem the premise is maintained to imply the conclusion in some sense other than merely because the former is false or the latter true, those were seen the reasons why the connection is considered to hold. Relatedly, the notion that a logical principle be true if, by whatever criterion, true under all truth conditions of its variables like *A* and *B* is fallaciously substituted for its truth regardless of what the variables stand for. This truth is the intent of those principles, meant to be true in, as said, all possible worlds.

The truth tables would even in compliance with their procedure not require the result of all truth combinations of their variables. This because the theorems, in implication form, are meant to assert that when the premises are true so are the conclusions. In Table 1 it is hence only required that by its arguments when $A \rightarrow B$ is true so is $'B \rightarrow 'A$, regardless of the truth of the last row. It happens that the theorems would be true in the remaining rows, those of false premises, under which the implications are likewise meant to hold.

To see what theorems so derived actually assert, however, it will be advisable to reexamine the table. In it, as in other truth tables, the theorem asserts through chosen symbols what is asserted underneath it. There its variables and their negations are either affirmed or denied in accordance with the first assumed combinations and laws of thought. In other words it is asserted by those marks that if *A* or *B* are true or false then they are and their negations are not, in effect restating the assumed or laws of thought. The rest of the marks assert whether or not combinations of the affirmations and denials of the variables are termed implications, as symbolized by the theorem. In other words the theorem says no more than that given certain truth combinations of *A* and *B*, those or those due to laws of thought hold, all nameable as in the theorem.

The same occurs in other truth tables, and it is consequently not surprising that logical theorems, thought to be demonstrated by them, be called tautologies. But the demonstration does not take place, even of, as remarked, laws of thought. Whereas the combinations of truth or falsity may, by a definition of symbols for them, resemble in table 1 the law of transposition, they do not prove it as it is intended to be understood. The actual law refers in its conclusion primarily to truth or falsity of a time other than in the premise. Instead the table refers to the same time only, the compass of the laws of thought. These laws in fact are confined to the same place as well, so as not to result in the conclusion of transposition even when of the same time but different place, the least such difference comprehended by that principle.

This is not to speak of the explicated revealing connections to which the theorems are expected to apply. Should the central implication be somehow revealing it would only be about the material implications of its premise and conclusion, not about others intended. Moreover while by the meaning of those implications and laws of thought the conclusion, since the required combinations for it result, does follow from the premise, it does not by the criterion of the truth table. By it the central implication is as noted true because of the independent truth values of the premise or conclusion, a criterion insufficient for deducibility of the latter from the former.

The theorems in the truth tables often resemble those valid in the usual sense, since they can in that event be considered offshoots of the others. Thus in the present theorem in Table 1 the material implications within the premise and conclusion signify only that, for instance, not both *A* and *'B* can at the time in question be true, the other truth alternatives diversified. But this condition obtains also in normal implication applied to a specific time, since "*A* implies *B*" was seen equivalent there to "Not both *A* and *'B*". The revealing connection discussed is applicable, because while *A* may be accompanied by *B* at all times, other things may not, but the connection may be mere coexistence. And by regular transposition, redundantly, if "Not both *A* and *'B*" is true at the time, so is "Not both *'B* and *A*". That is to say that as a consequence the curtailed premise in the truth table implies the like conclusion in it, and the same holds correspondingly for other theorems.

However, whereas theorems true otherwise may be true in accordance with truth tables, though because of expanded senses unproved by them, theorems true in accordance with truth tables can because of the same curtailment not be true otherwise, hence being false, since interpreted in the usual sense. Table 2 offers an example.

A	B	A	→	(B	→	A)
+	+	+	+	+	+	+
−	−	−	+	−	+	−
−	+	−	+	+	−	−
+	−	+	+	−	+	+

TABLE 2

The theorem could as before be by the criteria employed held to be true merely because when the premise is true the conclusion is, needing only the truth of the first and last rows beneath the theorem. But what would be a theorem should by now be manifest as of a familiar definition.

It is a definition by which if something, *A*, is true then everything, *B*, implies it, and which was indicated as objected to by the users themselves of truth tables. Table 2 indeed, as will now be clear, repeats, through its markings, that definitional statement. The conclusion is marked true whenever *A* in it, and in the premise, is. So are of that definition the other rows.

The supposed theorem does accordingly obviously not apply when the concluded is a customary implication, the connection which can be taken to be of interest in logical principles. That connection was expounded to require that not everything imply the implied. The theorem can be read to say that when something *A* is the case then everything *B* is accompanied by it, an accompaniment not suited for implication, and the theorem appears more absurd still if considering that most implications are about timeless laws, while the *A* as condition in it is of any one time. Perhaps most glaringly is the theorem false since implication is commonly taken to hold between things somehow closely associated as discussed, to have in conclusion *B* → *A* of the presumed theorem nothing to do with a fact of *A* in the premise.

That in truth tables one thing be held to imply another under all conditions other than if the first thing is true and the other false is defended by contending no difference from the other implications in practice. In both cases, it is argued, if it is known that *A* implies *B*, then at a time in question it is certain that not both *A* and *'B*, though any other condition may be true. That is to say that should at the time *'A* be true it is held merely a trivial convenience if hence by definition *A* implies *B*, since the law would not be in effect. The reasoning again commits, however, the ordinary fallacy of affirmation of the consequent, long cautioned about in logic itself. Because in either meaning if *A* implies *B* then at a time it need merely be true that not both *A* and *'B*, it does not follow that if at a time it is merely true that not both *A* and *'B* then *A* implies *B* in either meaning. That is the truth tables cannot, by deciding from merely not both *A* and *'B* one kind of implication for which the theorems are to hold, decide the same of an other kind.

The inappropriateness of truth tables deprives of an accepted procedure for deciding whether a supposed logical principle is valid. Such a procedure is understandably valued and, as indicated earlier (p.111 fifth par.), thought to be often impossible. But it was herein actually supplied by diagrams, and even when theorems were instead formally deduced, a like perception that they follow from others was seen utilized. It will be seen furthermore that, because the required principles are few, propositions stated in a symbolic language can be so connected that by scanning them, without the aid of diagrams, it can be decided what other propositions follow. The procedure as suitable for logic as a whole will be displayed upon surveying, next to preceding propositional logic, customary predicate logic.

The symbolic language used in that procedure can be quite simple, as it has as exemplified by form i (p.179) been for such as characteristic implication in propositional logic, but is not also in predicate logic. In it characteristic attribution is burdened by a complex symbolism, indicative of yet more excessiveness, attended likewise by inaccuracy.

Before considering the symbolism, it may be observed that the excessiveness and inaccuracy of such as at once assuming and denying the subject of a statement for supposed proofs in truth tables also enters diagrammatic proofs accepted in predicate logic.

As truth tables first listed all truth combinations of *A* and *B*, things connected in implication, so do these diagrams first depict all combinations of attributes *A* and *B* and their absences, things connected in attribution. How many the things connected depends on the theorem tested by the method, and the present diagram depicts the combinations when, in assuming in the theorem two connections before an inferred one, three attributes are given, *A*, *B*, and C. This occurs in discussed transitivity and syllogisms, for the last of which the diagrams are mainly used, by connecting *A* with *B* in one premise, *B* with C in another, and *A* with C in a conclusion.

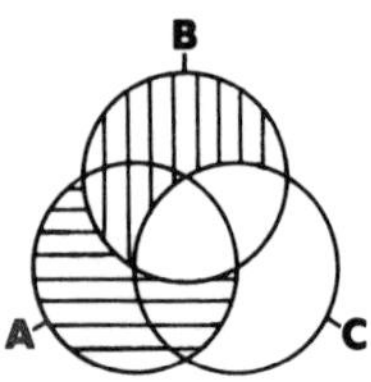

Correspondingly the circles in the diagram stand as marked for *A*, *B*, and C, with the area outside of either its negation as usual. The compartments resulting where the circles overlap, as well as the other areas when negations are included, then stand for the combinations mentioned. For instance the area outside the diagram stands for things neither *A* nor *B* nor C. An initial defect lies in these negations, because not all were seen to exhaust after affirmation all things. Of some things an attribute can be neither affirmed nor denied.

The diagram would thus be used to verify the transitivity principle (p.164). By its first premise it is determined that nothing is both *A* and *not-B*, and the area for that combination is shaded out (horizontal lines). Likewise by the second premise it is determined that nothing is both *B* and *not*-C, with the area shaded out (vertical lines). It is then observed that every *A* not shaded out is a C, to arrive at the conclusion of the principle. Before more it can here, too, be noted that e.g. the laws of thought are utilized without proof. Although "Nothing is both *A* and *B*", or " '(Some *A* is *B*)", can be said to mean "All *A* is

'(B)" (p.154 last par.), that the equivalence holds if *B* and *'(B)* are interchanged is an inference through *'('(B))*.

To proceed it can be observed that the unshaded areas of the circles depict the very premises as depicted in Figure III.7 (p.163), those areas as standing for the lettered entities sufficing for the conclusion in the first place. Therein can be found the inconsistent affirmation and negation of a subject at the same time. *A*, the subject of "*A* is *B*", is first signified by a circle, only to have a portion by shading repealed, and the same happens to *B*, the subject of "*B* is *C*". All of this is to say that the construction of all described combinations, and the subsequent deletion of some of them, is superfluous, as was superfluous the completion of all the rows in truth tables, were they of the desired utility. This may be the more appreciated on considering that when many circles or their substitutes are at issue the diagrams become impracticable.

They were thought an improvement over Euler diagrams (p.140 third par.) because seemingly disposing of the several believed required to disclose most conditions in theorems. The conditions in the present one were seen to admit four diagrams (p.163) for all pertaining connections, held to be wanting depiction. The now pictured diagram, however, is with that of Figure III.7 equally without three of those connections, e.g. the identity of *A*, *B* and *C*, and to supply them furthermore conceptually in the last depiction is, unlike in Figure III.7, hampered by the prearranged compartmentalization.

The same is accordingly the case in all such diagrams, which also are not as supposed the answer to disclosing spoken of existential import (e.g. p.150). As was remarked, under "some" in contrast to "all" the subject is unjustifiably restricted in logic to an existing one, since while "All *A* is *B*" is taken to signify that nothing is *A* and *not-B*, "Some *A* is *B*" is taken to signify that something is *A* and *B*. To so construe the meaning of the words has with other meanings of words been herein repeatedly pointed out to be an arbitrary matter, in this case particularly unsuitable for logical purposes, and in this case the peculiarity is that the sort of existence is not made clear, being applied to from a living one of a person to a mystical one of a number. The existence as regards "some" is in any event attempted to be worked into logical theorems, and in the diagrams now discussed a symbol for it is usually an x where some of one thing is premised to by overlapping be another.

In Figure III.9 (p.171) the overlap might thus be marked with an x, and indeed there is no hindrance to marking the more concise diagrams in this manner throughout if wished, for the same conclusions as in the more elaborate ones. As a matter of fact in the first diagrams the existence, if wished, could be understood from merely the partial overlap of two circles, with existence not admitted in full overlap of a circle, in "all" propositions. This cannot be done in the later diagrams, which for that matter would require regardless of existence a mark for "some" to avoid misreadings. Taking for example the premises "Some 'A is B" and "All B is 'C", chosen in the past for the very explanation of the diagrams now looked at, they can by diagrams herein used be pictured as at left. A conclusion is that some 'A is 'C. The other diagrams require the other depiction here. The only shaded area is, by the second premise, for things both B and C. As a result two partial overlaps of circles remain, none of which assures that some of one of the circles is of the other, existing or not, not to mention partial overlaps of circles with negations, or of negations with negations, these two kinds of overlaps figuring in the first premise and the conclusion. There is in consequence no choice but to mark the assertion of the first premise, that some 'A is B, regardless of existence. The conclusion sought, that some 'A is 'C, is, additionally, far from obvious. The first of these two diagrams, to be sure, has overlaps likewise not signifying connections, e.g. of A and B or 'B and 'C. But these are exactly the connections understood as undecided by the nature of the diagrams, which say no more than meant by overlaps of lettered circles. Should those connections be decided, appropriate marks can if need be be made, as were in Figures III.2 (p.144) and III.6 (p.160).

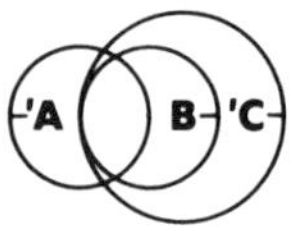

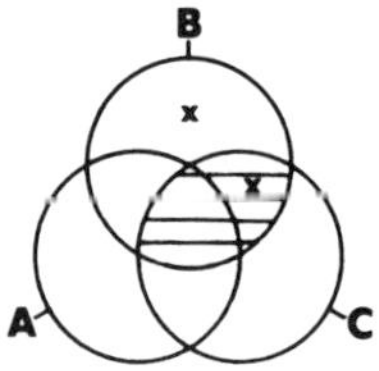

The foregoing notwithstanding, existential import is endeavored to be incorporated into the symbolism of predicate logic. In it

All *A* is *B*

would be symbolized by a less direct

ii. $(x)(Ax \rightarrow Bx)$,

read "For all things x, if x is A then x is B", and

Some *A* is *B*

similarly by

iii. $(Ex)(Ax \,\&\, Bx)$,

read "For something x, x is A and x is B".

The first of these—by speaking of things hypothetically A, not of A directly—suggests that there may be no A, and the second—by saying that something is A—declares that there is an A.

The existence in the last case is also signified by the E-like symbol, its parenthesized unit called existential quantifier and sometimes read "There exists something x such that". This quantifier and the universal one, of the parenthesized x in the other case, are meant to take the place of "some" and "all", but they refer, as seen, to x as a new subject, with A and B regarded as predicates, in after the quantifiers a reverse notation corresponding to one of mathematical functions.

The needless addition of these subjects is also argued required so as to distinguish them from those predicates, attributes. But as expounded in the first chapter (ca. p.38 through rest of chapter), no such distinction need be made. Things are indentified by attributes, and to say that a thing which is *A* is a thing which is *B* is no more than to say that an *A* is a *B*. And the addition of, generally quantified, variables like x for things as subjects is not an encumbrance alone. It is held that quantification of predicates like *A*, which normally are quantified subjects, belongs to logic of a higher order.

The ordering is related to the spoken of hierarchies of languages and classes, in belief that predicates somehow belong to a sphere beyond subjects, with a continuing order of predicates of predicates. The quantifiers discussed, however, are meant to already pertain to predicates, if *A* or *B* of the examples be so named. *(x)* and *(Ex)* speak in effect of all and some *A* respectively.

Their quantifying of things x instead results rather in unwanted meanings. "All" is not meant to be about singular propositions, those of a single *A*. Yet since the reference is to all things, hypothesizing some to be *A*, there may only be one *A*. Similarly "some" by referring to things in general, of which some are *A*, does not mean that all *A* may not be held to be *B*.

The hierarchical quantification of *A* or *B* as predicates, as do other quantifications, restates for the matter of that the understanding that the variables, as connoted by their name, stand for all things in the situation on hand. The axiom of mathematical induction (p.138 fourth par.) has thus been given in the form

iv. $(A)(a)(b)((A0 \,\&\, (Aa \rightarrow A(a+1))) \rightarrow Ab)$,

read "For all properties *A*, numbers *a*, and numbers *b*, if zero is *A* and if when *a* is *A* then *a* + *1* is *A*, then all numbers *b* are *A*". By quantifying all properties *A*, predicates, it is meant that the principle holds whatever the property may be. It is not meant that concerned are, as would be by the usual quantification, all things of a particular property, with *A* alongside standing for all properties. That it when used does, as in the preceding formula iv, is already understood by *A* as a variable.

The quantifier is hence redundant if not misleading, and so are the more frequently used ones for numbers. In iv it is equally understood by variables *a* and *b* that they concern any number in their place. The same redundancy occurs furthermore in the first of the two standard quantifications displayed (facing p., ii). By the variable x is already meant everything in the specified condition.

The second of those quantifications (facing p., iii) is correspondingly awkward. Not only x but *A* and *B* are variables which, as in theorems, stand for anything in whichever the situation. The traditional "all" and "some" does as indicated above not quantify those variables, but the specific thing they may among many stand for. In "All *A* is *B*" *A* and *B* speak of all kinds of things in that relation, and "all" speaks of all of a kind. In "Some *A* is *B*" *A* and *B* retain the universality of kinds, but "some", referring to those of a kind, does not. Accordingly, to use the last quantifier, along with the first, instead for variables, let alone ones more general than *A* and *B*, brings further disarray.

The use of the existential quantifier is also supposed justified by yet an additional workload imposed on the word "some". It has to do with relations other than that one thing is an attribute of another, relations alluded to (p.177 last par.) as basis of some systems of logic, although all deduction, as observed, can be achieved through the simple connections discussed.

One of the relations between two things would be symbolized by

v. $$(x)(Ey)(Rxy),$$

read "For all x and some *y*, x has relation *R* to *y*". The relation parallels the common universal proposition "All *A* is *B*", in which "some *B*" is tacit, which it can be with justice, since in the fact that *B*, *y*, is connected with each *A*, x, is implicit that some *B*, *y*, is, while no commitment is made as to whether all or another exact amount of them is in some way involved.

Despite that parallel, the relation *Rxy* in form v (this p.) is contrasted with those of *A*x or *B*x in ii and iii (p.186) by holding it to be dyadic, taking place between two kinds of things, and the others monadic, concerning only one kind of thing. Subject and predicate, represented by *A*x or *B*x, were observed, however, to likewise characterize two kinds of things accordable equal status, the two being of the relation that the first, or some of it, is included among the second.

In this relation furthermore the quantifications, thought to contrariwise serve the same function as in the relations now considered, do not. They were observed to redundantly or unsuitably quantify variables. In the present relations, however, the quantifications, though seeming to be of variables, are ones of all or some of a particular kind of thing represented by them. As in "All *A* is *B*", in "All x have relation *R* to *y*" all of a kind rather than all kinds referred to by *A* or x are meant. The appearance is false because x and *y* are used in place of *A* and *B*, in belief that it is not attributes that are dealt with.

It is thus erroneous to think that the relations presently considered expose an extension of the quantification used in predications like ii and iii and numerical iv. The present quanti-

fications are rather used in holding that through them, particularly those for "some", further logical distinctions can be expressed, as suggested on the last page. In scholastic logic it was noted that a statement of the form "All *A* have relation *R* to some *B*" can be taken to say either that each *A* has the relation to a different *B*, or that each *A* has the relation to the same *B*. The attempt was accordingly in modern logic to express the distinction by arrangement of quantifiers. It was felt that the second preceding interpretation, the sameness of *B* for each *A*, is clearer by speaking of *A* and *B* in reverse order, "To some *B* all *A* have relation *R*".
In the symbolism,

vi. $(Ey)(x)(Rxy)$,

"For some *y* and all *x*, *x* has relation *R* to *y*".

But the ambiguity of words does not obligate logic to symbolize every meaning. In the Middle Ages new logical consequences were sought by studying the subtleties of language, but as in other comparisons of words with fact, diversities in language do not signify diversities in logic. It would be observed about relations v and vi that the first follows from the second. But like other deduction this is true by the investigated standard logical principles. Since any *y* is by the meaning of "some" identical with some *y*, what is true of any *y* is true of some *y*. To wit if it is true that all *x* have relation *R* to any *y*, e.g. the same one, then they have the relation to some *y*.

In addition the arrangements of the quantifiers did not achieve the intended statements of sameness. The relations with the remaining arrangements are

vii. $(x)(y)(Rxy)$

and

viii. $(Ey)(Ex)(Rxy)$.

Exchanging somewhere *x* and *y* is not required. If exchanged either in the quantifiers or next to *R*, the relation will be passive, e.g. in v to all of one thing some of the other will have the relation; but the nature of the relation is beside the point, the interest being that any hold between things of quantifications as given. And if *x* and *y* are exchanged throughout, the result is merely a renaming.

The passivity of the second variable after *R* indicates that by vii is not meant mutuality of the relation, as in "*A* is identical with *B*"; such a relation would be given by adding an exchange of each *x* and *y*, a new statement since not independent, but not required here since of the same structure. Statement vii rather says that each *x* has the relation to each *y*, in a usual listing of all combinations of the quantifiers, as in previous combinations not necessarily required for the purpose. For the purpose of signifying or not by the arrangement that the same things of a kind are of a relation to things of another kind vii is not needed, for when all are of a relation to all, the same of each is always part, whatever the arrangement.

In contrast the notation employed is not adequate for the same purpose when some are of a relation to some, as in viii, which parallels the other common proposition, the particular "Some *A* is *B*". In viii, first quantifying *y* is to mean that the x have the relation to the same *y*. When the *y* may not be the same, they would accordingly be quantified after the x. Then the x, coming first, should be the same with respect to the *y*. As can be confirmed by the diagram, however, when the *y* are the same for the x, the x are for the *y*, and conversely of course, and hence it is never signified by the symbolism that the *y*, or the x, may not be the same, as they may.

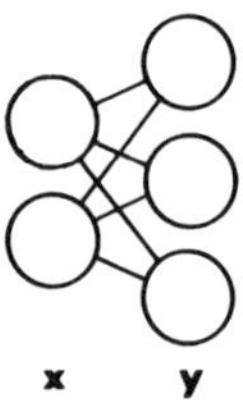

This result can as elsewhere be reached by customary deduction. By saying that the same thing is of a relation to a number of some other things is meant the same as merely saying that the thing, without speaking of its sameness, is of the relation to each of those things. Correspondingly, to say that some x have a relation to the same *y* means that each of those x has the relation to the same of each of those *y*, or by the last sentence simply to each of those *y*. By the same sentence therefore each of those *y* are of the relation to the same of each of those x, or simply to the same x. And since if one is the same for the other then the other is the same for the first, by transposition if one of these situations is not the case then neither is the other.

The additional overburdening of the term "some" by having it express beside spoken of existence sameness becomes thus a further barrier to its ordinary use, of quantifying a subject as not necessarily of "all", without regard to the sameness or existence.

Existence was seen (e.g. p.149 last par.) expressed as a matter of course independently of quantification, and plain signification of it is in fact available through customary symbolism. In propositional logic, in which variables stand for propositions, their truth is expressed simply by stating the variables. Variables were further, in theorems about them, seen applicable to any thing, its truth replaced by more general existence. And since the same variables were seen usable in predicate logic, existence in it can be expressed in the same simple way, by a variable alone. Quantification will be seen equally irrelevant to above sameness, as well as to distinctness, whose knowledge may be as desirable. Quantification can for that matter be largely done without altogether.

It was already observed how quantification of variables by

"all" is redundant, and how "some" is implicit in considering things, possibly negations. The latter quantification is usually made explicit only when the former is not necessarily the case but may otherwise be understood. It would be said "Some coal is browm" because "Coal is brown" would be understood to refer to all of it. This understanding suggests that not only variables but all universals, all words referring to more than one thing, could do without universal quantification, especially in a standardized logical language, where ambiguity is avoided.

In such a language the universals, names for particular kinds of things, were seen not even used but represented by variables, "All *A* is *B*" nonetheless not speaking of all things of the variable but all of the particular thing represented. There is obviously no problem in comprehending this, and neither should there be if the quantification is omitted, as done in implication. In it "*A* implies *B*" is understood to speak of all things of a kind as leading to some others, the variables in addition denoting all kinds to which the sentence may apply. Universal attribution can similarly be expressed by

A is *B*,

as was done on occasion herein before.

There is no need to worry about so-called indefinite propositions, like "Man is bearded", in which it may not be certain if all or some are at issue. It is the uncertainty by which things are qualified as some, which can for logical purposes be done by edict. If the speaker knows of the universality, the qualification can be omitted. The unqualifiedness of the above displayed expression also makes it useable for not only universals but individuals, as was implication in a broad sense.

As evidenced in this section, logical principles are often valid for multiple and single subjects alike, and the sole distinction will be disclosed to be that of the last section, that the complementariness of *B* and *'(B)* holds only for a single *A*. It does because an attribute denied of a single thing, as observed (e.g. p.143 second par.), is meant to be so fully, but not so with universal propositions. As in them, in their internally negative opposites the interest is in inclusive principles, not following from negation of internally affirmative ones, whereas the internally negative of a singular proposition is to merely state that the subject is other than stated by the internally affirmative, in equivalence to its negation. The equivalence was seen furthermore not to follow for the ordinary negative attribute, herein symbolized by *'B* as compared to *'(B)*. Similarly to the case of the universal *A*, the law that a single *A* is either *B* or *'B* does not hold unqualifiedly.

Most notable, since where the difference occurs it is of negated propositions, it is of little importance in customary deductions. For these deductions affirmative propositions, ones not negated and to which negated ones were in the last section seen convertible, will be found the ones of use.

These propositions were mentioned at the start of this section as of more interest, and they are the ones spoken of (p.183 last par.) as connectable in symbolic language, so as to enable easy inference. A suggestion of such inference is provided by the pursuits in general of man or animal. An affirmative proposition signifies knowledge that one thing may lead to another, which in turn may be known to lead to a further one and so forth, for inference of connections between remoter things. Deductions of this nature are made abundantly in all walks of life, including consciously deductive endeavors like geometry, without necessarily awareness of their conformance with logical principles. To avail oneself of the few basic principles can thus be regarded as preliminary to the predominance of other deduction, and it is primarily for that deduction that a simplified symbolism is of utility. Basic principles were observed to require conceptual substantiation instead.

Should it be insisted that they, too, be amenable to the symbolism, i.e. that the difference between universal and singular propositions be given by it, the difference can be additionally symbolized where of account. That is in an unquantified "*A* is *B*" *A* can normally be of any quantity, adding suitable symbolism if the quantity is wished specified. The difference for an individual *A* a logical exception, it is especially pointless to mark it where not needed.

It may be remarked that the difference between the singular and universal is thought to go farther. The belief was mentioned (p.161 fourth par.) that of something predicated of a subject there cannot only be one. Accordingly while it is traditionally acknowledged that "All *A* is *B*" implies "Some *B* is *A*", the inferred, predicating *A*, would be thought not to hold if there is only one. The belief was at that mention noted faulty, and an added reason is that when a single *A* is a *B* then some *B* is in fact the *A*, belief notwithstanding. The mistake is grounded on the discussed notion that subject and attribute are distinct, with the subject held an individual and the attribute a universal, although there can be many of the subject, or one of the attribute. The distinction between the individual and universal is further grounded on the discussed disputes about universals as independent of the individuals partaking in them. But universals, the words concerned, were observed meant to refer to the very individuals.

Omitting in accordance with the foregoing the universal quantifier to state "*A* is *B*", a symbolization of the same, analogous to that of implication (p.179, i), can be

ix. $A - B.$

It has apart from its extreme simplicity the advantage of providing for the mutuality of the relation, for identity, in its accustomed double line,

x. $A = B.$

Mutual implication, equivalence, may similarly by signified by the likewise known double arrow,

xi. $A \leftrightarrow B.$

Turning to particular propositions, those represented by "Some *A* is *B*", it will be recalled that they can be broadly taken to say

A can be *B*.

The linguistic utility lies in a corresponding symbolization, which can be

xii. $A/-/B,$

obviating quantifiers as prefixes, to facilitate the mentioned (e.g. facing p. second par.) connecting of premises to derive conclusions.

The strokes indicate qualification of the relation, as well as its reciprocity by their duality again.

In implication "some" was noted to be usually expressed only by negation of an opposite principle, but if need be the statement "*A* can imply *B*" can be considered, symbolized as $A/\rightarrow/B$.

The concern in the preceding regarding these symbolisms was the quantification of the subject, historically the one attended to, no doubt because of the interest in laws or their absence. They were observed to be about whether all of one thing are connected with another, the other mostly of interest without specific quantity. This may be held a reason why "some" is left tacit for it. Understandings of quantifications not made express extend to "all" as well, as indicated of variables and other universals, and they include moreover much more than would seem from the above.

There it is not explicit whether the displayed propositions symbolized are to stand alone or be part of others, such as logical principles. In the forms symbolized they indeed would be parts of others. For example in formula x it is not stated that all things are identical with all things, but as part of a longer statement the reference may be to any two identical things. The formula can also be viewed as representing any complete, likewise symbolized, deductive statement of identity, e.g. of a mathematical equality. The point was to assert disposability of the quantifications at issue in either case.

It is the first of these cases which is usually considered, without the thought that a more complex condition as a subject about which something is deductively true might also be quantified. Yet it is the last case that truly pertains to all instances of something. For illustration can be taken the law of transposition as symbolized in Table 1 (p.180),

xiii. $(A \rightarrow B) \rightarrow ('B \rightarrow 'A).$

Were it not the custom, as an instance of what is understood, not to quantify the *A* in implications, all *A* and all *'B* would be specified to be concerned, as done in attributions. It would not be specified, however, that all implications are referred to by the first one in the law, as likewise not done when laws are attributions, e.g. equations. But in present xiii it is only that first implication which unexceptionally applies to all instances. *A* and *'B* as about a kind are fully of all of it only when about timeless principles, while the law also applies to limited occasions regarding a kind. Still less unexceptional are the variables, noted in various usage also needlessly quantified. They on first use in xiii are only of things in the relation given, and on second use only of negations of these.

This does not take away entirely from the spoken of inclusiveness of variables and other universals. They were earlier spoken of as about all of the named things in the situations given, by which they are thus restricted. But it is still all that are so mainly understood, though only some might. It is understood that above xiii, unlike Theorem III.9 (p.171), refers to all of certain things under *A* when in the relation, not to some. Much more is understood, not merely in the symbolism, whose meaning can be codified for easy grasp, but in corresponding standard language, lacking the uniformity.

A statement in that language of the above law, more in keeping with xiii than its form in Theorem III.5 (p.159) and without even variables, may be "If one thing implies another then the negation of the second implies the negation of the first". In concord with the foregoing it is understood that the "if" applies unqualifiedly to all cases of the condition it speaks of, that, further, the "one thing" and the "negation of the second" apply to all cases of them at the given occasion, and that "thing" and "another" apply to all kinds of things in that relation to each other. In general by every universal, every word denoting more than one thing, as well as by every combination of them describing something universal, are in usage meant all of those things within the given restrictions, of which there may be none. If all are not meant, they can be expected to be quantified. Variegated language has exceptions as said, with indefinite propositions unclear about inclusiveness. Correspondingly inclusiveness, that all of a thing within perhaps a limit are meant, is often specified. But there is no need for the exceptions in an unambiguous symbolic language.

That is why it is redundant to speak in it of all, that meaning already contained in it where not otherwise quantified. The redundancy is particularly notable in mathematics, since in it quantification is in practice most frequent. An example was furnished by iv (p.187), and another, more like the preceding xiii in variables that are restricted, can be presented. It is of the discussed commutativity of multiplication, the principle quantified as

xiv. $(a)(b)(a \times b = b \times a)$.

There is no need for the quantification, since by the meaning of the variables the statement already speaks of all numbers *a* and *b* multiplied, and to be remarked is again that while the universally quantified variables are in fact restricted to those multiplied, the only fully universal part, referring to all instances without restriction, is the first multiplication as a whole, though not likewise quantified.

Variables can of course be fully universal too. As appears evident from what was said, those things are generally meant fully universal that are subjects of statements, possibly of ones part of other statements. This may again be attributed to interest in principles, as was original quantification (p.193 seventh par.), and in deductive principles that meaning again can be constant, dispensing with the quantification. Its omission was indeed seen inadvertent in principles like xiii and xiv, where the subjects are composite. But when the subjects are variables alone the practice can be forgotten. The same does not happen when the statement is an implication, as suggested previously. In the supposed theorem of the other table (p.182),

xv. $A \rightarrow (B \rightarrow A)$,

under *A* as subject all things, or all propositions, without restriction are understood, as are under *B*. But variables as subjects in mathematics would like other variables be quantified. This is more or less concealed in iv (p.187), where quantified subjects are *a* and *b*. Regarding it as well as xiii (facing p.) and xv (this page) it may be observed why subjects of statements part of other statements can be more inclusive in conclusions than in premises.

In xiii *A* concerns all of a kind, whereas in xv *B*, not being a repeat, concerns all things altogether. The reason is again found in what is meant. Principles are meant to assert something about each of the subject individually. Thus in xiii each instance of the premise implies individually the conclusion. Hence the subject within the premise itself is only about all of a kind as an instance named by *A*. However, in xv, since a conclusion in entirety applies to each instance of the premise, *B* names at once all kinds of things, namely all things since all of each kind are at issue.

It may also be noted that while in xiii *A*, though unquantified, names each time all of a kind, in iv *a*, though universally quantified, names each time a single number. A number can of course have many instances. A person has two eyes, two ears, etc. But as clear now, quantified are not all those instances, but all numbers. There is hence as suggested (p.187 fifth par.) additional inconsistency in quantification, which was designed for, in purport at least, not variables, but particular things they stand for. It might in fact with equal justification be required that particular numbers in similar use, too, be in mathematics universally quantified, due to their many instances. But as explicated, there is no need for such quantification in the symbolic language, including superfluously where in fact all things represented by a variable are referred to, as in the case of *b* in iv.

There the variable stands for the subject of the inferred. In an example of a mathematical variable for the subject of a whole statement, similar to last xv, that every number equals the product of two numbers, perhaps of itself and 1, would be quantified as in

xvi. $(a)(Eb)(Ec)(a = b \times c)$.

The quantifications are not only superfluous but in accordance with the foregoing wrong with regard to "some", the existential quantifier. "Some" is viewed as not necessarily "all", and "all" is applied, to repeat, also within restrictions. In present xvi *b* and *c* are restricted by the product that equals *a*, but although to accordingly quantify them would no doubt confuse they represent all numbers of that product, not merely some. It is rather the product that, at least regarding the number it equals, does not vary, and of which it might be said that some, not any, equals any number.

Even of that product or any other predicate, however, can it be said that, redundantly, all pertains to the subject that pertains to it, being restricted by it alone. In contrast as suggested (p.194 third par.), whereas what amount is in question regarding the predicate and other things not a subject is dependent on something else in the statements and hence cannot be less than determined by it, a subject is in this regard independent and hence can refer to less than necessarily all, it can refer to only some. Accordingly quantification by "some" in the sense of allowing less than "all" is suited again for subjects only.

The appropriatness of that quantification is thereby virtually eliminated in mathematics. Mathematics is not apt to state something about an unclear some of a subject. Even probability or improbability alone are weighted toward one side or the other, and normally the degree is specified. The unsuited use of the quantifier has due to its mistaken association with existence furthermore led to uncalled-for suppositions of existence. Many mathematical principles are accordingly called existence theorems, although merely stating that with certain things certain others are connected, the ones quantified "some", not as existing, but because of vagueness of amount. The statements as instanced by above xvi can to boot be viewed as universal ones, speaking "all" in the subject, which in contrast to "some" regarding it is not held to imply whichever existence.

"Some" was observed to in addition be called upon to try to denote sameness (e.g. p.189 first par.). The function was seen deficient, and as may be gathered from the preceding, the relations at issue can if needed be expressed without the quantification. Supposing they are of mathematics, they are formulated below in a not unfamiliar way. The relation of v (p.188), in which the sameness of the related to is undetermined, can be

xvii. $a\ R\ b.$

It can be read "All numbers *a* have relation *R* to a number *b*".

The relation of vi (p.189), in which the same is related to by all, can be

xviii. $a\ R\ b,\ (c\ R\ d) \rightarrow (a\ R\ d),$

read "All numbers have the relation to a number, and if a number c has it to a number *d* then all numbers do". If by vi be meant, as not made clear by the quantification, that the x may also have the relation to different *y*, then the strokes for "can" (p.193) can be used for

xix. $a\ R\ b\ ,\ (c\ R\ d)/\!\rightarrow\!/(a\ R\ d).$

"All numbers have the relation to a number, and if c has it to *d* then can all numbers".

Interposed can be a state of v not covered by the quantification and perhaps more likely than the last two, that all numbers have the relation to a distinct number, among them earlier spoken successors if in question (pp.137-138).

xx. $a\ R\ b,\ (c\ R\ d) \rightarrow {}'({}'c/R/d),$

to read "All numbers have the relation to a number, and if c has it to *d* then it is not true that a number not c can". The negation sign for logic as well as the strokes are made here use of for further purposes. A usual notation, used for successors and slightly lengthier, would be $a\ R\ b,\ (c\ R\ e)(d\ R\ e) \rightarrow (c = d).$

Corresponding to vii (p.189) is

xxi. $a \rightarrow (b\ R\ a),$

"All numbers *a* imply that all numbers *b* have relation *R* to them".

As to viii (p.189), seen to fail in distinguishing the sameness from its absence, it can first be given in an indeterminate sense, in likeness to xvii above.

xxii. *a/R/b,*

"A number *a* can have relation *R* to a number *b*". With, similarly to xviii, the relation to the same number, viii would be

xxiii. *a/R/b, (c R d) →'('c/R/'d),*

"A number can have the relation to a number, and if c has it to *d* then it is not true that 'c can have it to 'd." If similarly to xix those *a* may also have the relation to different *b*, viii is

xxiv. *a/R/b, (c R d) → ('c/R/d),*

"A number can have the relation to a number, and if c has it to *d* then 'c can". And if similar to xx the relation in viii be to distinct numbers,

xxv. *a/R/b, (c R d) →'('c/R/d),*

"A number can have the relation to a number, and if c has it to *d* then it is not true that 'c can".

The point in the last pages was to illustrate the needlessness of quantification where used in logic and related fields, and to generally establish a simple logical notation by which deduction can be performed as mentioned. For that deduction logical principles are likewise simple, and as evidence a few remaining ones are hereupon added to the former, together with further comments.

The entities of which logical principles were herein observed composed comprise basically no more than things viewed as undivided and represented by variables like *A*, and composites of things as connected by shared placement represented by symbols like the arrow "→" for implication, with possible negation of either whole units or things connected in them. Symbols were added for these negations, which can be held to include the concept "some", or "can", as negation of an opposite principle and symbolized on its own. Also symbols like parentheses were added to delimit units, and of importance now is that with the entities thus simply understood they can be easily listed, in order to determine from which follow which.

The list of undivided entities can be small, corresponding to those of the laws of thought as *A* and *'A*, and perhaps *'(A), ''A, '('A)* and *'(''(A),* more of the same leading to needless repetition. It is not difficult to see, as by diagram, that from any of these follows only what the laws of thought prescribe. No other undivided entity *B*, or composite *A → B,* or negation regarding these can be inferred.

A word about the laws of exportation and importation, which came into account with modus tollens (p.162). They respectively state that *(A & B) →* C implies *A → (B → C)*, and the converse. As a result modus tollens could be stated as *'B → ((A → B) → 'A)* or, exchanging variables and negations, *A → (('B → 'A) → B)*. There appears hence a consequence of *A* not part of the above. Instead, however, *B* was viewable as a consequence of *A* combined with *'B → 'A,* and the last unit is an additional assumption in both cases. Therefore for simplicity's sake only certain such arrangements will be specified. Since a statement was seen to mean the same with parts imported or exported, if a new letter, e.g. *B,* appears in the conclusion it should, with any unit it belongs to, be imported to the premise. The procedure is possible, since the new letter, with the unit, was indicated not to follow from a premise, but must be posited in a conclusion too, as above. The old form of modus tollens, *((A → B) & 'B) → 'A,* would correspondingly be restored. By the same token *'B* of the premise in this form can be exported to the conclusion, making for, as discussed, transposition, *(A → B) → ('B → 'A).* The object is to state as clearly what follows from units of two letters as from those of one.

The number of two-letter units used was seen more extensive than the other, in particular with respect to attribution rather than implication. It included in this respect not only the universal form, *A — B,* and negations of the whole or part of it as well as reverse sequences, but also the particular form, *A/—/B,* and negations and reverses regarding it. For the deductive purposes mentioned, however, much of the negations and reverses can be neglected. External negations especially were for these purposes said (p.192 first two pars.) to be convertible into their affirmative equivalents, by the laws of complements, an opposite converting not here required. And internal negations and reverses need not be considered in the units as independent premises, since the variables apply there to negations as well and with indifference to sequence. Consequently the main interest here is what conclusions not external negations may be drawn from the two in this paragraph symbolized two-letter units alone.

Such inferences were furnished in the first and last theorems of this section (pp.159, 171). In both cases the inferred was a reverse connection, the second found derivable through the first, and in accordance with the second of those principles another such conclusion, mentioned before (p.192 fourth par.), can be drawn from the premise of the first, mainly if of attribution. It is that

When A *is* B *then some* B *is* A,

because to speak of, all, *A* is by definition to speak of some *A.*

This principle can as easily be confirmed by a diagram of *A — B,* notwithstanding that it has been denied of not merely, as noted with its first mention, a singular *A,* but also a universal one, in conformity with the contention that whereas "all" may not signify the existence of the subject, "some" does. It need not be repeated that the distinction is uncalled-for, and due to it it is evidently also denied that *When* A *is* B *then some* A *is* B.

This added principle may also be considered, although of less account than the displayed preceding one, inasmuch as knowing specifically that, all, *A* is *B* makes the vaguer inference from it of little interest.

In consequence of transposition, that when *A* is *B* then *'(B)* is *'(A)*, follows on the same grounds also that when *A* is *B* then some *'(B)* is *'(A)* and some *'(A)* is *'(B)*. Put very simply, from "*A* is *B*", as to be seen, follows no more than, excluding external negations, " *'(B)* is *'(A)*" and corresponding forms of "some" for both connections in both directions.

The last of these forms quoted, "Some *'(A)* is *'(B)*" or " *'(A)* can be *'(B)*", is noteworthy as a consequence, because again implying that, revealingly as earlier expounded, not everything is *B*. If everything were, then not only all *A* but all *'(A)* would be *B*, with that consequence false.

That there is no other consequence of "*A* is *B*" can first be observed for any in question not a connection between *A* and *B* and their negations. As in the case of *A* alone and negations regarding it, it is evident, as by the diagram, that no other entity C or unit containing it can be inferred. Only units with *A* or *B* follow. Moreover it cannot be a unit with one of them alone, which would signify that when "*A* is *B*" is true then there is such a unit since, as in other implications, from the truth, the existence, of the premised follows the existence of the concluded, either perhaps a negation. But the connection between *A* and *B* was explicated not to require the existence of either, which therefore cannot be inferred. And a connection between units of the same letter, viz what follows from any one of them, was observed (p.198 next to last par.) derived only in accordance with laws of thought.

Only units used with *A* and *B* connected remaining, they beside the above are *A* — *'B*, *B* — *'A*, *'A* — *B*, *'B* — *A*, *A*/—/*'B*, *'B*/—/*A*, *'A* — *'B*, *B* — *A*, *'A*/—/*B* and *B*/—/*'A*. Keeping in mind that the present demonstrations apply to both attribution and implication, the negation signs are somewhat liberal. *'A* should strictly be *'(A)* in attribution. But since the issue is what does not follow from "*A* is *B*", or "*A* implies *B*", if something does not follow for *'(A)* it follows the less, by what was said, for *'A*. Thus among the few more things determined above to follow, those regarding *'(A)* do not for *'A*, unless transposition applies. In that event as in others of limited negation it is not too difficult to confirm that no more follows than with negation unlimited.

With that understanding of the preceding list of ten symbolized connections, the first six do not only not follow from *A* — *B*, but are impossible, as can be confirmed, except for the third perhaps, by the last diagram. The third connection once more expresses that not all is meant to be *B*, and its denial can be deduced from above following *'A*/—/*'B* by complement law, by which the rest of the six are from the known likewise denied.

The remaining four do not follow in the more usual sense, by which both they and their negations are possible. The negations of the first two are by complement law equivalent to the other two, and conversely, and hence if all four are possible none follows, since any that would would contradictorily make impossible another. The diagrams at right, complying with the assumed *A* — *B*, disclose each possibility. Specifically, the upper depiction is of *B*/—/*'A*, the lower of its negation in *B* — *A*, and *'A*/—/*B* and *'A* — *'B* follow respectively also by standard deduction.

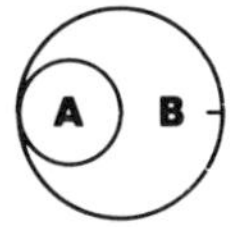

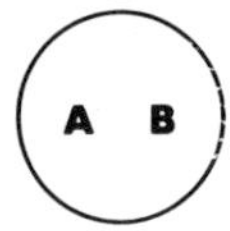

Coming to "Some *A* is *B*", or "*A* can be *B*", as a source of inference, less follows still. Only the converse by Theorem III.9 (p.171) does. On the same grounds as in the previous case, only the connections with *A* and *B* in each need as consequences be considered, despite the faulty position that the existence of *A* and *B* individually is implied. The units to be viewed are *A* — *'B*, *B* — *'A*, *'A* — *B*, *'B* — *A*, *A* — *B*, *B* — *A*, *'A* — *'B*, *'B* — *'A*, *'A*/—/*'B*, *'B*/—/*'A*, *A*/—/*'B*, *B*/—/*'A*, *'A*/—/*B* and *'B*/—/*A*.

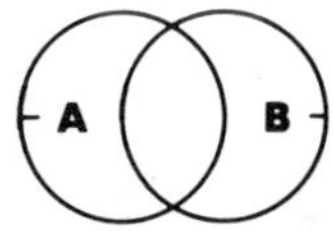

The first two are under *A*/—/*B* impossible, as seen by its diagram, or is deducible from the known by complement law. Of the remaining twelve the negations of the first six are by the same laws equivalent to the other six, and conversely, and hence again if all are possible none follows. The diagrams at right, complying with the assumed *A*/—/*B*, disclose each possibility. Specifically, the upper depiction is of *'A* — *B*, the lower requires its negation in *'A* — *'B* and *'B* — *'A*, and all other of the twelve units follow also by standard deduction.

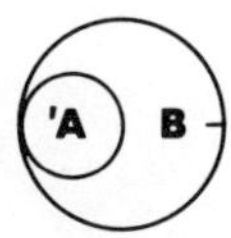

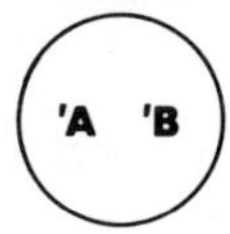

With respect to either of the two units, "*A* is *B*" and "*A* can be *B*", of which the consequences have in the foregoing been explored it may also be asked whether if combined with other units with *A* or *B* something follows that does not from the units separately. That something can was in fact seen regarding "*A* implies *B*" and *'B*, in modus tollens. But this combination and resulting *'A* were seen transformable into transposition, in which the first unit alone implies a like connection between the other two. The same transformations were seen possible with any two units implying something, and when one of them is thus an above tie between *A* and *B* and the other of an independent letter, what is implied by the last unit transported was already determined. Should there be more than one such independent unit, the same transportation and result apply. The question then is what follows from only combined units of the ties regarding *A* and *B*. By testing again through diagrams it can be established that whatever the number of the units what follows is still in accordance with the preceding. The testing is fairly brief, since the units with *A* and *B* are soon exhausted.

Consequences different from a combination of units than from them separately were also seen regarding complements. Thus from "Not all *A* is *B*" and "Not both some *A* is *B* and some *A* is *'(B)*" together but not separately follows "All *A* is *'(B)*", and likewise if *B* and *'(B)* are interchanged. The same was found not to hold when there is one *A*. Then the denial of "*A* is *B*" is equivalent to "*A* is *'(B)*", and conversely. This was the only logical difference between one and more *A* noted, and it may be confirmed as in the preceding that this is the only difference, with the externally unnegated connections here considered for deduction usable without regard to how many the *A*. More specifically, with only one *A* the same can be seen to follow and not follow from both "*A* is *B*" and "*A* can be *B*". By the latter it may seem that e.g. more is impossible, as that some *A* be *'B*, but since by not stating that *A* is *B* *A*'s singleness, or its "all", is not known, "some" not stated otherwise, the same possibilities remain.

In this survey of conclusions that follow or not from premises of two letters the letters, perhaps negated, were not treated as separate units, and it can further be asked what follows if they are. What follows from each was determined in the laws of thought, and no more can be seen deducible. Connections of premise with conclusion as well as connections within either were observed to consist in placement of one thing with another. And when in a premise two letters or their negations are not thus known to be connected, no conclusion of such placement can be, by diagram if wished, found reached other than for the separate letters by laws of thought. The different letters obviously could in absence of more knowledge be connected in any of the above ways.

The same inconclusiveness occurs when assumed are three or more letters of such independent units, simply because since no connection between them is known, any is possible. And when only two out of three letters are connected as described, a similar situation takes place. From $A \rightarrow B$ and C together follows no more than found to follow from them independently, with no connection between one and the other. Accordingly, to find what new conclusions can be drawn from three-letter premises, all three letters must be connected.

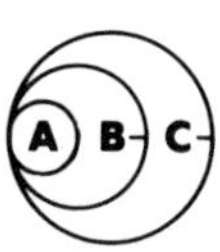

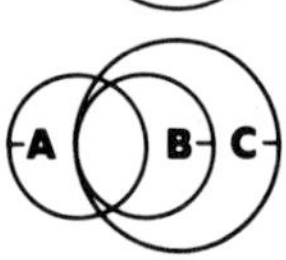

The by now most familiar such connection is the universal $A - B$ coupled with $B - C$, and one using the particular $A/-/B$ coupled with likewise $B - C$ was in certain forms mentioned also (p.164 sixth par., p.186 first par.).

The inference from the first of these of the transitivity, $A - C$, was furnished in Theorem III.7 (p.163) or the like principle for attribution on the page after, not to mention like visual confirmations elsewhere (pp.140, 184). A similar transitive inference from the other combination was indicated with its early mentions, namely that

When some A *is* B, *and* B *is* C, *then some* A *is* C.

This inference was noted to in fact be in accustomed manner deducible through the other. By the other any considered thing, for convenience named *A*, that is *B* is C, and hence since in the second combination a certain thing considered, some of any other *A*, is *B*, it is C.

There is a further transitivity implied by the first combination, apart from like implications by both of them on "some". Both imply "Some *A* is C" and hence "Some C is *A*". But the first also implies " 'C is '*A*", not only because *A* is C, but because 'C is '*B* and '*B* is '*A*, i.e. by transitive law reversed. The significance is that, knowing of transposition, in a sequence of implications from say *A* to *Z* it is as facile to infer by transitivity that '*Z* implies '*A* as that *A* implies *Z*.

Put simply again, a consequence of *(A — B)(B — C)* is transitive A — C, the other results following by mainly transposition or conversion as before, or by transitivity itself. By that transitivity was also seen *A*/—/C deducible from *(A/—/B)(B — C)*, and inasmuch as it may not be immediately clear what combinations result in transitivity, a simple rule can be applied. If each of a thing, *B*, of which there may be one, is of another, C, then anything, *A*, which is of *B* is of C. The deduction is in ordinary situations exemplified by the several times mentioned act of inferring an instance from a principle, *B* — C being the principle and *A* — C the instance, without normally bothering to state that *A* is a *B*.

To verify that no more follows from the preceding configurations of three letters than the spoken of, it can again be noted that neither a unit of one letter, perhaps repeated within the unit, nor any with a yet unused letter does, as happens however many letters are assumed connected. The first does not follow because, as pointed out (p.200 fourth par.), the existence or not of a thing *A* does not follow from the connections, and connections pertaining to it alone are decided by laws of thought. And the second does not follow because, nothing being known about the unused letter, anything about it is possible. For a similar reason, with connections of *A* with *B* and *B* with C no other connection can be concluded of *A* with *B* or *B* with C as a result of the combined premises. If assuming e.g. *A* — *B* first then, nothing being known about C, any connection of it with *B* is possible. This means that whatever the connection of *A* with *B* there can be any connection of *B* with C, and of course the opposite. But this means that whatever one con-

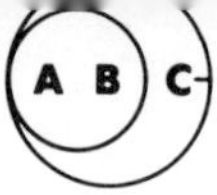

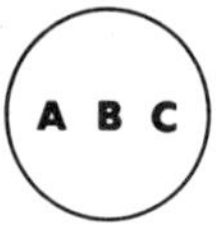

nection, or a series of them, none is implied of another, the other still of any enabled by its own nature.

In those configurations hence only connections that follow regarding *A* and C need be looked for, others having been determined.

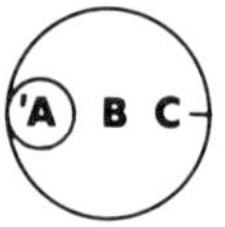

Of these connections the ones not found implied or precluded by *(A — B)(B — C)*, through transitive *A — C*, are, as with *A — B* previously, *'A — 'C, C — A, 'A/— /C* and *C/— /'A*. Since one half contradicts the other, if all are possible none again follows, and the first two diagrams here, complying with the assumed, disclose that result.

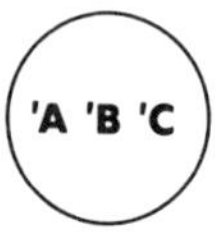

The connections not found implied or precluded by *(A/— /B)(B — C)*, through transitive *A/— /C*, are the also familiar *'A — C, 'C — A, A — C, C — A, 'A — 'C, 'C — 'A, 'A/— /'C, 'C/— /'A, A/— /'C, C/— /'A, 'A/— /C* and *'C/— /A*. That these contradictories are possible and hence do not follow is disclosed by the further two diagrams, which comply with the assumed.

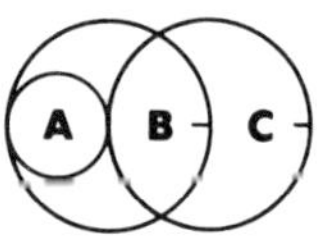

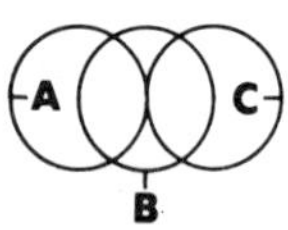

Considering the connections of "all" and "some" between *A* and *B* and between *B* and *C* without change of direction within the connections, the two configurations remaining are *(A — B)(B/— /C)* and *(A/— /B)(B/— /C)*, both pictured next. The question is whether any connection regarding *A* and *C* is implied by them.

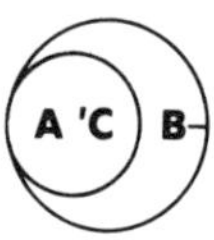

The complete list of the connections is *A — C, C — A, 'A — 'C, 'C — 'A, A — 'C, C — 'A, 'A — C, 'C — A, A/— /'C, C/— /'A, 'A/— /C, 'C/— /A, A/— /C, C/— /A, 'A/— /'C*, and *'C/— /'A*, and since one half contradicts the other, if all are possible none follows. The further two diagrams comply with the assumed in both configurations and disclose all those possibilities. Therefore none of them follows.

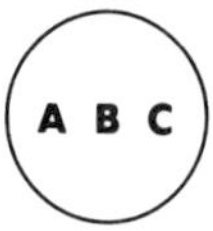

If configurations of other directions are considered, the remaining two are *(B — A)(B — C)* and *(A — B)(C — B)*, because, due to the indifference of letters or convertibility of "some", other changes in direction result in forms already given. For example *(A/— /B)(C — B)* results in *(C — B)(B/— /A)*, of a preceding configuration.

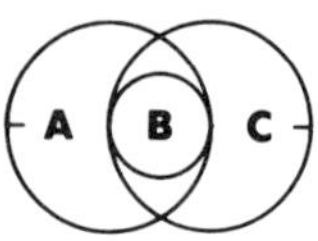

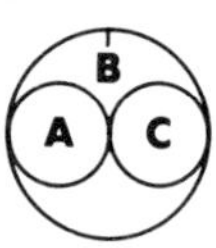

Of the two added forms, pictured next, the first one is seen to imply *A/— /C*. The same can be deduced in standard manner by the last two principles displayed (pp.199, 203), and the transitivity thus corresponds to the others in exemplifying an instance, *A/— /C*, of a principle, *B — C*. No other unit with *A* and *C* other than those found affirmed or denied through *A/— /C* follows, as confirmable in accordance with those remaining (this page fourth par.).

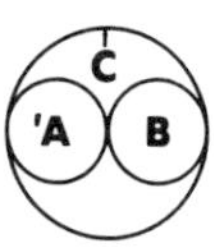

All of them are disclosed in the next two diagrams, which comply with the assumed *(B — A)(B — C)*. Hence none of

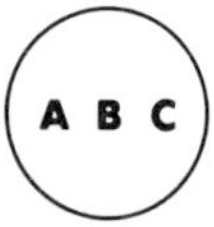

them, as before, follows. As to the last form, *(A — B)(C — B)*, it reveals itself to be transformable into the preceding one.

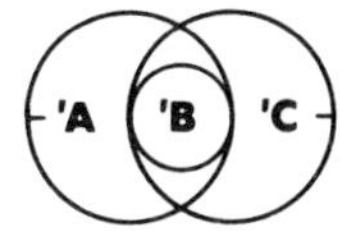

By transposition it becomes *('B — 'A)('B — 'C)*, and hence the same follows from it as from the other but for interchanged affirmation and denial of letters. To wit, a consequence is *'A/—/'C*.

Denial may also be combined with affirmation, to create further of these forms. But these are likewise transformable into former ones, or no connection regarding *A* and *C* follows. Only *B* has ground to be denied, while affirmed in its other mention, since negation of *A* or *C* does not alter the form. But for instance *(A — B)('B — C)* is equivalent to *('B — 'A)('B — C)*, an above form. The results are similar by like transpositions in the other forms except in *(A/—/B)('B/—/C)*, where not performable. But no connection for *A* and *C* follows from it, as can in the previous manner be confirmed by the diagrams here, which comply with the assumed.

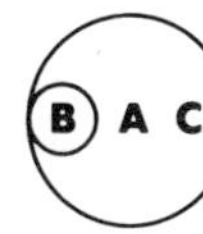

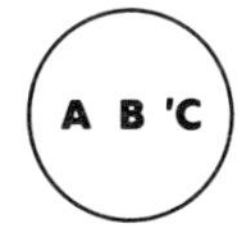

It may be further asked whether results not in accordance with the few listed principles do not follow if any of the above configurations are combined with other connections of *A* with *B* or *B* with *C*, as wondered about two letters only. That no more follows was for the most part answered (p. 203 last par.), it remaining whether a connection of *A* with *C* does, other than which follows from one inferred of them before. From it alone follows the same that does from such connection of any two letters, since the letters are indifferent, and the question hence is whether a connection of *A* and *C* follows in a novel way due to *B*.

It can by diagram with preceding ease, however, be determined that no connection in question of one thing, *A*, with another, *C*, results from a third thing, *B*, if each *B* is not connected, as in discussed form of a principle, with *C*, one of the other two things, of which some of the second, *A*, is also connected with *B*. It is the transitivity of acquaintance.

For these reasons no further principle enters also if an as yet not assumed connection of *A* with *C* is added, a connection more likely as a conclusion than additional premise. If for example to *A — B* and *B — C* is added *C — A*, the identity of *A*, *B* and *C* results by transitivities. From *B — C* and *C — A* follows *B — A* and hence due to *A — B* the identity of *A* and *B*; from *C — A* and *A — B* follows similarly the identity of *B* and *C*; and from these identities the identity of *A* and *C*. But no connection of either thing with another does not result from an exampled principle, since if deriving from a third thing, it does by transitivity, and if not, it does by the other laws.

The same reasoning by now evidently applies to configurations of four or more letters. Any connection between one and another follows either, through a further letter, by transitivity, or, through its own letters, by the other laws. And an unconnected letter, negations also considered, follows in accordance with laws of thought.

Unconnected letters, or their negations, when observed to follow in modus tollens otherwise (e.g. p.201 last par.), were seen connectable, to comply with the preceding. The reason is that these single-letter units do as noted (e.g. p.200 fourth par.) not follow from connected ones alone, and hence an unconnected one is a premise, transportable into the conclusion. Thus when a conclusion will not be such a resulting connection, it will as a one-letter unit follow by laws of thought from a like one in the premise. Confusion may though arise, because units of single letters—or by the foregoing (p.190 fifth par.) more generally the truth or not of propositions, or still more generally the existence or not of things—are often derived by way of logic other than laws of thought. Characteristically if known that *A* implies *B*, and *A* is found, *B* is inferred, casting doubt on the herein observed redundancy of modus ponens (p.162 last four pars.). In this case if *A* is transported the redundancy was seen explicit, and it should be added that since with another letter C instead in the one-letter premise no conclusion follows from both combined (p.202 fourth par.), modus tollens and modus ponens are the only possibilities. And the deceptiveness of language once again intrudes.

When a state is asserted in language without qualification of time, it is usually the present which is meant. As when saying that there is a solar eclipse. But when saying that when the moon comes between the sun and the earth then there is a solar eclipse, the meaning is timeless. The timeless statement is an example of "*A* implies *B*", and when added to its supposition is in modus ponens "and *A* then *B*", the meaning is equally timeless, for the principle is to as such apply to all times. What happens when a present state is, independently, asserted is in general rather a matter of an instance.

Because of the unqualifiedness of the statement, when *A* is stated respecting an occurrence, the same seems referred to as by that letter in "*A* implies *B*". But since the latter as a rule speaks of all times of *A* as times of *B*, and the former of this time of it, it is an instance of *A* and might be symbolized by another letter. It is not so symbolized, or a corresponding statement qualified, because the content is distinguished only by time, but it nonetheless plays such a logical part. The subsequent inference is by transitivity, which can take the form "If a time, *A*, is a time of *B*, and times of *B* are times of C, then that time, *A*, is a time of C", the time, as formerly, possibly a place. Accordingly if the present, otherwise expressed by *A*, is a time of *B*, it is a time of *C*, expressed by *C*, as presently existing, as would be done with *B*, the two alphabetically the former *A* and *B*, when on knowing the connection between them and that the present is a time of *A*, the present as a time of *B* is inferred. The concealment by language extends farther.

Through it an unqualified assertion speaks covertly not only of the present, but also of present knowledge of the asserted, in concord with the expounded relation of knowledge to reality. This should be clear from the very nature of inference, in which upon knowing one thing another becomes known. Accordingly when saying that *A* implies *B*, the purport is that when *A* is known, knowledge of *B* is ensured. This is especially notable when an instance of a principle is put as "If *A* then *B*". Meaning the present again, by "if" is meant, unlike by some of "when", that *A* is not known, by which to know *B*. That is to say it is meant, more pointedly than with the principle, that should *A* at any time be known, knowledge of *B* is ensured. In this case if it is also stated that *A*, namely that *A* is known, *A* is an instance in that sense. The present knowledge of *A* is an instance of knowledge of *A*, and hence knowledge of *B* is ensured. More can be said.

An instance may not be what might be called proper. As in former numerical cases, an instance of something may truly be identical with it. It can be that in "If *A* then *B*" at issue is not only a single connection but a single occasion on which upon making certain that *A*, one infers by the connection that *B*. The connection could be that if when a certain food cooking comes to a boil the heat is reduced then the food will be as desired. Then upon seeing that at the correct time the heat is reduced, by which one infers the desired result, the actual making certain of the needed condition is identical with the certainty assumed. The certainty first had the attribute of being assumed and then of being actual, i.e. it was like other identities characterized in different ways, and the attributes might again be symbolized by different letters, with e.g. *A* identical with *B*. The first connection would thus be "If *B* then *C*", but although the actuality *A* by transitivity ensures the actuality of *C*, it could not be stated as would be customary that if $A = B$ and $B \rightarrow C$ then $A \rightarrow C$.

Such a statement is not groundlessly called a conditional, with the "if" clause the condition for the "then" clause, but not necessarily true. The statement says that the conclusion is true provided the two premises are, without affirming either of the two. But the first of them was meant to assert the actuality of, affirm, *B*. The point is that the actuality cannot be put into a principle, which consists in a conditional. It should be first taken into account that the above $B \rightarrow C$, or "If *B* then *C*", is also a conditional, viewable as an example of premise $A \rightarrow B$ in modus ponens, as might in it above premise $A = B$ and conclusion $A \rightarrow C$ be viewed as respectively premise A and conclusion B. Then by $A \rightarrow B$ is not affirmed A and hence B, which rather are the subsequent intentions based on the conditional. Should the actualities be meant, then to restate in modus ponens that A and hence B would again be redundant. But $A \rightarrow B$ is meant to only assume, and should in such a principle subsequent A and B state actuality, that A and hence B are known, then they cannot at the same time be merely assumed in $A \rightarrow B$, but are known in it, for equal redundancy. Hence above mentioned present knowledge as a proper instance of one of the same thing does for transitive inference strictly not apply. Only knowledge of a particular time other than the present can be the instance of the knowledge assumed. And for the same reason in the last discussed non-proper instance, that of the identity of the assumed and the actual knowledge, the knowledge, of some particular time, cannot by a principle be stated at once as both assumed and actual. If stated as actual, being thus of the present, it cannot also be merely assumed, and if stated as assumed, being of another time, it cannot also be actual.

For the actuality to in regard to the conditional $A \rightarrow B$ be stated of A and hence B, as noted to be often done, the letters, as well as their connection, would stand as independent assertions, in what is called an argument form but is as a whole mistakenly likewise treated as conditional. The form may be "A implies B, and A; therefore B". There seems a return to modus ponens, but now stated is not a principle but a succession of things ascertained, not all of them at once, the symbolism serving to represent, not to prescribe.

Of interest is that such a deduction, when not of the proper instance in transitivity, cannot be made a principle, and modus ponens is hence of the same futility as were principles that, though not equally redundant, prescribe case inferences from principles (e.g. p.141 second par.). To through a connection infer one fact from another thus requires conceptual perception of the entailment in each case, and pertinent is that it takes place in accordance with listed logical law, by which the perception is of one thing coinciding with another, here by transitivity. To generalize this transitivity put in the discussed language of placement—actuality is the place of, the assumed, A; the place of, the assumed, A is a place of B; therefore actuality is a place of B.

The transitivity by which from the identity of an actual A with an assumed one, and from the implication by A of B, B is inferred can go as far as to concern actual and assumed existing knowledge. At issue is as usual not knowledge by someone else but by oneself or mankind collectively, since the interest is in that very possession of knowledge. And an *A* connected with *B* may not only be hypothetical but known, but not as so connected. A like situation occurred with an equality like 3 + 1 = 4 (p.137). Both sides of the equation were in a sense known, but although it may accordingly be known that 2 + 2 = 3 + 1, it may be known only by inference that in consequence 2 + 2 = 4. It was observed that in the process while something may be known, e.g. the second equation here, the knowledge may not be in consciousness, e.g. when affirming the first equation, so as to by it actually affirm the third one. Likewise when affirming a connection between *A* and *B*, knowledge of *A*, of its existence, may though possessed not be in consciousness, wherefrom to infer *B*.

Despite the subtle difference regarding *A* between its knowledge that is not and is in consciousness, when stating *A* and consequently *B* something else is meant by them than when stating their connection, though the language be the same. This is clear from the fact of inference alone, the inference of course being that *B* exists, inasmuch as *A* does. By virtue of that difference the inference was seen of transitivity, to like all deduction be made in accordance with not more than some of the basic logical principles given.

Whether something follows from something else can accordingly be decided in accordance with a rather few and simple principles, despite the contention that many logical and mathematical principles cannot be proven. The contention largely stems, as discussed (pp.111-113), from the mistaken belief that the statement "This statement is unprovable" is true and correspondingly unprovable, and it reached a field as extensive as mathematics in peculiar ways.

One of them is built on a system by which linguistic forms used regarding that statement are assigned numbers, whereupon on supposing to prove the truth of that statement, the proof is inferred to hold for those numbers. The numbers and especially mathematics are, however, irrelevant here. The supposed proof does not concern those numbers but things to which they are assigned. If a cause be numbered 1, and the effect 2, the consequence is not that the number 1 causes the number 2.

Irrelevant for another reason is the ascribing of unprovability due to that supposition to truths about all of an infinity of things, e.g. numbers. In support of the supposition that "This statement is unprovable" is true it is argued that every means of proof of the statement can be proven to fail, since its proof would contradict it. It is alongside argued that not all means of proof can be proven to fail, since the statement is otherwise proven unprovable and hence by its content proven, contradicting it again. But the meanings of "every" and "all" are the same, while contradictory things are said with regard to them in the last two sentences. Should there be doubt about the sameness, it is enough to exchange those words in the sentences, to see the arguments retained.

The second of these sentences actually reveals the earlier observed paradox unrecognized. It discloses that by stating the first one, a form of the customary proof alleged of "This statement is unprovable", the proof constitutes a contradiction of it. In lieu of that recognition it is maintained that there somehow is a difference between stating that something holds for all of a kind and that something holds for the first of them, the second, etc., as might be held said by speaking of every. Since unprovability is in the arguments, further, spoken of in terms of all attempted proofs that would fail, indefinite though their number may be, they would be viewed as infinite in number. It is correspondingly held that, as noted, truths about all of an infinity of things are not provable. In the preceding, however, the issue is the number, regarding a particular thing yet, of any proofs attempted, not the number of things to be proved.

There is more irrelevance. Inasmuch as it is thought that for the statement in question contradictorily all means of proof cannot be proven to fail but not the first, second, and the rest, it is believed, though the enumeration is but a way of speaking of all, that truths holding for an infinity of things can only be proven for particular ones at a time. This procedure is furthermore confounded with the one of proving something of a thing one step, rather, at a time, as conclusions are usually reached, by drawing from initial premises inferences that serve as further premises, and so on.

It is indeed possible through regular inference to find at one time that something is true of an infinity of things. If from an attribute certain things have in common, as by definition, another is inferred, it holds for an infinity of the things, since it does for anything of the first attribute.

In the disputing of provability regarding infinities the famous last theorem of Fermat, the 17th century mathematician, is often cited. It has to do with equations like those of the mentioned Pythagorean theorem (pp.86, 87), by which $a^2 + b^2$ equals c^2 when *a, b* and *c* are the sides of a right-angled triangle with the last side the longest. By Fermat's theorem the equation never holds if 2 is replaced by a higher natural number, with *a, b* and *c* likewise natural numbers. The provability of the theorem is questioned, because the numbers above 2 continue into infinity. It is acknowledged at the same time that with some numbers in place of 2, for instance 3 and 4, the theorem has been proven. But this is contrary to the generally proposed unprovability. A proof that the equation does not hold for 3 or 4 applies whatever the allied numbers *a*, *b* and *c*, and these continue likewise into infinity.

In point of fact, all logical principles, not only mathematical ones, apply to infinities. By applying to anything, they do to things of an infinity like numbers.

Utilizing then the not many basic logical principles, together with likewise uncluttered notation, there is a brief scanning procedure for deciding whether certain conclusions follow from given premises. The arrangement of symbols enables, as a matter of fact, a procedure more positive. Beside finding whether conclusions in question are entailed by the premises, the arrangement can be used for finding whatever is entailed by them.

This can be accomplished by combining them in symbolic form in a linkage resembling customary chains of equations and remindful of a sorites, a series of syllogisms stating all premises and omitting intermediate conclusions. The linkage differs from a sorites by, apart from employing only the symbolism, only once listing an attribute, a variable in general. The last indicates that the linkage also differs by its application to additional material, i.e. implication, by which it differs from chains of equations as well. It differs from both of those forms, further, by extending also in multiple directions, for multiple connections of a variable. It is illustrated by

$$\begin{array}{cccccccc} & & \mathrm{A} & & & & & \\ & & \downarrow & & & & & \\ \mathrm{B} & \to & \mathrm{C} & \to & \mathrm{D} & \mathrm{E} & \to & \mathrm{F} \\ & & & & & \downarrow & & \\ & & & & & \mathrm{G} & & \end{array}$$

With attribution marked in contrast to the arrow of implication plainly by a line, the general rule can be that, as in other reading, connections be read from left to right or from top to bottom, or, for more connections, inclined between those, namely from upper left to lower right.

A single train of reasoning is not apt to be as multidirectional as suggested. Illustrated is nonetheless beside such as separate implications by *A* and *B* of the same thing, C, a combining of two directions, implications, by C, should the implied, *D* and *E*, combined imply something else, *F*, with *E* alone implying G. The individual implications, or other connections, can thus be united in various ways, of importance being that they be appropriately linked, to facilitate deductions.

It will be obvious now that the deductions rely foremost on transitivity, the justification for linking one connection with another. It will be equally clear from what was said that transitivity between letters of any distance takes place wherever there is a continuity of implications. It can accordingly be from the depicted deduced for example that *A* implies *F*, or that *B* inplies *G*, true without need of *D*.

More can be deduced by also making use of transposition. Accordingly for example *'F* implies *'B*, or *'G* implies *'A*, true without *D*. Still more deduction is possible in view of convertibility of "some", of "can", as used mostly for attribution. Here the results are mainly that, taking into account that from "all" follows "some" as so-called subaltern, some *F* can be said to imply, be accompanied by, *G*, and the like is the case with *'A* and *'B*, as well as *D* and *E* since implied by *C*.

The four principles in the last two paragraphs referred to—transitivity, transposition, and perhaps conversion and subalternation—are virtually the required for standard deduction, as performable through the linkages. The laws of complements, seen the only other fundamental ones, were also seen to involve indirect, or external, negation, basically about what is known to be false rather than true, the laws translating one into the other. The known to be true was noted the interest in the deductions, and the complement laws, applied in life at least as much as a matter of course as are the others, thus serve the subsidiary role by which on reaching a denial one makes for those deductions an opposite affirmation, and on reaching an affirmation one does not lapse into its denial.

Other principles, even parts of the preceding, were seen consequences of the basic ones, with for example identity and equivalence signifying ties between *A* and *B* in both directions. This suggests further possibilities of the linkages. Beside using the same letter to end one statement and start another, it can be used for, beside a connection in the opposite direction, reverses in letter sequences that include occasions when negation is involved, as well as to state the denoted entity's discussed (pp. 206-209) existence or not, the knowledge of the same.

In mentioned identity and equivalence, or in $A/\!-\!/B$, the sequence can be reversed for any thus suitable linkage with another connection, as in $B/\!-\!/A - C$, and in the case of two statements like $A \rightarrow B$ and $C \rightarrow {}'B$ they similarly can by transposition of one of them be united, as in $A \rightarrow B \rightarrow {}'C$. When existence of an entity, or of its negation, is known, a simple mark like an underscore will do, as in

$$\underline{A} \rightarrow B \rightarrow C.$$

As explained, the knowledge or existence at the time is a form of an instance of knowledge or existence meant regarding the entity, *A*, to imply the same of what is connected with it, *B*. Consequently knowledge of the existence of the implied is by transitivity likewise ensured, as commonly understood, and the same is true of course of each succeeding linked entity, *C* or more. A simple mark for deletion will similarly serve when known is an entity's or its negation's nonexistence, as in

A→B→C̸.

In accordance with transposition then is ensured the knowledge of nonexistence of each preceding linked entity. These matters on existence and nonexistence apply of course as much to attribution as to implication, the first being part of the second.

Apart from availability of the linkages for both implication and attribution, the two can using the same variables be combined, as indicated before and given by

A→B—C.

The difference between the two connections was observed to be substantially that in implication one thing is accompanied by another within a distance if any that depends on the connection, and in attribution that distance is nil, the one thing being the other. In consequence, with attribution hence a form of implication, when the two are combined, transitivity of implication is in effect. This consequence is another understood as a matter of course, it being quite clear that if *A* implies *B*, and *B* is C, then *A* implies C.

It may be added that the transitivity also follows from an observed transitivity of attribution, by which if one thing is the same as another then what is true of either is true of the other (ca. p.166 last par.). This may be more apparent if the last displayed connections are interchanged, for

A—B→C.

Since *A* is the same as a *B*, and the *B* implies C, so does *A*. Not much harder is it to see that in the precedingly displayed since *B* is the same as a C, and *B* is implied by *A*, so is the C. The important is that however attribution and implication be combined, the implication is transitive.

While many known facts can for deduction be in linkages thus combined, it is not requisite that all reasons for that knowledge, itself often gained deductively, be stated in the same manner. Since the linkages are constructed for viewing how one thing is connected with another through transitivity, if a fact is not determined through it, there is no need to similarly depict the derivation.

Some statements in a linkage were, as in reversing a sequence, already seen derivable directly through other logical laws, which were few and simple enough to, along with the applied to, use unstated. Some of these, e.g. transposition and conversion, as well as transitivity itself are so used in fact for deductions from linkages themselves. Statements in a linkage may also be derived by transitivity, justifying perhaps also a linkage disclosing it. But more likely than not the deduction is a case inference, too brief to need depiction. As iterated, such deduction, from a principle, is an everyday process, often performed without stating either the likely familiar principle, "*B* implies *C*", or especially the specific connection, "*A* is a *B*", merely stating the instance of the principle, "*A* implies *C*".

Nondeductive determinations were treated elsewhere, some of them of definition, others of observation, and they are apt to become the facts combined in a deductive linkage, or be the basis from which those facts themselves are in preceding ways deduced. The last can take place principally when the determinations are quite general, the linkages serving mainly to combine particular facts.

They need hardly be used for additional logical principles, since things to be decided by means of logic were found to require no more than the principles listed. And if things subjects of logic are equally of certain generality, they may likewise require no linkage. Mathematics offers an example.

In its chains of equations, an application of linkage, parts, often numerical, are equated as a result of more general equalities, ones likely using algebraic variables. The particular equalities are, as above referred to, case inferences derived without stating the pertinent connections, here the general "*B* equals *C*" and specific "*A* is a *B*", to state the instance "*A* equals *C*". It is of interest that, although the inference is made without ado, it contains a complication similar to a preceding transitivity (last p. fourth par.). There implication by *A* of *C* is logically an attribute, resulting from the sameness of *A* and a *B*, or of *B* and a *C*. At present an attribute is the equality of *B* to *C*, because of which *A*, same as a *B*, is likewise equal to the corresponding *C*. For this inference thus equality is not about *B* and *C* as shared attributes identifying things (p.165 Theorem III.8), but is jointly with its object, *C*, an attribute of the subject, *B*. It is also noteworthy that, similarly to application of transitive or other logical law (p.141 third par.), the *C* inferred as equal to *A* is not any *C*, but one applying in quantity to *A*. From $a \times b = b \times a$ one does not conclude that 2×3, a case of the premise $a \times b$, equals $b \times a$, but 3×2.

Despite the complexity, such a result is derived with ease mentally, to set it down for a chain of equations. An inference is usually simpler still if of a case of such as a causal law or definition. The transitivity is likely of standard implication or attribution, and the implied or attributed may not be as specific. And as in mathematics, it is particular cases that mostly ask to be linked together.

In the large, general facts were observed in the last chapter to furnish the basis for dependence on things as realities, because it is through those facts that the things are known to be effectual. But it is eventually not the general facts that are the concern, but the particular instances, which when combined may lead to ultimate realizations. Having investigated those facts, laws governing reality, it is appropriate to as a result of them thus combine any specific determinations, and find what can be inferred.

The linking of the determinations in the symbolic form suggested may help to serve this purpose, and in the main has it been intended in this chapter to provide a stable foundation for deduction and the inquiries herein making use of it. Among these and relying also on ascertainments of the preceding chapters are the farther explorations following.

Chapter IV
THE TRANSCENDENT REGIONS

As indicated in the introduction, much of philosophy has increasingly denied the possibility of demonstrating any metaphysical facts, any what are thought of as unexperienced realities, let alone any that would transcend the material world as known to man.

The views were noted bolstered by the successes of observational sciences, and advances by science in general appeared to increase antipathy toward what were largely speculations. Deductive science itself, however, informs of the fallacy of the denial of the antecedent. If *A* implies *B*, it does not follow that *not-A* implies *not-B*. If realities held to be of experience, specifically ones of the natural world, are demonstrable, it does not follow that others are not. As noted also, all inferred, on which the preponderance of knowledge depends, is of the unexperienced.

The opinion that instead deductive truths, comprising the large part of inference, do not speak of reality can as indicated be attributed to the generality of logical or mathematical principles, which do not refer to particular realities that may be sought. It is one thing, however, to consider those principles in isolation, and another to confuse them with their application to actual problems. The significance of those principles lies in those applications, and they are indeed applied abundantly, whether by conscious reference to them or by compliance with them unwittingly. The first is done in profuse mathematics, and the second is indicator of the obviousness of logical fundamentals, whose instances are without knowledge of the principles perceived in particulars in question, unlike in induction, where the instance cannot be known without the principle. How pervasive the use of mathematics is for findings of realities would seem needless to say were it not for above contentions to the contrary. It need only be kept in awareness that quantities regarding things, such as distances through trigonometry, have been computed for millennia. How common in getting to know realities is utilization of logic was previously remarked regarding several theorems, beside the repeated observation of inferring by everyone of instances from principles by transitivity. Animals, too, avail themselves of that transitivity, in learning from repeated experience how to go about life, and they know likewise that in connected causations if, for instance, pushing at a tree will make it shake, and this will make it drop its fruit, then the first event will result in the last.

The knowledge of causation brings to the fore that man and animal make also other inferences of realities than deductive ones, to wit the inductive ones having to do with laws of nature. The point is that the acquaintance with nature as a reality, as consequential as expounded in the pertaining chapter, rests fundamentally itself on inference, on certainty of things not experienced.

There is in ordinary life thus continual and legitimate ascertainment of unobserved realities, as explicated in the last two chapters. Many of those realities were for that matter seen presupposed by the average man and scientist alike in their pursuits, to carry hence greater certainty than scientific findings. It is reliance on these findings that is primarily behind the emphasis on experience. The findings were moreover observed to be to a large measure of the conjectural nature of theories, which suppose at their foundation unperceivable realities. Whereas scientific assertions looked to are correspondingly subject to lack of substantiation, fundamental things presupposed by them were found to be to the contrary, among them ones called metaphysical.

Belonging to these were free will and a similar purposive independence in live organisms from physical and chemical laws. These as susceptible of demonstration about nature have been matters of most dispute. Matters that appear more remote than what is known as nature are furthermore equally susceptible of demonstration. The inquiry can accordingly proceed into realities that may be regarded as transcending nature.

Section 1
THE EXISTENCE OF GOD

It was observed in the first chapter that if something not linguistic is to be about an entity ascertained, it is necessary to have a concept of it, it is necessary to know what the meaning of the name applied to it is. In corresponding demonstration through discourse the meaning must therefore somehow be by language conveyed.

It is sometimes proposed that some concepts, as might be that of God, are ineffable, that they cannot be expressed or described in words. All concepts can be expressed in words, however, since any word can by choice be made to name a concept for that purpose. It is sometimes said that proper names do not have a meaning, and some dictionaries do not list them for that reason. But all a word needs for a meaning is that it designate something. Should the question of the ineffable be whether a concept can be described—that is, defined by usually a number of words to as presently of interest communicate the meaning—it was already expounded that all concepts admit of appropriate definition.

This is the more feasible if the concepts are of general acquaintance, as are those concerned in this disquisition. Yet it is contended that in particular the present concept emerging, that of God, is unknowable, because of his presumed otherness from all that may in the here and now be known by man. As explicated likewise, however, the use alone of a word, lest it be without meaning, presupposes knowledge of a concept behind it.

Knowledge of a concept of God is in accordance with the beginning of this section in addition requisite for attempting proofs regarding him, specifically his existence. It has instead inconsistently been put forward that it is possible to know that, but not what, God is. Essayed proofs of his existence supplied informal definitions nonetheless, and a further issue is whether a given definition is appropriate.

In conformity with previous remarks, definitions are sometimes adapted so as to enable an inference desired, which as a result does not pertain to what it was expected to. The definitions may not be of the expected for some other reason, and what is of account is that in each case the words defined are used equivocally, the subsequent reasoning misapplied.

With respect to the definition of God there is especial likelihood of misguidance, because the concept is variously infused with particulars of divergent beliefs. The definition can accordingly lose sight of the common concerns regarding God, concerns which it is in this writing the object to address, and which thinkers in general are presumed to have in mind. They are nevertheless neglected in mentioned proof attempts, which will in that light and otherwise now be reviewed.

FORMER ARGUMENTS

It may be noted that the definitions given with the arguments, sometimes by the same author, are disparate. They would accordingly not pertain to the same entity, they could in particular not all pertain to the common conception of God. On one occasion thus St. Thomas Aquinas, an above questioner of the knowability, gives nonetheless, in his believed five ways of proving God's existence, five respective definitions. Several of past arguments need correspondingly not be closely examined, because what they would prove would not be in accord with a satisfactory concept of God.

Such arguments are those called cosmological. Among them may be considered to be the first three of the referred to ones of Aquinas, and they maintain the existence of a primal, an uncaused, cause of all things. But the general concept of God can be held to require some power additional to that of first causation, a causation that may be as blind as most others appear to be, whether they themselves be caused or not. The proposal that a primal cause would be of greatest perfection, as advanced by Aquinas in his fourth way though not holding such attribute decisive below, is derived neither through natural nor logical law. The same is true of merely the contention that there is an uncaused cause, to briefly remark on the lack of soundness of the cosmological arugments besides.

In conjuction with them arguments called ontological and teleological form a triad of what appear the most debated regarding the existence of God.

Of these unduly the most seriously taken is the ontological one, associated with St. Anselm. Interestingly Aquinas questioned the definition commencing it, although it may be regarded as suited by connoting God to personify men's highest yearnings. The argument is

1.i. God is that than which nothing greater can be thought.

But, the argument proceeds,

1.ii. It is greater to exist in reality than in thought.

Hence, it is inferred,

1.iii. If God exists only in thought then he is not that than which nothing greater can be thought.

It is therefrom and from 1.i concluded that

1.iv. God exists not only in thought but in reality.

The argument though invalid has been falsely held refuted by Immanuel Kant. As did Hume before, he alleged that existence is not a predicate or attribute, that accordingly nothing is added to an object of thought by positing it to exist in reality. The understanding is that if the distinction in premise 1.ii above is thus unwarranted, what is inferred from it, and 1.i, does not follow. The distinction is irrelevant to the reasoning, however, not leading to the conclusion regardless.

The distinction can indeed be made, whether or not it be held namable as about an attribute. As noted more than once, whether or not existence be called an attribute is a matter of definition. And between a thing as a conception and as a reality there is more than a slight difference. The question as to fact or fancy is a principal one in human endeavors (p.25 last par.), with the greater importance accorded to things that exist in reality, not only in thought.

In consequence assertion 1.iii, which does follow from the two preceding it, is acceptable. As a matter of fact a similar assertion can be made with respect to most any definition of God.

As was observed about real entities like chairs (e.g. p.38 fifth par.), a thought of them is not one of them. It was observed also (p.39 fourth par.) that a thought of a reality conjectured, e.g. a quark, is likewise not identical with it, although the reality may not be certain either. Conjectured realities are many, all the assumptions, again, the truth of which is sought after in man's endeavors. Such an assumption is the existence of God. That is to say by God is envisioned a reality, not a thought, a thought of him not identical with him. Hence whatever the definition 1.i, the existence referred to in 1.ii is the assumption, and as in 1.iii accordingly if God exists only in thought then he is not the being assumed.

But as in the case of other assumed realities, the assumption does not imply the reality. The ontological argument faultily elicits conclusion 1.iv, by in accordance with the premises pitting existence in thought against existence in reality, overlooking that both remain conceptions, and equivocating the second of them with the actual.

In response to objection that something else of perfection, such as some island, may be imagined to exist though it does not, Anselm replied that whereas things other than God can be conceived not to exist, God cannot. The impossibility was further explained to mean existence that is necessary, in the sense that it is eternal. However, other assumed realities, whether assumed permanent or perishable, can likewise not be conceived not to exist, since contradicting, as above, the assumption of existents. To be precise, in questions of realities it is conceived that assumed existents may not exist, but in that case their concept is in practice deprived of one of the things by which it is formed, their existence.

The ontological argument has been thought recently revived on the basis of the just mentioned necessary existence as part of the concept of God. By that necessity if he ever exists then he always does, since an existence not eternal would by the definition not be of God, and if he ever does not exist then he never does, since any such existence not eternal would again by the definition not be of God. By this conception then, speaking of necessity and impossibility in place of "always" and "never",

2.i. It is either necessary or impossible that God exist.

But, it is argued,

2.ii. It is not known to be impossible that God exist.

Hence, it is inferred,

2.iii. It is not impossible that God exist.

In consequence and by 2.i. it is concluded that

2.iv. It is necessary that God exist.

The falsity of the argument is hinted at if the second premise is replaced by "It is not known to be necessary that God exist", leading to the opposite conclusion. The error lies in equivocating the two uses of "possible", or of "not necessary", referred to in the first chapter (p.37 sixth par.). The progression from 2.ii to 2.iii is fallacious, because while something may be possible in the light of man's knowledge, it may be impossible in fact, to never occur as in question.

Of the three mentioned types of argument for the existence of God the teleological may be of widest appeal. It is represented by the fifth above way of Aquinas, and it reasons from design or purpose exhibited in nature to a knowing designer beyond. It reasons by analogy, comparing the purposiveness of organisms to the similar purposiveness of a watch or of an arrow in flight. Both are produced by, in the persons of a watchmaker and an archer, beings of intelligence, of knowledge, whence it is surmised that the purposiveness of organisms has a comparable source.

At times the argument proceeds from considering a general order in the universe, ascribing a designing intelligence as cause. The concepts of order are sometimes opposing ones, however. In one sense what appears referred to is a uniformity as exemplified by laws of nature, and in another sense it is a utility of arrangement in contradistinction to what is looked upon as chaos due to the same forces of nature left to themselves. It is clearer consequently to consider in the argument the analogy with regard to purpose alone.

Analogy is inadmissible, however, as a form of inference. It constitutes what is known as the fallacy of undistributed middle, by which, in no more than unwarranted generalization, if some *B* are known to be C, it does not follow that anything *A* that is *B* is C. That and other lack of implication was treated more fully in the last chapter (p.204 fifth diagram for here), and here it would mean that because some things of purpose have a knowing author, not everything else of purpose needs to. The traditional teleological argument thus takes a leap from premises to conclusion without adequate connection. Yet, its major components are well-founded for an earnest inquiry into the existence of God.

Among the foregoing definitions of God, that of a power with knowledge in likeness to conscious man seems closest to the universal conception of a supreme being. And unlike the grounds adduced for his existence in other arguments, purpose in organisms, which pertains also to men and their preservation or interests, seems a reality of most concern as a possible manifestation of the workings of God. Both, knowledge and purpose, were explored earlier herein, and that the two concepts can be deductively rather simply connected so as to yield the searched-for conclusion will be found presently.

PROOF

In view of the observation that the universal concept of God can be taken to encompass the attribute of knowledge, it can be appreciated that he is accorded that attribute in major religions. But as indicated, a religion tends to embellish the concept with additional specific beliefs, not necessarily commonly shared. The disadvantage is that determination that a being of certain fundamental powers of concern exists is incumbered by specifying further attributes, of for instance how those powers are used. The search will rather be more advantageous if directed into the existence of a supreme being less narrowly defined, while the concern. The common concern indeed can be considered to be existence of a being of the fundamental powers nameable as sovereignty over man.

To be more explicit, the general conception of God can be considered to be of a being of the powers of man to a superior degree, such that he sees man's condition, has altogether knowledge of it and the conditions connected with it, and possesses the power to act accordingly. The attributes consisting in that knowledge alongside the power to bring it to bear, these traditionally expressed by the appellations of the Omniscient and Omnipotent, may in result be regarded as defining God.

Proof of the existence of God so defined is then undertaken here. While in doing so both attributes may be termed powers, whence the title of Almighty may be applied, it will be fitting to speak of the power of action as power, and of the power of knowledge as knowledge. Because there should be little question, further, as to the requisite power, with any of nature's events by which the requisite knowledge would be revealed presupposing that power by their presence, the inquiry will center on that knowledge.

Knowledge, in man, was earlier defined as awareness of something real (p.46 last par.), and the real as what is consequential in man's purposes (p.44 last par.), the two meanings suggesting, as also considered elsewhere (p.96 third par.), that the knowledge serves as a means toward fulfillment of the purposes. Viewing knowledge thus as a means, it admits of a more penetrating definition, one resting on seeing human knowledge and other of man's faculties in terms of their function, in keeping with the purposiveness of organisms in general.

What can in them be excluded as having function are entities which are the basis for it, namely the self and those ingredients of consciousness which are the ultimate purposes, objects of pursuit. But other parts of consciousness were seen as having functions in those pursuits. Passive perception supplies information on which the pursuits are based, and active will brings the pursuits into being. The processes may be intermediate, based on previous activity, and supplying further information.

The awareness as to which of the information one may be guided by, which of it represents reality, constitutes knowledge, whose function is correspondingly to be the guide in one's pursuits, to be the means, alongside one's power to act, toward fulfillment of one's purposes. Knowledge can in consequence be accordingly defined, inasmuch as it is its function which is of concern, not things extraneous to it, as may be acquisition of the knowledge through a material body.

In this larger sense, that goes beyond human attribute alone, knowledge is with power thus understood as the means to purposive activity, to purposive events, events that are, proximate or eventual, objects of purpose. And since a means is something by which something else is brought about, it can be designated a cause or its component. Knowledge can thus be defined as that which is with power the cause of purposive events.

There may arise questions as to the manner in which knowledge with power is a cause, since dissimilar from accustomed causation. But as observed regarding causation, such as causation of bodily motions by thoughts, its manner is irrelevant (e.g. p.62 second par.). Of account is that one event is always accompanied by another. In the case of causation by knowledge and power, the knowledge can be likened to a tool or material by the use of which something is effected, and the power, in being applied, can be likened to any such use. It suffices that these two factors be understood as that which is instrumental in producing purposive events.

The simplicity of the proof searched for should now reveal itself. It can be formally framed as follows, combining the foregoing definitions with previous observations, customarily a matter of course. It should be prefixed that when referring in the proof to the scope of the powers and of events caused by them, meant is a correspondence between these magnitudes, in concord with earlier observations on force as measured by result.

I.1. God equals knowledge with power of concerned scope.

I.2. Knowledge with power equals the cause of purposive events.

Hence, by I.1 and I.2,

I.3. God equals the cause of purposive events of concerned scope.

I.4. Purposive events of concerned scope exist in nature.

I.5. Events that exist in nature imply the existence of a cause of them.

Hence, by I.4 and I.5,

I.6. A cause of purposive events of concerned scope exists.

Therefore, by I.3 and I.6,

I.7. God exists.

The proof may be derived by means of a symbolic linkage as discussed (ca. p.211 through end of chapter).

$$\underline{P} \rightarrow C = K = G,$$

with definitions

P = the purposive events
C = their cause
K = the knowledge with power
G = God.

Because of the importance of the proof, some logical detail will be reviewed.

As discussed regarding linkages, which mainly connect particular facts, it is cumbrous that they be accompanied by listing of general facts that are bases. In the present case, while premise I.1 above is in the linkage repeated by the terminal equality, in the first equality there premise I.2, a general definition, is represented by the particular instance; and while premise I.4 is in the linkage repeated by the underscore of the first letter, in the implication there premise I.5, a principle of nature, is represented by the instance for purpose. Conclusion I.7 will thus be reached by seeing existence implied in the links on through the last letter, without intermediate conclusions I.3 and I.6, not dispensable where used if to ensure clarity.

Both forms of proof also combine implication with attribution, the last as equality. The equality occurs in premises I.1 and I.2 and conclusion I.3, the whole approximating a traditional categorical syllogism. Instead premise I.5 states alone an implication, an existence of what it connects stated in turn by premise I.4 and conclusion I.6, the whole approximating a syllogism called mixed hypothetical. And conclusion I.7 is derived by use of parts of each, I.3 and I.6, with existences connected through equality. The symbolic linkage similarly connects existences through all other connections.

More strictly by particular previous logical observations, in the first form of the proof the first of the three inferences is of a nature noted with respect to mathematical equations (p. 214 fourth par.); in I.2 the equality is the attribute of the subject, of which I.1 states a specific instance, I.3 stating the specific equality applying. The second and third of the inferences are of a nature observed to be mistaken for modus ponens (ca. pp. 206-208); in I.5 the implication is by a general condition, of which I.4 states a specific instance, I.6 stating the specific result; this statement of I.6 can similarly be viewed as about an actual existent, identical with the assumed one of the second of the equated in I.3, to ensure the actuality of I.7. The like occurs in the symbolic linkage, viewable as simply connecting implications.

As suggested by that linkage the reasoning, despite the apparent intricacies, provides little difficulty in practice, resting on common transitivity, by which one progresses from one of connected facts to another. Fact, existence, though in the last chapter assigned primarily to one only of the logics, is, as indicated before by finding the other logic part of the same, a question at the bottom of inquiries in general, so that even when the overt determination is only that something is of a certain nature, beneath is an interest in corresponding existence. In accordingly reasoning by successively connecting one thing with another, be the connections implications or attributions, it is natural to consider that the reality of one thing leads to the reality of another.

Yet an above formal procedure may needlessly complicate the deduction for a listener unaccustomed to it if of some length. If instead truisms are largely left tacit, as in mentioned enthymemes, it may be found easier to proceed from one statement to the next. The truisms are understood regardless, similarly to inadvertent application of logical principles in the preceding, and to interpose their statement can obstruct apprehension.

In the proofs above, as a truism could be regarded the definition of God, in I.1 and the ending equality in the symbolic linkage. But beforehand understood would be especially premises I.4 and I.5, and counterpart underscore and implication in the symbolized proof, as well as intermediate conclusion I.6. All these comprise in fact the basis for the popular teleological argument (p. 221 third par. through p. 222

second par.). It is remaining premise I.2, or the first equality in the linkage, which is the missing link in that argument and not as evident as the mentioned, with I.3 seen an intermediate conclusion corresponding.

In this light the worded proof can be informally abbreviated.

1. God is knowledge with power.

2. Knowledge with power, as in man, is that by which purposive doing is brought about.

Therefore

3. The purposive doing in living things is brought about by knowledge with power, namely God.

The first premise, a form of preceding I.1, was observed viewable as a truism, but it is given to affirm a meaning seen much obscured by diverse beliefs, and to state the attributes to be proven.

The second premise is a form of definition I.2, indicated as not necessarily evident. That the definition is appropriate is in the present premise briefly clarified between the commas.

The conclusion has, for continued brevity, two easily apprehended parts, one before the comma, and the other after.

It will be noted that for simplicity's sake other matters in this proof remain tacit beside I.3, I.4, I.5 and I.6 of the preceding, these four implicit in the conclusion now, including the concerned magnitudes. In the present first premise the concerned magnitude of the attributes is likewise understood, as is their identity with God. In the second premise an identity is more explicit, but less perhaps is that those attributes are causes, that may in the conclusion be inferred in conformance with nature's law. And in the conclusion implicit is, apart from the premises referred to, that the knowledge with power and consequently, as stated in likewise obviated I.7, God exists. All this can be held comprehended by a hearer of the demonstration, as were observed comprehended beside truisms complex meanings behind ordinary words.

It may yet be argued that assertions contained in the demonstrations, whether unspoken or express, may not be as acceptable as they appear. The spoken of scope of the attributes, even if great in totality, might be argued not to belong to the same power, but be divided among units as small as minutest parts of organisms, parts referred to in a previous chapter as thought to have purpose built into them (p.95 last par.). The extent of knowledge and power that could be then said to be present in them would be negligible, adequate only to their limited function. In similar confinement, even if a supreme being is a cause of things, he might be proposed not to exist today but only in the past, as held in some beliefs. The dependence on him as ministrant to human cares, in hope of which he is also called the One and the Everlasting, would by these hypotheses be ill-founded.

That the powers in question are of the concerned scope, however, is determined by observations preceding those regarding minute parts of organisms. They are the observations of the coordination of purpose in the organism's parts, directed toward the preservation of its whole, as well as the species. This phenomenon of far-reaching coordination presupposes its own cause, to wit the discussed powers appropriate to the purpose. It is this large-scale purposiveness of organisms which is seen to exceed, and have as part of its object, the conscious purposiveness of individual men or animals, which conscious purposiveness has as its part the motivating cares or feelings of the individuals possessing it. The knowledge and power at issue extend to all of these, as well as the surrounding world, utilized in behalf of the purposes.

The coordination spoken of betokens a single force or power, the power which thus coordinates and accordingly resides in the described capacities of knowledge and action. What constitutes a single entity was brought up (p.51 last par.) during the discussion of the self, noting that it is a matter of what is desired to be regarded as a unit. And in similarity to the oneness of the self as determined by the selfsameness of primary mental purpose, the oneness of God can be held determined by the selfsameness of projected purpose toward which different parts of the organisms and different powers of God as coordinator are directed.

The singleness and powers of God appear by the preceding determined with respect to only the purposes of particular organisms and their species. Considering man as an instance of these, however, the determinations are of the pertinence required, just as it was sufficient to ascribe reality to things by their consequentiality to man alone (p.46 second par.). As explicated, the concern regarding the nature of a supreme being is at the basis his sovereignty over man, even if not extending elsewhere. That power was found exhibited by jurisdiction over man's purposes, including elements of consciousness, and there is no other supreme power of purpose exhibited with respect to man. To elucidate, the only other purposive, not mechanical, forces known to affect men are other creatures or organisms. When the purpose is by the consciousness of the animal, a fellow sentient being, it is not of a supreme being in question. And when it is of the function of the organism, when a supreme being behind can be inferred, the purpose is known not to be directed at the interests of man, but of the organism.

Upon thus ascertaining a single supreme being over man, a

being that acts in accordance with man's interests, it may still be considered what the full extent of the deity's powers may be. For as signified by the common reference to him as all-knowing and all-powerful, it is of prevailing interest whether his powers may be unlimited, extending to the capacity to meet any of those interests, man's purposes.

Considering limitless power, the power of action, it has been interpreted as of actual predestination of all that ever occurs. The free will of man or animal would accordingly be precluded, as its earlier observed meaning as unimposed by any force would necessitate. But the unlimited power does not require its unlimited exercise. The will was indeed earlier herein found to be free, the freedom in point of fact seeable as bestowed upon man in virtue of God's power, in view of such as organs of sense perception and action, supplied in service of that will. Wondering how much farther the same God's power reaches than the control over man's organism, it may be taken into account that beside the ancestral connections of a species, or even the connections between all species proposed by evolutionary theory, organisms, not excluding plants, are so constituted as to be largely of dependence one on another. One of them can be or can provide the sustenance for another, setting the moral issue for the meanwhile aside. That their interests may be in conflict does not confute a common supreme being. The interests of members of the same family can be in conflict as well. Inorganic matter, furthermore, is likewise an object of dependence with regard to organisms. Not only in the life-sustaining sense applying to the elements of old, to water, fire, air, and earth, of which four the universe was thought to be composed. Also in the comprehensive sense by which all that has reality does because consequential to man, as set forth in this treatise.

This consequentiality of nature, in making significant the governance of all of it by the same laws, is further seen as established by the very purposiveness of man's organism. The organs of action and sense perception are made to affect nature and to perceive the results, as in frequent informing through pain or pleasure of influence on one's body. Acquaintance with the world at large, and consequently its presence as expounded, is to man for the matter of that given by way of the body's purposiveness. For the purpose of sleep or other requirements the world is removed from consciousness, possibly replaced by dreams or other images. Reality was indeed noted held to when unperceived be present because of its possible perception by man. The world and everything that occurs in it is together with other perceptions, all finding its realization in man's consciousness, in consequence the product of God's power. And his power can be said to extend beyond, toward capacity to meet any of men's purposes, in accordance with a plain process of induction. That the world with its laws of nature, including the living form's activities toward fulfillment of its purposes, extends beyond the present, whatever direction events should take, is already an ordinary induction, by which men's actions were observed to be guided. This is to say that under God's power fall, in concord with those purposive activities continued, all events that would be in man's interest.

As regards unlimited knowledge, it has been likewise questioned in the light of man's free will. It would be contradictory that God have foreknowledge of all future events, which would be predetermined accordingly, while man be given a choice in their determination. As implicit in that argument, however, the supposition that if man has a free will, the future accordingly undetermined, then God does not know all is equally contradictory. The recognition that if future events are known then they are determined discloses the understanding that knowledge is meant to be of the determined as reality or fact, in accord with knowledge as considered before in this writing. To affirm man's freedom to decide a future not yet determined and to also require that that future be the object of knowledge is hence inconsistent with that meaning of knowledge as about the determined. The question regarding God's knowledge is indeed that no fact, not what is not, be hidden from him. To these facts belong the intents of a free will itself, everything but the part of the future left undetermined, the determination of which, perhaps depending on man's use of free will, is in view of God's unlimited power nonetheless at his disposal. And that his knowledge as well is unlimited revolves around the same factors that play part in that power. That power was observed displayed by the purposive bringing to man's consciousness all reality, which finds its presence in that consciousness. In it was in fact seen to find its realization all that to man is. The realization was found to be either voluntary or involuntary, the first, unlike the second, of purpose which belongs to man's will rather than of that of the body. And by the preceding God possesses the power to fulfill either of those purposes, and he possesses that power, manifested in the organism's purposiveness, purposively. But by possessing the power to purposively fulfill all that may be purposed, that is the involuntary objectives in consciousness as well as the objects of man's volition, he possesses by the deeper meaning of knowledge, as means to fulfillment of purpose, all those means, to wit all knowledge.

Turning to the other question regarding the plenitude of what is demonstrated in the displayed foregoing proofs, to whether

God's existence as cause of purposive events is unceasing, the answer is supplied by the continuance of those events, taking again free will into account. Because of the free will of sentient beings, the course of things outside it, particularly of bodies of those beings themselves, is, by being subject to those wills, equally undetermined. Accordingly the response of those bodies or other organisms to the changes wrought is contingent upon those wills, to mean that only after their exercise is the specific purposive behavior of the organisms decided. As a result the existence of God as author of that behavior is a continuing one.

Remarkably, the fundamental disclosure of God's existence, underlying the substantially alike demonstrations of it so far presented, does not depend on the definition of God given, although those attributes are requisite. Nor does it correspondingly depend on the definition of knowledge, with power.

To demonstrate the existence of the God who has specifically the attribute of knowledge is universally comforting, because it connotes immediately that he is aware of man's concerns and may act accordingly. But because the desire is at heart for his power thus to act in behalf of man's purposes, the appropriate power of purpose, also, will define God.

The proof of God's existence based on such a definition retains the resemblance to the teleological argument. In that argument occasionally only a supreme designer is spoken of, without further particulars. His existence is alleged to follow from evidences of design. The notion of design, as suggested, is there ambiguous, having to do either with purposeful function, or order of some other kind. Sometimes the word is moreover meant to designate the product of a designer, to in circular argument make positing of design in nature assume a designer before inferred. The concept of designer is regarding his product comprehended in addition in a passive sense, as of one who fashions things, not who activates them. For these reasons and in compliance with present terminology it will be more fitting to speak of purposer and purpose than designer and design.

As an ingredient of the proof purpose, as an occurrence of appropriate scope in nature, was already considered in the previous demonstrations. And that instead of defining God by knowledge and power he may in the same active sense be defined as purposer, of likewise appropriate scope, was indicated in the preceding. To continue, similarly to the definition of knowledge and power but without the same need for preliminaries, purposer should without much dispute be definable as producer or cause of purposive events. Possession of this active power was explained as the interest in regarding a being as a purposer.

The present proof then proceeds along the same line as did the first one (p.224).

II.1. God equals a purposer of concerned scope.

II.2. A purposer equals the cause of purposive events.

Hence, by II.1. and II.2,

II.3. God equals the cause of purposive events of concerned scope.

II.4. Purposive events of concerned scope exist in nature.

II.5. Events that exist in nature imply the existence of a cause of them.

Hence, by II.4 and II.5,

II.6. A cause of purposive events of concerned scope exists.

Therefore, by II.3 and II.6,

II.7. God exists.

Not even the designation of God as purposer is required, furthermore, rendering parts of the proofs omissible. As remarked before the beginning of the first proof, force or power is determined in accordance with result, and presently it is indeed a power determined by purposive events of certain scope as effect that was observed the interest. The proof need consequently only begin by taking as starting definition from either the first or the most recent proof their first inference, I.3 and II.3.

III.1. God equals the cause of purposive events of concerned scope.

III.2. Purposive events of concerned scope exist in nature.

III.3. Events that exist in nature imply the existence of a cause of them.

Hence, by III.2 and III.3,

III.4. A cause of purposive events of concerned scope exists.

Therefore, by III.1 and III.4,

III.5. God exists.

Further reflection may go farther still in simplification. It is customary to query whether there must not be some purpose to nature, with the implicit understanding of a responsible power. Although such purpose is patently before the eyes of men, in the form of life as propounded, it manages to escape notice that that very phenomenon is one that is sought after.

While the significance of ordinary objects of knowledge, specifically nature's purposive events, can thus become obscured to the adult mind, it can be wondered whether a natural association of comparable events with a supreme being is not made by men, and animals, in their early stages of life.

Sentient beings do in fact become aware in their incipient experiences that something acts with regard to their interests. The source of that action may for the most part be the mother, but the young, learning very soon of causation, may not identify the originator immediately with her. Of importance is that there is a display of some thing's activities for the purpose of affecting the young's interests, and its concept of what performs these actions can be equated with that of a supreme being, although not yet, and in the case of an animal presumably never, known by a name. The question can be then what happens in the time between these primal perceptions and those of the grown individual.

It is in conflicting view proposed that the concept of a supreme being is a transference of the image of one's father. But as indicated in the preceding paragraph a transference can be seen to rather take place in an opposite direction. And apart from learning of something purposeful directed at itself and not yet known as a parent, the very young perceives as likewise purposeful other things as well. Not the least of these is its own body. In known curiosity about it the infant soon discovers that the body wants to, like other creatures in entirety, be treated well, at the cost of pain. This preservational purpose of one's organism thus becomes a virtual surrogate for one's own purposes, in animals thought to be of an instinct of self-preservation. And the world at large can be supposed to at first appear as equally purposeful. The playing of a kitten with objects as if they were animate is conspicuous in this regard.

But in time the inanimate character of a large part of nature is recognized, and to animals not even life in a plant may be evident, although they may retain a sense of purpose regarding their surroundings. With reference to one's own body and those of other individuals, they come to be identified with their owners, because of the close connection between the two. It is consequently not surprising that during growth one turns attention to parents and others of control as beings of purpose that affect one's life, while losing sight of the containing bodies and other organisms as purveyors of their own and, by supplying the powers of sentient beings themselves, overruling purpose.

Because of that association of action directed, well-intentioned or not, at one's interests with familiar persons or creatures, it is equally no wonder that a supreme being be expected to be revealed in anthropomorphic form. It may justifiably be assumed that God does resemble man in a sublime manner, if for no other reason than the thereby present embodiment of man's highest longings, as suggested previously. But as also expounded, the association of the relevant manifestations with their appearance as manlike actions is unnecessary for their establishment. The return to and uncovering of the fundamental attributes at issue is the foundation of the ascertainment of the existence of God, as represented by the foregoing proofs, progressing from connotation of more particular human qualities to the principal ones sought, and found in the purposiveness of life.

It may still be argued, in persisting skepticism regarding so important a proof, that life may yet be artificially created. Whatever possibilities exist, however, the furnished demonstrations could be invalidated only if the laws of nature failed to prevail, not to speak of the laws of logic. Should artificial life be possible, all power would not be placed into man's hands. Man does not create nature's laws, including those of live organisms, but is merely enabled knowledge of conditions in which they take effect. Creation of artificial life would accordingly only be creation of conditions under which life will enter, just as conditions can be maintained under which life is preserved. What causal laws characterize life and what is implied by them will not be demolished but constitutes reality on which everyone depends.

Section 2
FURTHER INQUIRIES

THE GOODNESS OF GOD AND MAN

So far these laws were determined to imply the reality of God as possessor of appropriate powers. It is naturally of concern how these powers are used—specifically, whether they are used in behalf of man's interests, whether God can be determined to be good.

The questions regarding goodness, or the good in general, have been major subjects of philosophical investigations, known under the names of ethics and aesthetics. As in the case of other subjects, the questions are on one hand about the nature of the thing discussed, that is to say what sort of conduct is ethical, or moral, and what an aesthetic experience, often termed the perception of beauty, consists in; the questions are on the other hand about the means by which those implicitly desired goods as ends can be achieved, although the means are sometimes identified with the subjects dealt with, with the ends.

It can at once be observed that what the nature of ethical conduct and an aesthetic experience is is again a matter of definition. Though both are designated as good, of that conduct only its final object, a well-being of the recipient, would be likened to that experience, generally meant to be satisfaction for its own sake, rather than gratification over something because it leads to something else. That satisfaction thus pertains to the purpose observed to characterize man and animal (e.g. p.50 second par.). But there need as with other definitions be no dispute about which entity called good is at issue, it depending on choice.

In aesthetics the entity of interest does differ from that in ethics foremost be needing to be only about the satisfaction, or a perceived thing causing it, not about action that has someone else's similar feelings in consideration. It differs in addition by having to do usually with, if not works of art, then other objects of satisfaction that are supplemental, not with critical ones, which are primary aims of morality. These satisfactions, concentrating on works of art, are correspondingly associated principally with those things that please through sight or sound, that have been termed the beautiful.

The designation of beauty in this connection has fallen into disfavor. It has long been acknowledged that works of art can deal with ugly subject matter, and it therefore seems inappropriate to regard them as beautiful. There is a difference, however, between a work of art and the content it represents, and it is the appeal of the work, not the content, which is referred to by the work's aesthetic value. What works of art are able to accomplish is to be pleasurable while the same may not be independently true of their subject matter. There is as a result no cause to abandon the term beauty, be it only a word. It is sometimes contended that neither beauty nor aesthetic appeal, nay any appeal at all, is required as a mark of art. But in that event a different meaning of a word, of art, is again adopted. If desired, anything else may be named art, but it would not be the subject contemplated.

This observation should not be mistaken for a frequent one opposite in purport, which expects of art that it depict a content. Content may not even be expressed, the requirement of art meant to be that it, among man's creations, please alone, in the above aesthetic sense. It may of course do so alongside some other function, insofar as that is something additional. Architecture can serve as example, and also illustrate absence of such as pictorial content. Neither is art for art's sake, if understood as emphasis on formal features independent of the perceiver, what is meant, with delight of the perceiver the test instead.

It could be maintained that in view of the profound truths art is often said to convey, at least some of it should be evaluated on the basis of content. But works of artistic merit often portray matters of discredited value, and the most serious facts can be presented in artless fashion, without it being decided to accordingly change the meaning of art. This is not to mean that what is appended to art is immaterial. If not intended to be self-sufficient then it certainly counts what else it performs, and it may be also appraised from that standpoint. As a matter of fact beauty can be an expression of the fittingness of that which is beautiful, as can for instance in nature appeal be a sign of benefit.

Nevertheless whether concerning art or more broadly the aesthetic, the meaning of the good in mind is of the satisfaction for itself, or of the perceived quality in a thing that directly elicits that feeling, not that has a less direct import instead.

This meaning has as indicated been taken issue with not only by denying that some sort of satisfaction need result from the thing perceived or that the thing need not be associated with some other matter, but also by denying that any perceiver response is of account, the value of the aesthetic object held to reside elsewhere. The contention is supported by pointing to the subjectivity of that response, which may differ from person to person, whereas an aesthetic object is viewed as being one objectively. It need only be repeated, however, that what is called aesthetic is a matter of choice, and of interest at present are things that cause certain satisfaction. If they do to no more than some, then so be it, but there is good reason to believe that things regarded as beautiful have at least potentially a general appeal, although particular tastes in such as foods may vary. The many differences encountered in responses can be to a large extent attributed to the disrelated indirectness of some appeal. A thing is often held beautiful because associated with some other.

Questioned is also the directness of the appeal with regard to literature. It is argued that being dependent on language as conveyor of meaning, its beauty is to be found in that meaning, frankly allowing that its aesthetic status may be in doubt. But similarly to a painting, the most beautiful subject matter can be described in poorest language, and a realization in literature is that language, as other things, can have its own beauty. The cognition of that is sufficiently displayed by rhymes in poetry. This formal attention belongs in fact to that also given to things of beauty in order to define them. Their formal aspect rather than the perceiver's favorable response would thus become the criterion of their aesthetic character, as would something else associated with objects of aesthetic appeal if accordingly defined. Such definitions of the beautiful can be seen unsuited if only because they by finding the objects to be of the appeal intimate it as the criterion after all. Moreover rather than stating what beauty is meant to be, they hypothesize the conditions under which it is brought forth. In accordance with a previous mention the beautiful as a sought after end is consequently confounded with the means to it.

The irrelevancy to it, to its perception, of many factors separate from it was noted above. And the search for what in the beautiful object itself, in its form in which perceived, accounts for its appeal is comparably not germane.

The elusiveness of any rules regarding such form is notorious, with formulas prescribing it known too well not to secure good works of art. Where rules have been attempted, they often have been lacking logically.

Cited in many ages as principal requirement for a work of beauty is unity, yet the word is as indefinite as noted of order (p.221 fourth par.), spoken of sometimes in place of it. The unity is explained by qualifying it as organic, through interdependence of all the parts of the work. It can accordingly be asked in what manner the parts are dependent on one another, and the answer can be found in the very meaning of the beautiful. As that which satisfies as explained, the beautiful must please by means of whatever formal parts it is composed of. If one part clashes with another, the import is that the work does not please in that manner, which is to say that one part is dependent on its compatibility with the other.

Into account is here taken the frequent reference to discord in art, particularly in a musical work. The matter may be likened to disquieting contents alluded to. By whatever standard sounds may be held discordant, they please together in the composition, for that is the criterion. Dissonance also finds its similitude in contrast, regarded in unison with repetition likewise an aesthetic requirement. The combination may also be known as theme and variation or simply sameness and difference. But the two need not come together for a thing to be beautiful. The beauty of geometric uniformity, exemplified by a square, has long been recognized, as has the appeal of nature's many irregular shapes, exemplified by a cloud. To say that the aesthetic must hence have either uniformity or irregularity would exhaust all things, since either attribute is the negation of the other, and all things are certainly not regarded as beautiful.

Requirements that beautiful things possess certain formal attributes usually furthermore engage in dual fallacy observed. One is an inference that because some things of those attributes are beautiful all are (the fallacy of undistributed middle), and the other an inference that because all things of those attributes are beautiful all beautiful things are of those attributes (the fallacy of affirmation of the consequent).

More apropos is that a protracted study of what formal attribute in things thus satisfies is beside the point, because what does is decided by direct perception of them. It would not be endeavored to instruct what in the taste of foods makes them pleasurable, placing a restriction on what they may taste like. It is to be understood that in question is not what in things may be desired by people for whom a product would by someone else correspondingly be prepared. In that case differing preference or need would be considered. As earlier regarding knowledge of meaning of words of one's own usage, or any knowledge possessed by an inquirer, the question is rather what in aesthetic objects appeals to their producers themselves. More generally the question as to what in beautiful things makes them appealing has to do with their appeal to oneself, and as one knows one's meaning of words without hypothesis, or has access to any of one's own knowledge, one need not investigate by given rules of form whether a thing has aesthetic value, for one can ascertain the same directly. The matter has bearing chiefly on the artist, the aesthetic form of whose work is accordingly not guided by rules, but by satisfying perception, granting the skills required.

In ethics the issues are of a similar nature. The original meaning of the ethical is oftentimes lost in efforts to formulate rules by which moral conduct should abide. That meaning was indicated to be and is herein considered as conduct in behalf of a well-being of other individuals, a well-being generally called happiness and to be sought for all mankind, as well as animals, within possible extent. As in other cases when determinations about a subject are confounded with it, however, through consideration of ways by which that happiness would be provided those of them that were found of a generality were adopted as definitions of morality in place of its fundamental meaning.

The results can be more disastrous than mere redefinition. When the means that may lead to human benefit thus replace it as ends, then on supposing them to be of higher value, human lives are often sacrificed for the sake of them. Such resulting actions then become in a turnabout the means to the misconceived ends, and in consequence further misconceptions can ensue. Seeing those actions as unconscionable, the oft quoted rule may be embraced that ends do not justify means. The use of the rule, however, can likewise bring about the opposite of the intended. If the end is the happiness spoken of and the means contrary to a referred to code, the results of prohibiting the means to the end can again be deplorable.

Whether it is the means or the ends that are important depends on what they are, in an example of how morality can be foresaken if dependent on rules.

The primarily important is that in accordance with the concerned meaning of morality equitable happiness be always the object. This purpose can itself be considered the decisive rule, as was in matters of fact the rule that an actuality be perceived appropriately to what is meant to make it one. Inasmuch as that purpose can be regarded as obligatory it can also be spoken of as duty, although that word has unfortunately been attached to the extraneous rules discussed. They are referred to as about duty for duty's sake, connoting a behavior which is aimless. And the point is that the behavior to be regarded as a duty is one aimed at other individuals' happiness.

The characterization of the aim of ethical conduct as that happiness is similarly to beauty criticized as platitudinous, as not designating the desires of everyone, or as forgotting that not everyone may find happiness in the same things.

That happiness be a platitude is of no relevance. Any confidence placed in what appear to be newly established facts is self-defeating if it rejects the existence of constants, on which all knowledge is founded.

That everybody's desire may not be happiness depends again on the meaning assigned to it. That meaning can herein broadly be taken to be the very fulfillment of one's desires. Happiness is by some equated with pleasure, which in turn is often assigned to sensory satisfactions. It is then argued that there exist other satisfactions or desirable things, such as knowledge. Concerned as said are things desirable for their own sake, and it can be questioned whether knowledge or other suggested goods belong to them. Anything so desirable, what is the ultimate object of desire by anyone, can regardless, however, be understood as meant by the satisfaction or happiness. It is the meaning by which desire is customarily connected with satisfaction, the object of the former being the latter. The two may not be in a sequence of time, desirability meant to be merely satisfactoriness itself, perhaps of a present state. Nor should the desirable be distinguished from the desired, under the notion that some do not know what makes them happy, desiring things undesirable. At issue is what makes individuals happy knowingly, not what someone else thinks their lot should be. In the same strain are of no concern allegations of unconscious desires, however discovered in absence of meanings outside consciousness, with conscious happiness the object.

That all may not be made happy by the same things seems the same question as the preceding on all wanting happiness. But now it is granted that all want happiness, satisfaction, and the query is whether what is satisfying to some is to others. As with beauty, however, the matter is not relevant to whether the happiness of fellow beings is the object of moral behavior. If a different thing brings happiness to each, the things sharing no other attribute, it is still the benefit intended, though its realization would be quite difficult.

But as it can be presumed that the beautiful is to a large degree the same for all men, so it can be presumed that with all men the immediate conditions for happiness are likewise to a large degree the same. Similarly to differences by regarding things as beautiful for reasons other than direct appeal, different desires can be held to substantially be for conditions expected to lead to those more fundamental in conducing to happiness. And because these fundamental conditions for happiness can be presumed to be considerably the same with mankind in general, they make feasible the discernment of means that may generally apply in seeking moral ends. Such a means is the universally sounded golden rule, that one should do onto others as one would have them do onto oneself. By having one's own desires as express criteria the rule can be seen as manifestly built on the assumption that the circumstances for happiness are the same for all. Less manifestly this assumption can be viewed as the foundation of other, more specific, rules as well, such as contained in the ten commandments, in accordance with which one would wish to be treated. As indicated, however, ethical rules as means may not be always appropriate for ensuring human happiness as end.

Even if the golden rule, expressing the basis for others, is interpreted to apply to only ultimate sources of satisfaction, these may not be uniform from person to person. As men can differ in their taste for a food, they can differ in their vision of an ideal existence. In this regard it may be recalled that the aims of morality are predominantly the satisfaction of more fundamental requirements than the sensuous ones that may be represented by preferences of the palate. The concept of happiness as the aim correspondingly warrants a yet more profound characterization in addition to the foregoing one. It is not the indulgence of momentary appetites which is of concern. Instead it is a comprehensive mental contentment, in which the senses, as signs of physical needs specifically, have a part, but which includes such intangibles as receiving love, or dispensing it, in reciprocal morality. This deeper meaning of happiness, of contentment, is easily perceived as a general one, inasmuch as grosser pleasures would be admitted not to bring happiness, contentment.

Recognizing the encompassing nature of happiness as compared to particular pleasures, the conditions for happiness may nevertheless likewise not be identical and the golden rule not apply unequivocally. The golden rule is nonetheless of exceptional value, especially with regard to tenderest feelings. Men regrettably often think themselves and perhaps those near to them to be of greater sensitivity than others, if not imagining others to be devoid of feeling altogether.

While rules in ethics can perform amiss, especially the more particular the conditions they would prescribe, there may be more general conditions for happiness that are commonly required, and to which a rule may accordingly apply. Aside from fulfilling others' more direct desires, one can provide means by which they can be fulfilled by their possessors. Among these means, next to physical ones, was indicated to be knowledge, acquired, in all learning of reality, through dependence on information received. Consequently in order that information one imparts be dependable, in accord with commonly sought trustworthiness, one should always be truthful. There are occasions of course when someone's knowledge of a truth is expected not to serve a good end, but in that case witholding the truth rather than lying is in order, since to allow for exceptions destroys credibility. But it should also not be thought that by observing a satisfactory rule one's obligations are always discharged.

The widely acknowledged exhortation that one should always be truthful, which includes keeping a promise if within one's powers and if any other required conditions are met, is one defectively justified in conjunction with the by many endorsed categorical imperative. In accordance with it one should act only on maxims one can will to be universal laws. It is argued that if, in a rule opposite to the above, it were a universal law that everyone in difficulty can make a false promise, then no promises could exist, since no one would believe them. It is concluded that one should will truthfulness a universal law.

Objectionable about this and conjoined arguments is that any purpose for the commended behavior is disavowed, in particular any benefit that may accrue to someone. Thus explanation is wanting why it is bad if a listener must disbelieve a liar, or if as a result promises cannot exist, not to mention that avoidance of disbelief through truthfulness is already a purpose.

Further the inference that no promise could exist as a result of disbelief has no basis, and it signalized a shift of attention regarding ethics from concern with benevolence to forms of non-contradiction. The suggestion is that false promises could not exist because contradictory. But they would merely be untrue, as is any statement inconsistent with fact. More pertinent is that the proposal that a contradiction or other logical falsity is immoral is out of keeping with the intended meaning of morality.

Furthermore even provided the reasons offered for not making false promises or lying are acceptable, the conclusion about truthfulness does not follow. If it is wrong that one should always lie, as was also posited, or that everyone in difficulty can make a false promise, it does not follow that one should never lie, or that a false promise cannot be made when in certain difficulty only or for some other reason, or that any of these cannot be done by only some.

On this ground it would seem that though it be found unacceptable that one should for arbitrary reasons lie or make false promises, there may be times when doing so could be justified. This view is in fact adopted by many, maintaining that for instance at one's deathbed one can be told a pleasant lie, since not verified. The requiring of that latitude, however, itself implants doubt about someone's truthfulness, to defeat its purpose.

More troubling than the arguments on particulars like truthfulness in prescribing the categorical imperative is the prescript in general. That it mean the same as the golden rule is with it expressly repudiated, and one can be at a loss as to what action be willed universal law, for one can so will most anything, including what is to one's own advantage. The indication is that the action be moral or, although the categoricality is to preclude a purpose, benevolent. But if the action is asked to be moral then the rule is circular, describing morality via morality, i.e. failing to be more illuminating so modified. And if the action is asked to be benevolent then it should by the rule be only taken if it can be willed a universal law. Therein lies the rule's injuriousness. It replaces action guided by humaneness with action according to prescribed procedure, the baleful consequences of which doctrinaire ways are legion.

The past approaches to ethics, as well as aesthetics, as an elaborate field on the order of a science can in fact be held ill-considered, similarly to before noted treatment of the human mind as if an unconscious mechanism, determining behavior in accordance with to be studied rules, discounting free will. The question of the concerned moral conduct is, as in the case of the beautiful, largely confused with its meaning, which not only informs of its sought after nature and is a matter of definition, but is understood by everyone, including children, as kindness. It is because the nature of moral conduct is thus common knowledge that people are held responsible for, supposing them ascertainable, acts of ill will but not acts of ignorance. As to particular acts that can be regarded as moral, it was already observed that certain fundamental conditions for happiness can be viewed as applying quite generally, as can the perception of certain things as beautiful. Corresponding to this view is again the golden rule, an expression of a natural comprehension that to be kind is to treat others as one likes to be treated oneself. Morality by consisting in the fostering of the happiness of others can in point of fact be viewed as founded on the conception that others, in their need for happiness, possess sensitivities like one's own. The golden rule correspondingly does not set up a procedure one must follow, merely speaking of like happiness to be striven for for all, just as a work of art may want to be of beauty by a shared meaning of the word, without requirements regarding the work's form. Beyond thus meeting the desires of everyone, a rule in a narrower sense would accordingly apply to everyone in every instance of the thing at issue. A rule that would apply to every aesthetic object beyond its appeal, or to each of a kind, was noted hardly formulable. When expanding appeal to the sphere of ethics, however, certain consistencies, extending to indirect connections, are observable in things beyond their production of well-being. Unlike the concerned results of certain kinds of pictorial or musical works, the tastes or smells of certain kinds of things can fairly regularly be determined to be pleasant or unpleasant. More broadly there are kinds of things, notably ones affecting the preservation of one's body, that are known to generally produce pleasure, as do nutrients, or pain, as do injuries. For such reasons provision of sustenance and shelter are regarded as foremost moral obligations. And of consequence is that these connections between certain conditions and resulting welfare have to do with sciences external to ethics. What conditions favorably or unfavorably affect the body is the province of medicine and by extension biology, physics, and so on.

Whereas it is rules of science, or rather laws of nature underlying it, that thus determine how moral objectives be attained, one can of course act morally without looking to scientific verification for each of one's moves. As expounded previously, scientific knowledge presupposes an ordinary knowledge of worldly reality, and within that knowledge falls acquaintance with man's and the animal's general needs such as mentioned sustenance and shelter. Furthermore in personal relations one is likely to know more about the other individual's situation than would a scientific thesis that speaks about everybody. This does obviously not mean that one has the ability to achieve every moral purpose, as does not science alone, both it and knowledge of individual need being correlates of each other. What matters is that one is equipped to act morally, in particular by means utilized for oneself in like situations, on the preceding understanding that certain basic requirements are the same for other beings.

As regards moreover not the intermediate requirements of such as the body, but the desired ends of the individuals themselves, their happiness, sciences are still less of dependancy. One simple way of learning what other persons desire is to ask them, for the concern as noted is what makes others happy in their own consciousness, not in the opinion of someone else. Even animals manage to communicate whether something pleases or displeases them, and men's tool of communication, language, was observed to be one of the common acquisitions through induction, and one whose understanding by science is presupposed in its ascertaining of human desires, if not presumptuously again telling others what their desires are. Another such common induction was observed to be, with the aid of language, that others share, beside one's bodily functions, the mental ones, along with corresponding experiences. To these experiences belong feelings, the satisfaction or dissatisfaction with circumstances, the objects of moral concern. Hence when particular communication is hindered one can use as guide, in likeness to the creating of art, one's own response to a contemplated condition, in moral pursuit of it for another being. Viz insofar as the conditions for happiness are the same one has to for their knowledge only rely on one's own feelings, without injection of scientific principle, and insofar as the conditions differ a principle is of no avail.

A person thus has a comprehension of what consists in moral action, which includes, alongside seeking of ultimate conditions for happiness of others, the affording of means by which they may themselves attain that end. Among these was seen to be knowledge imparted through truthfulness, and most moral action is in fact of furnishing such implements, as in providing circumstances for physical welfare, the receiver enabled then to make use of them. That action be so divided is in justice when considering that if one person be regardful of another's interests, the other would share in responsibility, each doing with regard to each as capacitated.

This mutuality suggests that men can also so arrange their lives as to benefit one another as best they can due to their developed competencies, such arrangements, larger than of the natural family, known as political units, chiefly states. Political theories abound, and by the foregoing important is that beside the fundamental goal of attainable happiness for all there ought to be a refraining from inflexible rules, in particular from imposing by government conditions not in accord with the people's desire. That desire once again, not someone's conception external to it, was noted the criterion of the circumstances for happiness, its political expression usually called democracy. Emphasis on this desire can be in conflict with both what are termed the political left and right. In one, the endeavor is for instance to abolish private ownership of property; yet it is doubtful that there are many who do not wish to treasure things as their own, with even animals resenting intrusion. In the other, individuals would be left to their own resources in fulfilling their basic needs, such as care for their health; but the very organizing by society begs for securing by it of everyone's essentials one cannot obtain alone. The focus is on bringing happiness in concord with shared wishes, rather than on implementing a conceived political system, the appropriate morality requiring by the aforesaid no further governance than the knowledge supplied by the particular expertise of those chosen to articulate and carry out those wishes.

The matter of morality being a commonly comprehended one, it appears mainly requisite to in informing of its attributes make known what the subject discussed, with largely avoidance of rules, unlike in searches for further attributes by principle of objects known. The searches regarding morality were indeed seen to revolve to a large extent around its definition. The question posed was noted part of that concerning the good, which has been held indefinable, because upon proposing a meaning, other things were found to be named good as well. But as reiterated, not only can a word be defined, but meaning is a matter of choice, and the choices can be several, resulting in different senses. Accordingly as indicated at the beginning of this section, there are diverse kinds of things referred to as good, accounting for the discrepancy about the word. As a good was noted to be designated an aesthetic experience or its object, the beautiful, as well as presently discussed ethical conduct and its objective, happiness. Good are called also the immediate circumstances for happiness, and anything that may by its workability lead to it. And good is the person who seeks these for others, who acts morally.

The last designation suggests that of interest is not merely that to seek the happiness of others defines moral conduct, but that it is a precept by which man should abide.

In keeping with the tenor of this book, or with expectations in general of supporting of statements made, it could be asked how the moral precept is justified. A longstanding contention is as a matter of fact that ascriptions of value in ethics or aesthetics cannot be substantiated, that they even lack truth or falsity, as mentioned in the introduction. As said there the contention is related to the questioning of facts not verifiable through the senses, and it is accordingly argued that moral injunctions are not statements of fact, the truth or falsity of which statements alone it is possible to establish. It is specifically argued that because moral injunctions say what ought to be, they cannot be inferred from what is.

The argument is again falsely dependent on language, however. To say that something ought to be done is similar to saying that something is necessary, both expressions sometimes substituted by phrases containing "must". And in both cases it is as before simpler to say "This must be done" than the what would be held true or false "If this is not done then the desired result will not be obtained." That result can for particular moral codes be considered to be the happiness spoken of. To hold then that these codes need no justification is equivalent to the mentioned hurtful proposal that they be observed for themselves, not as means to beneficial ends.

But at the base of the supposed unprovability of moral codes can be held to lie the thought that nature imposes no moral laws, unlike causal ones and perhaps those of logic. Thus it may seem that while the acknowledged laws cannot be ignored without risk, moral ones can since appearing arbitrary. But even if arbitrary, laws imposed by men can evidently not be ignored either. Children know that if not behaving they will be punished, and the like applies to laws of governments. Moral law is, however, not so arbitrary. Man-made laws or rules, including some called moral, can be contrivances of tyrants. But many result from the very same want prompting one to obey laws of nature. It is the want to be satisfied, to be happy. It is not only the inanimate that affects one's happiness, but animals and particularly other men as well, to give rise to assented to laws or rules aiming at happiness for all. Underlying is what in affinity with past usage may be termed a natural law of morality, of seeking the others' happiness. For one should if for no other reason seek it because as one cannot with impunity go counter to laws of nature, one cannot with impunity mistreat others.

One prefers to think that moral behavior is also appropriate under all circumstances, however, not only when recompense by others is at issue, and some may ask what the justification may be. Religion maintains retribution by God, similar to the responses of men. These are perceived as actions coming from outside oneself, but as suggested by the preference of moral conduct independent of circumstance, the motivation can also be found within one's own feelings.

The feelings are best known by the name of love. The word is like others used in various senses, and it is certainly not its meaning as much enjoyment of its object such as food that is here considered. In this sense the meaning can become the opposite of the intended, connoting selfishness instead of selflessness. In its pertinent use the word is likewise ambiguous. It sometimes and with no less importance does not refer to feeling but to action, as implied in the entreaty to love one's neighbor. The present meaning of love has to do with the feeling behind that action. It is love as a feeling of benevolence, of wanting the happiness of another. The feeling is sometimes called sympathy, referring to the sharing of another's gladness or distress, the meaning implicit in preceding love, by which happiness of another is desired by oneself as well as by the other. This feeling can accordingly be taken into account as motivation for morality, motivation that reaches farther than that of external requital, so as to be always present.

That sympathy be the ground for moral action has been contested as inappropriate because not everybody may feel sympathy or do so in equal degrees. Other grounds adduced for moral action, however, are likewise not certain to fit everyone. Whichever the rewards or punishments upheld to induce men to morality, their equal effect on all can similarly be questioned. It is true that men will often respond to coercion rather than performing the same action of their free will. But supposing the action a moral one and not some other, the implication is not that the person is void of sympathy. Instead it can be presumed that the person does not let such feelings interpose, under some notion of advantage derived. Coercion may prevent the assumed advantages, but being heedless of one's feelings may have a different result. Mankind is quite conscious of the many cases in which one's self-centeredness will subdue one's feelings of compassion. Of equal awareness is the affection in man's and the animal's care for their young. The last indicates that love, one's feelings for the interests of others, is as fundamental a function shared by sentient beings as are the other functions previously cited.

On finding one's own happiness the justification for acting toward the happiness of others, whether the reward is the internal one of love or the external one of requital, some might ask what the justification is for wanting to be happy. In the vein of the arguments that reasons cannot be given for morality, it is advanced that for some moral rules more general ones can be given as reason, and for those perhaps others, but that to escape infinite regress, a basic rule cannot be justified. On further thought it is admitted that a like issue can be raised in regard to all knowledge by asking for a reason why any claimed basis for it be accepted, and it is maintained that in real knowledge basic facts can somehow be agreed upon, without any more proof. But the throughout this volume found evasiveness of basic facts belies this belief. Objectivity versus subjectivity is moreover irrelevant. As also seen in what went before, knowledge does not depend on consensus, but on correct criteria. It will be well in this respect to examine justification.

Expressed as reason for something, it was earlier already found confused with cause. The cause of an event is sometimes called the reason for it, but so is its purpose if it has one. Furthermore the criterion on which a determination is based is called its reason likewise. For examples, as a reason for the finding of circulation of the blood may be given in one sense its movement due to the pumping of the heart, in another sense the function of distributing oxygen in the body, and in a third and incongruous sense scientific observation. A common ground can be detected. In determinations their criteria as reasons provide certainty, also present when knowing the function as reason of organic occurrences, and what events as reasons cause what others. The certainties were further seen to serve purposes of man, the purposes reasons, once more, for one's actions.

Among these kinds of reasons it is only material causation found to regress indefinitely, in conformity with the principle that all physical states have a cause. Even this infinity, however, is qualified. It is only required as long as the cause is physical. The free will as cause was observed to be uncaused. In the area of logic it was likewise observed that principles are not always based on broader ones, but can on their own be perceptually ascertained. Such ascertainment was in fact explicated to underlie all knowledge, with certain perceptions the criteria of truth, with no further confirmation. The adequacy was in places explained by equating description with explanation. No further reason after a decisive one also concerns its sense as a purpose, as in general indicated in a former chapter (e.g. p.50). In an organism the purpose of preservation could be held ultimate. But in man the ultimate purpose is consciously contentment, happiness, the eventual reason for intermediate purposes. It is sought for no other reason but itself, as observed in this section also with respect to its meaning, and hence, lest engaging in contradiction, requires no further reason. The obviousness may be made clear by stating redundantly that one is quite happy to be happy.

The possible attainment of satisfaction with no other end but itself was observed to (e.g. p.234 first par.) also characterize the good regarding beauty, as well as, when the satisfaction concerns the sought after happiness of others, the good regarding the person who by that endeavor acts morally. Corresponding to this meaning of goodness applied to a person is its meaning applied to God. By the goodness of God is meant that his purpose is the happiness of man and other creatures.

In searching accordingly for whether God is good it can be taken into account that it was through purpose itself as exhibited in organisms that he was found to be revealed. The remainder of nature does not behave purposively, whereby it might display either benevolent or malevolent intent. And the encompassing purpose of organisms was seen to be their preservation. This purpose was observed to in sentient beings be provided for also by, in cooperation with components of the body, those of the mind, including feelings of pleasure and pain, the feelings moreover extending in sympathy to the interests of fellow beings. Therefore insofar as preservation is the interest as road to happiness of man or animal, God is good.

The preceding may be viewed as a reply to what is known as the problem of evil. It is asked why if God is all-powerful and good does he permit pain. But in view of its function as a warning about bodily harm, pain is not synonymous with evil, on holding evil to connote ill intention. Yet it may be remonstrated that while the organism thus functions toward self-preservation, it cannot be said to, in the economy of a world in which one organism is sustenance of another, function toward preservation of others.

In answer it may serve to be remindful that it is in the end consciousness which determines the nature of reality, and whose contentment, even in the eyes of other individuals' sympathy, is of interest beyond a physical universe. The fortunes of this world are not necessarily the ultimate ones. It should be considered in this respect that conditions inordinate in anguish become removed from consciousness in forms like faint. But it may be persisted that if bodily existence is not the only one why should one suffer at all in connection with it, why should one, it may be asked, suffer altogether, and not be happy always.

The conditions for happiness may in this regard be again examined.

It was noted that by happiness is meant a comprehensive mental contentment, and the contentment may contain particulars which in themselves are grievous. Happiness can thus be compared to the mentioned work of art in which depicted particulars displease apart, but please as part of the whole. Indeed as may be also the case in a drama, what dissatisfies independently may become satisfying because of the anticipated outcome. This is in accord with the experience that not all that is painful is unhealthy, or that not all that is pleasurable is healthy. Man learns to renounce momentary satisfactions for more lasting ones. And that in the process the preliminary conditions become likewise satisfying is evidenced by the overwhelming majority of things that please as a means to something else, rather than for their spoken of own sake. Knowledge or money, prized in opposing ways and having not even direct physical functions, are prominent examples. Furthermore even failures and misfortunes represent and are valued as instructive experience. Any of these attitudes is expressed by the adage that all is well that ends well.

Still it may be protested why there should be troubling particulars, why all should not be trouble-free. Again those particulars can be compared to darker incidents in a literary or other composition. Beside the value of the incidents in the light of the larger work, the work cannot be fully appreciated without the incidents. In a broader context it is said that one cannot appreciate the good without the bad. In truth fulfillment unearned, attained without hardship, possesses for man no lustre. And the more lasting the ultimate fulfillment the more in imbalance is a sparsity of merit.

It may continue to be argued that although the worthiness appeals to the human sense of justice, things might be otherwise. Man might be happy under other conditions. But such argument is no longer relevant. At issue is what in fact is basis for man's happiness, and whether that basis is put at man's disposal, as signification of God's benevolence.

As disclosed in the previously said, man is furnished the very attributes that in confrontation with difficulties enable one to seek fulfillment of one's purposes, in consonance with the described preparatory conditions for man's happiness, to by the expounded imply God's goodness.

HEAVEN AND IMMORTALITY

The preceding observations call forth the conceptions of an afterlife and heaven, the circumstance of consummate fulfillment or happiness.

Because heavenly ideals may differ, because they should coincide with individual yearnings and be envisioned accordingly, little more need be said on the nature of heaven. It may only be noted again that desires can often be held to be alike in certain fundamental aspects, and therefore the same can be assumed in the present regard.

As complete realization of one's longings heaven is not thought to occur in this world. Neither a state of eternal bliss nor a temporal dispensation of justice is a culmination awaited in an individual's worldly existence. Consequently it is hoped that there is an afterlife, that human beings, and others, moreover are immortal.

The possibility of immortality, of survival of the self after bodily death, was indicated (p.12 third par.) to have been denied on the proposition that the self consists at least in part of one's body. The indication was given in connection with definition, which can be made to so characterize the self as to preclude the inference of immortality. As likewise observed (e.g. p.50), however, the self universally meant to survive the body is of course a disembodied one, often referred to as soul. This self was earlier described more specifically as an element of consciousness distinguished by a sensibility characterized by desire for happiness, attained perhaps in a future life and by the self newly embodied.

Granting that the self resides in consciousness, argument is also advanced that consciousness is in some manner identical with part of the body, the impossibility of which sameness, too, was explicated before (p.56 third and fourth pars.). Having to do with logical, intrinsic, rather than natural, extrinsic, connection is also the proposal made that mental entities devoid of a body are unintelligible. But one need only abstain from observing one's body to find that one's consciousness does not vanish, one's body indeed seen as only part of many objects of one's perception.

It remains to find that the existence of consciousness is not inexorably tied to the existence of the body without being part of it, that the mind, the self, indeed may always survive. It should at first be considered that the death of the body does not signify its disappearance, but its disintegration. This happens in conformity with conservation law, discussed in a previous chapter (e.g. p.74 last par.). Hence should the death of the body result in the death of the mind or self, the implication is likewise not that the mind or self disappears, but that it somehow separates into pieces. Indeed conservation law is as was expounded a fundamental inductive experience regarding the permanence of the world in its elementary material, as compared to ephemerals such as objects of dreams. Hence whatever in sentient beings the basic material of consciousness or the self, it, too, can be considered permanent. Unlike the case in organisms or other material entities, further, consciousness or the self are not meant to be of a particular arrangement of constituents. That is to say, they exist if their constituents, which need not be multiple, exist. In consequence, with the constituent, the material, of the self continuing to exist, so does the self.

Argument may continue by saying that conservation law applies to material things, but that it may not apply to the self, because no self has been observed to remain after death. In this regard it can be remarked that if the self does not remain, neither does reality, found dependent on one's possible perception of it (e.g. p.44 last par.). It could be replied that reality may not remain for the deceased, but it may for others. A rejoinder can be that since reality is as an ingredient of perception separately determined by each individual, it would cease to be each time an individual would, without the continuity ascribed to it. More of pertinence to answering the question whether worldly conservation applies to matter but not to mind can be found in the very continuity of worldly lives, of species.

As did induction of other minds depend not on constant observation of them, but on the observed constancy of other basic features in accordingly alike beings (ca. p.100 last par. through p.102 third par.), so does the induction that selves continue to exist not depend on their observation, but on the constancy of continuance of other like basic phenomena. The self when occupant of a living body was seen as a force which is the purposeful cause of certain of the body's activities, simultaneous with its other purposive activities, those of the organism. These signify the organism's life, and correspondingly when the organism dies, it is not only the self that ceases its activities in it, but the body's activities end as well. Yet the force which is the cause of the last mentioned activities does not cease to exist, manifesting itself in the offspring or other members of the species. It is the force herein identified with God. Viewing ther rest of nature equally by its activities, found to make it significant, the conservation of worldly entities, their continuation, is thus learned to in all known instances extend both, to those instrumental in events that are mechanical, to entities that may be called material, and to those instrumental in events that are purposive, to entities that may be called mental. Inasmuch as all laws regarding nature are inferred from constancy in all known instances, it can be concluded that the selves of man and animal continue to be.

Immortality alone may not be thought to provide happiness, nor, should it for some, may it be held to be the wish of all. Nevertheless it can as in the case of other fundamental feelings be presumed that contentful immortality is of deepest shared desire. Whether it be immortality or other objects of ultimate happiness that are pondered it is the goodwill of God that in accordance with the aforesaid ensures that the destination of the course of the trials of everyone be heavenly existence.

INDEX

THE FATE OF MIDAS and Other Essays

David Horowitz

Ramparts Press
San Francisco

Published by Ramparts Press, Inc., San Francisco, California

Library of Congress catalog card no. 72-85093
ISBN 0-87867-032-7 (cloth), 0-87867-033-5 (paper)
Printed in the United States of America

In the present historical context, the work of a radical intellectual is inevitably a lonely enterprise. For moral support, I would like to thank Peter Collier and Bob Kaldenbach, good friends during these years, who inadvertently made this book possible. Ralph Miliband and Isaac Deutscher gave me warm encouragement during the years I spent in England, and both exerted important intellectual influences on my work. Other intellectual debts are noted in the essays themselves. I also wish to thank Rhoda Slanger, whose painstaking editing of the manuscript helped to make these essays more intelligible than they otherwise might have been.

Contents

Introduction

This book is a fragment of one man's effort to understand the social framework of our time, and the possibilities for transforming it into something at once more rational and more humane. Most of the theoretical essays in this volume were written in the mid-sixties, when the American left was still hostile to any form of theoretical Marxism, and before "Marxism-Leninism-Maoism," in one variant or another, had been adopted as a hallowed canon by significant sections of its militant core. To my generation of the "new left," the substitution of Mao for Stalin in the Marxist pantheon would have seemed a poor parody of the tragic illusion of the old Communist left, which had all but ceased its activity after the famous Khrushchev Report in 1956.

My generation emerged as a political force at the end of the fifties, out of the debacle of that left and, in particular, its self-inflicted demoralization and defeat.* The characteristic premise of our radical consciousness was the recognition that the Twentieth Congress of the Soviet Communist Party, at which Khrushchev revealed the crimes and exposed the lies of the Stalin era, did more to unhinge and demoralize the American left than all the domestic repressions–from the Palmer raids to the McCarthy witch hunts–put together.

This conclusion was not drawn out of bitterness but was born of prolonged and agonized reflection. We lived through the McCarthy repression; many of our families and their friends suffered under it. We also witnessed the devastating effect of the Khrushchev revelations on the Movement of that era, and on its will to struggle. The lessons of the experience were painfully clear: a revolutionary movement can be tempered in the fires of political repression, but to have lived a lie, even naively, as most of the American Communist left did, is to be deprived of a ground to stand on, when events converge to force the inevitable reckoning. A truly revolutionary movement could not be built on the treacherous quicksand of revolutionary myth.

Out of this basic belief, we assumed our first task as a new political generation, of painfully restoring our sense of reality and reconstructing a revolutionary vision and hope. The very term which we chose to identify ourselves, "new left," was an effort to establish an identity free from the corruptions of the past. Some made this rejection of the past a political program in itself. Others of us thought that such a total

* In 1961, I wrote *Student,* describing and justifying the political emergence of this "new left," during the previous two years at Berkeley, including its anti-HUAC and anti-ROTC demonstrations and its efforts to end capital punishment. *Student,* which was probably the first book to have appeared either by or about the new left, was published by Ballantine in 1962.

gesture of rejection indicated a lack of realism and candor, and that only the effort to establish a real sense of continuity and difference would make possible the creation of a viable radicalism for the future. As part of this effort, we began to re-examine the whole left analysis that we had inherited. For if the theories and analyses had been false in respect to Russia, we asked, what validity might they have in any respect? In short, everything, for us, had been put into question.

For me, personally, the search for radical foundations led to a sustained inquiry into the history of the cold war. *The Free World Colossus,* which I wrote principally in the winter of 1962–63, in Sweden, was a radicalizing experience in itself. I had been prepared by the Khrushchev revelations and the subsequent invasion of Hungary for at least a partial validation of the liberal versions of this history in which American policy was seen to derive from the necessity of containing a Soviet expansionist threat. I found, instead, a firmer basis for a radical perspective than I had thought possible. The international power equation, that *ultima ratio* of political realists, was so structured throughout the first decade of the cold war, that not only were Washington's fears of Russian expansion and the Communist menace unreal, but to a large extent they had to have been actually fabricated. This fabrication, I surmised, must have served other policy goals besides containing Russian influence in Eastern Europe, and it was not hard to recognize these in Washington's program of counter-revolutionary containment in the Third World.

I deliberately restricted myself to a "behavioral" framework in *The Free World Colossus*—the pattern of policy as opposed to its causes—because I had no theory of causes at the time. That part of my radical inheritance was still in question. It was only four years later, having returned to the Marxist sources and having read extensively in the accounts of the Russian Revolution and its development,* that I attempted to formulate a revised Marxist theory of contemporary history in a book called *Empire and Revolution.* Utilizing the notions of "uneven and combined development," I tried to assess the impact of the Russian Revolution on the progress of international revolutionary development, and also to work out the complex relationship between the radical and conservative interests of the "revolutionary" nation state, a dilemma that Marxists had not formally analyzed before.

In the years between writing *The Free World Colossus* and *Empire and Revolution* (roughly 1963–1966), I spent most of my intellectual time and energy wrestling with Marxism's basic texts, especially *Capital,* and with the related economic theory.† The core essays of the present volume, in one version or another, were written in this period and are dominated by its concerns. These include the title essay, originally written as a critique of Marcuse's thesis of "one-dimensional" stability applied to contemporary capitalism; "A Note on Marx's Theory of Class"; and "Marx, Keynes and the Economics of Capitalism," which seeks to establish a common ground for the radical analysis of capitalism in the theories of Marx and Keynes. Also included is the essay on "Marx's Approach to the Political Economy of Capitalism," which was to have been the beginning of a book-length study but which time and circumstances never allowed me to complete. "Cor-

* Particularly helpful were the writings of Isaac Deutscher, whose acquaintance I had made and under whose influence I came while residing in London from 1963 to 1967.

† Most of the economic reading I did in these years found its way into the selections and bibliographies of *Marx and Modern Economics,* which Monthly Review published in 1968.

porations and the Cold War" combines the earlier interest in foreign policy with the new theoretical assurance, while "Marxism and Its Place in Economic Science" recapitulates some of the ideas which emerged from the studies of these years, although it was actually written in 1968 for an Economics Colloquium at the University of California, Berkeley.

My chief concern during this period and in these essays was to try to establish a firm theoretical ground for radical analysis; in particular, it was important to know how much of the theory remained viable after the Stalin debacle. I spent a long time, for example, trying to ascertain the precise relation between Marxist economic theory and orthodox economics. Having lived through the period when Lysenkoist biology was presented by the left as a radical truth to oppose to the false bourgeois biology of genetics, I was sensitive to the perils involved in so dramatic a claim and in so blanket a dismissal of academic knowledge. Thus, I wanted to be able to identify the perceptions and tools that Marxist economics shared and did not share with its academic counterpart, to understand in what precise sense it was "Marxist," and more importantly, in what sense it was "radical."

While I was occupied with these concerns in London, where I was working for the Bertrand Russell Peace Foundation, events were taking place across the globe which were to change the whole context of my work as a radical. In the United States, a new "new left" was being born, whose formative experience was not the collapse of a Marxist tradition, but the dramatic revolt of America's black ghetto communities and Washington's genocidal aggression in Vietnam. Where my generation of radicals was composed mainly of shaken-up sons and daughters of the old left, the new generation was composed mainly of the shaken-out sons and daughters of liberals and even conservatives, horrified by the racism and imperialism of their own American dream. For them it was not the left but the liberal God that had failed. While our generation groped through liberalism and "humanism" to a more complexly held Marxism, they leapt without hesitation from Mill to Mao. In part, this was because embracing the ideology of the victim seemed to them a moral act in itself; in part, because liberalism was so corrupted by its complicity in slaughter and oppression, so obviously a part of the problem rather than the solution, that even a vulgar Marxism seemed indisputably rational, relevant and reliable by comparison.

As a result of this development, the questions which had arisen for us about the adequacy of classical Marxism, let alone its contemporary offspring, did not concern the new radical generation, but seemed almost other-worldly, and even politically dangerous to them. Dialogues on any theoretical question were therefore not easy during the political upsurge of the second generation "new left," in the late sixties. The last three essays in this volume were efforts to speak across the gap at the beginning and end of a climactic phase of that political generation's development under the leadership of the Weatherman faction of SDS.

By spring 1971, Weatherman was a spent force, and the problem of revolution in advanced capitalist societies was recognized to be far more complex than previously supposed, far more difficult than the *moral* decision that such a revolution was necessary. Meanwhile, the accommodation of the People's Republic of China to the kind of "coexistence" policy that Peking had previously denounced as "revisionist" and "social imperialist" when practiced by Moscow, made it clear to most that the international dimensions of revolution were far more complicated than was suggested by the maxims in the little Red Book.

In the new context created by these developments, the concerns of the essays in this volume may perhaps for the first time seem relevant to both generations of the "new left." They are offered here as a contribution to the developing consciousness and cohesion of this left, in its efforts to forge itself into a serious and sustained movement for revolutionary change. If the past has anything to tell us about the future, it is not only that the struggle is likely to be a long one, but that if the struggle is not taken seriously in a theoretical as well as a practical sense, it may not succeed at all.

David Horowitz
Berkeley, California

Part 1

The Fate of Midas

. . . of two equal communities, having the same technique but different stocks of capital, the community with the smaller stock of capital may be able for the time being to enjoy a higher standard of life than the community with the larger stock; though when the poorer community has caught up with the rich—as, presumably, it eventually will—then both alike will suffer the fate of Midas. This disturbing conclusion depends, of course, on the assumption that the propensity to consume and the rate of investment are not deliberately controlled in the social interest but are mainly left to the influences of *laissez-faire.*

—John Maynard Keynes, *The General Theory*

* I wish to thank Paul Sweezy and Harry Magdoff for helpful criticisms of earlier versions of this essay.

Liberal Prophecy and Illusion

Surely one of the impressive ironies of the American crisis is that it has emerged in a period of unparalleled economic prosperity and at a time when the United States is at the very pinnacle of its career as a world power. This irony has not been overlooked by those seeking to understand events in the dominant liberal perspective of the day, but it has thus far been left unexplained. It is even questionable whether one can speak of an "American crisis" at all in connection with the liberal perspective, if one means to imply by that an integrated phenomenon rooted in the very structure of the American social and economic order. In the liberal view, the current disturbance of the status quo appears to be merely the cumulative result of a series of fragmented and only tenuously related troubles: a Vietnam "problem" here, a race and poverty problem there, problems of status insecurity throughout.

Not only has liberalism shrunk from a confrontation with the structural nature of the crisis, but it has been surprised by the appearance of the crisis itself. The intensification of the conflicts generated by the social "problem areas" and their eruption in civil violence at the surface of America's domestic order fly in the face of the liberal myth of slow but steady progress and come as wholly unexpected and inexplicable events. And this has led to a crisis in liberalism itself.

One has only to read the "consensus" pundits of the fifties—writers like Daniel Bell, Seymour Martin Lipset and John Kenneth Galbraith—to realize that the very assumptions of the postwar liberal faith—the transcendence of old-fashioned capitalism and capitalist class conflict, the "end of ideology" and the emergence of a pluralistically planned "new industrial state"—rule out the very crisis which is now irrevocably upon us. If this were the first time that liberalism had banged its head so firmly against the rock of historical events, the necessity of turning to other modes of analysis would not be so self-evident. However, the history of liberalism indicates that its incapacity is chronic and that the roots of its failure lie in the unshakable commitment of its spokesmen to the social and economic status quo.

Liberals of the Victorian era, basking in the sun of *Pax Britannica,* natural evolution and the free market economy, viewed their future as a golden age, promising Peace, Progress, and Increasing Social Sanity. A few souls among them, it is true, joined with the socialists in condemning the "residual" evils of industrial exploitation and the new barbarism of colonial expansion, but even among these, the inevitability of reform in white Christian democracy and the eventual, if gradual, elimination of these unwanted blemishes was an article of faith. Marxist unbelievers might warn against the mounting tide of capitalist monopoly and militarism, and the inevitable catastrophe of global warfare foreshadowed in the intensified struggle for world markets, but their "doctrinaire" clamorings could be safely ignored.

Until 1914, that is. In that inaugural year of the European slaughter the great white hope of nineteenth-century liberal civilization was shattered forever. But while the old complacency was shaken, the sustaining system, with its comforts, benefits and privileges for chosen strata, survived, and with it the necessity for renewed (and revised) rationalization. Thus the liberal mind emerged from the war with a doctrine whose thesis, if not basically different in terms of power and program, had nonetheless undergone a significant change.

For the first time, liberals were compelled to recognize that the basic features of the capitalist system, the great inequalities of wealth and power, the anarchic structure of the economic system, the cyclical spells of boom and bust, and the unchecked scramble for international markets were in fact grave menaces to social progress and order. Yet, however much the preceding disasters might have underscored the necessity of revolution, the liberal middle classes were no more willing to pay the price of such a revolution than they had been before. The impressive, if deceptive, performance of the economy under wartime planning and the equally deceptive postwar boom further helped prepare the ground in which a new faith could bloom. As the expansion of the twenties accelerated, the new liberals began to propound the notion of *an already achieved social transformation* and to hail the advent of a "new capitalism" in which wealth was alleged to be increasingly shared, production increasingly planned for social needs, and prosperity a permanent feature of economic life. As one prominent spokesman for this emergent ruling ideology proclaimed in a tract published on the very eve of the Great Depression: "Not merely will prosperity [soon] be stabilized, but the rule of class will for the first time disappear."*

The precipitous crash from the heights of this giddy optimism into the depths of the deepest abyss in capitalist economic history ought to have dispelled once and for all any illusions about the possibility for rational and humane social development under such a fundamentally flawed system. But while some liberals may have been tempted to abandon ship (even such apostles of "free enterprise" capitalism as Keynes began to talk about the necessity of a "somewhat comprehensive socialization of investment"), the mainstream of liberalism remained true to its faith. Indeed, the very voices that had heralded the phantom transformation of the twenties now began to praise the mild reforms and tinkerings of

* For a collection of such statements by prominent figures and groups of the twenties from Secretary of the Treasury Andrew Mellon to the President's Committee on Recent Economic Changes, see Lewis Corey, *The Decline of American Capitalism* (Lane, 1935).

the New Deal as yet another substitute revolution. In fact, the most salient characteristic of the New Deal was its utter failure to stimulate demand on the scale necessary to reflate the economy to its pre-depression levels. The very attempt to do so by government means had been abandoned by the Roosevelt administration when, with eight million still unemployed, the demand for war orders and the institution of wartime planning lifted the economy to hitherto unattainable heights. Meanwhile, the pastiche of partial reforms, mildly ameliorative social legislation (most of which had been projected earlier by the farsighted business executives of the National Civic Federation),* and war prosperity were built by liberal imaginations into a new revolutionary order. It was not long before the promise of permanently increasing economic affluence and perpetual social harmony that had apparently been laid to rest in 1929 was being resurrected in the cold-war fifties in an outpouring of ill-conceived enthusiasm which C. Wright Mills sarcastically dubbed the Great American Celebration.

Like its predecessor, however, this celebration was short-lived. The civil rebellions of the sixties in the black ghettoes, the threatening prospect of price inflation and world monetary crisis, and the escalation of the genocidal war against the peasantry of Vietnam abruptly dissolved the consensual order of American politics, deflated the Panglossian platitudes of the new liberalism, and prepared a shift politically toward the right and a further sharpening of social antagonisms and conflicts.

* See James Weinstein, *The Corporate Ideal in the Liberal State* (Boston: Beacon, 1968).

Liberalism, Marxism, and the Capitalist World System

Despite these repeated debacles of its world vision, liberalism remains in the current crisis the analytic framework in which all socially respectable (and academically "professional") interpretations of the social impasse must be set. An alternative approach exists in Marxism, but it is forced to lead an embattled existence underground—except in its official, ideological, and therefore safe, varieties.*

The contrast between the Marxist and liberal perspectives on twentieth-century capitalist development and the nature of the current crisis could not be more complete. To Marxists, the present crisis in American society comes as no isolated or unexpected event. It appears rather as a specific phase of the general crisis of world capitalism, which began with the monopolization and colonization movements at the turn of the century, erupted first in the barbarism of the first European World War, and has since established its permanent and pervasive character through the economic and political collapses of the interwar decades, their issue in the bloody engagements of World War II, and the emergence of the post-war cold war.

One of the chief features of the present phase has been the rise of the United States to pre-eminence in the capitalist world system, replacing England (and to a lesser extent France) as the guardian power of the international status

* The percentage of economists and sociologists familiar with the work of Marxists such as Maurice Dobb, Paul Sweezy, Paul Baran, Lewis Corey, Ernest Mandel, Harry Magdoff, Perry Anderson, and André Gorz is surely infinitesimal. A major theoretical work on economic development like Baran's *Political Economy of Growth* (Monthly Review Press, 1957) is virtually censored from the bibliographies of academic works on development, though its author was a highly respected professor at Stanford and well known to other academics.

quo. In this role Washington has necessarily emerged as the leader of a worldwide conservative coalition aiming to contain the anticapitalist revolution, which took root in 1917 in one of the most exploited and underdeveloped regions of the globe, and has been gaining ground in those regions ever since. It is this inheritance of a mortally challenged world system that explains more than anything else the paradox of America's present power and ultimate impotence, as so fatefully symbolized in the struggle over the destiny of Vietnam. In the two postwar decades the effort to contain revolution has cost the United States alone more than a *trillion* dollars of the national income. It has also resulted in the deaths of more than six million peasants in the exploited and awakening areas of the world at the hands of the U.S. and U.S.-Allied forces. The sheer magnitude of these figures indicates that they are not only symbols of the crisis in general, but expressions of its deepest causes, and that the crisis in American society is not separable from the crisis of its *world* system.

This "world system" is of course more extensive (and more complex) than the U.S. economic stake in it, but that stake is itself an impressive index of the increasingly international basis of the American social order. U.S. direct overseas investments now exceed the figure of sixty billion dollars. The sales of this overseas system is equal to 40 percent of the U.S. domestic output of mines, factories and farms, and accounts for more than 20 percent of the profits of U.S. nonfinancial corporations. The U.S. overseas economic empire is, in fact, the third largest economic unit in the world after the domestic economies of the United States and Russia.* In regions like the Middle East, Southeast Asia,

* Harry Magdoff, *The Age of Imperialism* (New York: Monthly Review Press, 1969).

and Latin America, the locus of a good many "international" crises, U.S. interests constitute *the* dominant economic unit; in other key areas, like the Indian subcontinent and southern Africa, U.S. interests share dominance with the corporations and financial institutions of other NATO powers, as the increasingly primary joint partners. It is not necessary, of course, that U.S. investments be the direct target of a revolutionary upheaval for U.S. investments to be threatened. Thus, what is at stake for American capital in Vietnam and in similar revolutionary areas is not simply the specific markets and resources of the countries in question, but the international status quo order–i.e., the whole structural environment, embracing economic, political, and social policies and institutions, that make it possible for U.S. capital to expand and grow throughout the region and the world.

So manifest is the importance of the U.S. overseas system to the emergence of international crises in the postwar period (and to the crises besetting American society at home) that it would seem to require no emphasis. Yet in the contemporary liberal perspective this system has hardly even begun to exist. Consider, for example, John Kenneth Galbraith's latest best-selling effort at a definitive analysis of what he calls "the new industrial state." Not *one* of the thirty-five chapters of his highly praised book even mentions, let alone analyzes, the U.S. overseas system or attempts to assess its ramifications. In other words, the most far-reaching postwar development in the American social structure, the globalization of American business, is simply *ignored* by the most widely acclaimed apostle of critical realism toward the corporate society. The American *imperium* is apparently not yet a subject for respectable discourse.

Non-Marxist social science in the United States was not always so willfully ignorant or so crudely apologetic toward American imperialism as it has come to be in the cold war years. In the thirties the distinguished (but now patronized) American historian Charles Beard had already drawn attention to the political implications of the stepped-up expansion of American capital overseas, following the First World War. For just as trade had followed the flag in the course of previous American overseas expansion, so the flag was invariably put at the services of American financial and corporate interests abroad. If the historical record was any indication, the risk of future overseas capital investments would be underwritten by the United States government itself and by the blood of its citizens pressed into service to defend them.* "The United States," Beard wrote, "through the investment of capital, has become a silent partner in the fate of every established order in the world."†

Capitalism and the Crisis of Abundance

The failure of liberalism to recognize the overriding significance of the American economic empire stems from its unwillingness to open its eyes to the *class* nature of American society. Similarly, its failure to understand the domestic roots of the crisis lies in a failure to see that the basic power division of society is indeed a class division and that this class division is tied to the social processes of accumulation, resource allocation and the distribution of goods and services. It is because liberalism fails to see the link between social power, social distribution, and social investment that it can fragment the facets of the current crisis, isolate them as

* Cf. the studies of American expansion and foreign policy by Beard (*The Idea of National Interest* [New York: Macmillan, 1934]) and William A. Williams (*The Tragedy of American Diplomacy* [New York: World, 1959]).

† Beard, *The Economic Basis of Politics* (New York: Knopf, 1922).

"problems," and project a solution that depends on the correction of errors of judgment and the reform of technical structures, rather than the root-and-branch overthrow of a basically maleficent, undemocratic, and obsolescent social system.

In attempting to arrive at a more satisfactory analysis it is useful to begin with a historical perspective.* For a long time an industrial economy is engaged in the process of industrialization, i.e., in the transition from non-capital-using to capital-using methods of production. During this transition, society's overall rate of consumption is low; its rate of saving for investment in yet more instruments of production is high. "Society," of course, is no homogeneous community where each labors for the benefit of all and takes his share according to some equitable principle of distribution and reward. Capitalist society is divided in a fundamental way into those who work for a wage and those who possess the capital to hire them (where "capital" means both surplus money and the instruments of production at which to work). During industrialization, it is the laboring class that tightens its belt, receiving a bare consumption minimum for survival, while the capital-owning class plows its surplus income (derived from profits) into new means of production and yet greater future income for itself. It is, thus, the unequal distribution of income which forces a low consumption rate on the great mass of the population, while providing the privileged few with a surplus (even after their lavish consumption requirements are met) to reinvest.

* The following argument draws heavily on Paul Sweezy's "A Crucial Difference Between Capitalism and Socialism" in Horowitz, ed., *Marx and Modern Economics* (New York: Monthly Review Press, 1968).

During the early stages of industrialization, demand for this investment surplus is generated primarily in the capital goods sector (plant, machinery, equipment, etc.) for yet more capital goods. As the productive powers of the economy increase and the period of industrialization draws to an end, however, the demand for further expansion naturally tends to slacken. As basic industries and communication systems come into being, the productive apparatus gradually becomes large enough to supply all the expansion and replacement demands of the industries in the consumption sector, while its own expansion demand diminishes to the vanishing point. The natural overall tendency of this development is toward what Keynes once called a "quasi-stationary community," where change "would result only from changes in technique, taste, population and institutions" rather than from the classical accumulation and industrialization process, involving saving and net investment.* There would still be progress in such a community–in the accepted sense of better-quality techniques, better-quality goods, and increased productivity–but such progress would take place as the result of the *replacement* of machines already in existence rather than as the result of *net* additions to the stock of capital (*net* investment).†

* The inevitability of such a development is sytematically argued in A. Murad, "Net Investment and Industrial Progress," in K. Kurihara, ed., *Post-Keynesian Economics* (New Brunswick: Rutgers University Press, 1954). The statistical evidence of a decline in net capital formation in the United States as an already existent trend is also discussed in this essay. Cf. also Magdoff, *op cit.*

† In the United States it is estimated that somewhere between one-third and three-quarters of the increase in per capita income of Americans in the postwar period was the result of technological progress rather than increased savings and investment. Cf. Edward Denison, *The Sources of Economic Growth in the U.S. and the Alternatives Before the U.S.* (Committee for Economic Development: New York, 1962).

The significance of the achievement of this stage in development–it might be called "full industrialization"–is that all the social energies and resources that went into accumulation (or investment in future production) could go into the realization of a humane and humanly wealthy social order in the present. The maldistribution of income, which restricted consumption for the many and generated an income surplus for the few, would no longer serve any social function,* as there would be no need for a net surplus, since the increase in production to cover population increases would result from the march of technical progress. Thus not only could the standard of living of the whole population be raised to decent levels, but there would be more time for leisure, for education, culture, and politics in the Aristotelian sense. "Given social production," wrote Marx, "the allocation of time naturally remains of the essence. . . . Just as in the case of a single individual, the all-sidedness of society's development, of its enjoyment, and of its activity depends on the saving of time. The economy of time, this is what all economy dissolves itself into–in the last analysis." In terms of our model, social income previously "saved" and "invested" in future production would be "consumed" in education and culture (in its broadest sense), environmental reconstruction and the uplifting of the social underclasses.

Thus, as a result of the previous accumulation of capital in the advanced industrial countries, human liberation, in the sense of a comprehensive redirection of social energies from the struggle for existence to the realization of a truly human culture, has become a real, practical historical prospect. But this prospect of liberation is foreclosed as a possibility by the class structure of capitalist society.

* Of course, industrialization, theoretically, could have been accomplished by other, less inequitable, means.

Already this is painfully visible in the United States. For the incredible powers of the productive organism in this richest of all countries make the problems of poverty, of environmental pollution and underdevelopment, of the disadvantaged underclasses and blighted cities, fully solvable with existing resources *within the present generation.* Not only could the $30 billion per year that has been made available for the slaughter of peasants in Vietnam be invested in such a program, but the utilization of existing capacity that is kept idle by the monopolistic structure of American capitalism would, on one estimate, double the manufactured wealth immediately available.*

The basic reason for capitalism's inability to make a rational and socially progressive adjustment to the onset of abundance is that under capitalist economic organization the end of production is not the fulfillment of human needs but the expansion of private capital. Social accumulation is private accumulation. In other words, the investment surplus (profit) which society no longer needs is also the *income* of the capital-owning class, the economic foundation of its very existence. Accordingly, any pressure to reduce and redistribute that income and reallocate the social resources which it commands is passionately and fiercely resisted. Indeed, this resistance has been historically built by the capital-owning

* According to Leon Keyserling, former chairman of the President's Council of Economic Advisers, the amount of output lost between 1954 and 1964 as a result of unemployment and underutilized plant facilities was $550 billion. This is a conservative estimate. An economist writing in the Marxist magazine *Monthly Review,* for example, analyzed idle capacity in the American economy and concluded that "American industry has enough idle capacity today to permit an almost instantaneous doubling of manufacturing output."–"Idle Machines," *Monthly Review* (June 1962).

class into the very economic, ideological, and institutional structure of the society which it dominates.

The resistance, of course, does not manifest itself directly as an opposition to the liberating program outlined above. A minority class which set itself in opposition to the raising of living standards, the eradication of poverty, the building of livable cities, the redirection of social energies to human cultural pursuits, would be swept into oblivion. Nor is there a conscious conspiracy on the part of capital owners to conceal their opposition to social liberation. As individuals, many would probably invite it. Their opposition as a class is not a conscious decision, but a function of the social mechanism. For it is a central feature of capitalism that the decisions about the overall allocation of social resources are ones that can never be directly confronted. There is no social economic plan, but the integration of a multitude of private "plans" through the market. An "invisible hand" organizes production and determines the allocation and distribution of social resources, so that in capitalism it appears as though the economy made decisions and ruled human beings. This is what Marx characterized as festishism, where human beings are ruled (as in religion) by their own creation.

Capitalism's adjustment to the onset of abundance should, therefore, take place through the mediation of the market. The offset to the decline in demand for continued *net* additions to the stock of capital would be accomplished through the price mechanism. As demand began to slacken, prices would fall; this in turn would bring about a falling rate of profit (or interest). The share of wage and salary earners in personal income would increase at the expense of the share of investors (capital owners) at the same time as the inducement to invest would decrease. These two influences would result in a reduction in the proportion of income going into savings (investment surplus) and an immediate rise in the real living standards of the wage-earning classes.

In practice, however, the price system in advanced capitalism does not work this way. As a result of monopolistic and oligopolistic concentrations of capital, prices are downwardly rigid: they rise, but in general, they do not fall. Now, as Paul Sweezy has pointed out, "what is often called the degree of monopoly (in the economy as a whole) is little more than a reflection of capitalists' success in putting up economic, institutional and legal fences around their profits." In fact, so preponderant has been the economic, social, and political power of capital in defense of its profits in all the capitalist countries that income shares have been kept remarkably constant since the end of the nineteenth century in the face of all redistributive forces.

The macro-economic result of this resistance is that capitalism, as it approaches abundance, is threatened, as Keynes put it, with "the fate of Midas." The richer a capitalist society becomes, the more it is faced with a critical problem of surplus capital absorption and hence with the prospect of stagnation, unemployment, and depression. What happens to an economy which generates an investment surplus that cannot be utilized is vividly recorded in the history of the American thirties. If profitable investment outlets cannot be found for the surplus; if society, whatever its real needs, cannot utilize its savings, returning them to the market as demand for yet more productive capacity and hence more consumption goods; then total income will contract and unemployment grow until savings fall to the level of investment. The monopolization of the economy intensifies the overall problem, not only by artificially maintaining the level of savings, but by retarding the introduction of innovations and thereby reducing the available number of profitable investment outlets.* Moreover, because of the expanding labor force and increasing labor productivity, the level of output and income at which there will be full employment is constantly increasing. Here the liberating promise of automation is converted into a boundless menace: To avoid *rising* secular unemployment, market demand must *increase* in proportion to the rate of increase of labor productivity plus the rate of increase of the labor force. Thus, the system is caught ever deeper in its web of contradictions, because the inducement to invest at a constant, let alone an expanding, rate, no longer exists.

The Crisis and the Keynesian State I: Theory

During the whole postwar period, of course, the threat of stagnation on the scale of the thirties has never materialized. This is because the system has managed to generate counteracting forces to maintain the rate of surplus absorption at prosperity levels. These counteracting forces, however, have necessarily operated within the framework created by capitalist class relations. The solution which they pose to the crisis of capitalist abundance is therefore no solution at all, but the crisis itself in a new form.

Private capital attempts to counteract the tendency to stagnation, viewed as a threat to profit margins, by *expanding* its normal domestic and foreign markets. The fruits of this latter effort can be seen in the phenomenal postwar expansion of U.S. capital abroad. While generating investment out-

* Cf. Joan Robinson, *The Accumulation of Capital* (London: Macmillan, 1956), p. 407.

lets and a vital export surplus,* it has also produced an interventionist and destructive foreign policy and in effect internationalized the American crisis. As for the expansion of domestic markets, the rigid and unequal distribution of income, which precludes a widening of the domestic consumption base, makes it necessary to induce those who already can afford to buy what they want, to want more and, if possible, to waste what they have already bought. This obscene objective is achieved primarily via the sales effort (underpinned by a vast credit liberalization and expansion of consumer debt). The immensely consequential nature of this enterprise can hardly be overstressed. Taking the whole of the sales effort into account, including, for example, the cost of annual style changes in the automobile industry, more money is spent on making Americans into "voracious, wasteful, compulsive consumers" than is spent on their entire education through the university level. Not the fulfillment of need, but the artificial creation of new desires; not education, but miseducation, at once moronizing and degrading, appear as the chief cultural contributions of advanced capitalism to human civilization.

The effort of private capital artificially to expand its domestic markets and forcefully to enlarge its international presence is not only socially wasteful, culturally pernicious, and politically destructive, but also economically insufficient.

* An export surplus has the same expansionary effect on the economy and on profits as a budget deficit. Without foreign markets "profits are conditioned by the ability of capitalists to consume or to undertake capital investment. It is the export surplus and the budget deficit which enable the capitalists to make profits over and above their own purchases of goods and services."—M. Kalecki, *Theory of Economic Dynamics* (Monthly Review Press, 1968), pp. 50–52. Purchases by the foreign affiliates of U.S. corporations account for 23 percent of all U.S. exports. See Magdoff, *op. cit.*

Consequently, the economic intervention of the state is required on an extensive scale to deal with the growing problem of "abundance." In this effort, the state theoretically has several options. It could, for example, dramatically shift purchasing power to the lower income units via progressive taxes and transfer payments and thus make effective the very real but powerless demand of the poverty-stricken, deprived two-fifths of the nation's population. Such tax laws exist, but in practice the tax system is widely recognized to function regressively,* and no significant income redistribution from capital owners to wageworkers and the poor has occurred as a result of state policies in any capitalist country. The reason, of course, is not difficult to divine. This kind of redistribution means a shift in wealth from a class which wields predominant political power—and in practice sets the guidelines for all state-administered programs—to classes which wield virtually none.

Moreover, the mainspring of the economic system—hence of the prosperity on which the survival of governments depends—is private investment. Thus, any injury to business confidence, such as would be caused by the enforcement of redistributive tax measures, would have a deleterious effect on the overall economic situation. In other words, assaults on the privileged sanctuaries of private capital (and property income generally) inevitably provoke spontaneous "retaliations" via a decline in current investment, a general shrinkage of demand and a corresponding drop in national income. As a result, across-the-board attempts to restrict corporate privileges and the prerogatives of wealth are not even attempted by governments except in times of exceptional national crisis.

* See Philip Stern, *The Great Treasury Raid* (New York: Random House, 1964); F. Lundberg, *The Rich and the Super-Rich* (New York: Lyle Stuart, 1968).

(When such crises pass, needless to say, capital mounts its counterattack and restores an equilibrium more to its taste.)

The same reasoning applies to the whole range of possible government purchases of the private product to meet needs in education, health, housing, culture, and recreation. A significant part of the payment for these goods and services must come from taxation of the wealthy, to whom they are already available, and thus would represent a redivision of the national income pie. Any attempt to correct the misallocation of resources and the resultant blight of the social environment on a truly significant scale would run head-on into the resistance of those forces whose own life-style with all its privileges depends on the maintenance of the status quo. At the other end of the scale, the redistributive limit is set by the need to maintain discipline over the labor force in the sectors which generate the social surplus. A rise in welfare benefits is always viewed by the managers of enterprise as a threat to the incentive system by which they maintain control of their workers. A break of the link between jobs and income would be tenable only in a system where social production was organized through social plans, rather than through private incentives in a market. In short, any attempt by the government to make up for the deficiency of demand which results from the inequalities generated by capitalist production relations must collide with the fact that these inequalities have their origin in a "private" and unequal organization of power which runs all through capitalist society and cannot be altered by any one set of institutions within it.

Striking confirmation of this analysis is provided by the experience of the welfare state in postwar England, where the expansion of welfare services has not brought with it any significant redistribution of income. This is because "the great mass of the working class and of the population as a whole receive back in services no more than they pay in taxes."* In the United States, resistance to welfare spending is certainly no less intense, and despite a dramatic expansion of federal expenditures, there has been no comparable increase in the realm of federal welfare. In 1939, 42.5 percent of federal expenditures was for education, health, labor, welfare, housing, and community development, whereas in 1965 the figure was only 7 percent.†

There is, however, one basic kind of government expenditure which performs the same economic function as consumption expenditures (thus sustaining total demand) and does *not* meet with resistance from the corporate interests, indeed is supported by them. This is *military* spending, which has the dual advantage of providing a virtually limitless market for the private product and also of performing a necessary service to the corporations which they could not provide for themselves—namely, the protection of their expanding investments and markets overseas. The huge arms budget is in fact *the* vital difference between America's economic performance since 1950 and the stagnation and depression of the 1930s, accounting for as much as 60 percent of gross investment in the pre-Vietnam war year, 1961. (It is, therefore, the vital difference for the *global* capitalist system.**)

* Anderson & Blackburn, *Towards Socialism* (Ithaca: Cornell University Press, 1965).

† Melman, *Our Depleted Society* (New York: Holt, Rinehart and Winston, 1965).

** This is because effective demand is linked through trade and finance, and the United States accounts for about half the economy of the so-called free world. On the role of arms spending in the Western world, *see* M. Kidron, *Western Capitalism Since the War* (Penguin, 1968); in the United States *see* Baran and Sweezy, *Monopoly Capital* (Monthly Review Press, 1966).

Baran and Sweezy have constructed an illustrative index of this relation. In 1939, they point out, the number of unemployed was 17.2 percent and the number of persons employed as a consequence of the military budget was 1.4 percent, or a total of 18.6 percent. In a comparable year, 1961, the respective figures were 6.7 percent and 9.4 percent for a total of 16.1 percent either unemployed or dependent for employment on military spending.

In other words, the so-called Keynesian solution to the stagnation and depression-bound system of the thirties in practice turns out to be not a welfare state, as liberal ideology proclaims, but a warfare state. A moment's reflection, moreover, will indicate why this should be so. Keynes showed that there is a natural tendency for capitalism to run into chronic stagnation, with permanent unemployment, and that capitalism is, by nature, highly unstable. In order to make up for private capital's failure to maintain the level of investment, Keynes argued that governments must undertake compensatory expenditures. But high rates of socially useful investment undertaken by the government may lead to a decline in the profitability of further investment in private enterprise. Thus "wasteful" government spending is more acceptable to investors than useful spending: "Two pyramids, two masses for the dead, are twice as good as one; but not so two railways from London to York" (Keynes). This explains the readiness of capitalist governments to spend money on armaments. For as the eminent Keynesian Joan Robinson has noted: "If there were no need for armaments, it would be necessary to make [socially] useful investments and so to encroach upon the power and independence of the capitalists. The capitalists therefore prefer a situation in which armaments do seem necessary. This cure, most of us would agree, is even worse than the disease, and on the basis of Keynes' reasoning it can be argued that capitalism will not save itself from the tendency to unemployment by any other means."*

Thus, in advanced capitalism, the rate of military spending has a strong, even irresistible, tendency to rise—first, because given the relative saturation of profitable markets and the stake of society's dominant class in maintaining its power, "wasteful" expenditures must be undertaken by the state on an ever-increasing scale to absorb the economic surplus (savings) and maintain a high level of output and employment; second, because as a result of the new technological level of the forces of production—and the complex and expensive nature of the research required to develop them—and of the monopolistic corporations' increasing control over the expanding Keynesian state, the "military-industrial complex" has become the focal point for the country's research and development funds;† and third, because the compelling pressure to expand overseas investment requires a vast network of bases, alliances, and generally mobile military forces for the dominant imperial power.**

In sum, the matrix of class power and interest which determines the normal path of capitalist social and economic development also exerts a formative influence over any attempts by the state to alter that path. For the state is not an institution suspended above society, but is itself a social

* "Marx, Marshall and Keynes," in Joan Robinson, *Collected Economic Papers, II* (Oxford: Blackwell, 1960).

† Nieburg, *In the Name of Science* (Quadrangle, 1965).

** This is an important point. The U.S. military umbrella makes it less necessary for a capitalist power like Britain to maintain a maximum level of forces; similarly the military-powered U.S. economic expansion buoys up the British economy at lower levels of British military spending.

institution, and the power relations generated by the existing economic order and its class structure may be modified, but not fundamentally altered, by the state.*

The Crisis and the Keynesian State II: Practice

A series of key economic decisions taken at the threshold of the present phase of the American crisis will illustrate these general observations and illuminate the specific way in which these structural relations manifest themselves at the political surface.

In 1961 a new administration calling itself the New Frontier had taken office in Washington. This new administration projected itself as socially aware, informed with idealism and sensitive as its predecessor had not been to the "other" Americas: the plight of the poverty-stricken underclasses, the suffering of the oppressed black communities, and the general blight of the social and human environment, which decades of unplanned urbanization and industrialization had wrought. Appropriately, the new administration was heralded as being the first to accept officially the Keynesian analysis and to acknowledge the power and responsibility of the state to deal with the demand problem via its own spending policies. The stage seemed set for a much-needed program of social reform, a beginning of the long-deferred and desperately overdue harnessing of the forces of the postwar prosperity to the task of promoting something like the general welfare.

It was not very long after its inaugural "honeymoon," however, that the Kennedy administration was faced with the

* On upper-class control of Washington in the postwar period, *see* G. William Domhoff, *Who Rules America?* (New York, Prentice-Hall, 1967).

necessity of making some hard political choices and laying its fine rhetoric on the line. A slackening of the economy on top of almost a decade of stagnation and sluggish growth made it imperative to take expansionary economic measures. The political question confronting the New Frontiersmen was what kind of measure it was to be. Initially the answer seemed to be a tax reform, which was to be combined either with a tax cut or an expanded program of federal expenditures to produce the required expansionary budget.

On the allocation side, the plugging of some of the more notorious tax loopholes which allow the very rich to escape the progressive intent of the existing tax laws would divert social resources away from the luxury sectors of the economy and make them available for those social areas and social groupings which lacked the necessities and amenities for a decent existence.

The second of the possible measures, a tax cut, would, if biased toward the lower income groups, broaden the consumption base and make goods from the private sector available to those in need of them. An increase in federal nondefense spending (the third possibility) would initiate the massive task of social reconstruction and rehabilitation made necessary by the past misallocation of resources under a system of production organized for private aggrandizement rather than social need.

The course actually taken by the New Frontier was simple and instructive. Under pressure centering within the administration in the person of Secretary of the Treasury C. Douglas Dillon (in private life one of Wall Street's leading investment bankers) and outside the administration in a committee headed by Stuart Saunders (head of the largest railroad in the country) and Henry Ford II, the promised tax reform was abandoned. Also rejected was any substantial expansion of federal expenditures on housing, urban development, conservation, environmental purification, education, and welfare. According to banker Dillon, in a speech presenting the administration's viewpoint, such expenditure might prove inflationary and could not be "justified on its own merit." The Kennedy administration had already increased the military budget by 16 percent, or more than $7 billion. And this at a time when U.S. missile and military superiority vis-à-vis the Soviet Union was overwhelming (i.e., according to Pentagon estimates, between five and ten to one).*

The measure finally adopted by the administration as being in the interests of the nation was the measure supported from the outset by Dillon and his friends: a tax cut. This was no across-the-board tax cut, however. As if to gild the lily, the Dillon-Ford interests pressed through a tax reduction sharply biased toward the corporate rich, since, they argued, if production were to be expanded, incentives must be given to the controllers of the means of production. (On the other hand, when the tax surcharge was put through four years later to stem inflation, it was an across-the-board surcharge, affecting all income categories equally.)

As a result of the tax cut, a family of four with a $3,000-a-year income received sixty dollars extra to spend, while a similar family with a $200,000-a-year income received $32,000 extra. Nor was this the end of the story. A series of steps to grant more liberalized depreciation measures to corporations effectively reduced corporate taxes between 16 and 23 percent, with the result that in the first five years of the Kennedy-Johnson administrations, corporate profits (savings income) rose 76.5 percent, while wages (consumption income) rose only 18 percent. The whole series of

* *The Free World Colossus,* chapters 23–25.

New Frontier measures represented a massive distribution of income from the poor to the rich, from consumers to savers, and while it inevitably put some immediate steam into the economy, it promised to deepen and complicate the long-term economic problem and its crisis. By 1965 slack was again being felt in the economy, and an imminent end to the long boom was being predicted in respected quarters when the escalation of the Vietnam war and the expansion of war expenditures from $2 billion to $30 billion annually spelled a temporary end to the recessionary movement.

The priorities expressed in the New Frontier spending and tax policies were as characteristic of the dominant forces of American society as was Dillon himself. Scion of the investment banking house of Dillon, Read & Co. and a director of the Chase Manhattan Bank, Dillon personified the most globally oriented interests of U.S. capital. There is certainly no mystery as to why the interests represented by Dillon, Read & Co. and Chase, with investments from Southeast Asia to South Africa, from the Middle East to the Cape of Good Hope, should regard the $30 billion (of public money) allocated for the counterinsurgency operation in Vietnam a justifiable expense a year or so after they had considered less than a third of the sum "too much" to spend for the rehabilitation of the most exploited and oppressed layers of American society.

However, these priorities could hardly be shared by the great mass of the American people. The black uprisings in the ghettoes of the American cities, the antidraft resistance, and the student rebellions are but the initial shock waves in what one day must become a popular earthquake against an intolerable social system: one that is richer than any in history, but cannot eliminate poverty or build a decent environment or even provide equality of opportunity for its citizens; a social system that can spend hundreds of billions to dominate the nonwhite peoples of the underdeveloped world and their resources and raw materials, but finds it difficult to shake free every penny it spends for the general welfare at home.

Because capitalism is by nature an exploitative system and the motive force of its development is not provision for social need, but the expansion of business profits, and because this expansion inevitably comes at the expense of the vast majority of the population and of the environment itself, the task of coping with the growing social catastrophe which its "progress" engenders is inevitably a Sisyphean labor. Indeed, even as capitalism's reaction to the revolutionary pressures generated by its exploitation of populations abroad is military violence, so at home the most basic and consistent response of the ruling powers to the social chaos which the system produces and to the revolts which its criminal priorities inspire is the extension of the mechanisms of repression and control. The democratic order itself threatens to become the first major victim of intensified class struggle.

Thus, the fabulous riches created by capitalism prove to be no more humanly usable than the riches created by the touch of Midas. To turn raw materials and human labor into capitalist gold requires the blood of millions of nonwhite peoples in the imperial realms and the labor and lives of millions of black and white Americans at home who have no stake in the imperial system, no real say in its governance, and who receive no essential benefits from its operation. This situation has already inspired an unprecedented disaffection among America's younger generations. For the technical-economic power to liberate America and all mankind is already available, and Americans are for the first time beginning to realize it. Before this liberation can take place, however, the technical-economic power to liberate must itself be liberated from the class that owns and controls it. To convert the menace of too much wealth and power for the few into the promise of enough for all, it is only necessary that the democratic principle be extended to the corporate and financial institutions of the social order. To do that is the task of the social revolution.

Corporations and the Cold War

Who makes U.S. foreign policy? The question is by no means academic, for the historical record shows that over the last fifty years and more, U.S. policy has consistently run in channels which are antagonistic to the most publicized ideals of the American Republic, issuing finally in the conflicts which we associate with the Cold War. Those ideals—enshrined in the Declaration of Independence—recognize the right of nations to self-determination, and of any oppressed people to overthrow by force the institutions of their oppressors in order to secure for themselves, after the example of the American Revolution, the rights to "life, liberty, and the pursuit of happiness."

Yet the record shows that as the United States has assumed the role of a great and then dominant world power, it has more and more consistently opposed the major social revolutions of our time, and in violation of the principle of

This essay was written as an introduction to *Corporations and the Cold War* (New York: Monthly Review Press, 1968).

self-determination, it has intervened militarily, diplomatically, and economically to crush or to cause grave setbacks to these revolutions, whether in Russia or Mexico, China or Cuba, Greece or Vietnam.

Nowhere has this pattern of policy been more evident, certainly, than in the American intervention in Vietnam. In 1945, the Democratic Republic of Vietnam was proclaimed in a document modeled on the American Declaration of Independence and at first recognized by the former colonial power, France. Yet when that power sought to reassert control of its former colonial territory, establishing a puppet regime in Saigon for this purpose, it found support in U.S. policy. Not only did Washington back France's illegitimate war of conquest with economic and military aid, but when the French failed, Washington itself took over the struggle to defeat the Vietnamese Republic through the quisling government in Saigon. Indeed, more than twenty years after the proclamation of Vietnam's Declaration of Independence, the Vietnamese peasants are still being assaulted by the U.S. armed forces in what has undoubtedly become the most ruthless and destructive intervention on historical record.

Nor is this counterrevolutionary expedition exceptional as U.S. Cold War policy, despite the unprecedented ferocity and unparalleled savagery of its execution. As already noted, it forms rather a consistent pattern with other U.S. interventions in Santo Domingo, Cuba, Guatemala, the Congo, the Middle East, China, Greece, and elsewhere during the Cold War years, and in Russia, Mexico, Cuba, China, and other countries earlier in the century. Indeed, counterrevolutionary intervention, which is at the heart of the Cold War and its conflicts, has been a characteristic of U.S. foreign policy ever since the United States embarked on a course of overseas economic expansion following the closing of the geographical frontier more than seventy years ago.

How is this counterrevolutionary policy, which runs directly counter to the high ideals of the American Republic, to be explained? How is it to be explained that the largest "defense" program of any nation in history (and of the United States in particular, which prior to the postwar decades never maintained a peacetime conscription army) is organized around the unprecedented concept of *counterinsurgency?*

These paradoxes can only be explained if it can be shown that there is a group wielding predominant power in the American polity whose interests run counter to America's high ideals, and which can impose its own interpretation of the American tradition onto the framework of policy-making in the state. If it can be shown that there is a *class* among the plurality of competing interest groups which enjoys a predominance of power and can establish its own outlook as a prevailing ideology, and if it can be shown that these interests are expansionist, anti-revolutionary, and tending to be militarist by nature, then an explanation of the paradoxical character of American policy will have been found and, beyond that, the sources of the Cold War conflicts and their permanence.

Such a "ruling class" can, in fact, be readily shown to exist. Its locus of power and interest is the giant corporations and financial institutions which dominate the American economy, and, moreover, the economy of the entire Western world. "In terms of power," writes one authority on the corporations (himself a corporation executive and former U.S. policy-maker), "without regard to asset positions, not only do five hundred corporations control two-thirds of the non-farm economy, but within each of that five hundred a still smaller group has the ultimate decision-making power. This is, I think, the highest concentration of economic power in recorded history." Moreover, "since the United States carries on not quite half of the manufacturing production of the entire world today, these five hundred groupings—each with its own little dominating pyramid within it—represent a concentration of power over economies which makes the medieval feudal system look like a Sunday school party."*

As this observer points out, many of these corporations have budgets, and some of them have payrolls which, with their customers, affect a greater number of people than most of the hundred-odd sovereign countries of the world. Indeed, the fifty largest corporations employ almost three times as many people as the five largest U.S. states, while their combined sales are over five times greater than the taxes the states collect.

In the last analysis, it is the dependence of men individually and collectively on the corporately organized and controlled economy that provides the basis of the corporate domination of U.S. policy, especially U.S. foreign policy. The basic fulcrum of this corporate power is the investment decision, which is effectively made by a small group of men relative to the economy as a whole. This decision includes how much the corporations spend, what they produce, where the products are to be manufactured, and who is to participate in the processes of production.

> A single corporation can draw up an investment program calling for the expenditure of several billions of dollars on new plants and products. A decision such as this may well determine the quality of life for a substantial segment of society: Men and materials will move

* A. A. Berle, Jr., "Economic Power and the Free Society" in Andrew Hacker, ed., *The Corporation Take-Over* (New York: Doubleday, 1965), p. 97. This is a collection of papers originally prepared for the Center for the Study of Democratic Institutions, Santa Barbara.

> across continents; old communities will decay and new ones will prosper; tastes and habits will alter; new skills will be demanded, and the education of a nation will adjust itself accordingly; even government will fall into line, providing public services that corporate developments make necessary.*

But this is not the whole extent of the power of the corporate investment decision. In the national economy, the small oligarchy of corporate and financial rulers, who are responsible to no one,† determine through their investment outlays the level of output and employment for the economy as a whole. As Keynes observed, the national prosperity is excessively dependent on the confidence of the business community. This confidence can be irreparably injured by a government which pursues a course of policy inimical to business interests. In other words, basic to the political success at the polls for any government, as to the success of its specific programs, will be the way the government's policies affect the system of incentives on which the economy runs—a system of incentives which is also the basis of the privileges of the social upper classes.

This does not mean, of course, that the business community as such must prefer a particular candidate or party for that candidate or party to be victorious. It means, much more fundamentally, that short of committing political suicide, no party or government can step outside the framework of the

* Hacker, *op. cit.*, p. 9.

† Berle, in Hacker, *op. cit.*, p. 91. Cf. C. Wright Mills, *The Power Elite* (New York: Oxford University Press, 1956), p. 126n: "As political organizations [the corporations] are of course totalitarian and dictatorial, although externally, they display much public relations and liberal rhetoric of defense."

corporate system and its politics, and embark on a course which consistently threatens the power and privileges of the giant corporations. Either a government must seize the commanding heights of the economy at once, i.e., initiate a course of social revolution, or run things more or less in the normal way, that is, according to the priorities and channels determined by the system of incentive payments to the corporate controllers of the means of production. This is an unspoken but well-understood fact conditioning politics in capitalist countries, which explains among other things why the pattern of resource allocation—the priority of guns over butter, of highway construction over schools and hospitals—is so similar in all of them. It also explains why, despite the congressional and parliamentary enactment of progressive tax laws in all these countries, the spirit of the law has everywhere been thwarted, and nowhere has the significant redistribution of income promised by these democratically ratified statutes taken place.

The sheer economic pressure which the corporations can exert over the policies of democratically elected governments is lucidly manifest in the experience of the Wilson Labour government in England. For, while owing its office to labor votes and labor money, this government was forced by "the economic situation," i.e., by domestic and international capital, to pursue precisely the policies which it had condemned as *anti*-labor while in opposition.

Of course, under normal conditions, and particularly in the United States, where no labor party exists, the corporations have less subtle means at their disposal for ensuring policies conducive to their continued vigor and growth. For

> all the political activities and functions which may be said to constitute the essential characteristics of the [democratic] system—indoctrinating and propagandiz-

> ing the voting public, organizing and maintaining political parties, running electoral campaigns—can be carried out only by means of money, lots of money. And since . . . the big corporations are the source of big money, they are also the main sources of political power.*

The means by which the upper classes maintain their privileged position and vested interests in countries where universal suffrage prevails vary with the differing traditions, social institutions, and class structures of the countries involved. They vary also with their historical roles. Thus, in the twentieth century, as the United States has replaced Britain as the guardian power and policeman of the international system of property and privilege, the corporate ruling class, with its equally expanding overseas interests, has less and less been able to entrust policy to indirectly controlled representatives and has more and more had to enter directly the seats of government itself.

In the postwar period, the strategic agencies of foreign policy—the State Department, the CIA, the Pentagon, and the Treasury, as well as the key ambassadorial posts—have all been dominated by representatives and rulers of America's principal corporate-financial empires. In addition, all the special committees and task forces on foreign policy guidelines have been presided over by the men of this business elite, so that on all important levels of foreign policy-making, "business serves as the fount of critical assumptions or goals and strategically placed personnel."†

* Paul Baran and Paul M. Sweezy, *Monopoly Capital* (New York: Monthly Review Press, 1966), p. 155.

† Gabriel Kolko, *The Roots of American Foreign Policy* (Boston: The Beacon Press, 1969), p. 26.

While the corporate-based upper class in general occupies a prodigious number of positions in the highest reaches of the "democratic" state, it need not strive to occupy all the top places to impose its own interpretation of the national interest on American policy. For precisely because the prevailing ideology of U.S. politics in general, and of the federal government in particular, is corporate ideology, reflecting the corporate outlook and interests, and because, therefore, the framework of articulated policy choices lies well within the horizon of this outlook, political outsiders may be tolerated and even highly effective in serving the corporate system and its programs.

There are two principal ways (in addition to those already discussed) by which corporate ideology comes to prevail in the larger political realm. In the first place, it does so through the corporate (and upper-class) control of the means of communication and the means of production of ideas and ideology (the mass media, the foundations,* universities, etc.). However, even this control, which is vast but not ubiquitous in ensuring the general predominance of the ideas of the dominant class, is not left to work at random. Thus, in Professor Domhoff's investigation of the American ruling class, he found that "in most instances" non-upper-class political leaders "were selected, trained, and employed in [special] institutions which function to the benefit of members of the upper class and which are controlled by members of the upper class." Such leaders, Professor Domhoff concluded, "are selected for advancement in terms of the interests of members of the upper class."

The second basic way in which corporate ideology comes to prevail, particularly at the foreign policy level, is by the

* See Horowitz, "Charity Begins at Home," *Ramparts,* April 1969; "The Billion Dollar Brains," *Ramparts,* May 1969.

very fact that the dominant reality of society is corporate, and therefore political "realism" dictates for any statesman or politician that he work within its framework and accept its assumptions. If the horizon of political choice is limited to an area in which the corporate interest is not directly challenged, because it would be both imprudent and impractical (utopian) to do so, if the framework of private property in the means of production is accepted as not realistically subject to change, then the "national" interest, which is the concept under which politicians and statesmen tend to operate (particularly in foreign policy), necessarily coincides with the interests of the corporations, the repositories of the nation's wealth, the organizers of its productive power, and hence the guardians of the material basis of its strength. In a class-divided society under normal (i.e., non-revolutionary) conditions, the national interest vis-à-vis external interests inevitably is interpreted as the interest of the dominant or ruling class. Thus, in a corporate capitalist society, the corporate outlook as a matter of course becomes the dominant outlook of the state in foreign affairs.

This is not to say that there is never a conflict over foreign policy which expresses a conflict between corporations and the state. Just as there are differences among the corporate interests themselves, within a general framework of interests, so there are differences between the corporate community outside the state and the corporate representatives and their agents in the state, resulting from the difference in vantage and the wider and narrower interests that each group must take into account.* But here, too, the horizon of choice, the framework of decisive interests, is defined by the necessity of

* We are dealing here with the United States. In countries where a labor party assumes government office, the relationship is more complex, but for the reasons outlined above the policy results are basically the same.

preserving and strengthening the status quo order of corporate capitalism and consequently the interests of the social classes most benefited by it.

What then is the nature of corporate ideology as it dominates U.S. foreign policy, and what is its role in the development of the Cold War? As a result of the pioneering work of Professor William Appleman Williams and his students,* these questions can be answered precisely and succinctly. The chief function of corporate ideology is, of course, to make an explicit identification of the national tradition and interest—the American Way of Life—with its own particular interest. This identification is accomplished by means of an economic determinism which takes as its cardinal principle the proposition that political freedom is inseparably bound up with corporate property, that a "free enterprise" economy is the indispensable foundation of a free polity (where "free enterprise" is defined so as to coincide with the status quo order of corporate capitalism, not with an outdated system of independent farmers and traders).

Starting from this root premise, the ideology, as articulated by American policymakers since the nineteenth century, maintains that an expanding frontier of ever new and accessible markets is absolutely essential for capitalist Ameri-

* William Appleman Williams, *The Tragedy of American Diplomacy* (New York: Delta Books, 1962); Walter LaFeber, *The New Empire, An Interpretation of American Expansion 1860–1868* (Ithaca: Cornell University Press, 1963); Lloyd C. Gardner, *Economic Aspects of New Deal Diplomacy* (Madison: University of Wisconsin Press, 1964). On the immediate Cold War origins, *see* also Gar Alperovitz (another Williams student), *Atomic Diplomacy: Hiroshima and Potsdam* (New York: Simon & Schuster, 1965).

ca's domestic prosperity,* and hence that the extension of the American system and its institutions abroad is a necessity for the preservation of the American, democratic, free-enterprise order at home. Originally formulated as an "Open Door" policy to prevent the closing of the external frontier by European colonialism, and to ensure American access to, and eventual domination of, global markets, this policy has become in the postwar period a policy of preserving and extending American hegemony and the free enterprise system throughout the external frontier, or, as it is now called, the "free world." From Woodrow Wilson's First World War cry that the world must be made safe for democracy, it was but a logical historical step to Secretary of State Byrnes's remark at the close of the Second World War that the world must be made safe for the United States. This is the core of America's messianic crusade: that the world must be made over in the American image (read: subjected to the American corporate system) if the American Way of Life (read: the corporate economy) is to survive at home.

If expansion (and militarism) had held the key not only to American prosperity,† but to American security as well, the postwar period would undoubtedly have realized Secretary of State Byrnes's ambitious goal. In the last stages of the war and the first of the peace, the United States successfully

* See the essays by Professors Gardner, Eakins, and Williams in Horowitz, ed., *Corporations and the Cold War* (New York: Monthly Review Press, 1968).

† On the ultimate connection between corporate capitalist prosperity and militarism, see Rosa Luxembourg, *The Accumulation of Capital* (New York: Monthly Review Press, 1968); Joan Robinson, "Marx, Marshall and Keynes," in *Collected Economic Papers, II* (New York: Oxford University Press, 1960); and Baran and Sweezy, *Monopoly Capital*, op. cit.

penetrated the old European empires (mainly those of France, Great Britain, and the Netherlands), assumed control of Japan and its former dependencies, and extended its own power, globally, to an unprecedented degree. By 1949, the United States had liens on some four hundred military bases, while the expansion of direct overseas investments was taking place at a phenomenal rate. Thus, while between 1929 and 1946 U.S. foreign investments had actually declined from $7.9 to $7.2 billion, between 1946 and 1967 they increased an incredible eightfold to more than $60 billion. It is this global stake in the wealth and resources of the external frontier that forms the basis of the U.S. commitment to the worldwide status quo (though it may not always provide the whole explanation for particular commitments or engagements). It is this commitment to the internal status quo in other countries (the State Department actually runs a course for foreign service officers and ambassadors called "Overseas Internal Defense") that renders Washington's expansionist program not the key to security but the very source of Cold War conflict, with its permanent menace to mankind's survival.

For the expansion of corporate overseas investment has to an overwhelming degree not produced beneficial results, and the status quo, of which the corporations inevitably constitute a dominating part, is almost everywhere a status quo of human misery and suffering:

> No one acquainted with the behavior of Western corporations on their pilgrimages for profit during the last fifty years can really be surprised that the . . . explosions now taking place [in the underdeveloped world] are doing so in an anti-American, anti-capitalist, anti-Western context. For many years these continents have been happy hunting grounds for corporate adventurers,

> who have taken out great resources and great profits and left behind great poverty, great expectations and great resentments. Gunnar Myrdal points out that capitalist intervention in underdeveloped countries thus far has almost uniformly had the result of making the rich richer and the poor poorer. . . .*

This has indeed been the undeniable historical consequence of capitalist corporate expansion, although this is not what one is led to believe by the orthodox theorists and academic model builders who function so frequently as the sophisticated apologists of the American empire and the policy of counterrevolutionary intervention necessary to maintain it.

In the writings of such theorists, the expansion of America's monopolistic giants and their control of the markets and resources of the poverty-stricken regions is presented as entailing the *net* export of capital to these capital-starved areas, the transfer of industrial technologies and skills, and the flow of wealth generally from the rich world to the poor. From this point of view, revolutions in the underdeveloped world which challenge the presence and domination of foreign corporations and their states are either misguided or sinister in intent, and contrary to the real needs and interests of the countries involved. Indeed, for those who maintain this view, revolutions are regarded as alien-inspired efforts aimed at subverting and seizing control of the countries in question during the period of great difficulty and instability prior to the so-called take-off into self-sustaining growth. This is the argument advanced by W. W. Rostow, former director of the State Department's Policy Planning Staff and

* W. H. Ferry, "Irresponsibilities in Metrocorporate America," in Hacker, *The Corporation Take-Over,* op. cit.

the chief rationalizer of America's expansionist counter-revolutionary crusade.

In fact, this view rests neither on historical experience, which shows the presence of foreign capital and power to have had a profoundly adverse effect on the development potential of the penetrated regions, nor on a sound empirical basis. Far from resulting in a transfer of wealth from richer to poorer regions, the penetration of the underdeveloped world by the imperialist and neo-imperialist systems of the developed states has had the opposite effect. As a result of direct U.S. overseas investments between 1950 and 1965, for example, there was a *net* capital flow of $16 billion *to the United States,* and this was just a part of the negative transfer. Similarly, when looked at in their political and economic settings, the much-heralded benefits of the advanced technologies transplanted into these areas, but remaining under the control of international corporations, also tend to be circumscribed and even adverse in their effects. Indeed, regarded in terms of its impact on total societies, rather than on particular economic sectors, the operation of opening the backward and weak areas to the competitive penetration of the advanced and powerful capitalist states has been nothing short of a catastrophe. For as Paul Baran showed in his pioneering work, *The Political Economy of Growth,* it is precisely the penetration of the underdeveloped world by advanced capitalism that has in the past obstructed its development and continues in the present to prevent it. Conversely, it has been primarily their ability to escape from the net of foreign investment and domination that has made a chosen few among these countries, like Japan, exceptions to the rule. Professor Gunder Frank and others have continued the work that Baran initiated, showing how foreign capitalist investment produces the pattern of underdevelopment (or "growth without development," as it is sometimes called) which is the permanent nightmare of these regions.

The view expounded by these writers, which is based on a thoroughgoing and concrete historical and social analysis, makes fully intelligible the fact of anti-imperialist revolution in the underdeveloped world and its inevitable conflict with the Western powers. Only this view can show revolution as the real full-blooded historical phenomenon that it is, rather than the implausibly contrived product of foreign-generated conspiratorial intrigue.* It also explains why communist and socialist revolutions have been so intimately and integrally bound up in the contemporary era with struggles for national liberation and self-determination. For the gateway to national political independence and economic development in the penetrated and dependent regions leads inevitably through the *class* revolution–i.e., the expropriation of the corporations' foreign and domestic agents who dominate the politics and economies of these countries, siphon off the national wealth, and prevent its utilization for overall national industrial development.

However, while the recent history of the Cold War can be seen to fall easily into this structural pattern of corporate expansion of the corporate system and the rising nationalist surge and counterrevolutionary intervention, the international conflicts of the entire postwar period present a somewhat more complicated problem for analysis. For in the early postwar years, the conflict between Russia and the United

* Perhaps the acme of absurdity in promoting the conspiracy theory was reached when President Johnson justified the intervention of thirty thousand Marines in the Dominican Republic in 1965 by the presence of fifty-three alleged Communists supposed to be behind the Dominican Revolution.

States over the peace settlement in Europe dominated relations between all states to an exceptional degree. Moreover, while this conflict was certainly related to the Open Door expansion of the corporate system and the rising nationalist and anti-capitalist revolutions in the underdeveloped world (from southeastern Europe to Asia), its domination by great-power politics and by the abrupt power shifts resulting from the war gave to it a different appearance and a character divergent in some ways from the conflicts of the later period.

This exception notwithstanding, the fanatical anti-communism which took root in this period and which has been such a central and consistent feature of America's messianic Cold War crusade fulfills a clearly discernible and indispensable function in corporate ideology and the success of the corporate program. For as a system which is by nature expansionist (from the sheer pressure of the world market and the competitive struggle to control it) and which generates nationalist resistance and revolt that must be countered and contained, the American corporate empire is beset by a real and basically insoluble problem: How can it justify the counterrevolutionary intervention necessary to extend and to preserve itself in terms of an American ideology of democratic pluralism and revolutionary self-determination? The corporate answer to this dilemma, arrived at early in American history, and in which anti-communism now plays the central role, is to present the intervention as a program of "containment" against a third threatening imperial force or party. Thus just as the U.S. thrust into the markets of China at the turn of the century was carried out under the cover of containing European colonialism, so the interventions in Cuba and the Philippines were presented as efforts to save those countries from the clutches of imperial Spain. The pre-communist origins of what has become a crucial ideological gambit in U.S. foreign relations are symbolized in the fact that when Bolshevism first triumphed in Russia, and there was no external communist power on which to blame the revolution, Lenin and Trotsky were presented as *German* agents, and U.S. counterrevolutionary intervention as an attempt to contain German imperialist expansion.* When the second major communist revolution was occurring in China, it could of course be presented by the State Department as a takeover by Russia, despite the substantial evidence available to document the rift between Stalin and Mao, about which the State Department was well aware. From then on, any communist revolution, no matter how nationalist in character or content, became in State Department White Papers the illegitimate offspring of "communist imperialism" centered in some conveniently located communist capital.

Historically, of course, there has never been a legitimate resistance or revolt from the point of view of the ruling power. American revolutionaries themselves were portrayed by their opponents as agents of the French. So it is, as part of an old historical pattern, that U.S. counterrevolutionary intervention in defense of the social status quo in Vietnam should be officially justified by portraying the Vietnamese guerrillas in the South as mere agents of their brothers in the North, and then by insinuating that the North is a puppet of Moscow or Peking. In this way, Washington, like all previous ruling powers, seeks to present its own role as that of the would-be protector of its intended victim, and in this case also as defending self-determination and therefore acting in accord with America's traditional ideals.

* Cf. William Appleman Williams, "American Intervention in the Russian Revolution, 1917–1920," in Horowitz, ed., *Containment and Revolution* (Beacon Press: 1968).

The increasingly violent contradiction between the American policies of expansion and counterrevolutionary intervention and American ideals has its roots in a past that long pre-dates the Cold War, although it is undoubtedly the Cold War ascendance of U.S. power that has made the contradiction so acute. This contradiction between American program and American creed reflects an equally important conflict between the structures of American social and political life, and the American democratic framework. For in a profound sense, foreign policy is but an extension of domestic policy: the inequality of privilege and power in American society mirrors (and serves) an even more insidious global inequality. Similarly, the gathering revolt against the corporate system at home is but one of the outward ripples of the post-1917 global revolutionary upsurge against the imperialist world system that America in part inherited and in part has taken over from the old European colonial powers. It should be clear from this that neither world history nor American policy, neither the Cold War nor the U.S. role in it, can be understood without a previous understanding of the class character of American society and the nature of the corporate system that underpins and structures it.

Academic Social Science and Corporate Empire

Consider the following organization. It has a budget exceeding $15 billion, or four times the gross national product of Cuba. More powerful than many sovereign states, it has a hundred fifty thousand agents, organizers and hired hands operating two hundred fifty sub-organizations in more than fifty countries. It is part of an international syndicate which controls the economic lifeblood of half a dozen strategic countries in the underdeveloped world. In itself it is a major political force in the key electoral states of New York, Pennsylvania, New Jersey and Texas, and it has close links with other syndicate members which are major political forces in California, Ohio, Louisiana, Indiana and elsewhere. Its agents and their associates occupied the cabinet posts of secretary of state in the administrations of Eisenhower, Kennedy and Johnson, and at the same time had influence in the CIA and other foreign-policy-making organizations of government at the highest levels. It has its own intelligence and paramilitary

An address delivered to the radical sociology caucus at the American Sociological Association meeting in San Francisco, 1968.

networks, and a fleet of ships larger than the Greek Navy. It is not a secret organization, but it is run by a self-perpetuating oligarchy whose decisions and operations are secret. And these affect directly, and significantly, the level of activity in the whole U.S. economy.

The organization is the Standard Oil Company of New Jersey, the successor firm to the original Rockefeller Trust. There can be no question as to the front-rank significance of this corporation in the American economy or in American politics. Yet, *there does not exist a single independent academic study of the operations of the Standard Oil Company, its relation to other interest groups in the American economy or polity, or its impact on American social, political or economic life generally.* Nor is this lacuna in the academic perception of corporate power unique.

If one were to name a handful of interests and interest groups exerting major influence on U.S. foreign policy, Jersey Standard all by itself would rank high on the lists, as would Standard of New York (Mobil), Indiana Standard and Standard of California. But Standard Oil is not an isolated complex in the corporate economy. In a more sophisticated view, the "interest group" which includes Standard Oil extends to the syndicate of oil majors, the network of family fortunes deriving from the Standard Oil companies and deposited on trust with the New York banks, the corporate law firms, and the closely interlocked directorates of financial institutions and industrial corporations which service and provide outlets for these base combines. This "interest group" includes the half dozen most powerful commercial banks in the world, the largest insurance companies and utilities, the most important investment banks and industrials; and its gross assets are larger than that of any country outside the United States. Not only is this far and away the most important "interest group" in the shaping of American foreign policy, it is a *determinant* group, exerting an influence greater than that of all others combined.

The foregoing assertion is based on considerable personal study of the subject and acquaintance with the modest but not insignificant body of nonacademic literature concerning it. By contrast, there is not a single academic social scientist who, on the basis of academic studies made within the framework of existing academic institutions, could challenge that statement with any authority. For neither this oil-financial interest group within the American ruling class, nor any major component of it, with one exception,* has so far as I can discover been subjected to an independent academic study of any length or kind. Not a book, not a monograph, not even an article.

So great and far-reaching are the implications of this vacuum in academic knowledge that a few illustrations suggesting the significance of the powers involved may be in order. From 1952 until his death in 1959, John Foster Dulles was secretary of state of the United States. Dulles was a senior partner in the law firm of Sullivan and Cromwell, corporate attorneys for Standard Oil. Dulles's brother Allen, also a senior partner in the firm, was director of the CIA for more than eight years, during which time the United States overthrew two governments, Iran and Guatemala, where Standard Oil and another Dulles client-firm, United Fruit, were at the center of national political crises, and invaded still a third, Cuba, where Standard Oil of New Jersey was not only the dominant U.S. firm, but in refusing to refine Soviet crude

* The oil industry has from time to time been studied as a pressure group, most notably by Robert Engler in *The Politics of Oil* (University of Chicago Press, 1967). But no attempt has been made to study in depth the operations of a particular firm, or the interlocks between oil, finance, institutions like the Council on Foreign Relations, and government agencies.

oil provided the critical issue in that country's initial conflict with the United States. One will look in vain in the *Social Sciences and Humanities Index* for a reference to the Dulles-Standard Oil law firm of Sullivan and Cromwell, or any of half a dozen equally important corporate law partnerships.

When John Foster Dulles died, he was replaced by Christian A. Herter, who had married into one of the original Standard Oil families and whose son is now a vice-president of Standard Oil of New York (Mobil). President Kennedy then appointed Dean Rusk, a former protégé of Dulles at the State Department who had become president of the Rockefeller Foundation in the same year in which Dulles resigned as chairman of the board of the Rockefeller Foundation to become secretary of state. The Rockefeller Foundation is a major stockholder (probably *the* major stockholder) in the Standard Oil Company of New Jersey.

When Rusk became secretary of state, Eisenhower's undersecretary of state for economic affairs, C. Douglas Dillon, was appointed secretary of the treasury, also a key foreign policy post. An investment banker whose firm services world-oriented oil companies, Dillon sits on the board of the Rockefellers' Chase Manhattan Bank. After leaving Washington he became president of the foundation-financed Brookings Institution, an important policy-formulating organization, and recently joined the executive committee of the Rockefeller Foundation. It's a small world at the top.

The big foundations, Carnegie, Rockefeller and Ford, in turn form the basis of a whole panoply of institutions which provide the institutional framework of foreign policy formulation. These include the Council on Foreign Relations, probably the single most important foreign-policy-formulating organization in the United States, in which David and Nelson Rockefeller, the Dulleses and Douglas Dillon have all played leading roles. Like the organizations and institutions already mentioned, the Council is not the subject of a single academic monograph. A rough idea of the importance of the Council on Foreign Relations–whose existence the professional sociologists and political scientists have managed to overlook–is suggested by Theodore White's report that on a list prepared for President Kennedy for staffing the State Department, sixty-three of the first eighty-two names were from the Council, which has only fourteen hundred members all told. In the Kennedy administration, the secretary of state and seven assistant secretaries and undersecretaries were Council members, as were four senior members of the Defense Department.

Academic social science overlooks not only the matrices of power and interest that on a *prima facie* basis are determinant forces in the shaping of American foreign policy, but the vast institutional consequence of the policy as well: the creation of an overseas empire.

This empire is founded on more than $60 billion in direct investments; its output amounts to the third largest economic unit in the world, after the domestic U.S. economy and the Soviet Union, and as Harry Magdoff has shown, in *The Age of Imperialism,* the demand in the capital goods sector generated by this empire and by the military machine necessary to defend it is the crucial factor in the postwar prosperity. Indeed, whether we look at the vast economic outlets, the unprecedented overseas military presence, including approximately three thousand bases and military installations, the trillion or so dollars of the federal budget spent on cold war programs to preserve and expand this presence, or the social consequences of this diversion of monies and energies into foreign wars and occupations, it is obvious that the empire represents a determining framework for the evolution and development of American society in the post–World War II period.

How would a conscientious and intellectually responsible social science proceed to study this empire? It would want to research the following:

1. The Economic Structure of the System
   a. U.S. corporate and financial interests overseas
   b. The benefits they receive from the inequitable structure of the international economy
   c. Their interest-group structure
   d. Their significance in the domestic U.S. economy; in the economies of the countries invested in
   e. Their influence on U.S. policy in Washington and the respective embassies
   f. U.S. federal economic programs (e.g., AID) as integral parts of the system (their economic function, their staffs, the special committees shaping them and the congressional lobbies backing them)
   g. "World" banking institutions and monetary institutions, their relation to U.S. banking interests and their policies as a reflection of these interests
2. The Military Structure of the System
   a. The shaping of U.S. military policy and corporate influence on military policy–special commissions, guidelines, civilian secretaries
   b. U.S. bases, installations and military alliances abroad
   c. The economics of base-building and military alliances abroad
   d. The specific corporate interests involved in base-building and supply operations
   e. The political influence in Washington and in the allied countries of U.S. corporations supplying the military and/or investing in the respective countries

3. The Political Structure of the System
   a. U.S. foreign policy and corporate interests abroad: the services provided to corporations by the State Department and other agencies, the positions taken by the government in regard to conflicts between host governments and the private property of U.S. nationals
   b. Special agencies such as the CIA, AID, etc., the influence of overseas corporate interests on them, especially in terms of providing their directorates; the coordination of, for example, CIA policy with corporate interests
   c. Policy organizations, such as the Council on Foreign Relations, the Committee on Economic Development, the Foreign Policy Association and the Brookings Institution, and ideology formation; their class basis and so forth
   d. Foundations and universities, their overseas programs, interlocks with corporate interests and so forth
   e. Influence of U.S. institutions in other polities
4. The Historical Development of the U.S. Overseas System
5. The Consequences of the System
   a. The economic, military and political consequences for the overseas areas
   b. The same for the United States
6. Comparative Overseas Systems

There are one hundred ninety-one centers of international studies and foreign affairs research in the United States and their activities are conveniently summarized in a directory published by the State Department. It is therefore possible to state categorically that *not a single one* of the topics listed above—which are vital to any serious, scholarly understanding of contemporary American society and foreign policy, as well as world politics and international development—is being systematically researched anywhere in the United States. In other words, on the basis of academically respectable and so-called professional scholarship, it is not possible to make any significant statements about the structure of the American social system and its directions, or of the international social system, and any statements that are in fact being made on the basis of academic efforts are contributions to ideology, not science.

One doesn't have to search for examples. The dominant academic theory of the power structure is still some version of pluralism, although the pluralist studies to date have all been of local communities and municipalities. In 1967, however, the pluralist thesis was formulated on the national level by the late Arnold Rose. His book, *The Power Structure,* was hailed by the *American Journal of Sociology* as a "splendid book" with both "a political and a sociological sophistication" which would "appear to be" a "complete" refutation of the "fanciful" notions of C. Wright Mills and other power elite and ruling-class theorists.* Rose's sophisticated political and sociological orientation led him to conclude that the "economic elite," outside the military supply industries, has no more influence on foreign policy than the workers organized into trade unions. (Only one member of the trade union movement has been appointed to the cabinet since the New Deal, and he lasted only three months.) Yet Rose offered no analysis of American foreign policy, its structure, or the personnel who direct it, and showed no knowledge of the existing literature on the corporate concep-

* Cited in G. William Domhoff, *The Higher Circle* (New York: Random House, 1970), pp. 311–312.

tion of the national interest. That such a book could be written by a self-respecting professional, let alone praised in a journal that pretends to serious intellectual concerns, is disgraceful. But it is only a small symbol of the disgrace of the sociological profession in general, whose ignorance of power in this country is matched only by its readiness to serve that power.

For the academic mind is not only vacuous in respect to the key social forces and institutions shaping American society and its relations with other peoples, it is also deeply and profoundly corrupt.

Thus, such integrated international studies as are in fact being conducted in the one hundred ninety-one centers on the one hand ignore even the possibility that there is a U.S. overseas system which in any way dominates the economic and political life of other peoples. At the same time, they provide the managers of that system with the most up-to-date techniques of administration and rule (as well as training potential administrators and technicians to implement that rule). Research into the political allegiance of national elites, the activities of local communist, nationalist and revolutionary groups, the principles of modernization without revolution, suggests the kinds of academic inquiries pursued in these centers.

This consistent bias in the assumptions and directions of research throughout the university system would be incomprehensible if one were attempting to understand it only in terms of random intellectual processes. There is nothing random, however, about the social forces that promoted the international studies concept, initiated the programs, and provided their financing. *All* of the international research centers now functioning in the United States university system, with one or two isolated and insignificant exceptions, were created by the corporate wealth which has been pumped out of the American overseas empire. *Every single one* of the eleven elite institutions of international studies, including more than ninety area centers, is funded by one ruling-class institution, the Ford Foundation, which has put more than $150 million into this kind of program. And every single one of them was initiated by either Ford, Rockefeller, or Carnegie, the prime movers of the whole international studies field. These foundations are actively run by directors of the international New York banks, the oil companies and Wall Street law firms, who move effortlessly to and from key posts in the State Department, the Defense Department and the CIA, as well. They are highly class-conscious, exceptionally sophisticated, and not likely to invest millions in research into U.S. imperialism and their own domination and exploitation of the underdeveloped world.

As the destruction of the Hispanic Institute at Stanford several years ago showed, no independent center of research can exist in the face of their active boycott and ill will. In short, institutional research on any significant scale is possible in this country only when it is initiated and funded by the ruling class, through its foundations and corporations (government agencies can be expected eventually to pick up the tabs for projects launched with private aid). Such crude realities, needless to say, never enter the analyses of the pluralist professionals (themselves significant beneficiaries of the largesse). For example, while virtually every voluntary policy association and independent policy or research institution of note, from the Council on Foreign Relations to the Brookings Institution to the Rand Corporation, exists by the financial grace of the big three foundations, and while the Rockefeller Foundation alone has been represented in every U.S. cabinet since the Truman administration and has numbered three secretaries of state among its top administrators, a respected professional like Rose can write, "Whatever the merits or defects of the philanthropic foundations, they cannot be considered great centers of power in the United States. This is especially true of the national philanthropic foundations, like the ones bearing the names of Ford, Rockefeller and Carnegie. Some of the local ones are much more powerful–e.g., the Kansas City Association of Trusts and Foundations." Is this sociology or satire? Such desperate ignorance in a work of serious pretensions speaks volumes about academic sociology and its vaunted standards. What is important to recognize is that Rose could get away with such fatuities only because the ignorance he flaunted is so general in the profession, while the possibilities of challenging it and establishing a countervision are so depressingly limited.

It is clear that the main barrier to serious social analysis in the universities is the failure of the academic profession to honor the pluralistic principle: to provide intellectual room for a critical dialectic to develop. In short, it is the absence of firmly established, certified and, above all, institutionalized radical traditions and schools. The inability of radical schools to establish themselves, in turn, is principally the effect of their *political* (rather than intellectual) inability to gain a foothold in the institutional framework of knowledge, to control university administrations, departments and funding sources for research on a significant scale.

The most important attempt to date to seize an administrative apparatus within the university structure was the effort by black militants to establish autonomous black studies programs. Although black studies programs have now been widely adopted, the crucial goal in the struggle–autonomy–was lost. That is, the militants failed to gain the ability to validate a radical definition of scholarship. In opposing the concept of autonomy, university administrators were able to enlist faculty support by invoking an alleged threat to some idealized notion of "academic standards," if autonomy were granted. The fact is that the same arguments were used twenty-five years ago against the international studies programs when they were first proposed, but the men from Rockefeller and Carnegie, with the *aid* of university administrators (usually from the same upper-class clubs), overrode all faculty objections. To this day, the international studies institutes are for all intents and purposes beyond faculty control or accountability.

Without an institutional base or funding source, it is virtually impossible for a radical perspective to establish itself as part of the "scientific" or "professional" academic canon. The work of Thomas Kuhn on the structure of scientific revolutions illustrates the obstacles nicely. As Kuhn points out, the acceptance (i.e., the social acceptance) of a paradigm marks a qualitative change in the development of any science. Until the paradigm is accepted and can be assumed, the individual scientist must in each work attempt to build his field anew, starting from first principles and justifying the use of each concept introduced. It is only when a textbook in his paradigm exists that he can abandon such elementary tasks, and begin his research where the textbook leaves off, and "thus concentrate exclusively upon the subtlest and most esoteric aspects of the . . . phenomena that concern his group." The hostile environment in which the radical or Marxist social scientist must work forces him back to first principles and prevents him from engaging in the prolonged study and collaborative research that leads to the more subtle, sophisticated and interesting aspects of his theory, and commands respect from other "professionals." Thus, contemporary Marxism can be dismissed as a candidate for serious academic concern not because it is subversive, but because it is "doctrinaire," "ideological," "hortatory" and in general unworthy of such high-class intellectual attention.

Even more obstacles are thrown in the path of the development of any radical perspective by the fact that paradigms structure not only the work of individual investigators, but also the very institutions within which organized research and theoretical activity take place. Thus, there is not even an academic field or department in which the systematic study of imperialism could be conducted within the present-day university. Only the imperialists of the Ford Foundation have the financial power to set up a new field or discipline and override the existing bureaucratic and professional privileges that normally operate to prevent any new definition of subject matter and procedures in the social sciences. In what academic department would it be considered legitimate to study and investigate the overseas systems in the manner suggested previously? Moreover, since the whole graduate program for training sociologists is oriented towards methodologies, research techniques, information and existing sociological literature that have little or no relevance to the study of imperialism, how is any member of the academic community to train himself in the techniques and school himself in the knowledge necessary to embark on such a study? It should be clear by now that what passes for social science in the university may be sophisticated, but in those areas which intersect the pivotal class struggles of the epoch, it is not serious. It is not science but ideology.

In the social analysis of ideology, it is not the origins of ideas in the minds of individual thinkers that must be explained, but the causes of their social dominance and institutionalization. And the means by which intellectual doctrines are developed, supported, propagated, and made generally dominant in the university are firmly in the control of forces external to the community of students and scholars. In vulgar brevity, *money* provides the power for sustaining, supporting and spreading ideas. In the university, money for research facilities, for time, for jobs, for disciples, sometimes for publication, for all the levers of prestige and power that are so integral to the operation of the academic enterprise, is the key to ideological hegemony.

With money you can promote an ideological perspective such as behavioralism, which, without the backing of Ford and Rockefeller, would never have had the opportunity even to develop or employ its methodologies, let alone rise to dominance in the profession. Or you can make possible the studies, conferences, publications, professorships and so forth that make a major force out of a doctrine as foolish and insubstantial as pluralism. Or you can create a major institutional revolution within the university system and a whole new center of academic power, as was done with the institutes of international studies in the postwar period.

One of the chief sources of patronage and research funds in the social sciences, and in many ways the only significant "planning" agency for the allocation of social science energies and research resources, is the Social Science Research Council. The Social Science Research Council portrays itself as an intellectual institution reflecting the views of its affiliated members–the American Sociological Association, the American Historical Association, the American Political Science Association, etc. In fact, the SSRC is the creature of the big foundations which finance and helped to create it. Its board is self-perpetuating; its executive officers form a permanent oligarchy of academic nonentities who happen to belong to the same upper-class club, the Cosmos, and have a penchant for staying in power for decades. Far from *reflecting* fashions in the academic professions, the SSRC *makes* those fashions in collusion with foundations that funnel the monies and put together the constituencies that can make a favored intellectual mode the dominating feature of the academic landscape. For example, the shotgun marriage of the OSS-CIA with the university community (a marriage that approaches its silver anniversary and is still going strong) was effected through skillful matchmaking and maneuvers on the part of the SSRC, which is as ubiquitous in its influence as it is elusive in respect to its intellectual basis and control.

There are, in short, no funds of any significant size available anywhere in the university system that are not under the control of the powers of the status quo, and specifically of the ruling class and its agents. This being the case, it is disingenuous to talk of scholarship, disinterested or independent social investigation and research, or "professionalism" (unless as a euphemism for intellectual prostitution).

The precondition for the development of any serious scholarship on an institutional scale is that the intellectual community take over the means of intellectual production and gain control over the allocation of its own research energies and resources. Academic liberation requires that no foundation or agency external to the university, i.e., not under the direct control of faculty and students, should fund any professor or any specific or specified project. All funding of research must be allocated by open bodies composed of faculty and students alone. No professor should consult or should be permitted to consult for any corporation or government agency for money or other means of remuneration, under pain of censure. The publication of texts and academic works must be brought under the exclusive control of academic cooperatives, however small, to ensure diversity and decentralization and to end the massive subsidy of conservative-liberal works by conservative university presses, foundations, corporations and the CIA. All administrators must be elected or appointed by faculties and students. Regents and trustees needless to say should be abolished.

In sum, the intellectual marketplace must be derigged. For

there are no standards now enforced by the so-called profession that can stem the corruption that has swamped the university over the years, submerging its high ideals under a sea of intellectual sludge.

One final note. While decrying the failure of the university to live up to its ideals, one must remember that it is a far more sinister institution in its present organization than this charge implies. For it is the dependable servant and willing provider of techniques, technologies, and technicians for the most rapacious empire in human history. It is not radicals who have politicized the university; the university is already totally political. What radicals must bring to the university is the commitment to oppose its subservience to power, to promote a better vision of the service in which its intellectual enterprise should be cast: as ally of the oppressed and exploited, as teacher of truth that is not for sale.

Part 2

Marxism and Its Place in Economic Science

In the last hundred years, the mainstream of economic science has been challenged by a variety of heretics—from Thorstein Veblen to John A. Hobson, from Major Douglas to Silvio Gesell. But none has sustained that challenge so long, or raised it to such threatening proportions for the security and self-confidence of the economic establishment, as Karl Marx. The footnotes and parenthetical asides of orthodox economics texts are peppered to this very day with instant refutations of Marx, and equally devastating sarcasms directed at his phantom disciples, whose specific arguments are rarely presented in any detail, and whose names (let alone works) are hardly mentioned. This is no oversight, but rather a subtle and extremely effective form of censorship, which is practiced in all academic fields and partly accounts for the fact that there are so few tenured Marxists in the academy today.

In explaining the awesome vitality of Marx, reference is often made to the existence of a global revolutionary movement which looks to his work for theoretical guidance. But this only puts the paradox another way. How can a century-old analysis provide the theoretical basis for the forces of change in the contemporary era? Conversely, how can the imposingly modern body of economic theory, with all its sophisticated techniques, appear to the revolutionary and radical forces of the world, whether in the rice paddies of Vietnam or the academic quadrangles of Berkeley and Harvard, so sterile, so conservative, and so irrelevant to the issues of our time?

The starting point of an answer to these questions lies in the recognition that Marxism and orthodox economics represent two complementary scientific paradigms. The Marxist paradigm is expressly constructed to analyze a system based on private capital and wage-labor. It is macro-economic and dynamic in character. It advances the notion that the central pivot of the present system is a relationship that is at the same time social and economic: namely, the institution of private property in the means of production. The orthodox paradigm, on the other hand, is basically static and oriented toward micro-economics. Above all, it abstracts from the specific differentiating characteristics of capitalist society in order to universalize its concepts and applications.*

The orthodox model is extremely useful as a framework for dealing with certain technical problems, such as the prob-

* Thus the Keynesian aggregates for analyzing national income are applicable to any economic society, whereas Marx's reproduction scheme is defined in terms of the fundamental division of the product between wage-earners and capitalists. Marx also disaggregates a producers' goods sector from a consumers' goods sector to give theoretical recognition to the fact that in capitalism the end of production is not the fulfillment of social needs but the expansion of private capital.

lem of optimalization and the analysis of market behavior both at the micro- and macro-economic levels. But given the lack of specificity in its primary assumptions and its failure to incorporate into the model the basic characteristics of a capitalist social economy, it is ill-equipped to analyze the structural determinants of the shape and development of that social economy. Insofar as the problems of capitalism do not stem from inefficiencies in existing markets, but from the influence of institutions *outside* the market (e.g., property and inherited capital accumulations) and therefore outside the purview of orthodox analysis, that analysis is relatively powerless to provide real understanding or insight. Hence its seeming irrelevance.

There is a certain irony in the fact that the nature of these two paradigms, and especially their complementary character, has long been recognized by serious, independent Marxists, but not by the proponents of orthodoxy. The presumably liberal neo-classicists and high priests of the academic establishment who pay homage to the values of pluralism continue to deny Marxism its place in the economic curriculum. Worse yet, orthodox economists (via a bastardized concept called the neo-classical synthesis) claim precisely that analytical range for their own analysis (namely the socio-economic system as a whole) that its very structure precludes them from claiming, thereby transforming their restrictively valid statements into generalized exercises in ideology and metaphysics. An ideology brooks no competitors, and Marxism is therefore kept well outside the bounds of academic respectability.

To economists brought up in the orthodox tradition, the foregoing will be far from self-evident, and a brief excursion into the history of economic doctrine may, therefore, throw some light on the problem—and at the very least indicate that one exists.

During the half century before the Keynesian Revolution, the marginalists were introducing mathematical rigor into economics and bringing it up to "scientific" status. Throughout this period, Marx and his disciples were looked upon with thundering scorn. "Nowhere," wrote Professor Alexander Gray in a standard text of the period, "is there in print such a miracle of confusion, such a supreme example of how not to reason" as in Marx. Even more famous, and more devastating because of its source, was Keynes's assault. "How can I accept a doctrine," he wrote in 1926, "which sets up as its bible, above and beyond criticism, an obsolete economic textbook which I know to be not only scientifically erroneous but without interest or application for the modern world." The irony of this was that Keynes himself, by returning to some of the abandoned macro-economic concerns of the classicial economists, opened the way to a reappraisal of Marx's contribution to economic theory.

For fifty years orthodox economists had regarded the economy as a self-adjusting mechanism with an inherent tendency to full employment equilibrium–quite in contrast to the Marxian picture, in which crisis was indigenous to the system. In 1929 reality forced its way into academic consciousness and stimulated Keynes's agonizing reappraisal of the received tradition. When the revisions were completed, it was apparent that, in Joan Robinson's words, "academic theory, by a path of its own [had] arrived at a position which bears considerable resemblance to Marx's system."* There were in both Keynes and Marx propositions to the effect that investment generates purchases without sales and

* Joan Robinson, *An Essay on Marxian Economics* (London: MacMillan, 1942). Joan Robinson is one of Keynes's most distinguished disciples and herself a major figure in the development of modern economic theory.

so promotes boom conditions, in both a repudiation of Say's Law, and in both the notion that the inherent tendencies of the system are toward something less than full employment equilibrium.

Given the realistic assumptions of the Marxian model, it is not surprising that Marx's business cycle theory should receive the high praise of so eminent and conservative an authority as Joseph Schumpeter. "In Marx," wrote Schumpeter, "we find practically all the elements that ever entered into any serious analysis of business cycles, and on the whole very little error. Moreover, it must not be forgotten that the mere perception of the existence of cyclical movements was a great achievement at the time."* Even more striking is the reappraisal of Marxian theory which some honest and honorable Keynesians undertook after Keynes's original macro-static analysis had been made dynamic by his disciples. In the words of Professor Kurihara, "[The] Marxian theory of capitalist development anticipates many modern long-run theories, namely the stagnation theories of Keynes and Hansen, the dynamic theories of Harrod and Domar, the 'cyclical growth' theories of Schumpeter, Kalecki, Kaldor and Goodwin, and Mrs. Joan Robinson's theory of structural under-employment."† Professor L. R. Klein even went so far as to describe Marx's theory as "probably the origin of macro-economics." (One cannot find any similar recognition, however, in Samuelson's currently standard textbook, *Economics.*)

What does this episode from the history of economic doctrine tell us, aside from the fact that Keynes and his fellow

* J. A. Schumpeter, *Capitalism, Socialism and Democracy* (New York: Harper and Row, 1950), p. 40.

† Kenneth Kurihara, *The Keynesian Theory of Economic Development* (New York: Columbia University Press, 1959), pp. 17–18.

academics read Marx superficially if at all? It tells us first that it was possible for several generations of economists, operating in what to all appearances was a completely liberal and open academic environment, to dismiss a major economist from serious consideration, and to exclude from its institutions an economic school whose analyses possessed far more insight into the macro-economic system than anything to be found in the orthodox tradition. Moreover, this exclusion was not made on the grounds that Marxism was subversive; the professors would not have permitted themselves such an illiberal stance. Rather, Marxism was regarded as unscientific, unprofessional and not up to the accepted academic standards.

In recalling this episode, the present generation of academic economists might perhaps be touched by a little modesty or shaken by a little self-doubt, in the midst of their own justifications for excluding Marxism from the academic community today. After all, the arguments for exclusion have not really changed that much. By exclusion of course I do not mean that an isolated Marxist who happens to be trained in *orthodox* economics cannot find an academic place. The situation is rather that there is no place in the academy for Marxian economics (*or* sociology) as such, whether in the pages of the *American Economic Review,* in the economic curriculum, or in the Departments of Economics themselves.

The continuing academic suppression of Marx and Marxism is a phenomenon that requires no active intervention, but takes place through the "normal" workings of the market. It is a suppression nonetheless. Many writers who took the time to ponder this problem in the wake of the Keynesian revolution came to the conclusion that the earlier exclusion of Marxism from the realms of legitimate economic science was the result of a misunderstanding. Pre-Keynesian orthodox analysis was primarily a static theory of economic equilibrium concerned with micro-economic problems, while Marxism was a macro-economic theory of dynamic change. Thus, the two belonged to different ranges of economic theory. Once this was recognized, the gap between them would cease to exist and a dialogue could take place. Mrs. Robinson, a Keynesian and a pioneer of modern price theory, even concluded her essay on Marxian economics with an observation that future progress in economics would depend on using academic methods to solve the problems posed by the Marxist model.

The paradoxical upshot of this understanding of the complementarity of the paradigms has been that Marxist economists have indeed recognized the utility of orthodox economics and have adopted in their own writings, for example, many of the tools of Keynesian income analysis. But there has been no such change of heart or perspective on the part of the orthodox economic establishment. Marx's theory is still described in elementary texts like Professor Grossman's as "primitive even for his own day." The works of Marx's disciples, their theoretical analyses and concerns, are disregarded and find no place in the main arena of economic thought.

The reason for this continuing gap between the Marxian and the orthodox approaches to the study of economic society is that Marxism is first of all a *class* analysis. Its paradigm is not framed in terms of profit-maximizing individuals or economic units in the marketplace. The Marxian focus is rather on the encounter between two socio-economic classes: owners of capital and wage-laborers. On the relationship of these two classes, the whole productive and distributive process turns; from it the power relations of the legal-political infrastructure of capitalist society develop and grow. The continuing schism between these two approaches to economics is accounted for by the inability of orthodox theory to assimilate the Marxian class analysis and its revolutionary implications.

Present-day orthodox economic analysis pays a great price, however, for its rejection of the Marxian model and class perspective. That price is a refined irrelevance which bears a generic resemblance to the situation in the pre-Keynesian era. In a recent critical essay Robert Heilbroner described the present state of affairs in stark terms: "The theory of economics, magnificent to behold, is considerably less impressive to use. It is true that it has given us a rough picture of how the market system works, both in allocating its resources and in determining the level of overall output. But beyond this conception, which can be taught with ease to a college freshman, the ramifications of economics have produced singularly little. . . . The beautifully finished portion called price theory fails to explain the pricing operations of the great corporations. International trade theory does not adequately account for the most important single fact about international trade–to wit, the failure of an international division of labor to shed its benefits on poor countries and rich countries alike. The theory of economic development does not tell underdeveloped countries how to grow."

In addition, "the distribution of wealth . . . is a central economic fact about which economic theory is mute. The effects on the distribution of income attributable to the process of growth is another, so that economics gives us no hint as to the disturbances and frictions produced by growth. . . The nature of class interests in a capitalist system is not mentioned in any textbook, so that nothing in the nature of political or social constraints bounds the free movement of the economic model."*

* Robert Heilbroner, *Between Capitalism and Socialism* (New York: Random House, 1971), pp. 119–22.

To Heilbroner's list of oversights, much more can be added. Orthodox economics does not credit the central expansionary roles played by federal military expenditures and private overseas investment in the postwar period; these are the cornerstones of the so-called Keynesian prosperity, fundamental not only in a quantitative economic sense, but also in their political ramifications. Also, the network of relationships which constitute American imperialism, a system which provides the political and economic framework in which international events take place in our time, does not come within the purview of the neo-classical synthesis.

In Heilbroner's view, the oversights in orthodox economic theory are not accidental, but result "from a fundamental failure of vision on the part of the modern model-builders, who do not see that the social universe that they are attempting to reproduce in a set of equations is not and cannot be adequately described in terms of functional relationships alone, but must also and simultaneously be described as a system of privilege. If a model of economic reality is to be relevant, in other words, it must portray both the functional relationships peculiar to the provisioning process and those stemming from the clash of interests generated by this very functional process itself."

Heilbroner goes on to ask: "Is it possible to construct a system that is at one and the same time a portrayal of functional relationships and of privilege?" Answering his own question, Heilbroner states, "There is one such system, Marxian economics." And, in a poignant recall of Mrs. Robinson's prescription more than twenty-five years earlier, Heilbroner concludes that "Marxian insights must be married to neo-classical techniques to produce an economic theory that is both elegant and consistent as a model and freighted with meaning as a theory of society."*

* Ibid, pp. 122, 124.

The orthodox theories which are summarized in the elegant equations of the mathematical model builders are too obviously restrictive in their assumptions and parameters to function successfully as ideology. When some effort to come to terms with social realities is unavoidable (as in writing basic textbooks or popular treatises, or offering political advice), orthodox economists fall back on the patchwork theory called "the neo-classical synthesis." The idea of such a synthesis originates with Keynes. Once aggregate demand is managed by Keynesian techniques, the neo-classical model supposedly comes into its own. In point of fact, this "synthesis" is not a synthesis at all. Or, put another way, there is no synthesis except by *ex cathedra* pronouncement. To be legitimate, such a synthesis would have to include a theory of the economy analytically linked to a theory of the state, since the management of demand by Keynesian techniques is a *political* process. Such an integrated analysis is possible, but it is called Marxism, not neo-classicism.

One of the supreme ironies here is that Keynes himself provided the basis for such a theory of the state, i.e., a theory of fiscal policy that would flow directly from a theory of the economy. By stressing the pre-eminent significance of the investment decision in determining the level of output and employment, and by illuminating the dependence of that decision on the expectation of investors, Keynes provided the key to a theory of fiscal politics which would show that the pattern of government spending as a policy must fall predominantly within the channels coincident with business interest. As Keynes put it, "economic prosperity is excessively dependent on a political and social atmosphere which is congenial to the average business man." A Marxist would only add that what is at stake is not the confidence of the *average* businessman, but rather, the confidence of the finance committees of the largest industrial corporations and financial institutions. On the basis of Keynes's insight and some elementary political observations, it is not difficult to work out an integrated theory of the relation between the economy and the state. But this is certainly not what is studied in courses on fiscal policy and public finance in the contemporary economics curriculum.

When we turn to the other side of the neo-classical synthesis we find not only a gap where a theory should have been, but a model that seems in every main particular constructed so as to invert the real state of affairs.

To the standard criticisms of the neo-classical model, its defenders have responded with one of two evasions. Either they have made epicyclic additions to their model, as in the theory of social costs, which is introduced to correct the identification of market value and real value, or they have added a general *caveat* to the effect that the assumptions of the theory prevent it from being applied "directly" to the real world. Clearly, it is about time that economists began asking themselves some pretty hard questions. The original architects of the neo-classical model were no doubt convinced that the markets they were studying were only deviating from perfect competition in a marginal and perhaps even remediable manner. They probably thought that the distribution of income would level out as the economy approached a post-accumulation stationary state. Moreover, in that pre-advertising era they may well have thought that the concept of consumer sovereignty was reasonably descriptive of economic reality. Can any honest observer of the present-day American economy entertain similar illusions? And if not, does it make sense to go on basing the main enterprise of economic analysis on a model which even its practitioners admit starts from a point so distant from the real world?

Admittedly, it is not merely inertia that has sustained this model so long, nor even its utility as conservative ideology.

Despite its distance from the concrete conditions of the capitalist economy, the effort to study the maximizing behavior of individuals in a perfectly competitive market has, as already noted, led to a highly sophisticated and even useful theory of economic *rationality* (the optimalization of means for the realization of given ends). This is a technical problem in any economic society and the orthodox techniques devised to solve it (from marginalism to linear programming) have a practical utility recognized both by corporate and government planning agencies. But to take a model designed for analyzing the general problem of resource allocation and apply it, as orthodox economists do, to the structurally distinct problem of understanding the shape and development of a specific economic system, is to abandon science for ideology. The end result is a confused, insubstantial and intellectually unworthy "synthesis." Around it, texts like Samuelson's *Economics* are written, and the standard liberal apologetics are built.

When we turn to the Marxist alternative, however, the path is not as clear as it should be. In particular, confusion exists as to what precisely constitutes the "Marxist" analysis, or in what sense, even, one can speak about a Marxist economics at all. This confusion exists both for Marxists and their critics.

The confusion stems in part from the historical role that Marxism has played as an official ideology in the Soviet Union and elsewhere, and in part from the historical development of orthodox economics, which underwent its revolution in perspective and technique shortly after the completion of Marx's work. Most of the controversy over the *economics* of Marxism has concerned the labor theory of value. Yet, the labor theory of value was not a *Marxist* contribution to economic theory; it was rather the orthodox value theory of the day. In defending or attacking the labor theory, therefore, one has to ask whether one is defending or attacking "Marxist" economics. Many serious students of Marx have concluded, as Professor Mark Blaug puts it, that "Marx's analysis of the structural development of capitalism at no point hinges on acceptance or rejection of the labor theory of value."*

The labor theory of value is not the only doctrine identified with "Marxist" economics which turns out to have a classical provenance. The theory of the falling rate of profit, for example, can be found in Smith and Ricardo; the theory of the concentration of capital can be found in James Mill; the theory of increasing misery has several orthodox sources; and so forth.

What, then, is the specific *Marxian* critique of orthodox political economy, and what is its special role? "Political economy," wrote Marx in a passage which suggests an answer to the problem, "proceeds from the fact of private property, but it does not explain it to us. It expresses in general, abstract formulae the material process through which private property actually passes, and these formulae it then takes for laws. It does not comprehend these laws, i.e., it does not demonstrate how they arise from the very nature of private property."

Marxist economics is then an economics which builds its model and selects its categories in such a way as to illuminate the manner in which the functional relationships (or laws) of the capitalist economy flow from and are shaped by the defining production (property) relations of capitalist society.

The Marxian analysis begins with the perception that the social institution of private property in the means of production (capital) results in investment surplus accruing to capital

* Mark Blaug, *Economic Theory in Retrospect* (Homewood, Illinois: Richard D. Irwin, 1962).

owners under conditions which dictate certain behavioral functions. As Heilbroner puts it: the Marxian model connects production functions to privilege functions. In short, the qualifications that may be brought in as an afterthought at the end of bourgeois analysis are placed at the very center of the Marxian analytical effort.

It is important to stress that the property institution, the fact that the majority of the population is barred from the ownership of capital (and thus from the means of subsistence), is what makes it possible for one class to appropriate a surplus. The existence of surplus value has nothing to do with the labor theory of value, as Lange has shown.* It is impossible, even, to derive surplus value from the labor theory of value. On the other hand, *every* orthodox theory of value is compatible with the notion that capital owners receive income as a monopoly price because of the basic division of society into wage-laborers (who lack access to means of subsistence or production) and capital owners (who supply capital for a "normal, historically determined margin"). In other words there is a *class* monopoly of the means of production. It is this monopoly that results in the social surplus (of production over consumption) as the income of the capital-owning class.† This income represents the bulk of society's savings. The control of it is crucial for analysis. Marx's focus on this control is what gives his analy-

* Oscar Lange, "Marxian Economics and Modern Economic Theory," in Horowitz, op. cit.

† It must be pointed out that this notion is quite distinct from the proposition advanced in some Marxist texts that capital has no scarcity value, or that the rate of interest would be zero in a socialist economy. Interest as an accounting device for allocating scarce capital resources can and must be distinguished from interest as the *income* of a social class.

sis the relevance which has been admired by non-Marxist economists like Robinson and Heilbroner, as well as by social theorists and historians in general.

The implication of the foregoing perspective on Marxist economic theory is that no particular doctrine or category can function as a criterion of Marxist orthodoxy. An analysis is Marxist when it is historically specific and locates the dynamic matrix of a social formation in its relations of production, which are *economic class* relations. There already exists, of course, a traditional corpus of Marxian theory which would logically form the starting point of any new analytical approach. But revision of the analytic tools and propositions of traditional Marxist theory is necessary if the theory is to develop as an intellectual doctrine. In principle, it may even be possible to create a theory which is "Marxist" in the restricted sense urged here, but which has little surface relation to the traditional Marxist categories and conclusions. Nonetheless, at this historical juncture the traditional Marxist paradigm is the only economic paradigm which is capable of analyzing capitalism as an historically specific, class-determined social formation. As such it provides an indispensable framework for understanding the development and crisis of the present social system and, as an intellectual outlook, would occupy a prime place in any scientific institution worthy of the name.

A Note on Marx's Theory of Class

"... it is the ultimate aim of this work to lay bare the economic law of motion of modern society ..."

Preface to *Capital*

The distinctive features of the Marxian sociology of capitalism are (1) that it defines an explicit relation between social structure and economic process, and (2) that it conceives the economic process *dynamically,* i.e., as a process of development.

This latter aspect is crucial to the whole conception, but the sociological critics of Marx have, without exception, ignored it—and thereby forfeited the relevance of their criticism. Outside the terms of reference which Marx laid down for his model, nothing can be easier for the critic than to prove a negative case. But from such proofs, nothing follows.

Despite the consensus among non-Marxian sociologists as to the hopeless inadequacy of Marx's two-class model, there is an area of contemporary study of society in which this very model, with its abstraction from the role of the middle classes, enjoys widespread acceptance even among orthodox practitioners. This is the field of modern economic dynamics (i.e., the theory of economic growth and development), where among the standard models used to determine the path of economic change are two-class models which divide society into wage-earners and profit-takers. From the point of view of what Marx was attempting to do with his analysis, viz., "to lay bare the economic law of motion of modern society," this is just the area in which the validity of his class model was crucial. That it is confirmed even by bourgeois theory and research testifies to the soundness of Marx's fundamental approach.

The concept of class provides the category through which Marx makes the vital connection between individual action and social role:

> I paint the capitalist and the landlord in no sense *couleur de rose*. But here individuals are dealt with only insofar as they are personifications of *economic* categories, embodiments of particular class relations and class interests."*

This is not to say, of course, that individuals cannot raise themselves, as individuals, above or beyond their class position and interests. Rather, insofar as they function *socially*, i.e., in terms of the social economy, they must function within the pattern laid down by the economic organization of society as determined by its mode of production. "My standpoint, from which the evolution of the economic formation of society is viewed as a process of natural history," wrote Marx, "can less than any other make the individual responsible for relations whose creature he *socially* remains,

* *Capital,* vol. 1, preface to the First German Edition (emphasis added).

however much he may subjectively raise himself above them."*

Thus, for example, the drive to accumulate capital, to amass monetary wealth beyond and indeed without any reference to possible consumption needs, is a "passion" that the capitalist shares with the miser. "But that which in the miser is a mere idiosyncrasy, is in the capitalist, the effect of the social mechanism, of which he is but one of the wheels." This mechanism, which imposes on the capitalist his behavior as a capitalist, is economic in character, although its basis—private ownership of the means of production—is sociological. The law which makes the capitalist's individual behavior conform to a class behavior is an economic law, the law of the market. He can ignore the law of the market, but the price will be his economic ruin, hence his elimination from the capitalist class. The condition of belonging to the class and enjoying its privileges and power is conformity to its pattern of behavior. In fact, therefore, it is only as the *objective* requirements of capitalist behavior become his *subjective* aim and the sole motive of his operations, that he is able to function as a capitalist, that is, "as capital personified and endowed with consciousness and a will."†

In this notion of a social role enforced on the individual class member by society's economic mechanism lies the first important consequence of the definition of class in terms of economic relations of production. This is a crucial difference between the Marxian model and, for example, the Weberian, in which the notion of class is conceived in terms of the market (the availability of typical "life chances")** and thus

* Preface, ibid. Emphasis added.
† *Capital,* vol. 1, p. 152 ("The General Formula for Capital").
** "Class, Status and Party" in Gerth and Mills, *From Max Weber.*

carries with it no imperative to socially consequential action. In fact, Weber recognized the existence of such an imperative in the pervasive rationalizing process of the capitalist market, but failed to incorporate this recognition into his stratification model:

> The capitalistic economy of the present day is an immense cosmos into which the individual is born, and which presents itself to him, at least as an individual, as an unalterable order of things in which he must live. It forces the individual insofar as he is involved in the system of market relationships, to conform to capitalistic rules of action. The manufacturer who in the long run acts counter to these norms, will just as inevitably be eliminated from the economic scene as the worker who cannot or will not adapt himself to them will be thrown into the streets without a job.*

The different significance which Marx and Weber attach to the "system of market relationships," the one placing it at the center of his sociological analysis, the other regarding it as a sub-system of a general, and in some sense *independent,* social system, reflects, in part, the difference between dynamic and static conceptions of the capitalist economy.

For Marx, the accumulation process which regulates social employment and consumption, and embodies the progressive development of society's material foundations (the basis on which all social institutions must rest), is the determinant factor in the evolution of capitalist society. For Weber, working with a different economic model—a model including in its assumptions consumer sovereignty, the self-adjusting rationality of the market, the primacy of exchange relations,

* *The Protestant Ethic and the Spirit of Capitalism.*

and the static hypothesis of given supply—it is the possession of goods and the power which derives from command over goods that is of primary importance for the concept of class. This power is also, of course, essential to Marx's conception. But for Weber it is *all* that is economically essential. *The question of social evolution is simply not seen, by him, in terms of the accumulation process.*

Incredible as this may seem, it is easily explained by the fact that the neoclassical economic theory, on which Weber based his analysis, did not itself recognize the question of *economic* evolution.* Thus, short of being a Marxist, or willing to accept some other heterodox economic theory, there was no way for Weber to be able to grasp the central role which capital accumulation plays in determining economic development.

The chief consequence of the shift from a static to a dynamic viewpoint is to alter the causal significance of the operative factors in the economic (and hence social) process. This was recognized by Schumpeter in *The Theory of Economic Development:* "Spontaneous and discontinuous changes in the channel of the circular flow [Schumpeter's term for a stationary economy] and . . . disturbances of the center of equilibrium appear in the sphere of industrial and commercial life, *not* in the sphere of wants of the consumers of final products." In other words, the determinant factors of long-term dynamic change in the economy are to be found in the sphere of production, not the sphere of exchange.

The reverse is true within the static equilibrium conditions

* E.g., see M. Abramowitz, "Economics of Growth" in *A Survey of Contemporary Economics,* 1952 and "The Theory of Economic Growth: A Survey," *Economic Journal,* December 1964. Talcott Parsons's characterization of the economy as an "adaptive" sector is based on a similar failure to grasp the autonomous role of the accumulation process.

of the circular flow (Weber's model). "We must always start from the satisfaction of wants, since they are the end of all production, and the *given* economic situation at any time must be understoood from this aspect." But: "*innovations* in the economic system do not as a rule take place in such a way that first new wants arise spontaneously in consumers and then the productive apparatus swings round through pressure. We do not deny the presence of this nexus. It is, however, the *producer* who as a rule initiates economic change, and consumers are educated by him if necessary; they are, as it were, taught to want new things, or things which differ in some respects or other from those which they have been in the habit of using. Therefore, while it is permissible and even necessary to consider consumers' wants as an independent and indeed the fundamental force in a theory of the circular flow, we must take a different attitude as soon as we analyze *change.*"*

It takes but a moment's reflection to realize the consequences of adopting this point of view: once we do so, the locus of determination of the whole range of social phenomena associated with production, distribution and consumption, including the all-important allocation of social labor-time, shifts from the exchange market and individual consumers (motivated by various status and prestige concerns) to the sphere of production, and thus the activities (mainly the investment activities) of an economic *class.*

It is in this nexus that the second feature of the Marxian class concept finds its justification. By defining class in terms of production relations, Marx is able to link a necessitated pattern of private behavior to the determining dynamic mechanism of society's economic development. Private accumulation of capital, under capitalist conditions, is social accu-

* *The Theory of Economic Development,* p. 65. Emphasis added.

mulation. Thus the Marxian concept of class at once yields determined lines of behavior for the individual capitalist and through him for the structure of action of the individual firm, and from thence to the development and functioning of the economy as a whole.

That Marx's sociological model has been subject to widespread misunderstanding can be seen at a glance in the fact that the Marxian concept of class is almost exclusively discussed in terms of the proletariat and its revolutionary potential, whereas the operative group in terms of the *functioning* and *development* of the capitalist system (the subject of Marx's major work) is not the proletariat at all, but the *capitalist ruling class.*

The sociological importance which Marx attached to the capitalist class in his analysis of the laws of motion of capitalist society is reflected in the shift in perspective from the early to the later works. In the early philosophical manuscripts, the system is viewed analytically from the point of view of labor and its self-alienation, whereas in the later work the subject is capital and its self-expression. To be sure, from the point of view of the revolutionary tendencies developing within the womb of capitalism, the alienation and exploitation of labor still occupies a central place. But the strategic factor determining the shape and evolution of capitalist society, in its normal functioning, is capital itself, and that social class which is its beneficiary and personification.

Marx, Keynes, and the Economics of Capitalism

When the accumulation of wealth is no longer of high social importance, there will be great changes in the code of morals. We shall be able to rid ourselves of many of the pseudo-moral principles which have hag-ridden us for two hundred years, by which we have exalted some of the most distasteful of human qualities into the position of the highest virtues. We shall be able to afford to dare to assess the money-motive at its true value. The love of money as a possession—as distinguished from the love as money as a means to the enjoyments and realities of life—will be recognised for what it is, a somewhat disgusting morbidity, one of those semi-criminal, semi-pathological propensities which one hands over with a shudder to the specialists in mental disease. . . .

> I see us free, therefore, to return to some of the most sure and certain principles of religion and traditional virtue—that avarice is a vice, that the exaction of usury is a misdemeanour, and the love of money is detestable. . . . We shall once more value ends above means . . .
>
> —J. M. Keynes in "Economic Possibilities for our Grandchildren"

On the surface, few thinkers probably appear more different, indeed more antithetical, than Marx and Keynes. This initial impression is reinforced, moreover, by the polemical atmosphere that naturally surrounds the work of two writers whose primary concern was the *modus operandi* of a system characterized by glaring inequalities of social wealth and power, and by gross irrationalities in the allocation of its human and material resources. Yet despite profound differences in analytical approach and programmatic conclusion, their respective understandings of the core process of the economic system of contemporary capitalism bear striking resemblances to one another.* By examining the convergent perspectives of such seminal thinkers, it may be possible to attain a more penetrating view of the social order and a clearer grasp of the principles of its transformation into something at once more rational and more humane. That, at least, is the assumption and hope of the present essay.

* The terms "economy," "economic process" and "economic system" refer to the activities involved in the production and distribution of material goods. The convergent views of Marx and Keynes do not extend to the "political economy" of capitalism, which includes the sociological dimension of the economic process. On this use of terms, see Oskar Lange, *Political Economy* (London: Pergamon, 1963).

i

Marx begins his critique of capitalism by distinguishing between the two forms of value of commodities, between their value to those who will use them, and the value they will bring in exchange. The value of an object in use is a *qualitative* value, individual and unique in character, and independent of the economic organization of society. Exchange value (which is, properly speaking, what is meant by "value" in an economic sense)* is, on the other hand, *quantitative,* and is the product of a definite organization of the social economy.

Exchange value arises only in those societies where there are independent units producing for a market, i.e., where there is a social division of labor, and people do not produce solely for their own consumption or for that of a self-regulated group, but for the consumption of independent others.

Once it is necessary to exchange on a considerable scale, it is necessary to have a quantitative standard by which the value of goods can be measured and compared. The standard, according to Marx, is the quantity of abstract labor time (socially necessary labor time) embodied in the commodities. This standard is embodied in a common commodity of exchange, which acts as a universal store and measure of value, a commodity called money.

As the independent form of exchange value, money expresses a *social* relation, namely that individual producers, each working in isolation, are in fact working for each

* When the word "value" is used by itself in the present text, its meaning is exchange value.

other.* Their exchange of commodities is an exchange of the products of their labor, and an expression of the mutual interdependence of ther individual labors as respective parts of the allocation of society's aggregate labor power. Each is dependent on the sale of his products for the money to buy the goods that he needs. Thus, a paradox arises: the *use-value* (to him) of his own labor and its product depends on its *exchange-value,* and this in turn on its ability to satisfy a *social* want.

Today what the individual produces may satisfy a social want, find a market, and be realized as an exchange value. But if tomorrow there is a surplus of his product in society, if the allocation of social labor has been such that there is no social demand for his product, then no matter how useful an object it may be, it has no *social* use, and consequently, no matter how much socially necessary labor time he has expended on it, no exchange-value. Thus his product is rendered useless to him, for he has produced it only to sell. In this way, the social division of labor stamps his production with a social character *despite* its private organization, and makes him utterly dependent on a *social* process over which he has no control.

Whatever the form of society, it is necessary to allocate the total labor of society in definite proportions to meet the requirements of social consumption. Where the divi-

* As Strachey once lucidly explained, "money *is* the unconscious expression, the fetish . . . of the social character of labour. 'The Social character of labour appears as the money-existence of commodities,' writes Marx. He means that under capitalism the only way in which the fact that we are all dependent upon each other's labour can be expressed, is that the tangible or intangible results of our labours should all be exchangeable one with another, by being all and each exchangeable with money." *The Nature of Capitalist Crisis* (London: Gallaucz, 1935).

sion of labor is extensive, but property is social, this allocation will take the form of a plan which balances the production of specialized producers with their consumption needs. In a society where means of production are privately owned, so that the interconnection of social labor is manifested in the *private* exchange of the individual products of labor, allocation cannot take place as the result of a conscious decision of the related producers or of their representatives. It takes place instead through the market, that is, through the operation of the "law of [exchange] value." The "social relation of production takes the form of an object [money] existing outside of individuals" whose relations to each other in production "assume a material character independent of their control and conscious individual action."*

Marx represented the exchange of commodities in what he called "simple commodity production" (pre-capitalist) by the formula C-M-C (commodity-money-commodity). He distinguished it from the circulation of commodities in a barter economy, which he represented (C-C) and where exchange took place directly between local producers and without the intervention of money. By contrasting these two economies he sought to emphasize the importance of the *continuity* of the exchange process in a money economy, where exchange

* "Since the producers do not come into social contact with each other until they exchange their products, the specific social character of each producer's labour does not show itself except in the act of exchange. In other words, the labour of the individual asserts itself as a part of the labour of society, only by means of the relations which the act of exchange establishes directly between the products, and indirectly, through time, between the producers. To the latter, therefore, the relations connecting the labour of one individual with that of the rest appear, not as direct social relations between individuals at work, but as what they really are, material relations between persons and social relations between things." *Capital,* vol. 1, p. 73.

is not local and where each specialized producer is utterly dependent on exchange for the satisfaction of his needs. For so long as production was privately controlled, it was by no means inevitable that the circulation process should in fact be continuous. If a break in the circulation should occur on a social scale; if the transformation of goods into money, or money into goods, should not be able to take place, a crisis would result.

In such a crisis, the basic contradiction between the private character of production and the social character of the labor in production (which only has value if social labor has been allocated in such a way that the product of the individual producer finds a buyer) expresses itself dramatically in the transformed aspect of money: "money becomes suddenly and immediately transformed, from its merely ideal shape of money of account [medium of exchange], into hard cash [store of value]. Profane commodities can no longer replace it. The use-value of commodities becomes value-less, and their value vanishes in the presence of its own independent form. On the eve of the crisis, the bourgeoisie, with the self-sufficiency that springs from intoxicating prosperity, declares money to be a vain imagination. Commodities alone are money. But now the cry is everywhere: money alone is a commodity! As the hart pants after fresh water, so his soul pants after money, the only wealth. In a crisis, the antithesis between commodities and their value-form, money, becomes heightened into an absolute contradiction."*

This contradiction is, of course, but another facet of the contradiction between utility and value. Real economic wealth is use-values, utilities, material things that satisfy human needs. Exchange-value and its crystallization, money, is a mere phenomenal form of value; it is the form that goods

* *Capital,* vol. 1, p. 138.

take in order that they may be exchanged. It is not itself "real" wealth, but a mere means of exchange. In commodity-producing societies, however, where production is not governed by a social plan, and thus where the allocation of social labor takes place through the operation of the law of value in the market, social production is and must be regulated not by use-value, but by exchange value, by the *money demand* for goods, rather than the real demand.

Moreover, whereas the use-value of every other commodity, as the object of a particular want, has a different value in different hands (e.g., it is valuable to the seller for the buying power it confers on him, to the buyer for its utility), money, as the commodity singled out to be the universal equivalent, is for that reason "an object of a *universal want* arising from the very process of exchange, and it has the same use-value to everybody, viz., that of serving as the depository of exchange value," of conferring the power of command over men and goods.* Thus, "money is not only *an* object of the passion for riches; it is *the* object of that passion." Moreover, since the passion for riches, as opposed to the passion for particular things, is possible only when "universal wealth" has been individualized in a particular commodity, money appears no less "as a *source* of the passion for riches."†

In sum, with the development of the circulation of commodities in exchange, there also develops the passionate desire to hold commodities in their abstract money form. "From being the mere means of effecting the circulation of commodities, this change of form becomes the end and aim."**

**Contribution to a Critique of Political Economy* (Chicago: Kerr & Co., 1904), p. 51.

† Ibid., p. 176.

** *Capital*, vol. 1, p. 130.

ii

Capitalism is a form of commodity production. It arises as a social system when a mass of laborers has been expropriated from ownership of any means of production and consequently appears in the market place under the compulsion to sell something in order to buy means of subsistence to survive. This "something" cannot be anything but the power to work, since the laborers have been divested of all means of production; they sell their labor power to an owner of means of production, that is, to capital (money). Capital buys their commodity, labor power, and then sells its products for more money than the cost* and thus increases itself in the process.

There is an immediately obvious and striking difference between simple and capitalist commodity production, which appears most visible in the formulas with which Marx describes their circulation processes. Whereas the formula for circulation in simple commodity production is C-M-C (commodity-money-commodity), the formula in capitalist commodity production is M-C-M′ (money-commodity-money, where M′ is greater than M). In other words, the

* This can be expressed in value terms by saying that capital buys labor-power at its value and thus acquires labor (the *product* of labor-power) below its value. The same idea, however, can also be put in straightforward empirical terms: ". . . Marx shows that the development of the capitalist system is founded on the existence of a class of workers who have no means to live except by selling their labor-power. Capitalism first expropriates the peasant and the artisan, and then exploits their labor. The possibility of exploitation depends upon the existence of a margin between total net output and the subsistence minimum of the workers. If a worker can produce no more in a day than he is obliged to eat in a day, he is not a potential object of exploitation." Robinson, *An Essay on Marxian Economics* (MacMillan, 1964), p. 17.

motive of *capitalist* exchange (hence of production, which appears as a mere element of the circulation process) is not another commodity–use-value, but more exchange-value, more *money.* *

In simple commodity production, exchange is a means of obtaining one product for another, thus it is "a means of carrying out a purpose unconnected with circulation, namely, the appropriation of use-values, the satisfaction of wants." The circulation of money as capital in capitalist commodity production is, on the contrary, "*an end in itself,* for the expansion of [quantitative] value takes place only within this constantly renewed movement [M-C-M′]."

The form of capitalist circulation, M-C-M′, is institutionally grounded in the social division between owners of means of production, on the one hand, and propertyless laborers on the other. The capitalist starts with money (M), buys means of production and labor-power (C), and then, when the production process is complete, reappears on the market with commodities to transform back into money (M′). Since both the starting-point and end-point of this process is money (M and M′), i.e., quantitative exchange-value, there would be no sense in the procedure unless there

* However, it is important to note: "The circulation from C-M-C does not simply disappear or become irrelevant with the coming of capitalist production. Indeed, for the great majority of people, the laborers, circulation continues to take the form C-M-C with all that this implies. The worker begins with a commodity, labor power, which at best has a very limited use value for him; he converts his labor power into money; and finally he uses the money to acquire necessaries and conveniences of life. This is C-M-C and the objective is an increase in use value. . . . It is therefore entirely mistaken to picture the worker as dominated by the profit motive or to imagine that he shares the capitalist's urge to appropriate 'ever more and more wealth in the abstract.' "–Paul Sweezy, *Theory of Capitalist Development* (New York: Monthly Review Press, 1962), p. 139.

was a quantitative difference between M and M′, unless the capitalist ended up with *more* quantitative value than when he began. "It is only insofar as the appropriation of ever more and more wealth in the *abstract* becomes the sole motive of his operations that the owner of capital functions socially as a capitalist, that is, as capital personified and endowed with consciousness and a will. *Use-values must therefore never be looked upon as* the real aim of the capitalist; neither must the profit on any single transaction. *The restless never-ending process of profit-making alone is what he aims at*" and must aim at lest other capitals drive his own from the field. Thus, the capitalist "shares with the miser the passion for wealth as wealth. But that which in the miser is mere idiosyncrasy, is, in the capitalist, the effect of the social mechanism of which he is but one of the wheels."*

This set of insights forms the kernel of Marx's analysis of capitalism, provides the basis of his critique of both capitalist exploitation and capitalist allocation, and is, as we shall see, the fundamental theoretical link between his analysis and that of Keynes. These insights constitute, moreover, so far as the economic mechanism of capitalist production is concerned, a thoroughly orthodox (post-Keynesian) view, though its full implications are rarely recognized. Thus, a volume in the series *A Survey of Contemporary Economics* published by the American Economic Association observes:

> [In capitalism] real assets and consumables, in bulk, if not in composition are valued not for themselves but for their monetary equivalent. All things are thought of as exchangeable and saleable, and therefore as convertible into money, the universal solvent. The money measure of goods becomes the *real* expression of their

* *Capital,* vol. 1, 152–3.

> value. Goods are money, and, from the viewpoint of capitalist motivation, it is from this equivalence that they derive their worth. In this view the classical distinction between real and money economics is effectively reversed. To the classicists . . . money was the means by which commodities are procured and services remunerated. Thus money-making is the way we get goods. All this, of course, is as it should be. But from the viewpoint of capitalist motivation, we do not make money to get goods. We make goods in order to get money.*

One consequence of this reversal of the relation between real and money economics, i.e., the transformation of circulation from the form C-M-C to M-C-M′, is that the potential for a disruption of the economic process is greatly increased. Even in simple commodity production the desire to expand wealth in its abstract form as money can conflict with the necessity of maintaining circulation because, as noted earlier, money acts both as a store of value and a medium of circulation. So long as commodity production remains simple, however, there is little likelihood that the kind of deep and pervasive crises experienced in capitalist commodity production would take place. On the one hand, the effects of individual hoarding, which are likely to be gradual anyway, can be offset by an increase in the total money supply; on the other, the fact that the circulation form remains C-M-C means that production is carried on basically for consumption, and consumption is a continuous process. In other words, Say's Law of Markets, which maintains that supply

* Moses Abramovitz, "Economics of Growth" in B. F. Haley (ed.), *A Survey of Contemporary Economics*, vol. 2 (The American Economic Association, 1952).

creates its own demand, may be said to hold true for simple commodity production (as a statement about the *probability* of crisis, however, and not about its possibility).*

The situation is quite different in capitalist commodity production, where the circulation form is M-C-M′, i.e., where the relation between real and money economics is reversed. Here the motive and aim which drives the economic process and causes circulation to be continuous is not consumption but the expansion of money-wealth. If anything should happen to curtail the prospective expansion of the money value of his invested capital, the capitalist would be induced to withdraw his money from industrial circulation, thereby causing a disruption, since his sole reason for putting money into circulation in the first place was to expand its value at the maximum possible rate. There is no other raison d'être of the circulation process in capitalism, no end such as consumption lying outside the process and governing it, which would be continuous.

In capitalist conditions, therefore, the expansion or contraction of production is determined by the money-return to owners of capital instead of being determined by the relation of production to social wants. "The capitalist mode of production comes to a standstill at a point determined by the production and realization of profit, not by the satisfaction of social needs."† In other words, production and consumption appear as mere by-products of the quest for wealth in its abstract form, *money*. The expansion of means of production (stock of capital) becomes an end in itself as the

* Paul Sweezy, *The Theory of Capitalist Development* (New York: Monthly Review Press, 1962).

† *Capital,* vol. 3, cited in Maurice Dobb, *Political Economy and Capitalism* (London: Routledge, Kegan Paul, 1960), pp. 116–17.

result of capital's drive towards its own self-expansion, and the system moves toward production for production's sake. The means of production are no longer mere means to expand the material life basis of society, but society itself appears as a mere means for the expansion of capital.* The very prosperity of capitalism is thus exposed by Marx as a human poverty.

Indeed, the whole critique of *Capital,* which opens with the observation that "the wealth of those societies in which the capitalist mode of production prevails, presents itself as 'an immense accumulation of commodities,' " can be seen as a critique of the capitalist *form* of wealth, of wealth regarded as an accumulation of commodities, an accumulation of capital, of *money* (each a different equivalent form of exchange-value). For, "when the narrow bourgeois form has been peeled away, what is [real] wealth if not the universality of needs, capacities, enjoyments, productive powers, etc., of individuals produced in universal exchange? . . . What, if not the absolute elaboration of his creative dispositions, without any preconditions other than antecedent historical evolution which makes the totality of this evolution . . . an end in itself? What is this, if not a situation where man does not reproduce himself in any determined form, but produces his totality?"†

The critique of the notion that wealth is capital, money, the institutionally grounded and all-pervasive notion of bourgeois society, lies at the heart of Marx's critique and analysis of capitalism, and to its sources he traces all the fundamental

* *Capital,* vol. 3, p. 245.

† Marx, *Pre-Capitalist Economic Formations* (New York: International Publishers, 1964), pp. 84–85.

paradoxes of the system. In the last analysis, it is only because the social production relation is embodied in an external object, money, that the needs of capital and its limitless expansion dominate the needs of human beings, that the act of human creation in the labor process entails the perpetual destruction of the humanity of the producers, that there can be poverty amid plenty, "crises of overproduction" amid unfilled wants, that there can be increasing moral degradation, ignorance, and brutality amid increasing scientific knowledge and material productive power.

The remedy which Marx proposes flows straightforwardly from the analysis: the social relation of individuals, which originates in the social division of labor, must be established directly in the process of production, and not indirectly through a thing, money, in the process of exchange. This can be achieved only through the social ownership of the means of production and the coordination of production with consumption through a social plan. Only then will the social relations between the producers be lucid, intelligible and under their control; only then can society free itself from "a mode of production in which the labourer exists to satisfy the needs of self-expansion of existing values, instead of, on the contrary, material wealth existing to satisfy the needs of development on the part of the labourer."*

iii

In comparing Marx's analysis of the capitalist economic process with Keynes's, the first and most important difference to be noted between them is methodological. For while Marx's analysis is always framed in terms of a historically specific socio-economic system, with concrete institutional

* *Capital,* vol. 1, p. 617.

characteristics, Keynes, like most non-Marxian economists, conceives his subject in ahistorical and unsociological terms, as an economic mechanism determined only by unchanging human psychology and various techniques and institutions which are always "given" and therefore untouched by the analysis.* For Marx, capital conceived as a social relation is considered prior to money in the analysis of capitalist conditions of production, and money is regarded primarily (though not solely) as a form of capital (i.e., as a means of hiring wage labor for production and appropriating the surplus social product).† For Keynes, however, money is an economic institution *per se,* the central determining institution of the modern economic system, which is therefore referred to as a "monetary economy."

Keynes's analogues to Marx's categories of simple and capitalist commodity production are what he calls Real Exchange and Monetary Economics. In a Real Exchange Economy, money is neutral; it is just a device for facilitating transactions in real things, and thus is important only in that it is more efficient than barter. In such an economy, since no one comes to market to sell unless he wants to buy, Say's Law holds and supply may be said to create its own demand. In other words, the assumptions of Real Exchange Economics are "precisely the same as those which will insure that crises do not occur."**

* For a lucid non-Marxian account of this difference, see M. Blaug, *Economic Theory in Retrospect* (Richard D. Irwin, 1962), pp. 245–248.

† *Capital,* vol. 2, part 1, and p. 116f.

** Keynes, contribution to *Festschrift für Arthur Spiethoff* (Munich, 1933), cited in Dudley Dillard, "The Theory of a Monetary Economy," in K. Kurihara (ed.), *Post-Keynesian Economics* (London: Allen & Unwin, 1955).

By contrast, a Monetary Economy is one in which "money plays a part of its own and affects motives and decisions and is, in short, one of the operative factors in the situation, so that the course of events cannot be predicted, either in the long period or in the short, without a knowledge of the behaviour of money between the first state and the last."* Commenting in 1933 on the absence of any satisfactory theoretical explanation of crises, in the canon of neo-classical economics, Keynes had written: "In my opinion the main reason why the Problem of Crises is unsolved, or at any rate why this theory is so unsatisfactory, is to be found in the lack of what might be termed a Monetary Theory of Production."† It was in an attempt to work out such a theory that Keynes wrote *The General Theory.*

The General Theory can be "summed up," according to Keynes's own account, by saying that "given the psychology of the public, the level of output and employment as a whole depends on the amount of investment."** What, then, determines the amount of investment? The answer provided by neo-classical theory,†† whose assumptions were those of Real-Exchange Economics, was "saving." Saving is but deferred consumption, the theory maintained, or investment in the future. Here we recognize Say's Law in perhaps its most crucial form: the supply of saving creates its own investment

* Ibid.

† Ibid. "Accordingly I believe that the next task is to work out in some detail a Monetary Theory of Production, to supplement the Real-Exchange Theories. . . . At any rate that is the task on which I am now occupying myself, in some confidence that I am not wasting my time."

** Keynes, "The General Theory of Employment," *Quarterly Journal of Economics,* February, 1937, reprinted in Harris, *The New Economics* (New York: Knopf, 1947).

†† "Classical" in Keynes's idiosyncratic terminology.

demand. If saving should be too high given available investment outlets, the rate of interest (which, according to the theory, is the "reward for saving") will fall, and consumption, *pari passu,* will rise. The system naturally and harmoniously adjusts the amount of saving/investment to coincide with output at full employment levels.

Such a theory was, of course, at violent odds with the obvious facts of capitalist development, and yet–it is salutary to remember–was academic orthodoxy for nearly half a century, while Marxian and non-Marxian economists (like J. A. Hobson) who rightly rejected its assumptions were contemptuously dismissed and relegated to the "underworld" of economic theory.* (The ideological overtones of this theory, moreover–particularly the justification of capitalist profit–are still very much in evidence in current textbooks and even current analysis.)†

Once it is recognized, however, that saving and investment in capitalist society are principally performed by capitalists and capitalist corporations, then the fallacy of the neoclassical argument immediately appears. This fallacy lies in the assumption that the principal motivation of society's effective economic agents is consumption, hence that consumption deferred today (saving) necessarily entails a decision to consume tomorrow, i.e., to invest. Put in other terms, it is the

* Both Hobson and Marx rejected Say's Law from the outset. Marx wrote: "Nothing could be more childish than the dogma, that because every sale is a purchase, and every purchase a sale, therefore the circulation of commidities necessarily implies an equilibrium of sales and purchases." For their rectitude and foresight, both were treated as "beneath the notice of a scientific writer" (Edgeworth) by academic orthodoxy.

† Cf. Joan Robinson, *Collected Economic Papers* III (Cambridge: Basil Blackwell, 1965), for critiques of various examples of reconstructed neoclassical doctrine.

fallacy of assuming that the increased desire to hold "wealth"–exchange value–is much the same thing as the increased desire to hold investments in real capital assets, i.e., to increase the production of use-values. Keynes's breakthrough from the vantage of orthodox economics came from seeing through the mystification that attributes to capitalist-investors the desire to increase use-values as such, rather than to increase the quantitative value of their capital:

> The absurd, though almost universal, idea that an act of individual saving is just as good for effective demand as an act of individual consumption, has been fostered by the fallacy, much more specious than the conclusion derived from it, that an increased desire to hold wealth, being much the same thing as an increased desire to hold investments, must, by increasing the demand for investments, provide a stimulus to their production; so that current investment is promoted by individual saving to the same extent as present consumption is diminished.
>
> It is of this fallacy that it is most difficult to disabuse men's minds. *It comes from believing that the owner of wealth desires a capital-asset as such, whereas what he really desires is its prospective yield [i.e., profit].* *

* Keynes, of course, did not distinguish between class patterns of economic behavior and this remains the primary deficiency in Keynesian analysis. Whereas Keynes's orthodox predecessors ascribed a consumption motivation to capitalist economic behavior, he attributes a capitalist motivation to the economic behavior of non-capital-owning classes. Since it is the economic activity of capitalists which is in fact determinant for the phenomena in which he was interested–changes in the level of output and employment–his confusion does not represent the kind of obstacle to analysis that the other confusion does.

From this straightforward observation–which, it may be noted, is built into the Marxian analytic structure (though it remained undeveloped by Marx*)–Keynes's General Theory flows. For if the primary interest of capital owners is not in consumption but in the expansion of the quantitative value of their wealth, i.e., in its prospective monetary yield, then the act of saving does not imply a decision to increase means of production, hence output and employment (and future consumption). For if the investment does not offer an attractive prospective yield, "there is always an alternative to the ownership of real capital-assets, namely the ownership of money and debts." When capitalists find it profitable to hold their wealth in its money form, that is, to withdraw it from industrial circulation, a crisis ensues.† Thus, "unemployment develops . . . because people [capitalists] want the moon–men cannot be employed when the object of desire [money] is something which cannot be readily choked off."**

At the heart of Keynes's theory then is precisely that disjunction between use-value and exchange-value that is the pivot of the Marxian analysis: the recognition that the driving force of the system, the source of its irrationalities, is the

* Marx's notes, collected as volumes 2 and 3 of *Capital*, actually provide the elements of a theory of effective demand (where neoclassical economics denied the very existence of the problem by appealing to Say's Law), but it is not developed there, and the Keynesian analysis thus constitutes an important addition to the theory of capitalist development. On the translation of Marxian categories into Keynesian aggregates, *see* S. Tsuru, appendix to Sweezy, *The Theory of Capitalist Development*, op. cit.

† The crisis is caused not by the quantity of money hoarded, but by the fact that the rate of profit falls below the rate of interest, which chokes off investment.

** *The General Theory*, p. 235.

quest for wealth in its abstract money form. In Professor Abramovitz's above-quoted formulation, "we do not make money to get goods. We make goods in order to get money." Or, as Marx observed: "The process of production appears merely as an unavoidable intermediary link [in the circulation process], as a necessary evil for the sake of money-making." To which Engels adds in a parenthesis with a distinctive Keynesian flavor: "All nations with a capitalist mode of production are therefore seized periodically by a feverish attempt to make money without the intervention of the process of production."*

iv

The parallels between Marxian and Keynesian analysis extend from these basic insights to common conclusions about the inherent cyclical tendencies of the economic system and its long-term secular trends.

The whole question of a theory of crises is a complicated one, and where Marx is concerned the complications are that much greater as a result of the unfinished state of the notes he has left. Nonetheless, one strand of his theorizing on the subject provides a particularly clear illustration of the links between his analysis and Keynes's. Here, Marx sees the conditions of *creating* surplus value as being directly contrary to the conditions of its *realization.*

As buyers of commodities, the workers are important for the market in which the capitalist is to realize his profit. But in order to maximize that profit, the capitalist seeks to depress the value of their commodity–labor power–to its lowest price. In short, since the capitalist buys labor power to make goods to make money, he tries to reduce his labor cost

* *Capital,* vol. 2, p. 56.

(and to raise prices) as much as possible. On the other hand, the money demand for the goods produced must come primarily from the same wages-bill, i.e., from what he has paid to labor. Of course demand expenditure is also forthcoming from capitalists investing in more means of production. But ultimately production remains production for consumption, and the profitability of such investment is determined, in the end, by the potential money demand for the consumption goods which will eventually be produced. The result is a chronic tendency to underconsumption in capitalist society, rooted in the self-contradictory aim of capitalists to expand their capital by developing the forces of production without limit, while at the same time restricting the *relative* consuming power of the population.

While Keynes does not focus on the relations of production as such, but deals in aggregates, his analysis lends powerful support to this thesis. In Keynes's analysis, the maldistribution of incomes arising from property results in a relatively low consumption schedule and relatively high savings, which must find an outlet in investment in yet more productive capacity if output and employment are to be maintained. At this point, Keynes adds an important dimension to the analysis by considering the tendency of the accumulation of capital goods to depress the profitability of producing still more capital goods, a tendency which increases the instability of the economy the richer it becomes in productive capacity, and which drives the system towards a "day of judgment" as the rate of profit declines towards zero.

> Each time we secure today's equilibrium by increased investment we are aggravating the difficulty of equilibrium tomorrow. . . .
>
> It is a curious thing, worthy of mention, that the popular mind seems only to be aware of this ultimate

> perplexity where *public* investment is concerned, as in the case of road-building and house-building and the like. It is commonly urged as an objection to schemes for raising employment by investment under the auspices of public authority that it is laying up trouble for the future. "What will you do," it is asked, "when you have built all the houses and roads and town halls and electric grids and water supplies and so forth which the stationary population of the future can be expected to require?" But it is not so easily understood that the same difficulty applies to private investment and to industrial expansion; particularly to the latter, since it is much easier to see an early satiation of the demand for new factories and plants which absorb individually but little money, than of the demand for dwelling houses. . . . every weakening in the propensity to consume regarded as a permanent habit must weaken the demand for capital as well as the demand for consumption.*

The obstacle to a clear understanding of the "threat" of saturated investment outlets, according to Keynes, is "an inadequate appreciation of the fact that capital is not a self-subsistent entity existing apart from consumption."† Here, although Keynes does not recognize the fact, theory merely reflects the existing conditions of production in capitalist society. For private ownership of the means of production, and private appropriation of the social product, in fact, di-

* *The General Theory,* pp. 105–6.

† The appeal to technical innovations to provide a way out of the impasse runs into the practical objections of the Kuznets data on net capital formation in the U.S. during the current technological revolution, and the theoretical objections of Sweezy, Steindl, Sylos-Labini and others.

vorces capital accumulation from the social conditions of its realization, as means and end of a single process, and in this sense actually makes of it "a self-subsistent entity existing apart from consumption." That is, capital accumulation, from the vantage of those whose decisions activate the process, is the *private* accumulation of capital, i.e., of money-value: the immediate incentive to accumulate, to engage the wheels of production, is not the existence of unmet consumption needs, but the prospect of expanding the value of capital.*

In other words, while capital accumulation as a *social* economic process is a means for creating *utilities,* use-values, i.e., for meeting consumption needs, as a *private* activity of entrepreneurs it is merely a means for expanding income, i.e., for creating quantitative exchange values. Hence it is that in capitalist conditions, the accumulation of capital, periodically and in the long run, appears paradoxically as an *obstacle* to accumulation; in Keynesian terms, "abundance of capital interferes with the abundance of output, old wealth is a barrier to the production of new wealth,"† or, as Marx put it, the *real barrier* of capitalist production is *capital itself.*"**

* This, of course, explains on the one hand why the production of automobiles and luxury items for the rich takes precedence over the production of schools and necessities for the poor, and on the other, why no production takes place in a depression when needs are high but the prospects for capital expansion are low. It also explains why the advent of "affluence" is regarded as a menace to growth.

† Dillard, "The Theory of a Monetary Economy," *op. cit.,* p. 23.

** *Capital,* vol. 3, p. 245.

V

What then of Keynes's concept of a "monetary economy" and its relation to capitalism? To answer this crucial question, it is necessary to treat Keynes's analysis of short-run changes in the level of output in closer detail.

In Keynes's analysis, the key decision to invest is based on the monetary yield that an investment project is expected to have over its lifetime (Keynes called this the *marginal efficiency of capital**), and the rate of interest at which money may be borrowed to finance the project. If the rate of interest (which Keynes, for illustrative purposes, once referred to as the *marginal efficiency of money*†) exceeds, or is expected to exceed, the prospective yield of investment, then investment will not take place and, other things being equal, there will be a corresponding drop in output and employment.

Now the marginal efficiency of capital, based as it is on expectations about the future of a market that is at best uncertain, is highly volatile; moreover, because the production of capital tends to raise its supply price (as pressure on the capital-goods-producing industries increases), and because the increase of capital itself depresses its rate of return, the marginal efficiency of capital has a long-term tendency to fall, and hence to fall below the rate of interest, thereby halting investment.

In the neoclassical theory, such a situation would never materialize under normal conditions. Arguing from the assumptions of Real Exchange Economics (including the full

* For our purposes it is equivalent to the *expected* rate of profit.

† Keynes, "The Theory of the Rate of Interest" in *Lessons of Monetary Experience, Essays in Honor of Irving Fisher* (New York, 1937), cited in Dillard.

employment of resources), neoclassical theory regarded interest as a reward for saving, that is, for abstaining from present consumption. In this view, a fall in the rate of profit, indicating a declining demand for investment, would be accompanied by a corresponding fall in the rate of interest (because of the decreased demand for savings) and hence an increase in consumption demand, which would take up the slack and maintain output at full employment levels. Thus, according to neoclassical orthodoxy, the rate of interest (the marginal efficiency of money) adapts passively to the marginal efficiency of other assets (which is to say that money is *neutral)* and does so in such a way as to regulate the balance of savings to maintain the level of output and employment.

Keynes, like Marx, rejects the notion that interest is a reward for saving and regards it rather as payment for the use of money, and more specifically, as a premium to induce money-holders *not* to hoard money; the rate of interest is then determined not by the supply and demand of savings and investment, but by the demand for *money* and the supply of money in circulation. The rate of interest is therefore *not* free to fall (since money cannot be produced by private enterprise) and hence does not passively adapt to the marginal efficiency of other assets, but rather "the marginal efficiency of other assets falls into line with the rate of interest."* In Keynes's theory, therefore, money "in its role as a store of wealth stands as a barrier to full production." Or more provocatively: "unemployment is caused by money."†

* Keynes, "The Theory of the Rate of Interest in *Essays in Honor of Irving Fisher,* p. 147.

† Dillard, op. cit. ". . . in the absence of money . . . the rates of interest would only reach equilibrium when there is full employment." *The General Theory,* p. 235.

This view of the strategic importance of money, via the rate of interest, in determining the level of investment, immediately raises the question, as Keynes put it, of "why anyone outside a lunatic asylum [should] wish to use money as a store of wealth?" In other words, why should it require such a high interest premium to induce people to lend money? "For it is a recognized characteristic of money as a store of wealth that it is barren; whereas practically every other form of storing wealth yields some interest or profit."*

Keynes's answer, his explanation of the rationality behind the desire to hold money, is the existence of "uncertainty" regarding the future: "The importance of money essentially flows from its being a link between the present and the future."† The possession of money "lulls . . . disquietude" about the future. The more uncertain the future state of the market (hence the value of capital assets and debts), the greater the propensity to hold wealth as money, the higher the premium required to induce people not to hoard it, consequently the lower the rate of return over cost on investments (since higher interest rates mean a higher supply price of capital), the greater the tendency of current investment to diminish and hence the lower the general level of employment and output. Such, in brief, is Keynes's explanation for fluctuation in a "monetary economy," that is, an economy in which money plays a *substantive* role, in which it is *not* neutral.

In framing his analysis so that it appears to ascribe to a technical institution–money–the evils of a system in which the prosperity of the entire society depends on the uncertain expectations of a small but powerful class for maximizing its wealth, Keynes betrays the ideological bias of his outlook.

* "The General Theory of Employment," *Quarterly Journal of Economics,* 1937, *op. cit.*

† *The General Theory,* p. 293.

Here the analysis turns away from the critique of capitalism as such and trains its fire on the financial and *rentier* aspects of the system. One expression of this approach, which also reveals its weakness in terms of Keynes's own analysis, can be seen in his praise of the monetary reformer Silvio Gesell as having more to teach the future than Marx.* Gesell propounded a stamped money scheme which would increase the carrying costs of money relative to its liquidity premium and thus bring down the rate of interest. But as Keynes elsewhere shrewdly observed: "If currency notes were to be deprived of their liquidity premium by the stamping system, a long series of substitutes would step into their shoes—bank-money, debts at call, foreign money, jewelry and the precious metals generally and so forth."† Indeed, "so long as there exists any durable asset, it is capable of possessing monetary attributes, and, therefore, of giving rise to the characteristic problems of a monetary economy."**

If this is the case, however, then the concept of a "monetary economy" defined as an economy in which there is an asset whose "liquidity premium is always in excess of the carrying costs"†† does not take us very far. Elsewhere, however, Keynes provided another definition, which offers a much more promising basis on which to build an analysis. "A monetary economy," he wrote, ". . . is essentially one in which changing views about the future are capable of influencing the quantity of employment [hence the level of income] and not merely its direction." For, if our knowledge of the future was calculable and not subject to sudden changes, "it might be justifiable to assume that the liquidity-preference curve was both stable and very inelastic." If such

* *The General Theory*, p. 355.
† Ibid., p. 358.
** Ibid., p. 294.
†† *The General Theory*, p. 239.

were the case "we might reasonably suppose that the whole of available resources would normally be employed."*

To make the implications of this approach clear, it is only necessary to consider the difference between debts and money as means of payment. Debts can only take the place of money as a means of payment in times of prosperity when the state of confidence is strong and the sale of commodities at profitable prices is assured. For it is in the commodity market that income will be earned to redeem the debts and make them good. So long as the commodity market is uncertain, which is to say so long as social production is not socially planned to balance aggregate supply and demand, periodic ruptures of industrial circulation and failures of confidence are inevitable. Hence cash will normally be preferred to debts and will earn an interest-premium. In such circumstances, the antagonistic relation between the rate of interest and industrial profit, between money and production, must necessarily appear.†

Money seems to lie at the root of the problem because money—as the independent form of exchange value—expresses the contradiction of private production in an exchange economy: that men's social relation in the division of labor is embodied in a thing, money, and not in the real relation of the producers through their collective control over the aggregate supply of social goods. That it is not money, as such, that causes the difficulties in Keynes's "monetary

* "The General Theory of Employment," *Quarterly Journal of Economics,* 1937, op. cit.

† Cf. Fan-Hung, "Keynes and Marx on the Theory of Capital Accumulation, Money and Interest," *Review of Economic Studies,* October 1939, reprinted in D. Horowitz, ed., *Marx and Modern Economics* (New York: Monthly Review Press, 1968).

economy," but money as *private property,* is evident the moment a socialist economy in which there are no privately owned means of production is brought under consideration. In such a system, the ownership of money would not be an alternative to ownership of means of production, and therefore, the desire to hold money assets could not provide a basis for withholding investment in real capital assets, thereby preventing the use of capital goods in production.*

We are now in a position to comprehend the identity between Keynes's monetary economy and Marx's capitalist one. For it is not money as such with which Keynes is concerned, but money as *capital,* as private property, as command over labor-power and hence as the motive and aim of social production. Keynes's analysis is an exploration of the consequences which flow from the fact that the social relation of production is embodied in a thing–money, which is itself a commodity, and therefore an object of appropriation by private individuals. The difference between the two conceptions is that Keynes begins his analysis with the fetishized thing, money, whereas Marx begins with the particular social organization of production that gives rise to this fetishism.

vi

Although, for reasons already indicated, Keynes's analysis does not explicitly recognize the strategic importance of capitalist property relations–the private control of social production–in giving rise to the characteristic features of a "monetary economy," his proposed remedies go significantly beyond mere monetary measures and do in fact constitute such a recognition. This appears, particularly, in Keynes's

* Dillard, *op. cit.*, p. 19.

declaration in favor of "a somewhat comprehensive socialization of investment":

> For my part I am now somewhat sceptical of the success of a merely monetary policy directed towards influencing the rate of interest. I expect to see the State, which is in a position to calculate the marginal efficiency of capital-goods on long views and on the basis of the general social advantage, taking an ever greater responsibility for directly organizing investment. . . .*

Keynes, however, never developed his critique to its proper conclusion. Although he is quite clear in his analysis that capital accumulation, even from the entrepreneurial point of view, is basically money accumulation, as Professor Dillard notes, "very little stress is placed on money as the objective to be desired from the *production* of real wealth as distinguished from money as an alternative form in which to hold wealth."† Whereas Keynes's concentration on the financial sphere led him to overstress the influence of the rate of interest,** his neglect of this aspect of the monetary motive of capitalist production led to fundamental ambiguities in his proposal for a comprehensive "socialization of investment." For Keynes did not mean by this an equally comprehensive

* *The General Theory,* p. 164.

† Dillard, *op. cit.,* p. 22.

** ". . . the rate of interest, though its movements tell in the right direction, is too weak an influence adequately to regulate the level of investment. . . . In the modern academic view, therefore, it seems that the importance of the rate of interest was very much exaggerated in the traditional theory, and that Marx was after all not much at fault in neglecting it altogether." Joan Robinson, *An Essay on Marxian Economics,* p. 70.

socialization of the means of production. Presumably, in Keynes's plan, the level of investment would be determined by the state, while the allocation, or at least the management of the investment, would be left to private decision. But—leaving aside the political problems of planning while the means of production are still in private hands—such a program would seem to assume the neutrality of money in what Keynes called the sphere of industrial (as opposed to financial) circulation, since the basis for increasing the total stock of capital assets would no longer be the ability to sell at a profit.

Professor Dillard has pointed out this potential inconsistency in Keynes's analysis and suggested the lines along which a complete and consistent Keynesian theory of a monetary economy would be drawn. Essentially this would involve extending the non-neutrality of money to the industrial sphere, thereby carrying out Keynes's own suggestion that money be related directly to the motives and decisions which determine employment and production.* "If the expectation of being able to convert real goods into money at a profit is the significant motivation of entrepreneurs in hiring labor," writes Professor Dillard, "it is pure euphemism to say that consumption is the ultimate purpose of production. A Monetary Theory of Production would stress pecuniary motivation."

The germ of such a theory is, of course, already present in Keynes's book,† and the suggestions made by Professor Dillard for developing it reveal further the striking parallel between Marx's and Keynes's understanding of the system.

* Keynes made this suggestion in the *Spiethoff* essay. Dillard, p. 27.

† E.g., in the treatment of effective demand: "effective demand corresponds to the [money] income, the expectation of which has set production moving." *The General Theory*, p. 299.

Since the individual producer who employs labor realizes his aim only when his output is sold for money on favorable terms, there is, observes Professor Dillard, "a clear contradiction between the meaning of money and goods in their respective roles as real and artificial wealth." For since "values are realized for the individual firm only if and when the conversion of goods to money occurs," it is evident that " 'real goods' appear to the individual producer as an *artificial* form of wealth until they are converted into money, which appears as real wealth to the individual producer." This, as we have noted before, reverses the role of money and goods in traditional economic theory. Whereas the mercantilists held that money was wealth, classical and post-classical economics have held that "*goods* are real wealth while money is a superficial embodiment of real wealth." Keynes instinctively sympathized with the mercantilists, because of his keen insight into the modus operandi of capitalism, but, as Professor Dillard notes, "he failed to reiterate or reintroduce this aspect of mercantilist thought."* Marx, on the other hand, did recognize the "truth" in mercantilist theory:

> The unceasing war of modern economists against the monetary and mercantilist system is mostly due to the fact that this system blabs out in brutally naive fashion, the secret of bourgeois production, viz., its subjection to the domination of exchange value. Ricardo, though wrong in the application he makes of it, remarks somewhere that even in times of famine, grain is imported not because the nation is starving, but because the grain dealer is making money. In its criticism of the monetary and mercantile system, political economy, by attacking

* Dillard, p. 28.

> that system as a mere illusion and as a false theory, fails to recognize in it the barbaric form of its own fundamental principles.*

Continuing his analysis of the relation of real to artificial wealth under what he calls "production on private account," Professor Dillard writes: "The unreal wealth (stocks of goods) of individual firms gains social recognition, only when it is sold, that is, converted into the unreal wealth of society (money). Real social wealth (stocks of goods) will be produced by entrepreneurs only if there is the expectation of transforming them into unreal social wealth (money). In brief, what is 'real' to society is 'unreal' to the individual producer; and what is 'unreal' to society is 'real' to the individual producer."

As Keynes notes in his *Treatise on Money*, the economic system abhors a stock of liquid goods, i.e., real wealth, because the carrying costs of stocks of goods stored for later sale "soon eat away . . . the (normal) value of the goods." (Dillard) Thus "every business transaction involves an embryo crisis which is averted if 'real' goods are converted into money." However, with embryo crises existing everywhere, with firms dependent on sensitive credit relations, a cumulative wave of liquidation may be set off, "motivated by the desire to hold the socially recognized form of wealth, that is, money."†

In crises, "the contradiction between individual and social forms of wealth" is more obvious than in prosperity. The desire to liquidate stocks becomes intense, and the inability to convert goods into money sets up a chain reaction punc-

* *A Contribution to the Critique of Political Economy*, p. 217; *Capital*, vol. 1, pp. 154–55.

† Dillard, *op. cit.*, p. 29.

turing the credit cycle and bringing the economy "tumbling down." Thus, Professor Dillard concludes, "the paradoxical position of money as the universally recognized form of private wealth which is not really wealth at all from the social point of view lies, in undeveloped form, at the heart of Keynes's Theory of a Monetary Economy."

To develop the thesis in a Marxist direction, it is only necessary to stress that the origin of these paradoxes is to be found in the specific relations of *capitalist* production. It is in capitalism that money is the socially recognized form of wealth (exchange value), the *private* pursuit of which governs the production of real wealth (use values). Money is the universal object of productive activity because the social relations of production are not embodied in a social plan, in the real connection of the social producers as self-conscious organizers of social production, but in a thing–exchange value–which can be appropriated and accumulated by private persons, specifically, by private owners of capital.

vii

Having established the congruities between the economic analyses of Marx and Keynes, it is important to develop a sense of the differences in their sociological and historical perspectives, in their understanding of the *political economy* of capitalism, as opposed to the relatively simpler issues of its economics.* These differences, moreover, are by no means irrelevant to their respective analyses of the evolution of the economic system itself.† For once the neoclassical concep-

* *See* note to p. 108.

† For important discussions of these differences see S. Tsuru, "Keynes vs. Marx: The Methodology of Aggregates," in Horowitz, ed., *Marx and Modern Economics,* and L. R. Klein, "Theories of Effective Demand and Employment" in *Readings in Economic Analysis,* vol. 2, 1950.

tion of a self-adjusting economic process is abandoned, together with the static viewpoint—and these are the main implications of the "Keynesian revolution"—the determinant forces in the development of the system inevitably become *sociological* in character.*

It is precisely in the realm of the sociological, however, that the differences between the two perspectives appear most sharply, and the relative strengths of the Marxian analysis are most apparent.

The sociological weakness inherent in Keynes's approach is exemplified in his attribution of the features of a "monetary economy" to the uncertainty of human affairs and the consequent necessity of lulling "disquietude" about the future. For these are factors which are universal in human society, and therefore ahistorical and socially unspecific. It has already been pointed out that Keynes was inconsistent in this approach, and that in his plea for a comprehensive socialization of investment there is, in fact, an explicit recognition that altering the social institutional arrangement would eliminate the uncertainty at the source of the system's malaise. But the framework of Keynes's analysis is firmly cast in unsociological terms, and the very ambiguity and inconclusiveness of his programmatic recommendations reflects this basic disposition of his outlook.

If the phenomena at the root of society's economic ills are, as Keynes in the main presents them, universal (mainly psychological) characteristics of human affairs, it is possible to conceive a solution that would not necessitate a social revolution. Such a revolution would be required only if it were necessary to alter power relationships which are institutionalized in the social order and secured by its moral, ideo-

* Cf. Eric Roll, "The Decline of Liberal Economics," *The Modern Quarterly*, January 1938.

logical and legal frameworks. If the economic problem is primarily psychological, or even logical, then all that is necessary is to analyze the problem and suggest a remedy and then move to have the analysis and remedy accepted by the political leaders in command of the state. This was the path Keynes took. Indeed, few have expressed its root assumption more provocatively than he. In the preface to *Essays in Persuasion* he described his "central thesis throughout" as being the profound conviction that the Economic Problem, "the problem of want and poverty and the economic struggle between classes and nations, is nothing but a frightful muddle, a transitory and an *unnecessary* muddle." And at the end of *The General Theory* he wrote, in a favorite passage of politician-professors, "soon or late, it is ideas, not vested interests, which are dangerous for good or evil."

The history of Keynes's own analysis in the three decades since these words were written, however, provides an extraordinary refutation of the proposition put forward and of the sociological assumptions which underlie it. For in the interim the ideas of *The General Theory* have passed from the status of economic heresy to a position of unchallengeable orthodoxy throughout the capitalist world. But the "Keynesian" policies of the various governments, left and right, labor and conservative, that have administered the capitalist states of the postwar period, bear little resemblance to Keynes's proposals for a solution to the Economic Problem.*

According to *The General Theory,* investment determines the general level of output and employment for the economy as a whole, while the decision to invest is based on the prospective returns to private capital. If the accumulation of

* Compare for example Keynes's remarks on p. 339 with the fiscal and monetary policies of successive "Keynesian" British governments in the postwar period.

capital makes capital less scarce (as Keynes maintained) and thereby lowers its return below the rate of interest, then investment will grind to a halt, causing a corresponding drop in the level of economic activity. In such circumstances "even a diversion of the desire to hold wealth [in its money-form] towards [real capital] assets, which will in fact yield no economic fruits whatever, will increase economic well-being."* In other words, if *useful* investment outlets become saturated (relative to existing effective demand, which depends in turn on the existing distribution of income) so that investment in real capital assets ceases to earn a return greater than the current rate of interest, employment and output can only be maintained if capital owners can be induced to invest in *wasteful* (but profitable) capital projects, and in particular, military construction, armaments and the like. " 'To dig holes in the ground,' paid for out of savings," wrote Keynes, "will increase, not only employment, but the real national dividend of useful goods and services."†

Keynes believed that once this analysis had been accepted, the "community" would not tolerate such a system any longer: "It is not reasonable," he wrote, "that a sensible community should be content to remain dependent on such fortuitous and often wasteful mitigations when once we understand the influences upon which effective demand depends."

The solution urged by Keynes was that the power of the state be used to depress savings and to control and stimulate investment, until capital was no longer scarce and owners of capital no longer able to appropriate an institutional rent. Keynes called this prospect the *euthanasia of the rentier*, and

* *General Theory*, p. 200.

† I.e., via the multiplier, initially the latter more than the former. Cf. *The General Theory*, p. 325.

expected it to do away with the most "objectionable" features of capitalism, which he thought could be accomplished within two generations. Nor was Keynes's prescription based merely on utopian longings for an ideal social arrangement. Given his analysis, it represented one of two practical and mutually exclusive alternatives, each implying a far-ranging set of consequences for the evolution of capitalist society. As the eminent Oxford economist J. R. Hicks pointed out in a contemporary review of *The General Theory,* if we accept Keynes's analysis, then "either we must accept something like the policy he advocates, of stimulating investment and repressing saving by changes in social organization; or our once benevolent science becomes a paean to destruction, whose heroes are earthquake, war, and conflagration, Attila and Genghis Khan, Great Raisers of the Marginal Efficiency of Capital and Creators of Employment."

This second alternative certainly describes, with discomforting accuracy, the direction taken during the last thirty years in the capitalist world. The sensible leaders of these communities have understood (thanks to Keynes) the factors on which effective demand depends, and have, despite Keynes's warnings, maintained an irrational system principally reliant on wasteful, not to mention deadly, mitigations of the declining marginal efficiency of capital. Without exception they have found in military enterprise the Great Raiser of the Marginal Efficiency of Capital, as Hicks foreshadowed. Thus the "muddles" Keynes fought against have been abandoned, his picture of the system has been accepted, but the system has not been changed, and the Economic Problem remains, indeed in more deadly form than before.

While Keynesians are left with only Original Sin or Human Folly to account for this pass in the evolution of the capitalist system, Marxians have, within the framework of their analysis, a basis for understanding what has happened. Unlike Keynes, Marx, as we have seen, anchored his analysis in the institutional framework historically specific to the capitalist system and in particular in the basic division of society's productive sector into laborers without means of subsistence and property owners sharing a class monopoly over the means of production. It is only this division which gives capitalists the effective power to advance money to wage workers for the purpose of appropriating the surplus part of their product (or in Keynes's terminology, to exploit the scarcity value of capital). In other words, it is only this basic relationship that bestows on money the power to expand itself as capital in the process of production and thus to give rise to all the features of a "monetary economy."

But this power relationship between capitalists and non-capital-owning classes does not and cannot end in the wage contract. It must be sustained by the ideological and legal framework of society and the apparatus of legal violence, in a word by the very state upon which Keynes's remedy depends. Here we find an explanation for the persistence of the system that Keynes exposed as being irrational from a social point of view. For to enact Keynes's program would mean to eliminate the income source of the most powerful social class, i.e., to liquidate its existence *as* a class. What may seem sensible, therefore, from a social point of view, does not seem at all sensible to owners of capital, and they naturally use every means at their disposal to thwart any programs which threaten their monopoly position and its privileges.

Their success in maintaining the ideological, legal and social structure which serves them, despite and even because of the expanded economic role of the "democratic" state, is attested by the constancy of the distribution of income, the growth of the industries of destruction and the parallel containment of welfare programs, the lack of any steps towards real (as opposed to merely "indicative") investment planning, and not least, by the continuing eclipse of Marx, whose basic model and insights could not have expected more conclusive if unwanted confirmation.

Part 3

Marx's Approach to the Political Economy of Capitalism

A proper understanding of Marxian political economy only begins with the recognition that the famous "Marxian" laws of capitalist development—the absolute general law of capitalist accumulation (the so-called "doctrine of increasing misery"), the law of the tendency of the rate of profit to fall, and the law of the increasing centralization of capitals—were for Marx the *data* and not the result of his analysis.[1] In light of all the Marx critiques and Marx defenses which have been built on the identification of Marxian political economy with these laws, such a statement at first seems incomprehensible. Far from being incomprehensible, however, it is readily established by reference to the appropriate texts and, this done, is easily seen to be essential for understanding what exactly a specifically *Marxian* political economy *is*.

1. Cf. R. L. Meek, "Karl Marx's Economic Method" in David Horowitz, ed., *Marx and Modern Economics* (New York: Monthly Review Press, 1968).

Let us consider, for example, the "absolute general law of capitalist accumulation," which holds that "the worker becomes all the poorer the more wealth he produces," that he "becomes an ever cheaper commodity the more commodities he creates," that with the increasing value of the world of things there occurs, in direct proportion, the devaluation of the world of men.

These particular phrases describing the law do not appear in *Capital* (though the relevant equivalents can be found there). They appear in the *Economic and Philosophical Manuscripts of 1844,* that is, in a text written when Marx was in his twenties, at the very beginning of his investigations.[2] Nor do these propositions represent, as some of the more superficial Marx-critics suggest, a mere projection of Marx's metaphysical preconceptions onto socio-economic reality. The passage just cited is prefaced with the remark, "We proceed from an *actual* economic fact" (emphasis in original)—and the manuscripts in which the passage itself appears are filled with long passages copied verbatim out of the standard texts on political economy of Marx's day:

"We have proceeded from the premises of [orthodox] political economy," writes Marx at the beginning of this particular manuscript. "We have accepted its language and its laws." On this basis, that is, "on the basis of [orthodox] political economy itself,"

> *in its own words,* we have shown that the worker sinks to the level of a commodity and becomes indeed the most wretched of commodities; that the wretchedness of the worker is in inverse proportion to the power and

2. Karl Marx, *Economic and Philosophic Manuscripts of 1844* (Moscow: Foreign Languages Publishing House, 1961), p. 69. The citation is from the manuscript titled "Estranged Labour" by the editor.

> magnitude of his production; that the necessary result of competition is the accumulation of capital in a few hands, and thus the restoration of monopoly in a more terrible form; that finally the distinction between capitalist and land-rentier, like that between the tiller of the soil and the factory-worker, disappears and that the whole of society must fall apart into two classes—the property owners and the propertyless workers.

In other words, according to Marx—the "young" Marx of 1844—the very laws which are usually identified with Marxian political economy as such, the laws of general accumulation and increasing centralization, are in fact contained and formulated in the non-Marxian, indeed pre-Marxian, political economy of the period.[3]

It is similarly easy to show that the other so-called Marxian laws are wholly orthodox in terms of contemporary political economy and can be found in any number of orthodox writings of the time. Not only, for example, did Adam Smith develop a theory of the falling rate of profit[4] but, in Marx's words, "this law [of the falling rate of profit] has been stated in a more or less accurate manner by Mr. Barton, Ricardo, Sismondi, Professor Richard Jones, Professor Ramsay, Cherbuliez, and others."[5]

Now it is certainly the case that when Marx applied himself to the body of orthodox economic theory, he refined and developed it. It is also true, consequently, that there are

3. The law of increasing centralization also appears in Engels's 1843 essay "Outcomes of a Critique of Political Economy" and in J. S. Mills's *Principles of Political Economy* (1848).

4. Marx, *Economic and Philosophic Manuscripts,* p. 41.

5. Karl Marx, *Value, Price and Profit* (New York and London: International Publishers, 1935), pp. 60–61.

important differences between the statement of these laws in Marx's early works and in the finished and unfinished volumes of *Capital.* But to take these formal refinements and revisions of essentially orthodox economic laws for the substance of Marxian political economy is surely unjustified and, at the very least, to lose sight of what is central and significant in Marxian theory.

There is, in any case, no need to speculate on the matter, for Marx tells us explicitly where, in his view, the inadequacy of orthodox economic science lies, and in what sense a new, or "Marxian," conception of the subject is required. Moreover, he tells us this also in the *Economic and Philosophic Manuscripts,* that is, at the point at which he was first formulating his general methodological outlook:

"Political economy proceeds from the fact of private property, but it does not explain it to us. It expresses in general, abstract formulae the *material* process through which private property actually passes, and these formulae it takes for *laws.*" Where political economy fails is that *"it does not comprehend these laws–i.e., it does not demonstrate how they arise from the very nature of private property."*[6]

It is a relatively straightforward matter to show that this critique of orthodox or "bourgeois" political economy remained consistent from the beginning to the end of Marx's analytic career. Thus, in Marx's first economic work, a polemic against Proudhon,[7] the basis of his critique was that "[Proudhon] has not perceived that economic categories are only abstract expressions of . . . actual relations and only remain true while these relations exist. He therefore falls into the error of the bourgeois economists, who regard these economic categories as eternal and not as *historical* laws *which*

6. Op. cit., p. 67 (emphasis added).

7. *The Poverty of Philosophy* (Chicago: Charles H. Kerr & Co., n.d.).

are only laws for a particular historical development . . ."[8] (emphasis added).

Twenty years later, in an obituary on Proudhon, Marx recalled with approval his early assessment of Proudhon's approach: "Instead of regarding the economic categories as theoretical expressions of the *historical* relations of production," he wrote, "[Proudhon's] imagination transforms them into 'eternal ideas,' existing before any reality, and in this manner he arrives, in a roundabout way, at the point from which he started, the point of view of bourgeois economy."[9]

It is not really necessary, however, to comb through scattered texts in order to arrive at a clear formulation of Marx's methodological orientation, his conception of a political economy different from, but integrally related to, the orthodox or *bourgeois* political economy of his day. For among his posthumous papers was found a sketch, written in 1857, that was to have served as a general methodological introduction to his main work, of which the four volumes of *Capital* were but one constituent part, and which was never realized in the form originally planned.[10] The purpose of the general introduction was to justify and explicate Marx's methodological approach to political economy in the form of a critique of

8. Letter to Annenkov, Marx and Engels, *Selected Correspondence* (Moscow: Foreign Languages Publishing House, n.d.), p. 45. Cf. R. L. Meek, *Studies in the Labour Theory of Value* (London: Lawrence & Wishart, 1956): "The central theme of *The Poverty of Philosophy* is that the economic categories–rent, profit, wages, exchange, value, division of labour, competition, money, etc.–are not absolute and eternal, but merely the abstract expressions of concrete, historical and transitory production-relations between men" (p. 145).

9. *The Poverty of Philosophy,* appendix 1, p. 195.

10. This sketch is reprinted in Horowitz, *Marx and Modern Economics.*

the orthodox approach of his predecessors.[11] In discussing the orthodox treatment of production as an economic category, Marx criticizes the economists for faulty abstraction on two counts. First, in establishing a starting point for their analysis, they abstract the individual producer from his social context with their famous "Robinsonades." Second, in attempting to analyze production *in general,* they abstract social production from its concrete historical development.[12]

11. Cf. Eric Roll, *A History of Economic Thought* (London: Faber, 1962), p. 258 et. seq.
12. Cf. Lange, "Marxian Economics and Modern Economic Theory" in *Marx and Modern Economics;* Mark Blaug, *Economic Theory in Retrospect* (London: Heinemann, 1962), p. 247 f.; Baran and Sweezy, "Economics of Two Worlds" in *Marx and Modern Economics.*

"Capital"

Capital, "the all-dominating power of bourgeois society," is the starting point of the analysis of capitalism. What is capital? According to orthodox political economy, capital is raw materials, instruments of labor and means of subsistence; it is *things* which are utilized to produce new materials, instruments and means of subsistence. These things are themselves the products of labor. Therefore, capital is accumulated labor which serves as a means of producing new products.[13]

But this definition is mere technology.[14] It abstracts from the definite character of capital in bourgeois society, as capital that hires productive labor power and earns a return. Capital is more than means of production in bourgeois society, it is itself "a social relation of production,"[15] an economic power which can govern productive labor power and appropriate a share in the product of that labor power.[16]

From where does capital derive its power of purchase over human labor-power? The Marxian perspective leads directly to an investigation of the social conditions that give rise historically to this peculiar feature of capital. By contrast, the orthodox or bourgeois perspective, which takes the given as the "natural," which identifies capital with a technical element of human activity that has existed from time immemorial, turns its back on the specific and transitory social content which capital has in the bourgeois epoch. Yet–in

13. Karl Marx, *Wage, Labour and Capital,* sec. 3; cf. Engels, *Anti-Dühring* (New York: International Publishers, 1934), part 2, ch. 7.

14. *Wage, Labour and Capital,* ibid.; "Introduction to the Critique of Political Economy," op. cit.

15. *Wage, Labour and Capital,* loc. cit. *Capital,* vol. 3, "The Trinity Formula."

16. Engels, loc. cit.

Marx's formulation—just as a Negro becomes a slave only under certain definite social conditions, so instruments and means of production, money and raw materials become capital only in the context of certain social relations. Torn from these relations, they are no more capital "than gold in itself is money, or sugar the price of sugar."[17]

What are the social relations which give rise to capital, that is, to the *relations* of capital to a sum of values which on exchange for labor power under competitive conditions earn a *net* return?[18]

The source of this most basic and wholly unique characteristic of capital under capitalist relations of production, is that its values are commodities of a special kind. For these commodities are the very conditions of labor, that is, of life itself (means of subsistence, means of production). Moreover, they are to be exchanged in the market with laborers who have no means of subsistence, no means of production of their own, who *must*, therefore, sell their productive labor power, rather than its product, and yield to the owner of capital a *net* return (surplus value).[19]

Marx's explanation of the source of "surplus value" or the owner's profit on capital was based, in accord with his general methodology, on a sociological analysis of the capitalist mode of production. However, in his economic writing generally, and in *Capital* in particular, Marx subordinated the sociological analysis on which his model rests to an answer to the question framed in terms of a particular theory of economic equilibrium, namely, the labor theory of value. This theory has since become the object of most of the at-

17. *Wage, Labour and Capital,* loc. cit.
18. *Wage, Labour and Capital,* loc. cit.
19. *Capital,* vol. 1, "The Buying and Selling of Labor Power"; *Wage, Labour and Capital,* sections 1 and 2.

tacks on Marx's analysis of capitalism, by critics who suppose that in revealing the inadequacy of the labor theory they undermine the very notion of surplus value and capitalist exploitation, which they presume to be derived from it.

In fact, however, the validity or lack of validity of the labor theory, as a theory of economic equilibrium, is of no consequence to the validity of Marx's answer to the question of how it is possible for capital to earn a return under competitive conditions.[20] In the first place, the *existence* of surplus value is not (and could not be) derived by Marx from the labor theory of value even in a strictly economic sense;[21] in the second place, the Marxian theory of surplus value and capitalist exploitation can be shown to be compatible with the principal orthodox theories of value, once Marx's sociological premises are granted.

Marx formulated the question about surplus value in the following way: "Surplus value must be explained on the assumption that commodities exchange at their values, or it cannot be explained at all."[22] In other words, as Maurice

20. This is not the same as saying that the labor theory of value has no practical utility. For such a claim, cf. Joan Robinson, *An Essay on Marxian Economics* (London: McMillan, 1964), p. 22, and Joan Robinson, *Economic Philosophy* (Penguin, 1962), ch. 1. For a reply, see Meek, *Studies in the Labour Theory of Value* and *Economics and Ideology*. Cf. also the controversy between M. Dobb and A. Lerner in *The Journal of Political Economy*, August 1939 and August 1940. See also discussion below.

21. Lange, "Marxian Economics and Modern Economic Theory," in Horowitz, op. cit.

22. *Capital*, vol. 1. Cf. *Capital*, vol. 3, p. 46 f.: ". . . in reality (i.e., in the world of phenomena) . . . surplus-value is given . . . as an excess of the selling price of the commodity over its cost-price; and it remains a mystery where this surplus originated—from the exploitation of labor in the process of production, or from outwitting the purchaser in the process of circulation, or from both." Cf. Hook, *Towards Understanding Karl Marx*, p. 167.

Dobb has noted, surplus value was taken by Marx to be "a *datum* which had to be reconciled with the theory of value, not deduced from the latter. The statement that bourgeois property-owners draw income that is unrelated to any productive contribution which they have made is evidently a *datum* given by experience, which for the purpose of his economic analysis was treated by Marx as a self-evident premise. . . . It was not a conclusion which had to be established *a priori,* by a chain of deductive reasoning, as some hidden premise latent in the theory of value."[23]

The fact that, within the free market, income from property ownership is "unearned" in the sense that it is not matched by some equivalent productive activity,[24] Marx explains by the existence of a particular institutional arrangement that converts labor power itself into a commodity. For labor power is a commodity whose "consumption," or use-value, is a source of exchange-value:[25] The cost of labor power (wages) is borne by capital, the product of labor power (finished goods) accrues to capital, and the value difference between them (minus rent, depreciation, etc.) is the income of capital.

23. Maruice Dobb, "Marxism and Economic Theory," *The Modern Quarterly,* vol. 3, no. 2, Spring 1948. Cf. also Dobb, *Political Economy and Capitalism* (London: Routledge, Kegan, Paul, 1937), ch. 3, where Marx's derivation is put in its historical setting.

24. The existence of unearned income is self-evident to others besides Marx, including those hostile to the labor theory—e.g., "Now it is self-evident, since some men live in idle luxury, that a laborer normally produces more than he consumes, and that this surplus goes to support idleness."—Bertrand Russell, *German Social Democracy* (London: Allen & Unwin), p. 25.

25. *Capital,* vol. 1, "The Buying and Selling of Labor Power"; cf. also *Engels On Capital,* pp. 31, 66.

The labor theory of value, therefore, is not designed to *posit* a phenomenon (i.e., surplus value and unearned income, or its necessary complement, exploitation), but rather to explain *how* unearned income can arise and persist in a free market situation. Indeed, the shoe usually designed for the labor theory by its critics turns out to fit the other foot. For it is the orthodox theorists who have been at pains to deny the evidence of experience, i.e., to deny that income from property is unearned, and to maintain "by a tortuous train of deductive argument" that this income *is* matched by an equivalent productive contribution.[26] It is they, therefore, who have been forced to posit the existence of a phenomenon, viz., "abstinence," or "waiting," whose basis in actual experience is dubious, to say the least.[27]

Not only is the labor theory not designed to posit the existence of surplus value; it is not necessary for an explanation of how this surplus value arises through exploitation. For if the primary significance which Marx attaches to the sociological division of the population in capitalist society (into owners of means of production and owners of labor power) is accepted, then all orthodox value theories can be shown to be compatible with the Marxian theory of exploitation. As the Marxist Oskar Lange pointed out: "If interest is explained by the marginal productivity of capital, it is only because the workers do not own the capital they work with that interest is the personal income of a separate class of people. If interest is regarded as due to a higher valuation of present than future goods it is only because the workers do not possess the subsistence fund enabling them to wait until

26. Cf. Dobb, "Marxism and Economic Theory," op. cit.; also *Political Economy and Capitalism*, ch. 5, "The Trend of Modern Economics."

27. Cf. Marx's revealing account of the first appearance of the abstinence theory in *Capital*, vol. 1, part 7, ch. 24, sec. 3, pp. 595–96.

the commodities they produce are ready that the capitalist advancing it to the workers gets the interest as his personal income. Just as in Marx's case it is because the workers do not possess the means of production that the surplus value is pocketed by the capitalist." In fact, the Marxian concept of exploitation is derived not from the labor theory of value but "from contrasting the personal distribution of income in a capitalist economy (irrespective of whether monopolistic or competitive) with that in an [economy] in which the worker owns his means of production."[28]

The division of capitalist society into owners of means of production (capital) and propertyless wage-laborers is, as Lange notes, the very cornerstone of the Marxian analysis of capitalism, providing not only the basis for its description of capitalist relationships, but the key to its investigation of the dynamics of capitalist development. In short, "the relation between capital and wage-labor determines the entire character of the mode of production (*Capital,* vol. 3, p. 857). For this reason, we shall consider more carefully Marx's own treatment of this sociological relation, and in particular his view of the concrete circumstances of its emergence.

The Capital-Labor Relation

The historical conditions for the existence of capital, according to Marx, are those which create a mass of "unattached" proletarians having no means of their own for producing their subsistence requirements, and which "hurl" these proletarians onto the marketplace to confront owners of capital, i.e., of means and money for producing and ob-

28. O. Lange, "Marxian Economics and Modern Economic Theory" in *Review of Economic Studies,* June 1935 (reprinted in Horowitz, op. cit.). Cf. Blaug, *Economic Theory in Retrospect,* p. 224.

taining the necessary subsistence. "The process . . . that clears the way for the capitalist system," wrote Marx, is that "which takes away from the laborer the possession of his means of production [e.g., the Enclosure Acts in England]; a process that transforms, on the one hand, the social means of subsistence and of production into capital, on the other, the immediate producers into wage-laborers. The so-called primitive accumulation [of capital], therefore, is nothing else than the historical process of divorcing the producer from the means of production."[29] With the polarization of the market into free laborers (in the double sense that they themselves do not form part of the means of production and that they do not own means of production) and owners of capital, "the fundamental conditions of capitalist production are given."[30]

The essence of Marx's sociological analysis of the capital-labor relation is that while the wage bargain appears as a free contract between legal equals, it is in fact not free,[31] and that this lack of freedom stems from a profound asymmetry of power and purpose embodied in what is formally a voluntary agreement.

This asymmetry manifests itself primarily, and most strikingly for Marx, in the fact that the worker bargains away

29. *Capital,* vol. 1, ch. 26, "The Secret of Primitive Accumulation"; cf. the often misunderstood passage in the *Economic and Philosophic Manuscripts* (p. 80), which finds its explanation in the above passage from *Capital.* "*Private property* is thus the product, the result, the necessary consequence, of alienated labor" (i.e., wage-labor).

30. Ibid. Cf. *Capital,* vol. 1, p. 170: "[Capital] can spring into life, only when the owner of the means of production and subsistence meets in the market with the free laborer selling his labor-power. And this one historical condition comprises a world's history."

31. Cf. *Capital,* vol. 1, pp. 176, 302.

more than he evidently *wants* to: indeed, so weak is the individual laborer vis-à-vis the capitalist that it is necessary to pass legislation to prevent the worker from "freely" bargaining himself and his family into *slavery*. At the end of the chapter describing the efforts of capital to push the working day to encompass the whole of the worker's life (and that of his family as well), Marx writes of the change in the worker's status before entering and after leaving the process of production:

> In the market he stood as owner of the commodity "labor-power" face to face with other owners of commodities, dealer against dealer. The contract by which he sold to the capitalist his labor-power proved, so to say, in black and white that he disposed of himself *freely*. The bargain concluded, it is discovered that he was no "free agent," that the time for which he is free to sell his labor power is the time for which he is forced to sell it, that in fact the vampire will not lose its hold on him "so long as there is a muscle, a nerve, a drop of blood to be exploited."

In order to protect themselves against this unlimited exploitation, laborers must band together as a class and "compel the passing of a law, an all-powerful social barrier that shall prevent the very workers from selling, by *voluntary* contract with capital, themselves and their families into slavery and death. In place of the pompous catalogue of the 'inalienable rights of man,' comes the modest Magna Charta of a legally limited working-day, which shall make clear 'when the time which the worker sells is ended, and when his own begins.' "[32]

32. *Capital,* vol. 1, ch. 10, "The Working-Day" (emphasis added).

The fact which the parliamentary reports cited by Marx record is that without legislation to restrict the power of capital in the wage bargain there is virtually no limit to what capital can compel labor to voluntarily sell itself into.[33] It can compel the worker to sell not only himself but his wife and small children into fourteen, sixteen, eighteen hours a day of dangerous, degrading, unsanitary, mutilating and literally death-dealing labor, all under competitive economic conditions and within a parliamentary-constitutional political framework.

In the previously quoted passage, Marx explains the paradox of free labor, which is really unfree,[34] by observing that the time for which the worker is free to sell his labor power is precisely the time for which he is *forced* to sell it. He is forced to sell it, because he must sell it in order to live. Divested of means of subsistence and of means of producing means of subsistence, he must use the time in which he could be producing for himself to produce for another. By contrast this "other" enters the market with means of production and money, not, like the laborer, to gain subsistence, but solely for the purpose of getting *more* value in exchange than he gives.[35]

There is, then, a profound asymmetry which characterizes the relative positions of capital and labor in the market, not only with respect to power but to the purposes for which

33. E.g., Marx cites the following revealing construction from a parliamentary report: "To permit, which is tantamount to compelling, to work 14 hours a day with or without meals, etc."

34. "Free labour (if so it may be termed) even in a free country, requires the strong arm of the law to protect it."–Parliamentary Report cited by Marx, ibid.

35. *Capital,* vol. 1, part 2.

they come to bargain: the capitalist comes as a self-dependent, that is, an *independent* dealer to exchange money and commodities solely in order to make more money; the laborer, as a dependent dealer to exchange labor power in order to eat.[36] It is this asymmetry that explains the fact of income accruing to capital. This is the very basis of the bargain the capitalist strikes with the laborer. If the potential for increasing his capital does not exist, if he can expect only an *equivalent* (i.e., after the process of production is complete and its products sold) in exchange for his capital, then he will withhold it: there will be no bargain, no investment.[37]

In sum, the reason that the possibility exists to expand capital in the market is, first, that there exists a margin between total net output and the subsistence minimum of laborers,[38] and second, that the division of society into owners of capital and propertyless wage-laborers means that capital can and will be used to hire labor power at a wage which is in fact less than the net value of the goods which the labor power produces. This is because the realization of such a margin, as profit, is *necessary* to induce the capitalist class

36. Ibid. Cf. also *Economic and Philosophic Manuscripts,* "Wages of Labour."

37. E.g., see Marx's discussion of the capitalist who finds, to his "astonishment," that after the process of production is over, "the value of the product is exactly equal to the value of the capital advanced." *Capital,* vol. 1, ch. 7, sec. 2, "The Production of Surplus Value."

38. "If a worker can produce no more in a day than he is obliged to eat in a day, he is not a potential object of exploitation. This idea is simple, and can be expressed in simple language, without any apparatus of specialised terminology. But it is precisely these simple and fundamental characteristics of capitalism that are lost sight of in the mazes of academic economic analysis."—Joan Robinson, *An Essay On Marxian Economics,* p. 17.

as a whole to hire labor power at all, while the laborers *must* find capital to hire them if they are to eat. This, then, is the sociological premise of capitalist exploitation in capitalist society and the meaning of Marx's statement that "capital is not a thing, but rather a definite social production relation . . . which is manifested in a thing and lends this thing a specific social character. . . ."[39]

The significance of this relation can readily be seen by comparing the Marxian theory of surplus value with modern orthodox theories of profit. For Marx, profit is a surplus whose appropriation is made possible by the basic division of society into owners of means of production and propertyless wage-laborers. Profit, as such, would exist even in conditions of perfect competition, even in the absence of innovation and change. Modern orthodox theories, on the other hand, tend to ascribe the very existence of profit either to monopoly conditions or to conditions of dynamic change. In the latter case, profit is regarded as the supply price of entrepreneurial risk-bearing, or innovation.

To establish the notion that net profit in a perfectly competitive market is possible only in conditions of dynamic change, orthodox theorists posit a stationary, or "circular flow," economy, in which there is no scope for innovation or enterprise. In such conditions, it is then argued, the earnings of entrepreneurs will fall to the level of managers' salaries, and no surpluses will accrue to employers of labor. For if they did, it is argued, the laborers would themselves turn employers and compete the surplus away.

39. *Capital,* vol. 3, p. 794. Cf. Engels's sarcastic jibe at the rising bourgeoisie: "You have destroyed the small monopolies so that the *one* great basic monopoly, property, may function more freely and unrestrictedly" (emphasis in original), in "Outlines of a Critique of Political Economy," *Economic and Philosophic Manuscripts,* p. 182.

On their own assumptions, such theories are not debatable; their logic is consistent and not open to dispute. The real question is whether the primary assumptions on which they rest are realistic in terms of the conditions of capitalist production. For the basic premise of all such theories is that there is *equal access to capital* on the part of all "wage-earners," employers and laborers alike. In Schumpeter's famous circular flow economy, for example, there are but two classes postulated, landowners and laborers, and landowners do appropriate a surplus precisely because they possess a class monopoly over the land. The difference between the Schumpeterian and Marxian models is simply that in the Marxian there is postulated, in addition to the land-owning class, a capitalist class which possesses an analagous monopoly over capital.[40]

The same point can be made in reference to the Wicksellian model of static equilibrium, in which profit appears as the reward of risk-bearing. In fact, as Joan Robinson points out, "the level of profits is supported by a scarcity of enterprise which is not due to the real cost of risk-bearing, but to

40. P.M. Sweezy, "Schumpeter's Theory of Innovation" in *The Present As History* (New York: Monthly Review Press, 1953), and R. L. Meek, "Karl Marx's Economics" in *The New Reasoner,* Autumn 1959: ". . . in most capitalist economies, which we should want to call 'competitive,' businessmen will expect to receive, and will usually in actual fact receive, over and above interest on capital, managerial salaries, etc., net profits at the rate regarded as normal in the industry, *even in the absence of such factors as monopoly and innovation.* For confirmation of this a glance at any manual of business management should be quite sufficient. . . . Marx's theory of profit is the only one in the field which in this vital respect is in full contact with reality, simply for the reason that it analyses profit in terms of, instead of in abstraction from, the capital-labour relation" (emphasis in original).

the scarcity of individuals who have anything to risk."[41]

Yet another, earlier formulation of this line of argument, which has the virtue of simply clarifying the issues and their relation to the specifically Marxian conception of political economy, was made by the Cambridge economist Maurice Dobb.[42] Most of the theories of the classical economists (we might add, of orthodox economists generally), Dobb noted, as well as much of liberal political philosophy, "would be admirable wisdom in a classless society." However, they are "not applicable . . . to a society based on . . . differential class advantage." One aspect of this inapplicability, writes Dobb, was indicated by Professor Cannan and Dr. Dalton, when they observed that economists had developed theories of distribution based on abstract *factors* of production, but not of distribution between persons and classes.[43]

To cite an instructive analogy, orthodox economists had found it necessary to develop a special theory of exchange between nations because national boundaries hampered the mobility of supply of resources. In other words, nations largely constituted "non-competing groups." Owing to differential advantages in international trade, one nation might obtain an abnormally high level of income. But similar considerations would seem to demand a special theory of exchange between classes as well, for mobility is "considerably ham-

41. *An Essay on Marxian Economics,* p. 56 et seq. Professor Robinson also disposes of the slightly different Marshallian version of this argument, on the same basic grounds.

42. "The Entrepreneur Myth" (1924) in Oskar Lange and Fred M. Taylor, *On Economic Theory and Socialism* (New York: McGraw-Hill, 1956).

43. Cf. Dobb's own discussion of marginal productivity theory in *Political Economy and Capitalism,* pp. 180–83.

pered by social distinctions, unequal educational opportunities, unequal money incomes."[44]

Professor Taussig had, in fact, suggested that social classes also constituted non-competing groups. "If this is so," writes Dobb, "a considerable part of the superior income of the richer class of society is to be regarded as an *institutional rent* or revenue,[45] due to restriction to a comparative few of the supply of persons performing the functions for which that class receives payment. The restriction is caused by the institutions of a class society. The 'rent' can be regarded either in its scarcity aspect, or in its differential aspect as due to the possession of certain differential class advantages. It was clearly this 'institutional rent' to which Marx was referring when he talked of 'surplus-value.' "[46]

The economic implications of the Marxian theory of surplus value, that is, of a theory which regards profit as symmetrical with rent rather than labor, can best be suggested by reference to Ricardo's critique of the landed interest in his theory of economic development.

In Ricardo's theory, rent was defined as a payment for "the use of the original and indestructible powers of the soil," and therefore, "no addition to the national wealth, but merely . . . a transfer of value."[47] The landlord did not provide a productive service for his payment: "The dealings between the landlord and the public are not like dealings in trade, whereby both the seller and the buyer may equally be said to gain, but the loss is wholly on one side, and the gain

44. *On Economic Theory and Socialism,* pp. 11–12.
45. "This term the writer owes to Mr. H. D. Dickinson. Mr. Dickinson, however, prefers to speak of 'restriction revenue.' " (Dobb's note).
46. *On Economic Theory and Socialism,* loc. cit.
47. David Ricardo, *The Principles of Political Economy and Taxation* (London: Everyman, 1962), pp. 33, 273.

wholly on the other." Moreover, in Ricardo's view, "the interest of the landlord is always opposed to that of the consumer and the manufacturer," i.e., to society's productive agents,[48] a fact of enormous consequence for the theory of economic development. For as accumulation progressed, diminishing returns on the land would, according to Ricardo, cause rents to rise, thereby raising the price of corn, i.e., the subsistence price of the laborer, and therefore his wages. Steadily rising wages would mean a falling rate of profits. Accumulation, therefore, because of the vested interest of a parasitic class in preserving its surplus payment, would generate a tendency to check accumulation, and this contradictory process would, in Marx's words, hang "like a doom over bourgeois production."[49] Ricardo therefore regarded the landed interest as inimical to economic progress, much as Marx was later to regard its capitalist successor.

While the analogy between capital and land is inexact,[50] it is strong enough to evoke interesting parallels between the Ricardian and Marxian theories of capitalist development, parallels which were undoubtedly in Marx's mind in framing his own analysis.[51] For if profit is not a payment for productive service, but a surplus analagous to rent, might not a similar antagonism of interests arise, a conflict between the capitalists' aim to preserve the value of capital and the requirements of the progressive development of the economic

48. Ibid., p. 225.
49. Cf. his discussion of Ricardo's theories of accumulation and consumption in Bonner and Burns, eds., *Theories of Surplus Value* (London: Lawrence and Wishart, 1951), p. 422.

50. Ibid., p. 288.
51. Cf., e.g., the following Ricardian formulation: "Is profit a creation of wealth, or is it not rather a transfer of surplus labor from the workman to the capitalist?" (ibid.).

system? Indeed, with the tendency of capitalist development towards increasing concentration of capital, i.e., increasing monopolization, and hence a situation increasingly analagous to that in which land "earns" a rent, might not a barrier to capitalist production, in the last analysis, prove to be capital itself?

The Concept of "Surplus Value"

We now turn to three points that have been raised in connection with Marx's discussion of the capital-labor relation and the appropriation of surplus value, which serve to illuminate crucial issues involved in the analysis.

The first of these questions the very necessity for employing an economic apparatus in the analysis, i.e., not merely the labor theory of value, but any theory of value. It is suggested by some writers that the real essence of the capital-labor relation is not economic at all, but purely sociological; that the source of the capitalist's ability to appropriate a surplus is not to be sought in the economics of the capitalist market, but solely in the fact of the "social power" available to owners of capital. It is this social power alone ("that constellation of forces–the role of government, the pressure of organization, superior bargaining power, tradition and customary practice–which are not a part of the competitive pricing process"[52]) that makes it possible for the capitalist to withhold a portion of the fruits of labor. Once it is recognized that not market, but social, forces yield the capitalist his surplus, the apparatus of value theory and all the barren disputes that attend its employment can be dispensed

52. M. Gottlieb, "Marx's Mehrwert Concept and the Theory of Pure Capitalism," *Review of Economic Studies,* XVIII, 3, no. 47, 1950–1951.

with, and the real core of the relation analyzed directly.[53]

However cogent this line of reasoning, Marx nonetheless conceived the problem of the surplus as first of all an *economic* problem, that is, as the problem of explaining how in a competitive society, where the majority of commodities normally sell at prices fixed in an impersonal market, incomes which assume the character of a surplus can be generated and can persist.[54] There are two basic reasons for Marx's insistence on formulating the problem this way.

While recognizing the general significance of social power, and indeed while stressing its particular role in determining wage levels and the conditions of production,[55] Marx regarded certain social relations, specifically the social relations of production, as a basic constellation of social forces, while other non-economic elements of social power he regarded as less basic, and generally as falling into line with this primary constellation. The *economic* rise of the bourgeoisie historically preceded the *political* dominance of the class and the establishment of bourgeois society generally.[56] Moreover, the dominance of the bourgeoisie as a class was guaranteed by its economic hegemony, by the evolution of economic relations, quite apart from its ability to secure its dominion

53. Ibid. Cf. also Engels's discussion of Dühring's "force theory" (in *Anti-Dühring,* op. cit.), which bears resemblance to Gottlieb's position.

54. R. L. Meek, "Mr. Gottlieb On Marx: A Comment," in *Review of Economic Studies,* XIX, no. 2, 1951–1952.

55. Gottlieb, op. cit. Cf. also *Capital,* vol. 1, especially ch. 10; and *Value, Price and Profit.*

56. For this line of argument cf. Engels, op. cit., p. 181 et seq. For a discussion by Marx of exceptions to this pattern, see the introduction to *A Contribution to the Critique of Political Economy* (Chicago: Charles H. Kerr & Co., 1904), "Production and Distribution."

in the political and social spheres.[57] Indeed, in England, political and social hegemony was attained only partially by the industrial bourgeoisie in the course of its "long" revolution.[58] (and to an even smaller degree subsequently in Germany).[59] Consequently, Marx regarded the social relations of production as fundamental, and other elements of social power as being derivative from and offering secondary protection or support to the primary matrix defined by these relations.[60] Thus, the fundamental source of surplus appropriation in capitalism, as in previous social formations, lay in the relations of production, and an adequate theory of the surplus, from a Marxian point of view, would have to be framed accordingly.

The second reason value theory cannot simply be discarded is that the market form which appropriation takes in capitalist society (and which value theory is formulated to analyze) is not peripheral to capitalism, but essential to its nature. It makes all the difference between one historical epoch and another that the laborer "voluntarily" bargains away his surplus in a "free" contractual relationship in capitalist society, whereas in feudalism the surplus is "taxed" from him, and in slavery not only his surplus but he himself is the property of his master.[61] Indeed, it is the *differentia*

57. Engels, op. cit., p. 205; Marx, Preface and Introduction to *A Contribution* (op. cit.).

58. Perry Anderson, "Origins of the Present Crisis" in *Towards Socialism* (London: Fontana, 1965); E. P. Thompson, "The Peculiarities of the English" in *The Socialist Register 1965;* and Anderson, "The Myths of Edward Thompson," *New Left Review,* no. 35.

59. E.g., Sweezy, "The German Problem" in *The Present as History.*

60. Engels, loc. cit. Marx, loc. cit. Like Marx, Engels recognizes exceptions to this order, but regards them as being severely limited in number.

61. *Capital,* vol. 1, p. 217, and *Capital,* vol. 3, p. 775.

specifica of capitalism that, in contrast to previous social formations, its root inequalities are enforced by free contract and free competition through the market, and not by naked force or institutionally sanctioned claims of status. To abstract from these features of the system, as the theory of "social power" does, is to abstract from what is essential and characteristic, rather than merely secondary or superficial.

A second question that suggests itself in connection with the analysis of surplus value is why the analysis should be framed in terms of the category "surplus value" at all. Rates of surplus value are not observable on the market. Workers seek to maximize wages; capitalists act in terms of rates of profit (i.e., in terms of returns on total capital, not merely "variable capital" or the cost of labor power).[62] Why go "behind" the market in this manner? If the behavior of the economic actors is determined by market phenomena (wages, interest and profits), what is the purpose of formulating a theory in terms of other categories which have no such operational content?

Before answering the question, it is important to note the enormous significance which Marx attached to precisely this kind of theoretical formulation. This is indicated in the mere fact that he titled his critical history of political economy *Theories of Surplus Value,* criticizing previous economists more or less on the basis of how clearly they understood the problems of the origin and generation of surplus value as the central problems of political economy,[63] and then according

62. In Marx's scheme, the rate of surplus is s/v, where s is surplus value and v is the variable capital (wages).

63. E.g., cf. Engels's description: "This section [of Marx's notebooks] contains a detailed critical history of the pith and marrow of Political Economy, the theory of surplus-value . . ." (Preface to vol. 1 of *Capital*).

to how well they solved these problems. Even more indicative, perhaps, is a letter which Marx wrote to Engels in January 1868 in which he described "the three fundamentally new elements" contained in volume 1 of *Capital,* which had just appeared. The very first of these new elements was "that in contrast to *all* former political economy, which *from the very outset* treats the particular fragments of surplus value with their fixed forms of rent, profit, and interest as already given, I first deal with the general form of surplus value, in which all these fragments are still undifferentiated–in solution, as it were." (Letter of January 8, 1868)

The reason for Marx's procedure emerges clearly in the course of the analysis of profit, rent, and interest in volume 3 of *Capital.* In particular, if interest and profit are treated (as they are in orthodox theory) only as they appear in the market, and not in their general form as a surplus, then the source of their generation and appropriation is effectively obscured. Interest appears as a property of capital, profit as wages of enterprise.[64] To rest in these appearances, however, is to remain on the surface of bourgeois reality and to obscure the social relation on which these phenomena rest.

While "interest-bearing capital" earns a return for the lender, it does so only because he lends it to another person who "throws it into circulation, turns it into a commodity as *capital,*"[65] that is, uses it to employ labor and create surplus value, i.e., profit. "Loaning money as capital–its alienation on the condition of it being returned after a certain time–presupposes, therefore, that it will be actually employed as capital. . . ." The real cycle made by money as capital (i.e., through the production process), "is thus the premise for the legal transaction by which the borrower must return the

64. *Capital,* vol. 3, ch. 23, "Interest and Profit of Enterprise."
65. Ibid., p. 337

money to the lender."[66] Interest, therefore, "appears originally, is originally, and remains in fact merely a portion of the profit, i.e., of the surplus-value, which the functioning capitalist, industrialist or merchant has to pay to the owner and lender of money-capital whenever he uses loaned capital instead of his own. If he employs only his own capital, no such division of profit takes place; the latter is then entirely his." Indeed, insofar as capital owners employ their own capital in the reproduction process, they take no part in determining the rate of interest. "This alone shows that the category of interest–impossible without determining the rate of interest–is alien to the movements of industrial capital as such."[67]

There is nothing generically "Marxian" in this view of interest, taken by itself. Thus Adam Smith wrote: "It may be laid down as a maxim, that wherever a great deal can be made by the use of money, a great deal will commonly be given for it. . . . The progress of interest, therefore, may lead us to form some notion of the progress of profit."[68] More recently, rejecting the notion that the rate of interest measures the rate of discount of the future, because individuals prefer consumption now to consumption later, Professor Robinson has argued:

66. Ibid., p. 343.

67. Ibid., p. 363. The *rate* of interest, for Marx, as for Keynes, is essentially a monetary phenomenon. Cf. Blaug, *Economic Theory in Retrospect,* p. 265, and Fan-Hung, "Keynes and Marx On the Theory of Capital Accumulation, Money and Interest" in *Marx and Modern Economics* (op. cit.).

68. *The Wealth of Nations* (New York, 1906), p. 87, cited in Joseph M. Gillman, "An Evaluation of John Maynard Keynes," *Science and Society,* vol. 19, p. 107.

> The rate of interest is normally positive for a quite different reason. Present purchasing power is valuable partly because, under the capitalist rules of the game, it permits its owner (directly or by lending to a business concern) to employ labour and undertake production which will yield a surplus of receipts over costs. In an economy in which the rate of profit is expected to be positive, the rate of interest is positive.[69]

Since interest, in its phenomenal form, appears as the property of capital, the other part of surplus value, "profit of enterprise," necessarily appears as coming "not from capital as such, but from the process of production," and in particular from the *organization* of production. Moreover, since "the process of production, separated from capital, is simply a labour-process . . . the industrial capitalist, as distinct from the owner of capital, does not appear as operating capital, but rather as a functionary irrespective of capital, or, as a simple agent of the labour-process in general, as a labourer, and indeed as a wage-labourer."[70]

Thus profit, in orthodox analyses, is treated as a necessary payment for wages of superintendence or management, and the function of the industrial capitalist is treated as symmet-

69. Joan Robinson, *The Accumulation of Capital* (London: McMillan, 1958), p. 395: "A positive rate of interest being established, for every individual owner of wealth the present value of purchasing power exceeds its future value to the corresponding extent. It is then proper to arrive at the present value of expected future income by discounting it at the appropriate rate of interest. This has nothing whatever to do with the subjective *rate of discount of the future* of the individuals concerned, though it is true that a comparison between his subjective discount rate and the rate of interest obtainable may be said (if he knows how to express himself in such terms) to influence his saving habits."

70. *Capital,* vol. 3, pp. 374–75.

rical with wage-labor, in other words, as independent of capital and its specific social attribute under capitalist production relations–i.e., as "property commanding the labor-power of another."[71] In abstracting from the social-property relation embodied in capital, the analysis treats the whole process as a purely technical phenomenon, and the function of the capitalist consequently acquires an implicit justification as a technically required aspect of the organization of production.

In his own discussion of the treatment of profits as the wages of management, Marx points out that whereas the labor of supervision is indeed technically required "wherever the direct process of production assumes the form of a combined social process," the function of supervision nonetheless has a dual aspect which must not be overlooked. On the one hand, wherever many individuals cooperate, there is required "a commanding will" to organize and unify the process. "This is a productive job, which must be performed in every combined mode of production."[72] On the other hand, there is a different kind of necessity for supervision arising in all those modes of production which are "based on the antithesis between the laborer, as a direct producer, and the owner of means of production," i.e., which involve the appropriation by the owner of the means of production of part of the producer's surplus.[73] The greater this antithesis and

71. Ibid., p. 374.
72. Ibid., p. 376.
73. Ibid. Cf. Marx's parallel and illuminating historical discussion of the same phenomenon in the chapter on "Cooperation" in volume 1: "[since] . . . the control of the capitalist is in substance two-fold by reason of the two-fold nature of the process of production itself,–which, on the one hand, is a social process for producing use-values, on the other, a process for creating surplus-value–in form that control is despotic." And: "The control exercised by the capitalist is not only a

antagonism, the greater the role of supervision as a dominating authority, which, indeed, reaches its acme in the slave system.

This dual role of the supervisory power in the productive process in class societies is analagous to the dual function of the state, which also attains its clearest expression in its most despotic forms. For in despotic states, "supervision and all-round interference by the government" clearly involves both "the performance of common activities arising from the nature of all communities, and the specific functions arising from the antithesis between the government and the mass of the people."[74] Supervision is both regulative and integrative, in a technical sense, and authoritative and dominative, in a class sense.

At this point in his argument, Marx notes a further interesting and revealing analogy. On the one hand, ancient writers on the slave system blurred the distinction between the two sides of the work of supervision, and combined them in theory, even as they were inseparably combined in practice. On the other hand, the same theoretical course is taken by those "modern economists, who regard the capitalist mode of production as absolute." Moreover, just as modern apologists of the slave system (in the United States) use the necessity of the work of supervision to justify slavery, so, notes Marx, the orthodox economists utilize it to justify the wage system.

---

specific function, due to the nature of the social labour-process, and peculiar to that process, but it is, at the same time, a function of the exploitation of a social labour-process, and is consequently rooted in the unavoidable antagonism between the exploiter and the living and labouring raw material he exploits." (pp. 332, 331).

74. *Capital,* vol. 3, pp. 376–77.

The Negro, according to the Southern argument, had the strength and power to labor, but was denied, by Nature, the intellect to govern his labor or the will to perform it. But Nature provided him with a master to coerce that will and make him useful. Thus it was not injustice to leave him in his natural (slave) condition and give him a master to govern him, "nor is it depriving him of any of his rights to compel him to labor in return, and afford to that master just compensation for the labor and talent employed in governing him and rendering him useful to himself and to the society."[75]

As Marx observes, the same kind of argument can be (and is) used in relation to wage labor. For like the slave, the wage laborer must be put to work and ruled over in the work process. Assuming this relationship of "lordship and servitude," it is certainly proper "to compel the wage-laborer to produce his own wages and also the wages of supervision, as compensation for the labor of ruling and supervising him," or, in the words of the apologists of slavery, "just compensation for the labor and talent employed in governing him and rendering him useful to himself and to the society."[76]

In developing the argument that profit, like interest, is merely part of an appropriated surplus, despite the fact that it appears to arise from production, and therefore that it appears to be a necessary payment for some function performed in production, Marx abstracts from the market situation in which the production process takes place. Consequently, Marx fails to consider the alleged function of the entrepreneur as the organizer of production *for the market,* which provides the principal source of modern justifications for profit (e.g., as the reward for risk-taking or inno-

75. The statement was made by a lawyer in the United States named O'Connor, and is cited by Marx, *Capital,* vol. 3, p. 378.

76. Ibid., p. 379; cf. vol. 1, p. 332.

vation).[77] This gap is implicitly bridged, however, in the clinching point of Marx's general argument, where the discussion takes an intriguingly "modern" turn.

For Marx points to the growing divorce of ownership from the work of supervision as substantive proof that the profit the capitalist receives is payment for no necessary function performed in the production process. The modern corporation,[78] developed with the credit system, has the "increasing tendency to separate [the] work of management as a function from the ownership of capital, be it self-owned or borrowed." Similarly, cooperative factories, where "the manager is paid by the laborers instead of representing capital counterposed to them," prove that "the capitalist has become no less redundant as a functionary in production than he himself, looking down from his high perch, finds the big landowners redundant."[79] Thus in capitalist corporations, as in cooperative factories, "the wages of management both for the commercial and industrial manager are completely isolated from the profits of enterprise."[80] Hence the profits of enterprise accruing to industrial capitalists as industrial capitalists in no way represent necessary payments for a necessary function performed in the process of production.[81]

77. Cf. Frank H. Knight, *Risk, Uncertainty, and Profit* (1921); Joseph Schumpeter, *The Theory of Economic Development* (New York: Oxford University Press, 1961); Roll, *A History of Economic Thought* (op. cit.).

78. "Joint stock-company," in nineteenth century terminology.

79. *Capital,* vol. 3, pp. 379–80.

80. Ibid., p. 381.

81. Cf. Joan Robinson, *Economics, An Awkward Corner* (London: Allen & Unwin, 1966): "The notion that property carries obligations which justify privilege is contradicted by the separation of ownership from control in modern business." Cf. also Robinson, *An Essay on Marxian Economics,* p. 18.

Summing up the entire argument with respect to interest on money-capital and profit on industrial capital, Marx writes: "Since, on the one hand, the mere owner of capital, the money-capitalist, has to face the functioning capitalist, while money-capital itself assumes a social character with the advance of credit, being concentrated in banks and loaned out by them instead of its original owners [i.e., since interest-earning capital is also managed by functionaries], and since, on the other hand, the mere manager who has no title whatever to the capital, whether through borrowing it or otherwise, performs all the real functions pertaining to the functioning capitalist as such, only the functionary remains and the capitalist disappears as superfluous from the production process."[82]

Thus, from a sociological point of view, the employment of the concept of surplus value allows Marx to put the social power relation which capital represents[83] at the very center of his analysis. The immediate and most important consequence of this, analytically, is to establish the correct order of priority between technical and class relations. For embodied in the surplus-value analysis is the recognition that the role of the capitalist in production is determined not by his relation to the technical process of production, as orthodox theory implies, but by his control of capital: "It is not because he is a leader of industry that a man is a capitalist; on the contrary, he is a leader of industry because he is a capitalist. *The leadership of industry is an attribute of capital,* just as in feudal times the functions of general and judge were attributes of landed property."[84]

82. *Capital,* vol. 3, p. 380.
83. Under capitalist conditions: private property in the means of production, and a market for free wage labor.
84. *Capital,* vol. 1, p. 332 (emphasis added).

We have touched here on an extremely important methodological point. We have seen that the orthodox analysis, by focusing on a technical relationship between capital regarded as means of production and the labor required to operate capital, in effect excludes from consideration the historically conditioned social power relationship of capital itself. In this, as previously noted, lies the essence of the distinction between Marx's sociological economics and orthodox economics. Thus, as Marx writes in his discussion of "Revenues and their Sources" in volume 3 of *Capital:* "capital-profit (profit of enterprise plus interest), land-ground-rent, labor-wages, this is the trinity formula which comprises all the secrets of the social production process." But the formula remains opaque to orthodox analysis, which regards capital (considered simply as a sum of values, means of production) as the source of "profit" (profit plus interest), land as the source of ground-rent, and labor as the source of wages. (Moreover, since interest, in orthodox analysis, appears as the specific product of capital, and profit as wages of enterprise, the orthodox formula reduces itself to capital-interest, land-ground-rent, and labor-wages, where profit, "the specific characteristic form of surplus-value belonging to the capitalist mode of production," is conveniently eliminated.)[85]

In orthodox theory, these "alleged" sources of wealth "belong to widely dissimilar spheres and are not at all analogous with one another." Moreover, they are conceived in ahistorical, asocial form, so that capital, "a definite social production relation, belonging to a definite historical formation of society,"[86] is identified with capital as such, a thing, a sum of values, which is then represented as being a source of more value than it is worth. Similarly, labor as a general activity in

85. *Capital,* vol. 3, p. 794.
86. Ibid.

production is identified with *wage*-labor, and land with landed *property,* both of which, "like capital, are historically determined social forms; one of labor, the other of monopolized terrestrial globe."[87]

In this perspective, bound as it is by the horizon of capitalist production relations, "since wage-labor does not appear as a socially determined form of labor, but rather all labor appears by its nature as wage-labor . . . the definite specific social forms assumed by the material conditions of labor," i.e., the produced means of production (capital) and the land, "directly coincide with the *material existence* of these conditions," that is, with the general form of these conditions in the labor process, "independent of its concrete historically determined social form, or indeed independent of *any* social form."[88] In other words, in this view, the socially changed form of the conditions of labor in the capitalist epoch–i.e., the conditions of labor "*alienated* from labor and confronting it independently" as monopolized means of production (capital) and monopolized land (landed property)–appear to coincide with the unchanging "existence of the produced means of production and of the land in the process of production in general."[89] Capital and produced means of production become (in such a perspective) identical terms, as do land and land monopolized through private ownership. "The means of labor as such which are by nature capital, thus become the source of profit, much as the land as such becomes the source of rent."[90] The independence of the conditions of labor from labor, the "unique form of this independence with respect to wage-labor" in capitalist con-

87. Ibid., p. 795 (emphasis added).
88. Ibid., p. 803 (emphasis added).
89. Ibid., p. 804 (emphasis added).
90. Ibid., p. 804.

ditions, becomes "a property inseparable from them as things, as material conditions of production, an inherent, immanent, intrinsic character of them as elements of production. Their definite social character in the process of capitalist production bearing the stamp of a definite historical epoch" is conceived to be "a natural, and intrinsic substantive character belonging to them, as it were, from time immemorial, as elements of the production process."[91] Consequently, the *general* roles played by the forces of nature, the produced means of production and labor as a general activity in the production process, appears to be expressed in the specific respective shares (profit, rent and wages) claimed by them as *property* in capital, landed *property* and *wage*-labor under capitalist conditions of production.[92] (Just as products appear "naturally" to confront the producer "as an independent force in capital and capitalists—who actually are but the personification of capital—so land becomes personified in the landlord and likewise gets on its hind legs to demand, as an independent force, its share of the product created with its help").[93]

It is true, of course, that this is the way the sources of revenue appear to the capitalist, the landlord and the wage-laborer themselves in capitalist conditions of production. That is, to the capitalist, capital appears as his actual source of revenue, as does land to the landlord (and the wage-laborer gets the full value of his labor power). But "the finished form which economic relations manifest upon their surface in actual existence, and consequently the representations of them out of which the bearers and agents of these relations seek to develop a clear idea of them . . . are quite different from the

91. Ibid., p. 805.
92. Cf. Dobb, *Political Economy and Capitalism,* pp. 180–83.
93. *Capital,* vol. 3, p. 804.

inner form which is essential but hidden. . ."[94] Despite appearances, it is only the social relations of production, the property relations in means of production and land that permit the capitalist to appropriate the surplus labor of the laborer, and the landlord to attract a portion of that surplus for himself, while the wage-laborer is left, under the title of wages, a portion of the value he has created in order to reproduce himself.[95]

Thus, while the economic actors may regard their revenues in this "reified" way, it is a vulgar economic science that does "no more than interpret, systematize and defend in doctrinaire fashion the conceptions of the agents of bourgeois production who are entrapped in bourgeois production relations. . . . all science would be superfluous if the outward appearance and the essence of things directly coincided."[96] Yet this is precisely the picture presented by (post-Ricardian) orthodox economic science: in its "trinity" formula–capital-interest, land-rent, labor-wages–"we have the complete mystification of the capitalist mode of production, the conversion of social relations into things, the direct coalescence of the material production relations with their historical and social determination. It is an enchanted, perverted, topsy-turvy world, in which Monsieur le Capital and Madame la Terre do their ghost-walking as social characters and at the same time directly as mere things."[97]

94. Ibid.

95. Ibid., pp. 801–802.

96. *Capital,* vol. 3, p. 797. Cf. Letter to Kugelmann (11 July 1868): ". . . the vulgar economist thinks he had made a great discovery when, as against the revelation of . . . inner interconnection, he proudly claims that in appearance things look different. In fact, he boasts that he holds fast to appearance, and takes it for the ultimate. Why, then, have any science at all?"

97. *Capital,* vol. 3, p. 809. Cf. Dobb, op. cit., ch. 5.

The task of an authentic science would be to demystify this system, to destroy "this false appearance and illusion, this mutual independence and ossification of the various social elements of wealth, this personification of things and conversion of production relations into entities, this religion of everyday life."[98] The whole structure of *Capital*, which moves in its analysis from the social relations embodied in the immediate simple productive process (volume 1) to the more complex and concrete forms of capital and its movements until it approaches "step by step the form which they assume on the surface of society, in the action of different capitals upon one another, in competition, and in the ordinary consciousness of the agents of production themselves,"[99] reflects this project and enterprise.

In an essay on Marx's earlier *Contribution to A Critique of Political Economy,* Engels made an observation which casts an illuminating light on this methodological perspective. Political economy, Engels noted, begins with commodities, i.e., with the exchange of products, whether by individuals or communities. A commodity is a commodity, however, "solely because a *relation* between two persons or communities attaches to the *thing,* the product, the relation between producer and consumer who are here no longer united in the same person." This, Engels observes, is a particular example of a fact "which runs through the whole of economics and which has caused utter confusion in the minds of the bourgeois economists: economics deals not with things but with relations between persons, and, in the last resort, between classes; these relations are, however, always *attached to*

98. Ibid.

99. *Capital,* vol. 3, p. 26. On the structure of *Capital,* cf. Sweezy, *The Present As History,* pp. 11–20; Lange, *Political Economy,* pp 100–18; Meek, "Marx's Economic Method," op. cit.

things and *appear as things*" (emphasis in original). This "interconnection," which, according to Engels, was recognized in isolated cases by other economists, "was first discovered by Marx as obtaining for all economics. . . ."[100]

The use of the concept of surplus value to analyze a phenomenon not appearing directly in the actual market, but only in the simple immediate production process, finds its sociological justification, then, in the following way: it puts the relations between social classes, between men as producers, back into the economic process, as its underlying basis. It is the concept through which the sociological and historical dimension of the economic process is revealed.[101]

Before leaving this discussion of surplus value, it may be helpful to probe somewhat more deeply the relation between the sociological analysis embodied in the concept and the economic analysis of volumes 2 and 3 of *Capital,* at least in a general way. This will be more easily accomplished if we focus on a secondary conceptual relationship, namely, between the *rate* of surplus value, s/v, and the *rate* of profit, $s/c+v$, where s is surplus value (the excess of net product over wages), c is constant value (depreciation plus raw materials) and v is variable capital (the wages bill).[102]

The rate of surplus value, s/v, which is a ratio of the time in which the worker works for the capitalist to that in which he works for himself, is "an exact expression for the degree of exploitation of labor-power by capital, or of the laborer by the capitalist."[103] (It should be noted in passing, however, that in the absence of certain simplifying assumptions, e.g., a

100. Marx and Engels, *Selected Works,* p. 374.

101. Cf. Dobb, op. cit., ch. 2 and 3; and Sweezy, op. cit., pp. 128–30.

102. *Capital,* vol. 1, ch. 8 and 9; Robinson, *An Essay on Marxian Economics,* p. 65.

103. *Capital,* vol. 1, p. 218.

general equality of rates of exploitation in all branches of production, s/v must be treated as an aggregate, and that for the actual individual enterprise, s/v is, in Marx's sense, a "purely theoretical abstraction.")[104]

Interesting insight into Marx's intent in formulating this ratio is revealed in his discussion of various alternate formulas for the rate of surplus value. Thus, he rejects the formula $s/s+v$, or surplus value over the value of the product (the value created), despite the fact that, economically, this formula expresses the same situation as is expressed in the one actually adopted,[105] and moreover, that this is a functional relationship that might actually appear in capitalist accounts. Marx's reasoning is as follows: "The habit of representing surplus-value and value of labor-power as fractions of the value created [$s/s+v$]—a habit that originates in the capitalist mode of production itself . . . conceals the very transaction that characterizes capital, namely, the exchange of variable capital for living labor-power, and the consequent exclusion of the laborer from the product. Instead of the real fact, we have the false semblance of an association, in which laborer and capitalist divide the product in proportion to the different elements which they respectively contribute towards its formation."[106] The difference between the formulas is

104. Rudolph Schlesinger, *Marx: His Time and Ours* (London: Routledge & Kegan Paul, 1950), p. 116 f.; Sweezy, p. 65.

105. ". . . the formulae II [$s/s+v$, or surplus value over *total* labor time] can at any time be reconverted into formulae I [s/v] or surplus value [necessary labor time]" (*Capital,* vol. 1, p. 533).

106. "All well-developed forms of capitalist production being forms of cooperation, nothing is, of course, easier, than to make abstractions from their antagonistic character, and to transform them by a word into some form of free association. . . . H. Carey, the Yankee, occasionally performs this conjuring trick with like success, even with the relations resulting from slavery." Note by Marx, *Capital,* vol. 1, p. 533.

thus a *sociological* difference, the one obscuring, the other revealing the underlying relationship of classes and, as we shall see later, the general relation between human labor in capitalist society and its productive apparatus.[107]

However, while sociologically it may be crucial to put the relationship between surplus and necessary labor at the center of analysis, or at least to express this relationship with utmost clarity, the same cannot be said automatically from an economic point of view. Not only may other ratios be more important economically, but (as in the case of the rate of profit) they can change independently of changes in the rate of surplus value, and even in its total sum.[108]

Marx's discussion of the rate of profit and its relation to the rate of surplus value is interesting in that he explicitly recognizes that the rate of surplus value is "invisible"[109] and has no effect on the calculation of the capitalist: "The capitalist does not care whether it is considered that he advances constant capital to make a profit out of his variable capital, or that he advances variable capital to enhance the value of the constant capital; that he invests money in wages to raise the value of his machinery and raw materials, or that he invests money in machinery and raw materials to be able to exploit labor."[110] The capitalist is only interested in the excess of value (s) at which he sells his commodities to the *total* capital ($c+v$) advanced for their production, although it is true that the nature of surplus-value impresses itself con-

107. Cf. Robinson, *An Essay on Marxian Economics,* p. 22.

108. *Capital,* vol. 3, ch. 3; cf. Marx's letter to Engels, April 30, 1868, which gives a summary account of the contents of volume 3.

109. "Surplus-value and rate of surpus-value are, relatively, the invisible and unknown essence that wants investigating, while rate of profit and therefore the appearance of surplus-value in the form of profit are revealed on the surface of the phenomenon" *(Capital,* vol. 3, p. 43).

110. Ibid., p. 41.

stantly upon his consciousness during the production process, "as his greed for the labor time of others" reveals.[111]

Moreover, and more importantly, Marx recognizes that economically it is incorrect to ignore the differences between the rates of exploitation and profit, and to reduce the observable phenomenon of profit to its more fundamental "essence"[112]: "It is altogether erroneous, as a study of the Ricardian school shows, to try to identify the laws of the rate of profit with the laws of the rate of surplus-value, or vice-versa."[113]

But if the laws of profit rates must be studied as such, and are not merely derivative of the laws of surplus-value, in what sense may the latter be said to be the "unknown essence" of the former? Sociologically, the answer is straightforward and in accord with the whole tenor of the previous discussion. If all parts of capital appear equally as the source of excess value (as in the formula for the rate of profit, $s/c+v$), then the critical social relationships embodied in capital are obscured, for "capital appears as a relation to itself."[114]

Economically, on the other hand, there would seem to be three grounds for regarding the rate of surplus value as the "unknown essence" of the rate of profit. First, if the labor theory of value is adopted, then the appearance of profit can only be explained on the basis of an analysis of surplus value, and it becomes necessary to explain the rate of profit on the basis of the rate of surplus value (the so-called "transformation problem"). Second, the rate of exploitation may be shown to be historically prior to the rate of profit and to provide an explanation for its normal levels, as Joan Robin-

111. Ibid., p. 43–44.
112. See preceding footnote.
113. *Capital,* vol. 3, p. 45.
114. Ibid., pp. 48, 45.

son has recently suggested.[115] Finally, since in conjunction with other ratios, in particular the organic composition of capital, c/v, the rate of surplus value in fact determines the rate of profit, then, provided certain technical relationships obtain (in particular, a labor-saving bias in the trend of technical innovations), the rate of exploitation may have a long-run effect on the rate of profit and hence the economic operation of the system. (In fact, the technical trend has failed to materialize, with the consequence that the ratios remain indeterminate in the long run, and thus s/v remains thus far an economically invisible and non-functional relationship, in the capitalist system.)

The point that should emerge from this discussion is that the social dimension of the capital-labor relation, as expressed in the surplus-value analysis, while related to the economic dimensions of the system is not at every level co-extensive with them, and that Marx recognized and accepted this. Indeed, the argument of volumes 2 and 3 of *Capital* constitutes an implicit recognition that the model of the system's essential relationships contained in volume 1, while providing the determinant matrix of the system, is not sufficient to describe its operation or reveal its laws of motion, and that it is therefore necessary to integrate these core "Marxian" relationships with an economic model that incorporates economic forces and categories as they appear on the surface of reality, that is, as they appear in orthodox economic theory.

Surplus Value, Income and Exploitation

It is to disclose the implications of the institutional framework of the capitalist system that Marx treats all income

115. Joan Robinson, *Collected Economic Papers* (Oxford: Basil, Blackwell, 1965), vol. 3, pp. 178–80.

from property as surplus value. For, as Lange has pointed out, the substantive function of Marx's distribution theory is to contrast incomes arising in an economy of independent equal producers (simple commodity production), and by implication a socialist economy, with incomes arising where the means of production are monopolized, through the institution of private property, by a particular class which confronts propertyless wage-laborers in the market.[116]

Now, the relatively straightforward and generally indisputable sociological point embodied in Marx's distribution theory has been thoroughly confused, as previously suggested, by Marx's adoption of the labor theory of value and the subsequent abandonment of that theory by orthodox economists. For although Marx's theory of surplus value is not (and cannot be) formally derived from the labor theory of value, in Marx's own presentation the two tend to appear inseparable, and indeed Marx himself, by insisting on the "barren" character of capital, helps to make them appear so. This has the effect of taking the argument out of the social sphere, where its significance for the specifically Marxian analysis of capitalism lies (Adam Smith was a labor theorist, but not a Marxist), into the domain of formal and highly abstract economic argument, where its relevance to the Marxian analysis is at best a tenuous one.[117] While it may

116. Lange, "Marxian Economics and Modern Economic Theory" (op. cit.).

117. Further confusion is created by those critics of Marx who interpret the labor theory in Marx's formulation as a version of natural rights theory designed to insert a moral argument into what is ostensibly a purely economic analysis in order to claim that all income from property is theft and the whole product rightly belongs to labor. E.g., A. D. Lindsay, *Karl Marx's Capital* (London: Oxford University Press, 1937). The answer to this interpretation has been succinctly put by Blaug: ". . . however much every sentence of *Capital* radiates moral zeal, Marx did not write three volumes to furnish a *positive* demonstra-

have made sense for Marx to formulate his sociological analysis in terms of the orthodox value theory then current, it makes no sense now to tie together two arguments—the economic utility of the labor theory of value, and the sociological (or socio-economic) validity of Marxian distribution theory—where there is no need in fact to do so.

For the above-mentioned confusions arise precisely because arguments that are separate and independent have been treated as interconnected and interdependent. The argument that capital is productive is not at all the same as the argument that capitalists are productive.[118] Similarly, the argument that labor is the sole source of exchange value is different from, and *not* a necessary premise of, the argument that *income* from property rewards no service performed by the recipient but is a function of the economic role and social power of his property.[119]

In other words there is a distinction between the theory of profit or interest as a distributive share, and profit or interest as a necessary cost payment to enable production to proceed in an economically efficient manner, i.e., as a rational accounting device. The first of these implies a theory of social

---

tion of a *normative* proposition. The labor theory of value may be associated with definite moral sentiments, but it does not rest upon them. At bottom, its appeal is to science, not to ethics" (*Economic Theory in Retrospect,* p. 221). Cf. also Meek, *Studies in the Labour Theory of Value,* p. 215 et seq.

118. "Whether we choose to say that capital is productive, or that capital is necessary to make labour productive, is not a matter of much importance. What is important is to say that *owning* capital is not a productive activity" (Robinson, *An Essay on Marxian Economics,* p. 18).

119. "Capital is . . . the governing power over labor and its products. The capitalist possesses this power, not on account of his personal or human qualities, but inasmuch as he is an owner of capital" (*Economic and Philosophic Manuscripts,* pp. 36–37).

or socio-economic relationships; the second implies a theory of relationships which are predominantly technical or economic. The difference between them may be suggested by contrasting Marx's theory of interest with the theory of Böhm-Bawerk.

Like Marx, Böhm-Bawerk regarded land and labor as the only primary factors of production, treating capital as produced means of production that merely transmit value to the product. Moreover, he denied that the existence of interest was owing to any personal activity of the capitalists.[120] On the other hand, Böhm-Bawerk not only rejected the labor theory of value, but argued from the premises of the "subjectivist" marginal utility theory. Starting from these premises, Böhm-Bawerk argued that because there exists a subjective disposition to prefer present to future consumption, capital-using methods of production, which are "roundabout" or time-consuming, are also value productive. In other words, interest on capital is the price paid for overcoming the time discount between present and future goods. As such it is a general economic category, a means of allocating resources between current and future consumption, and hence would appear even in a socialist economy, i.e., in the absence of private ownership of capital.[121]

120. Cf. Blaug, pp. 225–26, where this line of argument is suggested.

121. E. v. Böhm-Bawerk, *The Positive Theory of Capital,* 1923, pp. 365–67; Blaug, op. cit., p. 227. Cf. Joan Robinson: "The association of the rate of interest with capitalist exploitation has made socialist planners shy of using it. And, as we have seen, the rate of return which emerges from the Walrasian model has no particular authority. Yet the notion of a 'cost of waiting' has a commonsense meaning in a planned economy. When output is growing, there is a technical superiority of present over future resources, because present resources can be invested to increase future productivity. Thus the growth rate of the economy itself measures the cost of waiting."–"Consumer's Sovereignty in a Planned Economy," *Collected Economic Papers III,* p. 78.

While maintaining, in contrast to the labor theory of value, that interest was a necessary cost payment (viz., to pay the "cost" of waiting), this line of argument did *not*, as previously noted, necessarily imply that such *income* on capital was an "earned" distributive share. Böhm-Bawerk explained capitalists' receipt of surplus-value by the fact that while surplus value is produced by land and labor alone, it accrues only after the passage of time. Thus, in place of Marx's argument that workers get the value of their labor-*power* but that the actual *labor* they perform exceeds this value, Böhm-Bawerk argued that they get the *present* value of their future output (discounted at the rate of interest) but not its *future* value, which is greater. The difference between present and future values is pocketed by the capitalist as interest (under competitive conditions) because he can afford to wait, while the workers, who own no capital or means of subsistence of their own, are economically dependent on capital owners and are therefore compelled to pay the premium for present goods.[122]

Thus, starting from diametrically opposed theories of value,[123] it is possible to end up with essentially similar

122. Blaug, op. cit., p. 226, also p. 449 et seq. Needless to say, the "Marxian" implications are not so clear in Böhm-Bawerk's own formulation; he lays stress, for example, on the necessity of waiting as the cause of the "economic dependence" of the workers, when it would be more correct to stress the class monopoly of land and capital as the cause. Cf. N. Bukharin, *The Economic Theory of the Leisure Class,* pp. 124–25.

123. For critiques of Böhm-Bawerk, from the point of view of the labor theory of value, see Bukharin, loc. cit.; Dobb, *Political Economy and Capitalism,* p. 151 et seq.; and the essay by Hilferding in Paul M. Sweezy, ed., *Karl Marx and the Close of His System* (Augustus M. Kelley, 1949).

theories of distribution.[124] Moreover, while regarding interest as a necessary cost payment, even under socialism, [125] it is possible to recognize that income from property is "unearned." To adopt such a position is to imply that under a socialist organization of production there would be no income from property, but that all surplus value would not accrue to the laborer.[126] Both Marx and Engels made clear their agreement in principle with such a position. As Engels wrote, "there is no social state possible in which the laborer could receive for his own consumption the total value of his product." Even in a socialist society "there still remains the necessity for an accumulated social reserve fund, and then the *laborers,* that is to say *all,* would remain in possession and in enjoyment of the total product, but each isolated worker would not enjoy the integral product of his own labor."[127]

124. In fact, as indicated in the discussion earlier, the evolution of industrial forms makes the whole question of value irrelevant to this issue: "The academic economists, by treating capital as productive, used to insinuate the suggestion that capitalists deserve well by society and are fully justified in drawing income from their property. In the past, a certain superficial plausibility could be given to this point of view by treating property and enterprise as indistinguishable. But . . . nowadays the divorce between ownership and enterprise is becoming more and more complete, and . . . the typical entrepreneur is . . . indistinguishable from *rentiers,* who employ salaried managers to run their concerns. Nowadays, therefore, it seems simple to say that owning property is not productive, without entering into any logic-chopping disputes as to whether land and capital are productive, and without erecting a special analytical apparatus in order to make the point."—Robinson, *An Essay on Marxian Economics,* pp. 18–19.
125. For a discussion of the problem from a labor theorist's point of view, cf. Dobb, "Discounting the Future" in *An Essay On Economic Growth and Planning* (London: Routledge and Kegan Paul, 1960).
126. It is also to recognize that interest is not a Ricardian surplus, *sensu stricto.* Cf. Blaug, op. cit., pp. 226–27.
127. Introduction to 1884 edition of *The Poverty of Philosophy,* Kerr edition, p. 24; cf. Marx, *Capital,* vol. 1, p. 235.

Similarly, Marx, in his marginal notes on the Gotha program of the German Workers party, criticized the implicit demand that labor's cooperative produce, i.e., the *total social product,* should be distributed among the laborers, "that in communist society every worker must receive the 'undiminished' Lassallean 'proceeds of labor.' " For, from the total social product must be deducted: first, depreciation costs to replace the used-up means of production; then funds for net investment to expand the means of production;[128] and finally, reserve funds "to provide against accidents, dislocations caused by natural calamities, etc." These deductions Marx describes as an "economic necessity," their magnitude being determined by purely economic considerations (i.e., "according to available means and forces, and partly by computation of probabilities"), but as being "in no way calculable by equity." Böhm-Bawerkian interest naturally would come under this heading.[129]

After these deductions, there remains that part of the total product that is actually destined for consumption. From this there must now be deducted "the general costs of administration not belonging to production," the costs of public goods and services (schools, health services, etc.), and finally "funds

128. When Blaug writes that "On Marx's definition . . . 'exploitation' means positive net investment" (op. cit., p. 226), he is right, *provided* this investment occurs under capitalist relations of production. Although Marx's terminology (e.g., describing surplus value as "unpaid labor") unfortunately seems to suggest that " 'exploitation' can cease only when the whole current net output of labor accrues to labor as current consumption" (Blaug), it is evident from Marx's comments on the Gotha program, and his remarks elsewhere, that *production* relations and not *distribution* relations provide the key to his concept of exploitation. All this merely indicates further how the labor theory of value serves to confuse Marx's sociological analysis.

129. This is especially clear in respect to Joan Robinson's remarks on the concept of interest under socialism (cf. note 121, above).

for those unable to work." Only after all these deductions have been made is the total product then divided among its producers for their consumption.

From these remarks it is evident not only that the Marxian analysis of exploitation is compatible with theories of value other than the labor theory, but also that an emphasis on distribution *to the laborer* is a misplaced one. The important distributional fact under capitalism is the fact of appropriation by a non-productive class *which controls the conditions, instruments and purposes of labor.* Indeed, the emphasis on conditions of labor, on the control of social capital, is paramount for Marx. Thus in another marginal note on the Gotha program, Marx decries the statement that "labor is the source of all wealth" ("wealth" here standing for utilities, *not* values). For such a statement, in the first place, is not true (nature provides the material for labor), and in the second place, draws attention from "the *conditions* [of labor] that alone give [it] meaning" (emphasis added). In fact, since "labor depends on nature, it follows that man who possesses no other property than his labor power must, in all conditions of society and culture, be the slave of other men who have made themselves the owners of the material conditions of their labor. He can work only with their permission, hence live only with their permission." Hence it is a "mistake" to make a "fuss" about "so-called distribution" and to "put the principal stress on it." The capitalist mode of production rests on the fact "that the material conditions of production are in the hands of non-workers in the form of property in capital and land, while the masses are only owners of the personal condition of production, of labor power." If, however, the elements of *production* are distributed in this manner, "then the present-day distribution of the means of consumption results automatically." Conversely, "if the conditions of production are the cooperative property of the workers themselves, then there likewise results a distribution of the means of consumption different from the present one."[130]

This distribution, as noted, does not entail full rights for each worker to the "undiminished proceeds of labor." The Marxian concept of exploitation (from a purely distributional point of view)[131] does not flow from the notion that labor is the sole source of value, but from the recognition that income from capital and land is income from *monopolized* means and conditions of production; it is privately appropriated income that is social in origin, and it is appropriated by a class which has taken no part (i.e., has expended no effort or talent) in creating it.[132] This sense of exploitation may be preserved even if a value theory is adopted in which interest appears as a "natural" and necessary economic phenomenon, although Marx's attachment to the labor theory of value prevented him from recognizing this. The labor theory, in fact, tends to confuse the issue by regarding all surplus labor as "unpaid" labor, and therefore implying that in a non-exploitative system labor would receive its "undiminished proceeds," an implication that Marx clearly rejected.

130. *Critique of the Gotha Program,* FLPH (Moscow, n.d.).

131. In fact, it is probably incorrect to speak of a "Marxian" concept of exploitation that is purely distributional, as is evident from Marx's references to "so-called distribution." For Marx regarded the relations of production to be primary and determinant, and hence the concept of exploitation is seen, by him, in terms of these relations. However, the above formulation may help to clarify the meaning of the concept of surplus value as Marx applies it to the incomes of landlords, industrial capitalists, and *rentiers.*

132. Actual wages of management are, of course, not part of surplus value.

The heart of Marx's theory must be seen in terms of *production,* not distribution relations. From this viewpoint, labor is exploited so long as there exists a class monopoly over its instruments and conditions, hence its product and purposes. This is the sociological significance of Marx's theory of surplus value, stripped of its purely economic labor theory form.

Part 4

Bertrand Russell: The Final Passion

Towards the end of his life, Bertrand Russell spent most of his time in Plas Penrhyn, Wales, in an ample but not opulent house set high on a cliff, with a spectacular view of the Glaslyn estuary below. He came down to London rarely, the wearying six-hour trip and the pressure of appointments presenting hardships he could bear less and less as time went on. Because of a kink in his throat, and the inadvisability of an operation at his advanced age, he was already living on a wholly liquid diet, which he roguishly supplemented with seven Red Hackle scotches a day.

I met Lord Russell on one of the increasingly rare occasions when he was spending a few months in London in his Chelsea flat. It was on a crisply clear day early in the fall of 1965, and I remember feeling anxiety and agitation as I searched out the number I had been given among a row of indistinguishable and modest red-brick houses. A compulsive early arriver, I walked around the block several times after

This article was written for *Ramparts* magazine March 1970 on the death of Bertrand Russell.

locating his flat in the hopes that others would have arrived by the time I got there, and I could slip in unnoticed. Finally, I knocked weakly on the door.

It was opened by a diminutive, incredibly frail and fragile-looking white-haired old man. A mixture of feelings came up like a blush—awe, humility, admiration, and most of all, a sense of unbridgeable distance. He smiled, amused at my confusion but also so warm and friendly that he had already overcome the worst of it, although I never did manage to conquer that sense of being where I didn't belong, of not being remotely capable of stepping across that awesome gap—a gap created by time, by culture and by forces of history that I could only dimly imagine.

I followed Lord Russell's slow steps down the corridor, past the portraits of his ancestors: Lord John Russell, his grandfather, who presided over the famous Reform Act of 1832; William Russell, who, as he pointed out later with a puckish twinkle in his eye, had opposed authority and had his head cut off. The short walk was obviously a great burden on him, and it alerted a Bellowesque guilt in me. ("Jesus, Lord Russell, you didn't have to come all the way to the door just for me.")

Later, when I got used to Russell and his routine, I was to realize that these efforts—the arduous trek down the short but seemingly endless hall, the pouring of tea for everyone from what appeared more a cauldron than a teapot in those frail, bony hands—were, for him, part of a fierce struggle against the failing of the life force, against time which had not beaten him over all the generations, although it had beaten down those he had known, loved and fought. *("I believe,"* he had written, *"that when I die I shall rot and nothing of my ego will survive. I am not young and I love life but I should scorn to shiver with terror at the thought of annihilation. Happiness is nonetheless true happiness because it must come to an end. Nor do thought and love lose their values because they are not everlasting.")* On that first day, however, after we got settled and began talking, one thing quickly became clear: the physical decline was deceptive; the mind which peered out through those at once sad and twinkling eyes was keen and resilient.

The gathering which I had come to attend was a meeting of the members of the Bertrand Russell Peace Foundation to discuss plans for setting up an International War Crimes Tribunal to investigate America's war in Vietnam. The room was filled with people who were under thirty, and more likely under twenty-five—all born after Russell had attained more than twice that age. In the political actions in which he engaged during the last years, it was always thus: we who served him and laid plans with him always looked at him across a full lifetime.

A memoir by Ralph Schoenman, his former secretary, captures it well: "We are separated by sixty-four years. His talk is studded with Lenin, Victoria, Poincaré, Mill, Browning, Wilde—'How close were you to Bakunin, Bertie?' 'Not all that close, but then I wasn't well acquainted with Methuselah either.' "

The meeting was one of those interminably windy sessions familiar to anyone who has been in on the organizing of anything. It veered off on a dozen tangents, all the time increasing for me the incongruity of the afternoon—the legendary Lord Russell, godson of John Stuart Mill, holding court with these youthful activists and entering their circumambulatory discussions about organizational details and structures of the forthcoming Tribunal. Russell was concerned that the plans should not be too grandiose and appear ridiculous in the outcome. One long digression of the afternoon concerned possible sites for the Tribunal, and elaborate speculation as to whether any government would allow it.

Russell was heavily inclined to doubt the will or ability of any officials—Russian, Swiss or Third World—to be hospitable to a project which they wouldn't control and which would undoubtedly get them into hot water with the United States.

This skepticism—which turned out to be simple realism—was a feature of Russell's intellect that was to impress me again and again in the brief period in which I was a director of the Bertrand Russell Peace Foundation. Russell's incapacity for illusion—that ingrained sense of doubt which was his inheritance from the age of Victoria—was an essential characteristic of his being. In a BBC interview on his ninety-fourth birthday, Russell had been reminded that many of his critics were claiming that the youngsters who had followed him in his nuclear protests were just young and irresponsible, and that when they got to be over thirty, they would become conservative and respectable and abandon him. What did he think? Russell, whose actions had foreshadowed and inspired the upsurge of mass protest in the sixties, replied: "Yes, that's probably true." Could I, I would ask myself many times after hearing this story, put my life energies into the political struggle if I did not really believe I was helping to shape a future majority, if I was not confident of the ultimate triumph of reason and justice?

There was on the other side of Russell's profound skepticism, however, an equally profound romanticism. Among his books was a whimsical one-sentence work which he had written in his eighty-ninth year, called *History of the World in Epitome.* It began with a picture of Adam and Eve and ended with a photograph of the atomic bomb. "Since Adam and Eve ate the apple," read the text, "man has never refrained from any folly of which he was capable." He had a passionate love for this same wicked, folly-ridden creature, man. Some called it quixotic but Russell was well aware of the monstrous cruelties his passion encompassed. He was like those favored figures of Shakespeare's imagination, romantic skeptics who, like Hamlet, were disgusted by the animal in man and the vanity in his works, yet recognized him as the noblest of creations. It was in this ability to embrace antitheses that the compelling magnetism of Russell lay. You had in Russell's presence at once awesome tradition, genius, and age, and from the very center of all these humbling radiances, a ninety-year-old imp who would puncture the illusion, the pomp and heroic vision with a deflating barb. As his old friend Leonard Woolf once remarked of Russell, "It is very rare to be a Socrates and a Puck at the same time."

Nothing was more alien to Russell than posturing, and nothing more devastating to pretension than his own searing vision: if there is a lesson in his life, it is that in the last analysis, the truly heroic can arise only on the ground of the relentlessly real.

* * *

"In his youth he did work of importance in mathematical logic, but his eccentric attitude toward the First World War revealed a lack of balanced judgment, which increasingly infected his later writings." So Russell wrote of himself in a mock obituary which he composed in 1937. But this whimsy became, in the eyes of editorial writers in the great Western newspapers, reality, and their abuse of the political writings and activities of his last years was unstinting. These culminated in an incredible viciousness directed against the last great effort of his life—the pitting of his intellect and final energies against the American destruction of Vietnam.

From the editorial page of the *New York Times,* under the headline "Corpse on Horseback," C. L. Sulzberger "informed" readers that Russell had "outlived his own conscious ideas and [become] clay in . . . unscrupulous hands." The tragedy of the War Crimes Tribunal, Sulzberger continued, "cannot fairly be laid at the door of the wasted peer whose bodily endurance outpaced his brain. . . ." This was written in May 1967, a week before Russell's ninety-fifth birthday, when the Tribunal was in session, and while Lyndon Johnson was still president of the United States. It was written before the revelations about the massacres at My Lai and elsewhere, and before the great revulsion against the war which broke forth in the massive Moratorium demonstrations. Even now, however, the consensus of obituaries on Russell is that this last gesture (referred to variously as a "mock trial" or the "notorious trial") was something to be ashamed of, a final unfortunate surrender to the naiveté, caprice and inconsistency which characterized his involvement in social affairs.

Such a distortion is easily conjured out of the press symbols of Russell's career. To see Russell clearly across the near century of his life, however, is to comprehend the inner consistency of his stance, from his resistance to World War I, through his nuclear protests, to his last defense of Vietnam's revolutionary peasants—this final act, the hardest, the most courageous, the most important gesture of all.

Russell's very first book was a critical account of German Marxism (with an appendix by his wife Alys on Marxism and the woman question). His first venture into politics saw him stand unsuccessfully as a candidate for Parliament with women's suffrage as one of his main planks.

In *Roads to Freedom* (1918), Russell outlined a program of guild socialism and laid down the two principles of reform in international relations which became the all-consuming cause of the last decade-and-a-half of his life: "First, the avoidance of wars, and, second, the prevention of the oppression of weak nations by strong ones."

It was the *Practice and Theory of Bolshevism* (1920), written on his return from a trip to revolutionary Russia where he met Lenin and Trotsky, that established Russell's reputation as an early anticommunist. What he had written about this crisis in world history, however, was something quite different from what his reputation as a "liberal anticommunist" might suggest. "I believe," Russell declared at the outset, "that Communism is necessary to the world, and believe that the heroism of Russia has fired men's hopes in a way which was essential to the realization of Communism in the future. Regarded as a splendid attempt, without which ultimate success would have been very improbable, Bolshevism deserves the gratitude and admiration of all the progressive part of mankind."

It was the method by which the Bolsheviks were attempting to establish socialism that caused Russell's doubts. What he reacted to most negatively in this "method" was its fanatical intolerance and its welcoming of class war and its hatreds which the counterrevolution had, he conceded, made necessary. With the advent of Stalin came the institutionalization of the worst elements and tendencies in Bolshevism as he had witnessed them in 1920. It was only after Stalin's death, and the subsequent changes in Soviet policy, that Russell's view of Russian communism became less censorious. In this he was greatly influenced, as were many other socialists, by the writings of the Marxist biographer of Trotsky, Isaac Deutscher, whom he later chose to serve on the War Crimes Tribunal.*

Prior to Russell's invitation, Deutscher had not participated in a political action since the 1930s, when he had been expelled from the Polish Communist party (whose entire central committee later perished at Stalin's hands) for "exaggerating the dangers of Nazism" and similar Trotskyist

* In fact Russell had been in touch with Deutscher previously, and Deutscher used to visit him at his house in Richmond in the early fifties.

sins. Denounced as a Marxist revolutionary by the right, as a spokesman for Wall Street by the Communists, and as a Stalinist apologist by the Trotskyists, Deutscher had lived the last thirty years of his life in political isolation for his principles, a situation which Russell understood well.

I remember how moved Deutscher was when we brought him the invitation from Russell, and how deep was the respect which this classical European Marxist expressed for the English empiricist's life and work. The Russell-Deutscher relationship subsequently provided one of the most touching and fulfilling moments in the Tribunal proceedings. On November 13, 1966, the Tribunal met for the first time in closed session in London. Russell appeared and read a brief statement asserting the need for such a Tribunal "composed of men eminent, not through their power, but through their intellectual and moral contribution to what we optimistically call 'human civilization.' " When he finished, there was a respectful silence as he turned, and with his usual slight annoyance at the hands that went out to help him, began the slow, aching, proud steps that would take him to the door. I understood the silence—again that awesome gap between the figure and his audience, though this was a group considerably closer in age and in distinction than most—but I felt it still and especially inadequate. And then Deutscher rose and addressed him for all the others, for the French philosopher Jean-Paul Sartre, for the Yugoslav historian Vladimir Dedijer, for the eminent mathematician Laurent Schwartz and the rest. Deutscher, who orally dictated his epic historical works, had the most literary and finely architected speaking style of anyone I have ever heard, and now his Central European accents filled the room as he told Russell what a magnificent and courageous task he had undertaken, what a beacon of hope he was to the young, what a light to the oppressed, and what a debt of gratitude was owed to him. The old man nodded, visibly moved, and then turned again to make his slow way out.

* * *

Each of the principal Tribunal figures was, like Russell, one of those displaced intellectuals that had been cast into the twilight zones of politics because of his commitment to the Enlightenment ideals that capitalism and imperialism had made impossible, and that the Stalinist revolutions had betrayed. There was Sartre, the president of the Tribunal, who had traveled from existentialism to Marxism, but because of his fierce and principled independence had been compelled to live a political career under attack from Communists and liberals alike. And there was Dedijer, the chairman, a thrice-wounded Communist partisan, once one of the four top leaders in Yugoslavia, who had been cast into internal exile for defending Milovan Djilas, even though he did not share Djilas's views.

These men, and most of the other Tribunal members, were Marxists, it is true, albeit independent ones. Russell's intellectual distance from Marxism, however, has been exaggerated (on occasion even by himself). Where the basic divergence really lay was in Russell's stress on psychological factors as motive forces in history, and even more profoundly in his skeptical outlook, which was both philosophical and constitutional: "Throughout my life," he wrote in the second volume of his *Autobiography,* "I have longed to feel that oneness with large bodies of human beings that is experienced by the members of enthusiastic crowds. The longing has often been strong enough to lead me into self-deception. I have imagined myself in turn a Liberal, a Socialist, or a Pacifist, but I have never been any of these things, in any profound sense. Always the sceptical intellect, when I have most wished it silent, has whispered doubts to me, has cut me off from the facile enthusiasms of others, and has transported me into a desolate solitude." These lines were written apropos his antiwar activities during the First World War, when he worked with "Quakers, non-resisters and Socialists" as an ally, but not a comrade. He would tell the Quakers that some wars were justified, and the Socialists that he opposed the tyranny of the state, and get suspicious looks from both.

World War I and its aftermath had deepened Russell's skepticism to the point of despair. "The optimist now," he wrote in 1948, "is the man who thinks it possible to hope that the world will not get worse; to suppose that it may get better in any near future is scarcely possible except through willful blindness." In the last two decades that Russell lived after these words were written, and especially after the development of the hydrogen bomb in 1953, he dedicated his political energies not only to the end that the world should not become a worse place to live, but that it should not cease to be a place to live altogether. In 1954, he concluded a radio broadcast on the hydrogen bomb by saying, "I appeal to you as a human being to human beings: remember your humanity, and forget the rest. If you can do so, the way lies open to a new paradise; if you cannot, nothing lies before you but universal death." In 1955 he initiated a joint manifesto of scientists from both East and West (a radical departure for the times) warning against the dangers of nuclear annihilation. From that time on he became the intellectual symbol of the struggle against the bomb.

In 1957 he launched the Pugwash conferences of East-West nuclear scientists, which had an important influence on the subsequent development of the nuclear test ban, and in 1958 helped to found the Campaign for Nuclear Disarmament, which he served as president. In 1960, when the CND and its Aldermaston marches were at the height of their popularity, he resigned as president to lead a campaign of mass civil disobedience under the auspices of a "Committee of 100." Early in 1961, Russell led a sitdown of five thousand people at the Ministry of Defense. Later in the year he addressed a meeting in Hyde Park, which was stopped by the police. Russell was arraigned with other members of the Committee for inciting civil disobedience and was sent to Brixton prison for seven days. (He had previously spent six months there for his opposition to World War I.)

This frail eighty-nine-year-old had replied with a firm "No I won't" when the magistrate offered to exempt him from jail if he pledged himself to good behavior. When the sentence was pronounced, cries of protest went up from the onlookers. This gesture of concern wounded the old man's pride. "It angered me," he said. "I knew that it was well-meant, but I had deliberately incurred the punishment and, in any case, I could not see that age had anything to do with guilt. If anything, it made me more guilty. The Magistrate seemed to me nearer the mark in observing that, from his point of view, I was 'old enough to know better.' "

In October 1962, the Cuban missile crisis brought mankind to the brink of disaster that Russell had fought so long. The crisis over America's former neocolonial dependency, coupled with the steady escalation of U.S. intervention in Indochina, brought to a climax a change in Russell's sense of the priorities involved in mankind's survival. In many ways this change represented a return for him to his perspective when he first raised his voice in rebellion during the 1914 War which, he noted wryly on his ninetieth birthday that year, had been the war to end peace.

Nineteen-fourteen marked for him a dividing line not only between eras, but between worlds. A phrase in a diary note he set down a week before his birthday in 1950 expresses the almost preternatural significance of that date for him. Writing of the marital difficulties of his children he says: "They were born after 1914, and are therefore incapable of happiness."

* * *

During the years of his opposition to the First World War and his consequent isolation, there was one figure who stood out above all the rest in Russell's admiration and foreshadowed his own future course. E. D. Morel was a liberal crusader against the atrocities being committed by white Europeans in Africa, particularly the Belgian Congo, and was the founder of the Congo Reform Association. A major theme of Morel's work was that the bestiality, violence and aggression of European imperialism in Africa had come home to roost in the European conflict. For this, he was (in Russell's words) "more than any other opponent of the war . . . attacked by politicians and the press," and was eventually thrown in jail, where "he suffered an injury to his health from which he never recovered," dying in 1922.

Russell himself recognized the economic, as well as the moral and political, interaction between imperialism and the World War, and in 1934 finished his book *Freedom and Organization* with the following admonition: "The same causes that produced war in 1914 are still operative, and, unless checked by international control of investment and of raw material, they will inevitably produce the same effect, but on a larger scale. It is not by pacifist sentiment, but by a world-wide economic organization, that civilized mankind is to be saved from collective suicide."

For a considerable period, coinciding with the early Cold War, Russell had thought that Stalin's tyranny was taking an expansionist turn, patterned on the Napoleonic episode after the French Revolution. Since the mid-fifties, however, like many others, he had changed his views and recognized the essential conservatism of Stalin's foreign policy. Nuclear weapons had made the ambition of global empire a possibility, but it was the "free world" empire of the United States, with its thousands of overseas bases, and property rights to most of the world's natural resources, that was expanding across continents and oceans, intervening in underdeveloped countries and raising threats to world peace. "As my researches into the origins and circumstances of the war in Vietnam showed, the United States was embarking upon military adventures which increasingly replaced war with Russia as the chief threat to the world. The fanaticism of America's anti-Communism, combined with its constant search for markets and raw materials, made it impossible for any serious neutral to regard America and Russia as equally dangerous to the world." So Russell wrote at the end of volume 3 of his *Autobiography,* adding that, "For people in the West, this was most difficult to admit, and again I experienced the silence or opposition of those who had come to accept my views of the previous decade."

There is a control in these words, a suppression of personal bitterness and pain wholly characteristic of the man, which gives no hint of the vicious weapons of attack that were wielded against him in his last years, the wounds he suffered, or the anguish of the battle he fought. Even now, one can only guess at their measure. To attend the press conference announcing the War Crimes Tribunal, for example, Russell, now a few months shy of ninety-five, undertook the long trip to London in the dead of winter. Caxton Hall, where the conference was held, has a winding staircase which must have seemed interminable to the old man as he mounted it at a snail's pace to confront the glaring inquisitorial klieglights and the hatchet faces of the world's press jammed in intimidating, hostile numbers in the inadequate room. For his attempt to lend an aged hand to the Vietnamese, the most distinguished living philosopher in the West was featured in the august *New York Times Magazine,* which described his entry thus: "A stir, a bustle, a craning of necks; he comes! *He* comes? Say rather, without disrespect, *it* comes. . . . The man who has now become the holiest relic the international left possesses is to be unwrapped and shown to the populace."

It was not only the West that dealt blows to Russell at this hour. Because the Tribunal was independent, and because the uncompromising terms of its mandate would make cooperation with the United States more difficult, the Communist countries had disapproved of the Tribunal from the outset. By their silence, the Soviet and East European press assured a minimal awareness of the Tribunal's findings in the white sectors of the world where that awareness was needed most.

From its inception, the Tribunal had no real base of support, beyond the agreement of the Vietnamese to cooperate. The money to finance its $200,000 costs came almost entirely from Russell himself, who had only a modest annual income from books. As a young man he had given away his inheritance, and the controversies which arose over his antiwar activities and liberated views on sex made university appointments scarce. Readers of the *Autobiography* know what a struggle it was for him for decades to live on royalties from his books, so that it was a poignant and touching irony that when the advances on the *Autobiography* brought him a small fortune for the second time in his life, he gave it all to the War Crimes Tribunal.

It is difficult to know how deeply the unscrupulous reporting of the prestige press in the West, along with the lack of immediate success of the Tribunal, affected Russell. His ninety-fifth birthday took place just after the first Tribunal session. In contrast to his ninetieth, when an orchestra had played in his honor and he had been toasted by lords, ladies, old distinguished friends and celebrated intellects, this one saw him once again isolated, probably more than he had ever been. The Tribunal had deprived him of being regarded affectionately as a remarkable antique from the Victorian era, to be trotted out for annual celebrations. He had done something that old men aren't supposed to do: he had rebelled against the respectability his age and achievements guaranteed him. As a younger man, he had raised his voice against the bourgeois morality that stifled sex, and now he protested against the morality that sanctified official murder.

The battle which Russell had chosen to enter in his last years was infinitely bloodier and dirtier than the previous ones he had come through so well. In part this was in the nature of the contest. It was as though a revered prince of the Philistines had taken his stance by the side of David and slung verbal thunderbolts at the giant. To oppose in its own citadel white Western civilization, to take up the cause of the niggers of the earth, to lay the finger of blame on the technological Goliath, the "last best hope" of liberal democracy, as it committed mass murder in the rice paddies of Southeast Asia—this was to court devastation. And thus, the media of the Western world entered a loose conspiracy to take revenge against Russell by portraying him as a senescent, bird-like and wrinkled creature who should have done himself the favor of dying when his reputation as a humanist and philosopher was unsullied by such follies as intruding in global politics on the side of the weak and oppressed.

But there was another, more personal, cross which Russell had to bear into the conflict. In his last triumphant battle as the head and inspirer of the "Committee of 100," he had stood forth as advocate and antagonist and led his troops in his own person into the fray. Between then and the Tribunal the body had begun to give up. No longer could he speak extemporaneously before the public: the eyes had weakened, and read only with immense effort under the television lights;

the voice was thinner and seemed at times ready to disappear forever; the dignified stride had collapsed into an unseemly shuffle; and the face often became slack, giving a false impression of vacuity that the incomparably quick mind still burning inside must have found especially painful to bear.

History has already vindicated the public acts of Lord Russell's last years: the historical record will show that the War Crimes Tribunal—the climax of what began as a lonely crusade—correctly characterized and identified a war of atrocity, a war conducted to maintain imperial dominance in Southeast Asia, a war representing the archetypal conflict of the age and the chief threat to mankind's future survival. But history will not show the inner struggle of the man who initiated this Tribunal. It will not record the triumph of an heroic will that could not hear the cry of suffering without attempting to answer, or the passionate concern for human survival that moved an old man to put himself in an international pillory before the greatest power in the world as the defender of a peasant people and its struggle to be free.

For most, Lord Russell will be remembered as the great mathematician and philosopher, the man whose life encompassed the transition from Victorianism to the modern world, the friend of men as various as Alfred North Whitehead and D. H. Lawrence. But for me, the image was formed on that first day in Chelsea: the arduous shuffle, the pixy smile, the brittle bowed movements, the kind, wise face which hid the anguish of its own struggle.

To have known him is always to be humbled by the courage, the immense guts of the old man, and the sustaining calm of the inner vision: "An individual human existence should be like a river," he had written, "—small at first, narrowly confined within its banks, and rushing passionately past boulders and over waterfalls. Gradually the river grows wider, the banks recede, the waters flow more quietly, and in the end, without any visible break, they become merged in the sea, and painlessly lose their individual being. The man who, in old age, can see his life in this way, will not suffer from the fear of death, since the things he cares for will continue. . . . I should wish to die while still at work, knowing that others will carry on what I can no longer do, and content in the thought that what was possible has been done."

Isaac Deutscher: The Man and His Work

i

Throughout his life Isaac Deutscher remained a lonely, if towering, figure on the political and intellectual landscape of his time. This is not to say that his genius lacked recognition: his talents were so formidable that they compelled recognition. But despite his achievements as a renowned biographer, historian and Marxist, he was, in a deeper sense, a leader without a following, a shepherd without a flock. Like Trotsky, the protagonist of his biographical masterpiece, who became a "prophet unarmed" in postrevolutionary Russia, Deutscher was for most of his life a political stranger in his epoch, "condemned to hurl the lightning and thunder of his words into the void."

This is the introduction to *Isaac Deutscher: The Man and His Work* (London: MacDonald, 1971). An earlier version served as the text of a eulogy delivered at a memorial meeting for Isaac Deutscher held at Gandhi Hall, London, October 1967.

A survivor of the classic period of Bolshevism, with a revolutionary vision too piercing and authentic to meet the standards of Stalinist and anti-Stalinist orthodoxy, Deutscher was long condemned to the isolation of a political heretic. But with the birth of a new revolutionary left in the years since the Soviet "de-Stalinization" of 1956, Deutscher's work has stood apart from the discarded sectarian curios to serve as a vital link between revolutionary generations, between the traditions and achievements of the old revolutionary left and the new.

The New Left began as a healthy reaction against the stultifying doctrinal hang-ups of its elders, proudly unconcerned with foreign social systems and theories. This ingenuousness, important in its time, has increasingly given way to a strong impulse toward revolutionary internationalism. And this restores the experience of the Russian Revolution to central relevance again, not as an historic clash between the policies and personalities of Trotsky and Stalin, but as a primary watershed of a continuing revolutionary development. The Russian paradox—between classical Marxism, which is a theory of revolution for industrialized, formally democratic capitalist societies, and the actual birthplace of the revolution in pre-industrial, autocratic Tsarist Russia—this paradox has been repeated over and over in the succeeding era, in China and beyond.

The enigma that absorbed Isaac Deutscher's genius, the contradictions and tensions manifested in the Trotsky-Stalin split, between European and non-European Marxism, between "post-scarcity" and scarcity economies and cultures, have revealed themselves to lie at the heart of revolutionary internationalism: the attempt to forge a worldwide revolutionary front in an unevenly developed and nationally divided world. A theory was needed which would be adequate to the times.

Deutscher's account of the Soviet development, through his biographies of the two epochal figures in whom the conflict was polarized, provided such a theory, though it was not articulated in any formal way. Schematizing was alien to the style of Deutscher's Marxism and to his sense of human and social complexities. Marxism for him was not a dogma, but a method to be used with all the subtlety and nuance demanded by life's infinitely various textures. He was always fond of pointing out how much richer in complexities was the Marx of the historical works on Louis Napoleon and the class struggles in France than the Marx of the celebrated Preface to the *Critique of Political Economy,* who briefly summarized the principles of his outlook. It is an impressive measure of Deutscher's Marxism that the quality of his work is immediately apparent to the layman whose eye does not sketch out the sources of its architecture, but whose sensibility can appreciate a masterpiece when it sees one.

In his own life, Deutscher in a sense lived the dialectic he grappled with in his works. He joined the Polish Communist party in 1926 at the age of nineteen. As the revolution in Russia began to succumb to the chauvinism and backwardness of its national environment, Deutscher joined the Trotskyist Opposition, which was struggling to arrest Bolshevism's departure from traditional Marxist and socialist norms. In 1932 he was expelled from the party for "spreading panic about Nazism." The liberals and social democrats were held to pose the primary political dangers. During the next years he continued his opposition, attempting in vain to stir up resistance in the left to the mass terror in Russia and the infamous purge trials in which the Leninist old guard perished, virtually to a man.

In 1938, however, when, convinced that the Third International was morally dead, Trotsky launched its "successor," Deutscher demurred. "The creation of every one of the earlier Internationals," argued Deutscher at the time, "constituted a definite threat to bourgeois rule." This would not be the case with the Fourth International, because no significant section of the working class would respond to its manifesto and it would become a mere collection of sects. It was necessary, he maintained, to wait for a new upsurge of revolutionary forces.

Deutscher was thus cut off even from the defeated Trotskyist Opposition. It was at this point that his lonely sojourn began, a sojourn that Deutscher's genius transformed into a unique contribution to the international revolutionary movement and its future regeneration. Having belonged to those whom Stalin had defeated, Deutscher set out systematically to examine why Stalin had won, why the revolutionary development had taken the course that it did. Ultimately, Deutscher came to see Stalinism differently from Trotsky, who emphasized the Machiavellian usurpation and bureaucratic betrayal of the revolution. For Deutscher, the incipient degeneration of the revolution was already manifest when both Lenin and Trotsky were in the full vigor of their leadership and power, and was the result of the isolation of the revolution and the autocratic backwardness of its national setting. Moreover, Deutscher saw in Stalinism not merely a Thermidorian bureaucracy, subverting and arresting the revolutionary development, but a bureaucratic revolution, itself carrying through that development, though in a distorted form, with the barbarous means and the primitive outlook of its native surroundings.

For this, Deutscher was made a heretic and an outcast from the left: damned by the Stalinists for maintaining his Marxist ideals and outlook against the debasement of the revolution, and denounced by the anti-Stalinists for affirming that the brutally realized achievements of Stalin *were* revolutionary, however truncated and disfigured they may have been.

Deutscher resisted the temptation to cut through the tangled ambiguities of the Russian Revolution with a sharp slogan. But neither was he seeking to mediate between old enemies with a scholastic formula of revolutionary sin and grace. He was set apart from those, including Trotsky, who were trapped in a dualism that Deutscher knew must be understood in order to be transcended.

What is now usually called the "new left" became such by detaching itself from the "old" during the de-Stalinization period in Russia three decades after Lenin's death, and the first eruption of the Trotsky-Stalin conflict. This historical conjuncture was by no means accidental, for it was only the dethronement of Russian Stalinism after the Khrushchev report that made space for the new movement, liberating it from the tutelage of Soviet Marxism and its subordination to Soviet policies. "New left" means, in effect, the left beyond Stalinism (and Trotskyism), and *that* (within Marxism) is the meaning of Deutscher's work as well.

ii

Deutscher, the biographer of Stalin and Trotsky, left no autobiographical statement. Yet in fragments of his work, which like all art contain a large element of introspection, we can see reflected the essential features of his own character and achievement. A decade before he died, Deutscher gave a lecture titled "The Message of the Non-Jewish Jew" in which he discussed six Jewish heretics, who were also great revolutionaries of modern thought, including Spinoza, Marx, Rosa Luxemburg and Trotsky. As Deutscher so often used a literary image to bind up complex themes in his larger works, so he began this lecture with a symbolic story: When still a child, he had come across a scene in the *Midrash* which had gripped his young imagination. It was from the narrative of Rabbi Meir, the great saint and pillar of Mosaic orthodoxy, who took lessons in theology from a heretic bearing the nick-name *Akher,* the Stranger. Once, on a Sabbath, Rabbi Meir had gone out on a trip with his teacher, and as usual they had become engaged in deep argument. So intently had Rabbi Meir listened to the words of wisdom falling from heretical lips that he failed to notice that he and his teacher had reached the ritual boundary which Jews were not allowed to cross on the Sabbath. At this point the great heretic indicated to his pupil, the Rabbi, that they had reached the boundary, whereupon the Rabbi turned and went back to the Jewish community, "while the heretic rode on–beyond the boundaries of Jewry."

So intrigued was the young Deutscher by this story, that when he was thirteen (and still an orthodox Jew) he began to write a drama about Rabbi Meir and the heretic Akher, and tried to find out more about Akher's character. For the boy was deeply impressed by the figure of Akher and the enigmas which his story posed to an orthodox viewpoint. "Why," the boy wondered, "did Rabbi Meir take his lessons from the heretic? . . . Who was he? . . . He appeared to be in Jewry and yet out of it. He showed a curious respect for his pupil's orthodoxy when he sent him back to the Jews on the holy Sabbath; but he himself, disregarding canon and ritual, rode beyond the boundaries. . . . What made him transcend Judaism?" These were the questions that agitated the young Deutscher.

In retrospect, it is not at all surprising that the adolescent boy, who was to renounce his own religious upbringing shortly afterwards, should have been impressed with the heretic Akher, nor that the biographer of the heretic Trotsky should, a third of a century later, still be compelled by the wisdom of the haggadic tale. Indeed, how well the figure of Akher fits Deutscher himself. For Deutscher was also the heretic of communism who in the post-Stalin decade became a teacher, mainly to rank-and-file communists, but to not a few "rabbis" of communism as well. "To those of us," wrote a former communist miner after Deutscher's death—"to those of us who were groping, in the '50s, for an explanation of the brutally irrational distortions which had cramped the life of the socialist movement, the almost lone voice of Deutscher came as a blinding revelation."

And Deutscher was no less the heretic-stranger, who appeared to be in communism and yet not in it, to be of communism and yet not of it, and who, like Akher, showed a curious respect for his pupils' orthodoxy, and a care lest they wander beyond the boundaries of Marxism and of communism, and become lost.

And it was Deutscher who, alone among European socialists, was invited by the American New Left, to whom his Marxism itself was then heretical, to address them at their great antiwar teach-ins. And it was Deutscher who proclaimed at Berkeley to this New Left the urgency of giving back to class struggle its old dignity, and of restoring meaning once more to the idea of communism. Listen again to the voice of Deutscher's communist pupil: "For so many of us, he was a regenerator of hope. In him we found the link between humanism and socialism which allowed us to rediscover Marx himself and our own history." The very essence of Deutscher's work was the transcendence of communism, in the Hegelian sense; of preserving the best, the real achievement, of the old, even while surpassing and annulling it towards the new.

Hand-Me-Down Marxism and the New Left

The rafters of the Chicago Coliseum had hardly ceased to reverberate with the chants of the rival factions, when the ghost of Karl Marx was being heaped with blame for the SDS debacle. "Alas," mourned establishment pundits in ill-concealed triumph, "the New Left has finally gone the primrose way of the Old. Marxism has at last cursed it with factional wars and historical irrelevance. The apostles of ultra-democratic revolution and 'power to the people' (the most incendiary notion in the modern world) have shown themselves ready, if inept, practitioners of the art of political manipulation. The idol-smashing revolutionary vanguard has again been revealed as a latter-day religious cult prostrating itself before patron saints and overseas meccas, while suppressing the heresy of thought with mind-gluing incantations from holy scriptures. R.I.P."

But the smug obituaries are, to say the least, premature. The "movement" is first of all larger than any of its organizations. The virility of the New Left, the sheer vitality of its actions and the deep, deep roots of its culture of rebellion will surely bypass the martinets of any Bible-toting, icon-worshiping elite, should such a group seek to impose its Law—whether from the closeted cells of a Maoist sect or through the once open forum of SDS. For the time being at least, this remains the revolution that can't be taken over.

Nonetheless, the still unfolding fate of SDS—until now the central organization of (white) student struggle—cannot remain a matter of indifference to the radical movement from which it draws its strength and which, in turn, it inspires. Too much of the tried and tested leadership, too much of the best and most militant energies of the left are caught up in the current enthrallment of SDS for the outcome not to have significance for the movement as a whole.

What is at the source of SDS's descent into a politics at once so claustrophobic and incomprehensible as to virtually insure the isolation and defeat of those who adopt it? A politics so antagonistic to the imaginative, open spirit and creative action that has informed and powered the New Left since its emergence from the ashes of the Old a decade ago? The present vanguard seems to have forgotten that the New Left had to midwife its own birth precisely *because* the old line-toeing, Lenin/Stalin/Mao-quoting vanguard had finally encased itself in a sectarian, sterile solitude where it had only its own self-righteousness for company.

One can readily appreciate why liberals would rush to attribute the difficulties of America's New Left (and the demise of the Old) to "Marxism." Liberalism's Great American Celebration of the Fifties had all but disappeared in the Great American Disintegration of the Sixties. The bankruptcy of the liberal world-view has become more and more self-evident with each new stage of the social crisis. Who can still put credence in the basic tenets of the postwar liberal faith: the essential harmony and pluralistic democracy of America's "affluent" society, the alleged solution of the fundamental problems of the Industrial Revolution, the end of class-based struggle and its revolutionary ideologies? If the new generation has absorbed one lesson, it has been that of the vacuity of liberal analysis, the hypocrisy of liberal preachment and the collusion of liberal practice in the imperialist and racist world system of U.S. corporate capital.

How lucid Marxism—with its focus on the inequities and irrationalities of the status quo—now looks in comparison to the soothing obfuscations of the liberal mind. For what is Marxism but the recognition of the class pivot of history and the class basis of social oppression, coupled with a clear commitment to one side of the social struggle: the side of the oppressed against their oppressors? Far from being a handicap, the discovery of Marxism by the movement has put within its grasp the possibility of becoming a serious revolutionary force for the first time. A long-range perspective on real social tendencies (not illusory promises, superficial harmonies and surface stabilities) is essential to the development and success of any movement for social change and transformation, and it is Marxism above all other ideologies that has shown itself capable of providing such a perspective for the capitalist era.

But there is Marxism and there is Marxism. A Marxism which is developed in a concrete social context, which is flexible, open, and unafraid to re-think its revolutionary perspectives according to specific conditions, and which fashions its language as a means of communication, analysis and mobilization, rather than employing it merely as ritualistic invocation, can be just the powerful instrument that a revolutionary movement requires.

But there is also Marxism of the hand-me-down variety, where an ideological perspective and vocabulary developed in a different epoch or a different political-cultural environment is transposed whole and adopted as an all-embracing wisdom.

This attempt to don the ideological garments of the victims of imperialism and their vanguard may satisfy many egos and assuage much guilt, but it doesn't help to build radical constituencies and revolutionary forces in the United States. Yet such a direction appears to be developing in SDS, where both major factions at the Chicago convention spoke in the language of Maoism and put forth a Maoist model of the world revolutionary process as their own.

The self-styled Marxist-Leninist-Maoists of SDS would do well to remember that the New Left grew out of two bankruptcies—not just liberalism, but old-line Marxism as well. The failure of Marxist (or Marxist-Leninist, or Marxist-Trotskyist) vanguard parties to build revolutionary movements in the advanced capitalist countries is an historic fact that no revolutionary can afford to ignore. The "Marxist-Leninist" groups which exist in these countries have either isolated themselves as sterile sects, or transformed themselves into basically reformist organizations like the Italian and French Communist parties. A careful analysis of these failures will show that hand-me-down Marxism and overseas mecca-watching played a significant role in each.

Can Maoism, the new vogue in SDS ideology, itself provide a reliable guide to the causes of the impasse in Western revolutionary Marxism? There is little reason to think so. According to Maoist theory, the key to all contemporary developments in the international revolutionary movement is Khrushchev's denunciation of Stalin in 1956, which marks the emergence of "modern revisionism" and its doctrines of "peaceful coexistence" and "peaceful transition" to socialism (in certain "favorable" circumstances). But the historical record shows that the reformism of the Western Communist parties (not to mention most of those in the Third World) predates Khrushchev's denunciation of Stalin by at least two and probably three decades, as does the promulgation of the so-called "modern revisionist" doctrine of peaceful coexistence between the systems.

Of course, this is not merely a case of error in historical interpretation on the part of the Chinese. The fact is that the Chinese Communist party, in order to pursue its ideological struggle with the Kremlin, has deliberately rewritten the history of even its own movement to obscure the role of Stalin both in obstructing the Chinese Revolution and in transforming the Communist parties in Europe and elsewhere into reformist organizations.

A theory such as Maoism, in which the answers to key questions are based on the rewriting of history, can hardly provide a sound guide to revolutionary practice in the long run. Sooner or later the manipulation of facts will lead to a gap which cannot be bridged by administrative measures and historical legerdemain. Perhaps the gap will not be as large as that which developed in the Stalin era and which discredited and disoriented a whole revolutionary generation in the West. However, the very existence of the gap will prove crippling to a party which tries to build a revolutionary program across it, for *integrity* is a basic weapon in the revolutionary arsenal, just as the ability to grasp real social relationships and forces is its greatest strength. A revolutionary movement thrives on candor just as surely as a ruling class lives by deception.

The penchant for ideological manipulation is not peculiarly Chinese. To some extent, any revolutionary party which achieves power in an underdeveloped country must itself become a ruling stratum. The problems of industrialization, education and democratization (including the liberation of internal nationalities) still lie before it, and it must deal with these problems in the face of encirclement and armed hostility from imperialist forces. Moreover, the urban proletariat in such a country is itself so underdeveloped as to be incapable of providing the leadership prescribed for it in the classic Marxist conception. Historically, therefore, the revolutionary party has tended to substitute itself for the revolutionary class and, as a consequence, to resort to the techniques of manipulation and deception reminiscent of (but by no means equivalent to) the techniques used by the ruling classes of old. (The practice tends to vary: in some revolutionary countries, like Cuba, the level of revolutionary candor has been extraordinarily high;* in others such as Russia, the reverse has been true.) In any event, because of these distortions, the attempt to transplant uncritically such revolutionary ideologies into the revolutionary movement in the United States serves to weaken the movement in a profound way.

A further element of distortion in the official ideologies of underdeveloped revolutionary regimes is introduced by the contradictions arising from the conservative character of the nation-state itself, a factor which has received little attention from Marxist theoreticians to date. Thus China's support for the reactionary military dictatorship in Pakistan (and its silence during the repression of working-class strikes and student demonstrations after the fall of Ayub Khan) may be understandable from the point of view of the state interests of China and the diplomatic support it received from the Ayub regime; but from the point of view of the international revolutionary movement, which Peking aspires to lead, it can only be seen in a very different light.

These are not academic points. The "weatherman" statement of the majority faction in the new SDS leadership (non-PL) is built around the strategic concept of "people's war" as laid down by China's Lin Piao. The concept envisages a united people's front of Third World liberation forces encircling the principal metropolis of imperialism—the United

* Three years later, this unfortunately seems to be less and less the case.

States. The concept is derived from China's own revolution, which was fought as a national war of liberation against the Japanese and progressed from its peasant base in the countryside to the towns.

The inadequacy of such a concept for a world characterized by uneven levels of development in which nationalism and its offspring, the nation-state, are still vital historical factors, needs no emphasis. One has only to look at the contradiction between China's policy and Pakistan's revolution, or even more obviously at the Sino-Soviet split (neither the Soviet Union nor the Sino-Soviet split receives any mention in the fifteen-thousand-word global analysis called "weatherman") to see how abstract and unrealistic such a projection can be.

No doubt, a consistent perspective in the Maoist vein can still be constructed by ignoring the tensions between revolutionary policy and *raison d'état,* and by assigning the Soviet Union to the imperialist camp (a ploy which makes a mirage both of the arms race between Russia and the U.S. and of their military support for opposing sides in revolutionary struggles such as in Vietnam and Cuba). There are obviously more things on revolutionary earth than are dreamt of in Maoist and "weatherman" philosophy; these are things, moreover, which a revolutionary movement ignores at its peril.

The main consequence so far of SDS's new-found orientation is its essentially fifth-column mentality and its largely negative vision of revolution in its home environment. It is not surprising that Lin Piao and the Chinese should see the struggle against U.S. imperialism in negative terms (get off our backs), but the transposition of this attitude to the supposed revolutionary vanguard inside the imperialist powers renders it self-defeating, not to say absurd. Thus the "weatherman" program in effect proposes approaching

American workers with the argument that everything they possess is plundered from the Third World (a false proposition in any case: it is the imperialists who benefit and the workers who pay the costs of imperialism), and that a revolution should be made in this country so that they can give it back.

No revolution was ever built on a negative vision. Moreover, there is no reason even to attempt to build the American revolution as a negative act, a program of social demolition. At a time when the industrial engine has reached a point in its development where it opens up a vista of material plenty and free time for all, America's imperialist system saddles its people and all mankind with militarism, war, pollution, deprivation, exploitation, racism and repression. America now possesses the means to a humane, livable, democratic future for all its citizens, but only if they are ready to seize the means of production and overthrow the system which dominates their lives just as surely as it dominates the lives of those in the Third World who suffer under its aggression and rule. That is the revolutionary foundation and the internationalist bond as well. It is certainly true that the liberation of the Third World will hasten the liberation of the U.S. But it is no less true that the American revolution is the key to the liberation of mankind. This is the insight that was missing in Chicago; let us hope that it returns to SDS before long.

(August 1969)

Revolutionary Karma vs. Revolutionary Politics

It has been almost two years since SDS went "revolutionary," splitting into Marxist-Leninist sects and Weatherman guerrillas. They haven't been good years for anyone; and on balance they haven't been good for the left at all. To be sure, there is still a growing *culture* of revolution, which is what people usually mean when they refer to the "Movement"—a profound and reflective alienation of the spirit from a system cancerous with racism, exploitation and its own aggressive expansion. The present government has done everything in its power to increase this disaffection. It clings to an imperial war for which it has no popular support and which it has pledged to give up. It is so dependent on racist political alliances that even the liberal disguise of civil rights tokenism is no longer sustained. It is unable to hide the costs of capitalist prosperity, which have been dramatically revealed by the ecology movement; and the long economic boom is over, welfare rolls mounting and budgets shrinking and the strains in the economic system impelling the government flagrantly to create the longest recession since 1933 and the highest unemployment in eighteen years, while 30 percent of the nation's manufacturing capacity stands idle.

But just when all these forces have converged to create the most fertile field for radical organizers since the Great Depression, they are virtually absent from serious politics. Not only is there no national organization of the left with any breadth of composition and program, but the main motion is in other directions: towards new "lifestyles" rather than new constituencies, towards political communes and collectives rather than parties and coalitions, towards underground violence rather than aboveground organizing. What appears to be lacking is not only the ability but the very *will* to mobilize the new energy of discontent and to convert it into a real force against the system.

In this new culture of lifestyles it has become fashionable for the group to mercilessly criticize individuals and their "bourgeois" failings. But there has been no similar impulse toward self-criticism at the organizational level. This, of course, has never been a notable feature of "vanguards"; but the growing disparity between the potential for organizing on the left and the vacuum of organized radical action (notwithstanding a rash of bombings and other militant gestures by small groups) has become impossible to ignore. If all this was not clear before, it is now that the most celebrated of the revolutionary vanguards, Weatherman, has seized the time to call for a change of political course in an underground communiqué which even for its unspoken admissions took a lot of courage to issue.

"New Morning–Changing Weather" opens with reflections on the heaviest event in Weatherman's brief and mercurial history. This is the "townhouse explosion" of about a year ago in which three young Weatherpeople were accidentally killed while manufacturing "anti-personnel bombs" to be used in what the statement describes as a "large-scale, almost random bombing offensive." The object of the offensive was "to hurt the pigs materially" because a previous firebombing attempt using less heavy technology had failed to do so. The contemplated "offensive" was evidently connected with no other objective or planned political action. According to the new communiqué: "The townhouse forever destroyed our belief that armed struggle is the only revolutionary struggle. It is time for the movement to go out into the air, to organize, to risk calling rallies and demonstrations, to convince that mass actions against the war in support of rebellions do make a difference. Only acting openly, denouncing Nixon, Agnew and Mitchell, and sharing our numbers and wisdom with young sisters and brothers will blow away the fears of the students at Kent State, the smack of the Lower East Side, and the national silence after the bombings of North Vietnam."

Anyone familiar with the development of Weatherman will be immediately struck by the tragic ironies which echo through this passage, the more so in that the politics which it advocates are such an obvious imperative now, as they have been thoughout Weatherman's existence. For it was Weatherman that, as a leadership faction in SDS, collaborated in the destruction of the only national youth organization capable of carrying out the actions it now calls for. It was Weatherman that blazed the trail to the political underground where it presently exists in hunted isolation. And it was Weatherman that defined the political context in America as a "war" situation, projecting itself as a white combat force behind the lines. Moreover, the awful accident in the townhouse followed by only three months the famous Weatherman "War Council" in Flint, Michigan, where Charles Manson became a heroic symbol and "the heavier the better" was enshrined as the criterion for revolutionary action. Yet despite all this the new statement declares that as a result of the accident "the future of our revolution has been changed decisively."

One may legitimately ask two questions. The first is why it took a year, during which bombing was celebrated as the revolutionary way in a series of communiqués, to come to this realization. The second question is perhaps more answerable: how is it possible for an accident, however tragic and painful, to lead to such a momentous result, unless the direction of revolutionary action was irresponsible and unpolitical in the first place?

But in the most characteristic aspect of the Weather Bureau statement there is no effort to analyze the politics of the problem or even to recognize the need for such an analysis. Weatherman's self-conception as a vanguard doesn't require its leadership to justify itself in political terms. Analysis is reserved for "academic ideologues"; and a revolutionary *ethos* becomes its own justification.

As if to emphasize the immunity of its political modus operandi from critical inspection, the Weatherman communiqué says that the tendency to consider "only bombings or picking up the gun as revolutionary" is a "military error"—seeming to imply that it is not political. But of course it not only *is* political, it goes to the very heart of the Weatherman strategy. By defining the situation inside America as a war situation very early in its career, Weatherman chose a politics that inevitably forced it underground as an organization, where it has now become aware—in the words of the communiqué—"that a group of outlaws who are isolated from the youth communities do not have a sense of what is going on, cannot develop strategies that grow to include large numbers of people, have become 'us' and 'them.' " If this political impasse is to be avoided by future vanguards, then its sources must be understood.

To say that Weatherman "chose" a politics that forced it

underground is not to ignore or deny the tremendous repression that the State has unleashed on all organized rebellion and dissent in America, but only to draw the proper balance between objective and subjective factors in one particular case. Virtually from the outset, Weatherman projected *itself* as an outlaw vanguard, and undertook actions, such as the Chicago "Days of Rage," which drew little political support but were seen as a proving ground for future combat forces, with "victory" being defined as having demonstrated that the enemy's military could be assaulted in open street-battle by a psyched-up "revolutionary" attack force. In short, going underground, becoming an outlaw band of urban guerrillas, was less an alternative forced on Weatherman than an *ideal* of revolutionary struggle to which they themselves aspired.

It is relatively easy now, as it was at the outset of Weatherman's career, to see the errors which were to lead them to such political bankruptcy and personal grief. In the first place, there was a drastic underestimation of the strength of the enemy. At this stage and with the present activated forces, the barricades of ruling-class power cannot be taken by revolutionary storm. American revolutionaries are dealing with the strongest power structure in the world, not one of its satrapies in some outlying outpost of the empire. In the second place, Weatherman overestimated its own strength, or more accurately the potential of the forces it was attempting to catalyze—principally the white youth ghettos to which it still refers as apparently its only revolutionary constituency. For it remains to be shown that the values of the Woodstock Nation will lead in practice to a sustained revolt against the dominant culture and its power structure. That there is no necessity in such a development is clear in the non-program articulated in Charles Reich's *The Greening of America,* where the mechanism of social change (as in all traditional religions) is an evangelical approach towards a changed consciousness. The third, and perhaps most important, political error committed by Weatherman, as already indicated, was in calling for a "war" against the American State in the absence of any support for armed conflict or any understanding of the class terms of such a conflict, so that the revolutionaries would be seen as potential allies by oppressed Americans rather than as fifth-column aliens, cardboard figures in the classic nightmares of the witch-hunting right.

All this said, it must be added that the political confusion which Weatherman exhibited from the outset, and which was recognized immediately within a large part of the Movement, had no effect on Weatherman's ability to exert a profound influence on the most energetic and intelligent cadres in SDS and the Movement generally. Moreover, the key to the present paradoxical situation and impasse is contained in this very admiration. For it was the *moral* example Weatherman set, the audacity and courage, the ability to live up to a revolutionary ideal, that reduced potential critics to silence and inspired its imitators, just as it was the *moral* dimension (rather than any intellectual substance) of its argument for war inside the mother country that carried conviction. For if Vietnamese are dying and their land is being destroyed by American power, by what bizarre structure of justice in the universe does America expect to be exempted from the consequences of its deeds and have the war stop at its borders?

Weatherman itself was always primarily a moral rather than a political phenomenon. The desire to achieve political results by gaining mass support was always distinctly secondary to the necessity of proving that "white-skin privilege" could be overcome, that the sons and daughters of "Amerikan" affluence could dare to die for their Asian brothers. In essence, the townhouse explosion was a moral witness, like that of the Quaker Norman Morrison, who burned himself and is now memorialized by the Vietnamese. The religious, not to say Kierkegaardian, overtones of the last preparation of the townhouse collective are deafening: "At the end, they believed and acted as if only those who die are proven revolutionaries. Many people had been argued into doing something they did not believe in, many had not slept for days. Personal relationships were full of guilt and fear." The tragic subordination of the political to the ethical, of reason to faith, led directly to the disaster: "The group had spent so much time willing themselves to act that they had not dealt with the basic technological considerations of safety. They had not considered the future: either what to do with the bombs if it had not been possible to reach their targets, or what to do in the following days." This oversight was not the result of mere carelessness, but reflected the priorities of the group. What was significant for them as revolutionaries was not the political consequence of the deed, but its *karma.* What was important was the *will* to bomb. Revolution here has almost ceased to be a strategy for social change and has become instead a yoga of perfection.

The religious mode of revolutionary action is not exclusive to Weatherman but has already become an important tendency in the Movement. As the commune or collective becomes increasingly the life-unit of young revolutionaries, it is likely that the tendency will be intensified. For this reason, the dangers of confusing the moral and the political must be recognized and overcome if the left is not to isolate itself utterly and inflict its own defeat. It is not that communes should be abandoned, but merely that the principles of spiritual transformation and political struggle should not be confused.

Consider the experience of a former member of a Berkeley political commune where this distinction was not recognized:

"The communal hierarchy was calibrated in units of 'revolutionary-ness.' To be on top was to be the most revolutionary. There were basically two paths of ascent. If one felt confident enough, one took the direct path, trying to establish oneself in fairly traditional terms of what it means to be revolutionary–disciplined, energetic, militant, self-sacrificial, etc. The indirect path was better suited for the less confident. This path consists in redefining what it means to be revolutionary usually in more personal and cultural terms." Thus even self-sacrifice can be a way to supremacy, given the present structure and social meaning of action. For no party or vanguard, commune or collective can transcend the environment in which it was born and is destined for an indefinite time to function. This indeed is the historical premise of the political-social revolution, which seeks to create the social space in which the utopias of the spirit can come to fruition.

"Like any other presently existing social unity," the ex-communard observes, "a commune, regardless of how revolutionary it is, is permeated with hierarchy, competition and domination. There are structural incentives which induce psychological violence. There are real things to be won and lost. The collective interest of revolutionaries is not much more harmonious than that of any other social group. And this is the real heartbreaker. After running from the terror of functioning within bourgeois social institutions and finally ending up in the libertarian wing of the Movement, I discovered that the dynamics of in-groups and out-groups, of pecking orders and advancing yourself at the expense of yourself as well as others, is–although more confusing because of its political garb–every bit as brutal as was my adolescent peer group, a prototype of bourgeois social barbarism."

The parallels between the situation inside the commune

and those present in many parts of the Movement are clear. The "most revolutionary" rise to the top of a hierarchy—despite much cant against "elitism"—in both cases. This is the critical paradox of the religious striving for perfection when introduced into the social/political struggle: that the values become inverted, that the quest for purity leads to corruption, that the attempt to incarnate the pure communist spirit leads directly to the resurrection of bourgeois barbarism. For the revolutionarily virtuous naturally assume the mantle of a priesthood, and the priesthood soon flaunts the old vices: self-righteousness, arrogance and privilege.

From the revolutionary vanguard which serves the people in the name of the revolutionary ideal, to the inquisitorial vanguard which indicts the people for failing to live up to the ideal, the transition is swift. The slogans "fight the people" and "trash the mass movement"—notorious ideological detritus of the Weatherman episode—are but the audacious formulations of a mood that is present wherever a "true" communist casts his eye on an unpurified white-skin-privileged child of the bourgeoisie.

All this is not to assert the independence of politics from ethics, but merely to call attention to the proper relationship between the two. Many who presently confuse the relation derive their revolutionary guidelines from precedents which they conceive to have been set by the Chinese and Vietnamese. Yet the principle of the primacy of the political is evident (even to a fault) in both revolutionary experiences. Thus, for example, when the Red Army was put under a strict moral code in regard to its treatment of civilians, that was precisely so that it could be recognized by them as the servants of their interests, their guardians as opposed to their oppressors. In short, the purpose of the stringent moral code was not to set them off from the masses, but to give them access to the masses, and win their confidence. When treated correctly, the moral superiority of the revolutionary is one of his principal weapons in the political struggle, and ultimately the source of his material superiority.

Contrast this with the new revolutionary militants. Already the moral-religious quest for the revolutionary ideal, without regard to the specific political context, has caused the left to forfeit its real moral superiority in the struggle. The willingness to adopt the rhetoric of war, of random violence ("blasting caps to the Capricorns," comments one of the underground papers in which the Weather Bureau communiqué appears), may in some absolute moral scale demonstrate the personal liberation of these revolutionaries from complicity in America's genocide, and may symbolically invade the imperial sanctuary. But in the time-bound realm of the political and in the atmosphere of moral ambiguity through which most people trudge, it has only lost the left its necessary role as a protector, as guardian of the human concern and antidote to the killer system.

If groups like Weatherman and the revolutionary hucksters and hipsters who have followed in its wake have done nothing else, they have helped to create a climate in which members of the Movement–let alone potential allies–no longer feel confident of their vanguards, but in fact feel threatened by them, morally if not physically. Perhaps the most damaging effect of the Weatherman syndrome is that even those who would neither join nor endorse them still accept them as the true revolutionaries. Whatever else they were they are certainly a hard act to follow. Now the workaday political organizing that must be done will seem only the shadow of an act, compared to the setting of a bomb. People have to regain confidence in the legitimacy of their politics.

The Weatherman communiqué itself points to this lesson.

It notes that Terry Robbins, who died in the townhouse, had previously prepared the political groundwork for the student awakening at Kent State, which came to fruition in the student strike against the invasion of Cambodia. No bombing offensive that Terry Robbins and his few comrades could have carried out could have matched, in real practical aid to the revolutionaries not only of Indochina but all of the Third World, the political work that he did in raising the anti-imperial, antiwar consciousness at Kent State. The imperial system is global and its margins are thin. Political struggle which denies Washington the ability to take on any intervention it deems necessary–perhaps Chile tomorrow, South Africa the day after–may be the critical factor in the destruction of the empire and the ultimate, practical survival of mankind. But it can only accomplish these ends if it can organize large masses of Americans–white as well as black and brown, straight as well as hip, worker as well as student, old as well as young.

"Serious politics," Lenin once remarked, "begin where millions of men and women are; where there are not thousands, but millions." Or, as another Lennon, John, recently said, "Let's own up now and see who's who, who is doing something about what, and who is making music and who is laying down bullshit."

(February 1971)

Trotsky and the New Left

One important lesson that the American New Left has learned to its cost over the last decade has been the wisdom of Lenin's dictum, that "without revolutionary theory, there can be no revolutionary movement." During its brief existence as a political presence, the New Left witnessed the release of vast political energies of change, and itself led massive political protests against the war in Vietnam. At the same time, however, it was unable to create a viable political instrument of its own, or to develop and sustain itself as a coherent political movement. Running the gamut from an initially "anti-ideological" posture to a feverish embrace of sectarian Marxisms and anarchism, the New Left entered the 1970s as a tendency without organization, a movement without direction—or, rather, with such a diversity of directions as to constitute a mere drift in the social and political currents of the time, rather than a driving force of revolutionary change.

* This essay originally appeared as an introduction to *Trotsky: The Great Debate Renewed* (St. Louis: New Critics Press, 1972).

In both its initial desire not to be continuous with any past or tradition, to create itself *ex nihilo,* and in its sudden impulsive adoption of prefabricated ideological constructs and political identities, the New Left revealed its peculiarly American roots. For America is itself the "new nation," willfully created: a unique rupture in the historical process. It is a land without a visible past, or more accurately, where the past is constantly being erased by the technologies of commerce, and the market's cult of the disposable, the obsolescent, and the new. To invent theory as one goes along, to conjure identities at will (and abandon them when they prove inadequate) is wholly American, and in the true tradition of its pragmatic gospel. Likewise the search for ready-made replacements for worn-out theories, the expedient appropriation of ideologies that have worked for others.

But have they? And if so, to what extent? Under what conditions? And in what context?

To revolutionize a social order, it is as necessary to understand the process of revolution as it is to understand the structure of the status quo. The revolutionary movement, no less than the social order which it seeks to change, *is* what it has been; and what it is, moreover, sets the limits of what it can become. A revolutionary theory that does not understand the conditions of revolutionary success—not only the errors of failed revolutions, but the failure of successful revolutions—does not begin to be adequate to the task at hand.

At the gateway to any attempt to establish a critical understanding of modern social revolution stands the figure of a man so "controversial" thirty years after his death that within his own country his name is expunged from the record of the revolution he led, while except for a small idolatrous segment, the revolutionary movement generally has not begun to assimilate his revolutionary role. The progenitor of virtually all revolutionary Marxist critiques of Communist revolutions and revolutionary states, vilified by Stalin as a renegade, counterrevolutionary wrecker and Fascist agent, and eventually murdered by his henchmen, Leon Trotsky was in reality one of the most extraordinary revolutionary figures of all time.

In order to lend persuavesiveness to the comments that follow, it should be noted that the present writer in no way regards himself as a "Trotskyist." Further, he considers the sterility of organized Trotskyism to be an integral part of the tragedy of international Marxism in the epoch of the Russian Revolution and its aftermath. In its long, intimate polarization with Stalinism, for example, the main Trotskyist movement in the United States (YSA-SWP) has come to practice a politics which bears uncanny resemblance to the politics of the Communist Party, USA, in the heyday of its anti-Trotsky fervor. Most ironic of all is the YSA-SWP's enthronement of the principle of "ideological homogeneity" as a doctrine of party orthodoxy, since this was the essence of Stalinism's original triumph over Trotskyism: to render all organized dissent within the Communist movement *heresy,* and by so doing establish that monolithic frame which became its hallmark, and which destroyed the ability of the international revolutionary movement to think and theorize, and ultimately to develop its praxis as a revolutionary vanguard.

The only significant actor in the Russian October of 1917 to play a major role in the revolution of 1905, Leon Trotsky personally contributed more to the Bolshevik conquest of power than any other Bolshevik leader with the exception of Lenin. So, far from being an alien in the ranks, as Stalinist historians have portrayed him, Trotsky was a man whose extraordinary talents and genius were matched by such utter integrity of purpose and dedication to the revolution that, in the midst of the civil war, Lenin authorized him, as organizer and head of the Red Army, to issue without prior consultation or approval any order that he deemed necessary to defend the Bolshevik regime.

It was Trotsky who, as a brilliant orator and the president of the key Petrograd Soviet (a post to which he was elected both in 1905 and 1917), mobilized the mass support for the Bolshevik party. Trotsky's part in these historic days has been summarized by Sukhanov, a non-Bolshevik eyewitness of the events: "Tearing himself from the work in revolutionary headquarters he would fly from the Obukhovsky factory to the Trubocheny, from the Putilov to the Baltic shipyard, from the Riding Academy to the barracks, and seemed to be speaking simultaneously in all places. Every Petrograd worker and soldier knew him and heard him personally. His influence–both in the masses and in headquarters–was overwhelming. He was the central figure of those days, and the chief hero of this remarkable page of history."

If his public activity were the sum of Trotsky's role in the October Revolution, it alone would have ranked him as one of its most important figures. But it was, in a sense, only the beginning of his contribution. It is one thing to be a popular leader, a *vox populi* giving expression to the pent-up sufferings and rage of previously silent masses, inspiring this new social force to seize the historical hour and redress epochal grievances and injustice. It is quite another, however, to be the leader of a vanguard party. Behind the scenes, in the highest councils of the Bolshevik party, while Lenin was in hiding, it was Trotsky who carried the fight to endorse Lenin's summons to insurrection. The opposition to the proposed seizure of power was formidable, and at first included not only Zinoviev and Kamenev, but the bulk of the party leadership. Furthermore, when the struggle was won, it was Trotsky who emerged as the master tactician of the actual insurrection. For Trotsky was president of the Petrograd Soviet, the very center of the popular revolutionary power, and as head of the Military Revolutionary Committee of the Bolshevik party it was he who chose the timing and determined the tactics of the insurrection, planned its strategy, and carried it to its successful conclusion.

To seize power was an extraordinary accomplishment, but to hold power was even more difficult. The fledgling regime was internationally isolated by the failures of the European revolutions and domestically weakened by four years of world war. Now it was faced not only by the revolt of the disinherited classes of the old order, but by the military intervention of the dominant capitalist world powers as well. In this new struggle, which was to last three interminable and extremely bloody years, Trotsky's role was again unparalleled. For it was he who created and organized the Red Army, and, as its commander, led it to victory.

With victory, and the consolidation of Bolshevik power, the second phase of Trotsky's career began. It was this phase that produced the epochal controversy over "Trotskyism," which persists to this day. From 1923 to 1929 Trotsky was the principal leader of the Bolshevik internal oppositions, which developed in the face of policies undertaken by the regime that seemed to depart from the traditions of Marxism and Bolshevism, and the revolutionary program of October 1917. These oppositions eventually came to include most of the figures of the "Old Guard" of Lenin's party, including Zinoviev and Kamenev, who had at first sided with Stalin against Trotsky.

After 1929, the year of his exile and the consolidation of Stalin's absolute dominance of the party, Trotsky became the sole voice opposing Stalin's policies among the original revolutionary leadership. "Throughout these twelve years, from 1929–1940," writes Trotsky's biographer Isaac Deutscher, "no voice could be raised against Stalin in the USSR; and not even an echo could be heard of the earlier intense struggles, except in the grovelling confessions of guilt to which so many of Stalin's adversaries had been reduced. Consequently, Trotsky appeared to stand quite alone against Stalin's autocracy. It was as if a huge historic conflict had become compressed into a controversy and feud between two men."

To what extent the policies of Stalin were "betrayals" of the revolutionary ideals, and to what extent they were necessary accommodations to the social situation in which the revolution found itself, constitute the essence of the controversy over Trotskyism. The issues span the entire range of modern revolutionary problems, including the relation between national struggles and the international revolution, between revolutionary administrations and the laboring classes, between revolutionary democracy and revolutionary stability, between the efforts to promote the growth of the forces of material production and the need to develop revolutionary consciousness in the new order. Every significant Marxist (and even non-Marxist) critique of Communist practice in these areas, from that of Mao Tse-tung to Fidel Castro and Che Guevara, owes a debt to Trotsky's analysis in his polemic against Stalin. His was not only the first major attempt to come to grips with these questions, but in many ways is still the most penetrating and profound.

On the other hand, his mistakes, both theoretical and practical, were serious and must not be overlooked. Among the most important was the too simple analogy he drew between the bankruptcy of the Second International and that of the Third, and his parallel reduction of the crisis of the revolutionary movement in the Stalin period to that of a crisis of revolutionary leadership. This, he felt, could be cured by the creation of a new international, guided by the classical principles of Bolshevism under Lenin. Within this framework of analysis, however, there is no way to explain adequately the triumph of the Yugoslav, Chinese, and Vietnamese revolutions, which followed World War II, under Stalinist auspices. The fact that they were led by maverick Stalinists (and opposed by Stalin) does not resolve the dilemma; if Stalinism could produce mavericks like Mao, Ho and Tito–who were all in turn opposed by *their* domestic Trotskyists–then wherein lay the necessity of a Fourth International? At the very least, it is impossible to sustain the political parallel between the Communist International and the International of Social Democracy that is so central to Trotskyism. All this is not to say that the heart of Trotsky's criticisms of the policies of the Comintern–in Spain, in Germany, in China–were not correct: by and large they were. It is only to underscore the importance of viewing Trotsky's critique as a necessary point of departure for analysis, and not an adequate theory and program in itself.

It is the very failure of the non-Trotskyist left to assimilate Trotsky's insights and to accept him as a figure in the mainstream of the revolutionary tradition that makes the continued vigor of Trotskyism as a sect possible. It is an important aspect of the effort to build a viable, non-sectarian revolutionary tradition that Trotsky be restored to the honored position his life and contribution warrant, and that his theoretical insights be critically confronted and understood.

CONTENTS

PREFACE

Sucrose is the organic compound commonly known as table sugar and sometimes called saccharose. The molecule is a disaccharide composed of glucose and fructose with the molecular formula $C_{12}\ H_{22}\ O_{11}$. A white, odorless, crystalline powder with a sweet taste, it is best known for its nutritional role, but its applications cover a wide array of disciplines. This book examines how sucrose plays an important role in different scientific areas. The research on sucrose represents important scientific challenges, whose solution has wide impact on a variety of issues. From a conceptual point of view, this research stands at the crossroads of many scientific sectors, such as physics, chemistry, biology and food science and has implications in several disciplines, e.g., pharmacology, toxicology, nanotechnology and medicine.

Chapter 1 – Metal content in intermediate an in byproducts of sugar technology is important due to some of them are used in animal or in human nutrition. Numerous metals are necessary for the human organism, but in large amounts they are toxic. The metals, which are found in sugar beet, might exist in molasses and in dietary fibers from sugar beet and through it, they may be incorporated into human food. The aim of this work is to investigate the application of different sample preparation methods for determining the content of certain selected metals using atomic absorption spectrophotometer. It is determined the content of macro- and microelements in composite samples of sugar beet, dried sugar beet pulp, molasses and sugar. The division of each metal through the technological procedure of sugar production, from the row material through the intermediate products, to the final and byproducts is also determined. Experimental data proved that for determining metal content in sugar beet pulps both sample preparing methods could be used equally. Molasses has the highest content of potassium, about 37000 mg/kg, followed by sodium and calcium with 9000 and 3000 mg/kg, respectively. From original iron content in sugar beet there is appropriately only half of it left in dietary fibers (130 mg/kg - 180 mg/kg). From the analyzed microelements the most present in dried sugar beet pulp as in molasses is iron with average content about 150 mg/kg.

Polycyclic aromatic hydrocarbons (PAHs) are fused-ring aromatic compounds, very important group of persistent organic pollutants present in the air, in water sources, in the soil, in sediments, in animals and plants in various industry products. Traces of these substances have been found in various food products. Most of them are very mutagenic and carcinogenic because of the ability of its metabolites to react with DNA inside the cell. Until industrial revolution, there was a balance between forming of PAH and natural degradation of PAHs. PAH, s has little but almost the same amount. With development of industry and intensive communication this is the misbalance in environment and the speed of PAHs deposition are increased. The mentioned substances are mainly formed during incomplete combustion of such are coal, gas and oil. By wet and dry deposition, they are maintained in all kind of matrix of living sources. The war in the Serbian Republic in 1999 destroyed large amounts of crude oil and derivates have consequence of possibility to carry PAHs into nutrition (food) chains.

Industry plant, such as sugar beet could be contaminated by PAHs by deposition from air and/or by transport and drying.

The aim of the technology of sugar-beet manufacturing is to produce sugar from row material under optimal technologogical and economical conditions. Among main product, sugar crystal, byproducts are molasses and sugar beet fibers. Sugar-beet fibers, mainly used as animal feed, are dried in filter dryer with rotational drum. Dryers could be heated by gases from their own heater, which are set for one kind of fuel or for heating could be used gases from their heating house, which passes through adequate plants to remove ash and soot. This is the reason why it is expected in dryed sugar beet fibers the amount of PAHs to be high. Determination of PAHs in different sources from environment natural sources is complex and difficult. Difficult is due to PAHs are present in very little amounts and due to their present in complex matrixes which contains hundreds of different kind of organic compounds in different range of concentrations. Problems at identification are due to great number of PAHs izomers. Due to the reason mentioned above it is necessary to carry on the sample-preparing and the clean-up. The precision of the results is very influenced by sample preparing method.

In this work is examined the presence of PAHs in sugar and in sugar beet fibers. PAHs are examined by method which is recommended for thes type of matrix, with some changes due to characteristics and complexity of samples. Beside PAH content in mantioned products os sugar factory, it is determined the reproductibility of the used method. For these experiments samples are used from two sugar factories from Vojvodina wich are representative for given areas.

At sugar and sugar beet fibers samples preparing as extraction agens are used methanol, cyclohexane and dimethilformamid. The identification of PAHs are carried out using gas chromatography with flame ionization detector.

Chapter 2 – The aim of this chapter is to report some experimental findings on the dynamical effects induced by the addition of homologous disaccharides, i.e. sucrose and trehalose, to hydrated proteins. On purpose Elastic Incoherent Neutron Scattering (EINS) data, collected by the IN10 ILL spectrometer in the T=20 K ÷320 K temperature range, on dry and hydrated Lysozyme, also in the presence of disaccharides, are reported and discussed. Furthermore, Fourier Transform InfraRed (FTIR) spectroscopy data are reported in order to show the bioprotective effectiveness of trehalose connected with the application of an extremely low frequency electromagnetic field, at 180 μT.

In particular, the neutron scattering results highlight that the dynamical transition, registered at about T=220 K in hydrated Lysozyme, in the presence of disaccharides is shifted to a temperature of T=255 K; on the other hand, FTIR spectra show an increase of the CH_2 group spectral contributions at 1921 cm^{-1} and 1853 cm^{-1} after 3 hours of exposure, and that such effect is not observed after the addition of disaccharides at the same exposure conditions.

Chapter 3 – The role of disaccharides as bioprotectors is intimately connected with their interaction with hydration water. To investigate this issue, depolarized light scattering spectra of aqueous solutions of sucrose have been recorded in the range 0.3 GHz – 30 THz by combining the use of a double monochromator and a multipass Fabry-Perot interferometer. The spectra give us information on both the rotational diffusion of a single sucrose molecule and the effect induced by this solute on the picosecond dynamics of water. In particular, two distinct relaxation processes have been identified, and assigned to hydration and bulk water molecules. The mobility of water localized within the sugar hydration shell is found to be lower than the mobility of water in bulk. The number of molecules involved in the slower dynamics and the extent of retardation are quantified and discussed in comparison with the results recently obtained for other mono and disaccharide solutions.

Chapter 4 – Strawberry impregnated with sucrose was used for the jam preparation, and the effect of various impregnating conditions on the stability of anthocyanins in the jam was examined. The amount of sucrose in impregnated strawberry depended on the concentration of sucrose solution and the operation time for the impregnation. It was kinetically indicated that the impregnation of strawberry in advance of the jam preparation stabilized anthocyanins in the jam. The rate constants by the Weibull model for the color deterioration of the jam impregnated with sucrose and the degradation of anthocyanins in the jam were estimated, and the relationship between the two rate constants was observed to be almost linear.

The antioxidative ability of the strawberry jam correlated with the amount of anthocyanin in the jam. It was shown that the impregnation of strawberry with sucrose was effective for improvement of functional stability of strawberry jam.

Chapter 5 – During the past few centuries humans have transformed from rear to voracious consumers of sugar. The present chapter sheds light on the questions of why we did increased our sugar consumption and what effects sucrose intake can produce on our mood and mind. Once consumed, sucrose sends signals to the brain via specialized taste receptors and glucosensing mechanisms. Sucrose intake activates in the brain the primary gustatory pathway and the brain reward system, which recognizes sweet taste of sucrose as rewarding. The role of the sweet taste system is to detect potentially high-energy sweet food that normally is relatively rare in the nature. The glucosensing mechanisms stimulate or inhibit food intake according to the energy needs. Because of the scarcity of sweet food in the nature, seeking this type of food requires some effort. Therefore, once such a food is found and consumed, this effort would be awarded by the brain reward system. These sophisticated systems work properly when their functions are not compromised by the unlimited availability of sweet palatable food, which may counteract the precise mechanisms controlling food intake. The experimental results obtained in animal models have shown that seeking and consumption of the regular non-sweet foods activate the medial hypothalamus which is directly related to the control of energy homeostasis and stress response. In contrast, seeking and consumption of sucrose inhibit the activity of the medial hypothalamus, but strongly activate the brain reward areas. This sucrose-induced shift in neuronal activity results in consumption of more and more palatable sweet foods at the expense of regular low-energy foods. Repeated overeating of sucrose can alter the neurochemical state of the brain reward regions, promoting sucrose craving and triggering sucrose binge-eating episodes. On the other hand, a sucrose-induced decrease in the activity of the medial hypothalamus directly affects the response of neuroendocrine system to stress. The stress-induced neuronal expression of stress neuropeptides as well as the release of plasma stress hormones is blunted by sucrose consumption. This 'anti-stress' effect of sucrose may explain overconsumption of sweets during stress even in the absence of hunger or needs for calories. This chapter reviews the neuronal effects of sucrose that from one side is beneficial by giving us energy and helping to relieve stress, or, from the other side, it may be detrimental by leading to uncontrolled craving for sucrose, eating disorders and obesity.

Chapter 6 – Sucrose is an important macronutrient that provides humans with a source of energy. Sucrose most important advantages include low cost and easy availability. Aiming to modify the rheological properties of a system, sucrose addition has been investigated and has shown to be successful in several areas. In the food area, sucrose is very important, as it can be used as an ingredient or a preserving agent and its effect in rheological properties is investigated in order to obtain, for example, information about differences in food texture. Sucrose has also been employed as an emulsifier in oil-water emulsions that reduces the interfacial tension, denoted by viscosity changes. The ceramic area has also used sucrose to adjust the forces between the particles that compose the dispersions since sucrose provides steric hindrance, hydration repulsion or electrosteric stabilization. Ergo, the objective of this chapter is to present literature examples regarding sucrose addition and its effect on the rheological properties of the mentioned areas.

Chapter 7 – Carbohydrates are the most abundant organic compounds on the world. Consequently, sucrose is a molecule abundant and inexpensive. The products of sucrose hydrolysis are glucose and fructose, which are used in the food industry. The sucrose derivatives, such as esters and ethers, have interesting properties due to the presence of lipophilic and hydrophilic moieties, provided by sucrose and alkyl chain. Traditionally, these reactions are carried out over homogenous catalysts, which are widely used in chemical processes to synthesize fine and bulk chemicals. However, they have serious drawbacks of hazards in handling, difficult separation and production of toxic waste. Solid catalysts can replace the homogeneous ones for simpler and environmentally more benign processes. Heterogeneous catalysts have been used in hydrolysis, esterification and etherification reactions of sucrose. In this work, the use of different solid catalysts for the conversion of sucrose (by hydrolysis, esterification and etherification) will be reviewed.

Chapter 8 – *Annona cornifolia* A. St.-Hil. is a small annual perennial tree found in the Brazilian savannah and is popularly known as “araticum-mirim”. The ripe orange fruit pulp is sweet and aromatic. The green fruit is popularly used in the treatment of ulcers. Sucrose octaacetate was obtained from the ethanol extract of *Annona cornifolia* seeds by acetylation with pyridine and acetic anhydride, and purified using column chromatography (silica gel and Sephadex LH-20). In a previous study, the antifungal activity of sucrose octaacetate was detected against the pathogenic fungus *Paracoccidioides brasiliensis*. *P. brasiliensis* isolates (Pb-18, Pb-11, Pb-01, Pb-B339, Pb-8 and virulent Pb-18) were susceptible to sucrose octaacetate. In the present work, the possible cytotoxic activity of sucrose octaacetate was evaluated by studying its effects against human tumor cell lines, including melanoma (UACC-62), renal carcinoma (TK-10) and breast cancer (MCF-7), using the sulforhodamine B assay. Sucrose octaacetate showed a cytostatic effect at 59.32, 63.98 and 32.51 μg/mL against the UACC-62, TK-10 and MCF-7 cell lines, respectively. In summary, this study provides evidence of the cytotoxic effect of sucrose octaacetate from the ethanol extract of *Annona cornifolia* seeds and also reports on the bioactivity of this compound for the first time. These results represent a step toward the use of this product as a drug candidate.

Chapter 9 – Sucrose plays an essential role in Nature as part of the CO_2 assimilation pathway in the biosphere. In plants, sucrose is important for the allocation of carbon resources, and participates in a regulatory network that coordinates metabolism and development. Its metabolism is coordinated with the expression of photosynthesis-related genes by a feed-back regulation, and a sugar signaling pathway. Also, sucrose is accumulated in response to environmental stresses and its degradation has been associated with a high demand of carbon and energy in sink tissues.

In the last decades, several studies on sucrose degradation in plants brought to light novel trails on carbon trafficking and the metabolic paths leading to the regulation of gene expression. However, recent findings point to an intricate relationship between sucrose metabolism and the whole plant physiology. This review is focused on the elusive Alkaline/Neutral-Invertase (A/N-Inv) isoforms. These enzymes have been long believed as cytosol-exclusive proteins that hydrolyze the disaccharide for general or maintenance functions in plant cells. Nevertheless, the story has changed in the last few years when novel subcellular localizations and essential functions have been demonstrated for A/N-Invs. From being neglected as unimportant proteins, these enzymes became leading actors in sucrose catabolism with significant roles in root morphogenesis, photosynthetic apparatus biosynthesis, and abiotic stress adaptation.

The aim of this chapter is to present a detailed and updated discussion of the most significant findings on the physiological properties of A/N-Invs. Also, the authors incorporate this group of invertases into the metabolic paths leading sucrose into the different circuits that govern carbon partitioning, storage and regulation of whole plant metabolism.

In: Sucrose
Editor: Salvatore Magazù

ISBN: 978-1-62417-984-6

Chapter 1

METAL AND POLYCYCLIC AROMATIC HYDROCARBON CONTENT OF PRODUCTS IN SUGAR PRODUCTION

Zita Šereš,* Biljana Škrbić, Dragana Šoronja Simović, Biljana Pajin, Ljubica Dokić and Djordje Tadić

Faculty of Technology,
Department of Carbohydrate Food Engineering,
University in Novi Sad, Serbia

ABSTRACT

Metal content in intermediate an in byproducts of sugar technology is important due to some of them are used in animal or in human nutrition. Numerous metals are necessary for the human organism, but in large amounts they are toxic. The metals, which are found in sugar beet, might exist in molasses and in dietary fibers from sugar beet and through it, they may be incorporated into human food. The aim of this work is to investigate the application of different sample preparation methods for determining the content of certain selected metals using atomic absorption spectrophotometer. It is determined the content of macro- and microelements in composite samples of sugar beet, dried sugar beet pulp, molasses and sugar. The division of each metal through the technological procedure of sugar production, from the row material through the

---

* E-mail: zitas@tf.uns.ac.rs.

intermediate products, to the final and byproducts is also determined. Experimental data proved that for determining metal content in sugar beet pulps both sample preparing methods could be used equally. Molasses has the highest content of potassium, about 37000 mg/kg, followed by sodium and calcium with 9000 and 3000 mg/kg, respectively. From original iron content in sugar beet there is appropriately only half of it left in dietary fibers (130 mg/kg - 180 mg/kg). From the analyzed microelements the most present in dried sugar beet pulp as in molasses is iron with average content about 150 mg/kg.

Polycyclic aromatic hydrocarbons (PAHs) are fused-ring aromatic compounds, very important group of persistent organic pollutants present in the air, in water sources, in the soil, in sediments, in animals and plants in various industry products. Traces of these substances have been found in various food products. Most of them are very mutagenic and carcinogenic because of the ability of its metabolites to react with DNA inside the cell. Until industrial revolution, there was a balance between forming of PAH and natural degradation of PAHs. PAH, s has little but almost the same amount. With development of industry and intensive communication this is the misbalance in environment and the speed of PAHs deposition are increased. The mentioned substances are mainly formed during incomplete combustion of such are coal, gas and oil. By wet and dry deposition, they are maintained in all kind of matrix of living sources. The war in the Serbian Republic in 1999 destroyed large amounts of crude oil and derivates have consequence of possibility to carry PAHs into nutrition (food) chains.

Industry plant, such as sugar beet could be contaminated by PAHs by deposition from air and/or by transport and drying.

The aim of the technology of sugar-beet manufacturing is to produce sugar from row material under optimal technologogical and economical conditions. Among main product, sugar crystal, byproducts are molasses and sugar beet fibers. Sugar-beet fibers, mainly used as animal feed, are dried in filter dryer with rotational drum. Dryers could be heated by gases from their own heater, which are set for one kind of fuel or for heating could be used gases from their heating house, which passes through adequate plants to remove ash and soot. This is the reason why it is expected in dryed sugar beet fibers the amount of PAHs to be high. Determination of PAHs in different sources from environment natural sourcrs is complex and difficult. Difficult is due to PAHs are present in very little amounts and due to their present in complex matrixes which contains hundreds of different kind of organic compounds in different range of concentrations. Problems at identification are due to great number of PAHs izomers. Due to mentioned above it is necessary to carry on the sample-preparing and the clean-up. The precision of the results is very influenced by sample preparing method.

In this work is examined the presence of PAHs in sugar and in sugar beet fibers.

PAHs are examined by mathod wich is recommended for thes type of matrix, with some changes due to characteristics and complexity of samples. Beside PAH content in mantioned products os sugar factory, it is determined the reproductibility of the used method. For these experiments samples are used from two sugar factories from Vojvodina wich are representative for given areas.

At sugar and sugar beet fibers samples preparing as extraction agens are used methanol, cyclohexane and dimethilformamid. The identification of PAHs are carried out using gas chromatography with flame ionization detector.

INTRODUCTION

Raw Materials and Products in Technology of Sugar from Sugar Beet

The basic raw material in the sugar industry is sugar beet. The by-products of the industry are molasses, which is a raw material used in other technological processes, and sugar beet pulp. All the elements or compounds contained in the raw material, i.e. sugar beet, as well as the by-products of the sugar industry, namely sugar beet pulp and molasses, are recycled in the human organism through fodder, or more specifically, animal meat, or thorough the product of consumable crystal [1].

Mineral matter is essential for a normal development of sugar beet which, while growing, obtains it from the soil. The composition and the content of the mineral matter in sugar beet vary depending on the sort of sugar beet, the soil, climatic conditions, the method of growing and the supplements used. The quantity of mineral matter, determined as ashes, normally constitutes from 0.4% to 0.6% per beet [1]. In the course of the technological process of beet processing the metal content is distributed between by-products and the product.

In addition to being used as animal feed, the dried sugar beet pulp is used as an additive in human diet for it is rich in nutritive fibers. Moreover, it has a good capacity of binding certain metal cations [2]. Therefore, the pulp is expected to have an increased metal content.

Molasses, a by-product in which all non-saccharic compounds accumulate following the crystallization of sucrose, contains approximately 30 %/SM of non-sugars (other than-sugar elements) of organic and inorganic origin. Out of it, around 11.5 %, calculated on dry matter, of non-sugars are inorganic salts most of which are potassic salts. As to the microelements, iron is the most dominant with 170 mg/kg [3].

Quality Requirements

Sugar Beet

Sugar beet (Figure 1) needs to be undamaged. It must not be attacked by mold and dry rot, especially by wet rot. Sugar beet must meet the requirements specified in national standards (Table 1) [4].

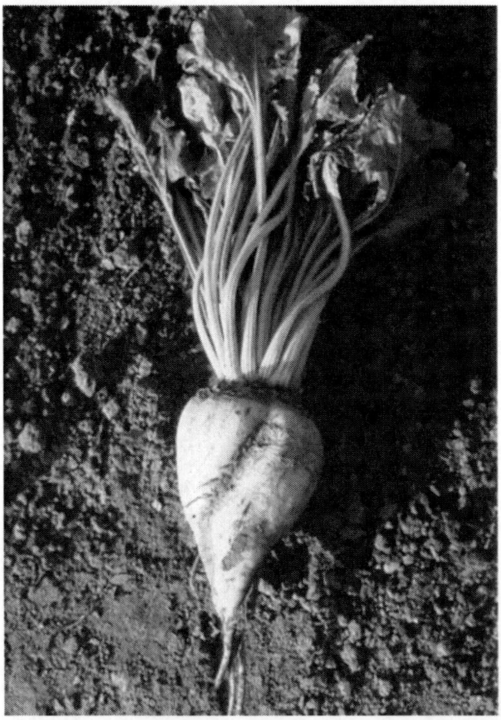

Figure 1. Sugar beet.

Table 1. Defined properties of sugar beet according to national standards

Parametar	%(m/m)
Mechanical damage	maximum 15
Thawed roots	maximum 2
Wither roots	maximum 2
Rotten roots	maximum 0.5
The presence of animal beet	not allowed
Polarization (sucrose content)	minimum 14.5
The content of inorganic impurities (clay, sand, stones, etc.).	maximum 15
Content of organic contaminants (weeds, straw, leaves, etc.)	maximum 0.25

EXTRACTED PULP

Extracted pulp (Figure 2) is obtained as a by-product after extraction, and its quantity is defined by the quality of beets. By its structure it is complex colloidal capillary porous entity [5]. The chemical composition of the extracted pulp is shown in Table 2 [6]. Extracted pulp can also be raw material for extraction of pectin, araban and cellulose [6, 7, 8]. The most significant possibility of utilization of the extracted pulp is its use in animal feed and in production of additives assigned to food industry, as dietary fiber concentrate[9, 10, 11, 12].

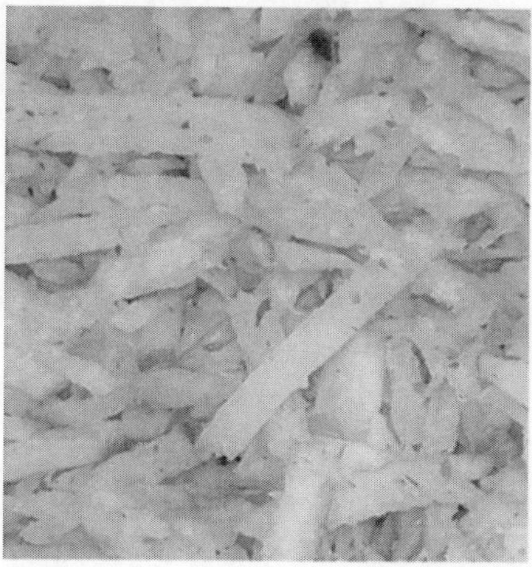

Figure 2. Extracted pulp.

Table 2. Average chemical composition of extracted sugar beet pulp

Chemical components	content [%/dry matter]
Hemicelulose (mostly araban)	26.0
Pectin	24.0
Celullose	23.0
Proteins (according to the Kjeldahl Nx6,25)	9.0
Sucrose	6.0
Lignin	4.5
Non-soluble mineral compounds	3.0
Fat	0.5

Due to the high content of water extracted the pulp is further processed by pressing to dry matter content of 16-23% [13, 14], and for longer storage period it is dried to dry matter content of 87-96% [5]. Table 3 shows the requirements that must be met by dry pulp (Figure 3) [12].

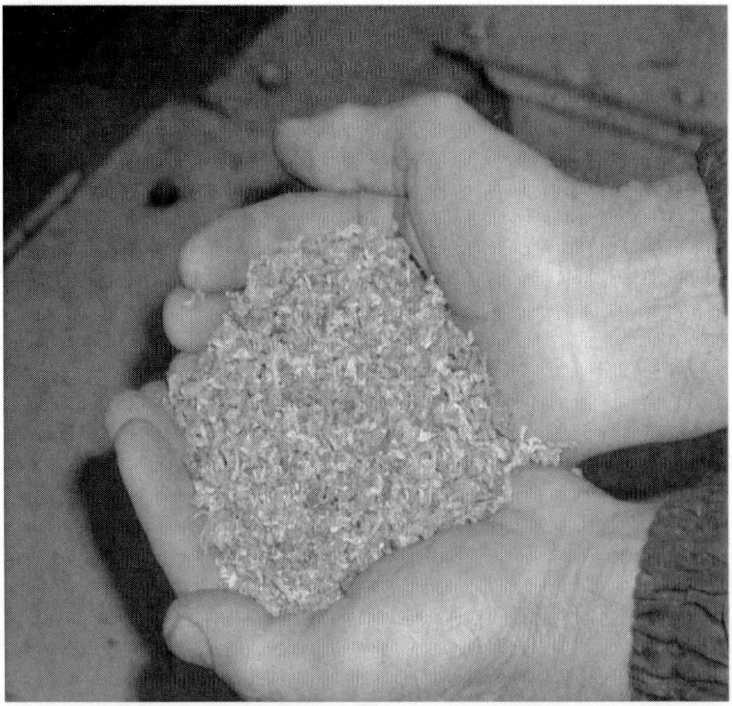

Figure 3. Dry pulp.

Table 3. Defined characteristics of dry pulp according to national standards

Product	Proteins [%]	Humudity [%]	Sucrose [%]	Ash [%]
Core	> 8	< 12	-	< 7
sugar beet dried pulp with molasses	> 8	< 14	> 10	< 8
sugar beet dried pulp with stillage of molasses	> 8	< 14	-	< 8

Molasses

In the sugar industry molasses (Figure 4) is generated in the last degree of multi-stage crystallization of thick juice obtained in the processing of sugar beet. During technological process about 4% of molasses is gained calculated on sugar beet. Molasses is a thick, viscous, dark liquid that contains a large amount of sucrose, which can not be isolated by further crystallization [5].

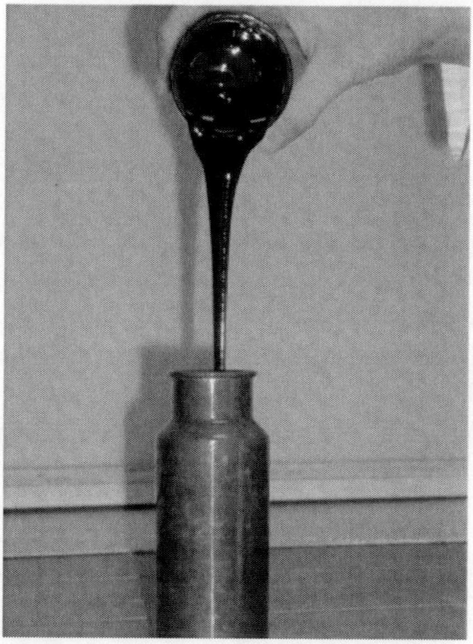

Figure 4. Molasses.

Table 4. Average chemical composition of molasses

Organic compounds	content [%]
Sucrose	51.0
Raffinose	1.0
Invert	0.5
Proteins	5.0
Glutamine acide	4.0
Betaine	6.0
Other N – compounds	1.5
Organic acids	1.5
Other organic acids	1.5
Mineral compounds	content [%]
K_2O	4.30
Na_2O	0.90
CaO	0.26
MgO	0.14
SiO_2	0.10
Al_2O_3	0.07
Fe_2O_3	0.02
CO_3^{2-}	3.50
SO_4^{2-}	0.55
Cl^-	1.60
PO_4^{3-}	0.06

The formation of molasses in the technological processing of sugar beet affects the physical and chemical factors. Physical factors are manifested in the increase in viscosity due to the presence of large amounts of nonsaccharose compounds, which affects the reduction of crystallization rate of sucrose, while the chemical factor is considered as increasing the solubility of sucrose because of the presence of nonsaccharose compounds, mainly on the basis of formation of easily soluble additive compounds.

Table 4 shows the average chemical composition of molasses [15]. According to national standards the molasses as a by-product of sugar technology must meet certain requirements (Table 5).

Table 5. Defined physical and chemical properties of molasses according to the national standards

Parametar	Value
Dry matter content [^{o} Bx]	minimum 76.3
Sucrose content [%]	minimum 46%
pH at 20 ^{o}C	7.0 – 8.0
SO_2 [%]	maximum 0.1%

Sugar

Sugar (Figure 5) is one of the few food products that come on the market in almost chemically pure form. Sugar is purified and crystallized sucrose with a clearly defined quality, provided by Yugoslav Standards [16]. Characteristics of edible sugar, defined according to national standards, are shown in Table 6 [17].

Table 6. Defined properties of sugar according to national standards

Parameter	I category	II category	III category
Ash [%]	maximum 108.0 – 117.0	maximum 270.0 – 288.0	
Colour [ICUMSA]	maximum 22.50 – 26.25	maximum 45.00 – 52.50	
Colour at Saccharoflex	maximum 2.00 – 2.25	maximum 4.50 – 5.00	maximum 6.00
Moisture [%]	maximum 0.1		
SO_2 [mg/kg]	maximum 15		
Sucrose [%]	minimum 99.7		
Invert [%]	maximum 0.04		

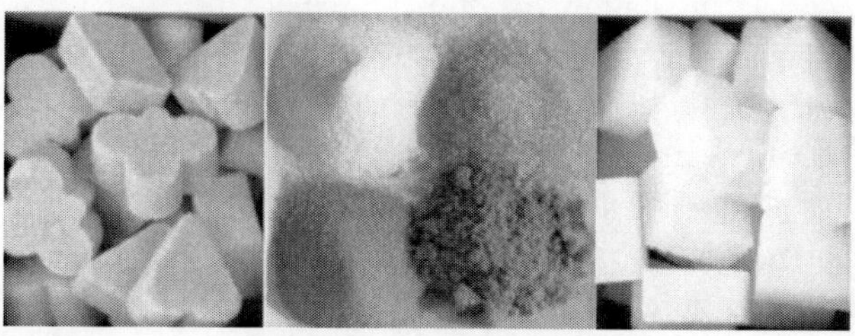

Figure 5. Sugar.

METAL CONTENT OF PRODUCTS IN SUGAR PRODUCTION

Controlling the content of metals in sugar is highly important since sugar is a significant ingredient in many food products and plays a fundamental role in the diet of little children and the elderly. Researches worldwide are thus focused on devising and discovering adequate methods for the determination of metals and on varying the metal content both in the products and by-products of sugar technology and in the soil in which the beet or cane has been grown, depending on the influence of various factors [18; 19, 20]. The content of metals in sugar beet, dried sugar beet pulp and molasses is not defined by the national book of regulations, which refers to technological parameters only [21].

According to the national regulations, the maximum content of copper, lead and arsenic allowed is defined at the level of 1 mg/kg [22]. The Codex Alimentarius Commission prescribes the maximum limit allowed for arsenic, copper and lead in sugar of 1 mg/kg [23].

The Hungarian regulation [24], in compliance with that of the European Union, prescribes the maximum limit allowed for arsenic – 0,1 mg/kg, quicksilver – 0,02 mg/kg, lead – 0,5 mg/kg, cadmium – 0,02 mg/kg, copper – 2,0 mg/kg and zinc – 3,0 mg/kg.

The aim of the work was to evaluate the content of K, Na, Ca, Mg, Cu, Zn, Fe in samples of sugar beet, dried sugar beet pulp, molasses and white sugar, and to investigate the application of different sample preparation methods for determining the content of metals using atomic absorption spectrophotometer.

The division of each metal through the technological procedure of sugar production, from the row material through the intermediate products, to the final and byproducts is also determined.

Many metals, including heavy metals, are essential, though toxic in larger quantities. The accumulation of toxic metals in the environment is continuously increasing.

Consequently, one of the key environmental problems is the determination of the content of metals in all food products and raw materials that are involved in the production of food and food chain. For obvious reasons, a great deal of attention has to be dedicated to all the issues that are directly related to human nutrition. [25].

Polycyclic Aromatic Hydrocarbons

Polycyclic aromatic hydrocarbons (PAH) represent a significant group of POP (persistent oganic pollutants), i.e. chemical pollutants. These are organic pollutants that can have toxic and carcinogenic effects. Their presence was detected in air, water, soil, sediments, plants and foodstuffs. PAH occur from incomplete combustion process (combustion of wood, fossil fuels) and in the process of carbonization of organic matter. At room temperature PAH exist in the solid state, they are very chemically inert and insoluble in water due to high molecular weight. They have expressed hydrophobic character. In the ultraviolet and the visible spectrum PAH absorbe a light [26, 27]. Because of their properties such as low solubility in water, high molecular weight and high boiling temperature, PAH exist in nature for a very long time and can not be chemically or biologically degraded, so they are considered as persistent [28]. In developed countries the POP content in various foods is regulated by low. There are several international conventions dealing with the POP content in the living world [28].

Table 7. Physical properties of some polycyclic aromatic hydrocarbons

Compunds	Molecular mass	Vapour pressure at 25°C, [Pa]	Solubility in water at 25°C, [g/l]
Naftalene	128.2	2.4	1.25 – 3.4×10^{-2}
Acenaftilene	152.2	1.3×10^{-1} – 1.3×10^{-2}	3.420×10^{-3}
Acenaftene	154.2		
Fluorene	166.2		8×10^{-4}
Fenantrene	178.2	9.06×10^{-2}	4.35×10^{-4}
Anthracene	178.2	3.20×10^{-2}	5.9×10^{-5}
Fluorantene	202.3		2.6×10^{-4}
Pyrene	202.1	9.20×10^{-5}	1.33×10^{-4}
Benzo(a)anthracene	228.3	1.47×10^{-5}	1.1×10^{-5}
Krizen	228.3		1.9×10^{-6}
Benzo(b)fluoranthene	252.3		2.4×10^{-6}
Benzo(a)pyrene	252.3	7.33×10^{-7}	3.8×10^{-6}
Indeno(1,2,3-cd)pyrene	276.3		
Dibenzo(ah)anthracen	278.3		4×10^{-7}
Benzo(ghi)perilen	276.4	1.33×10^{-8}	3×10^{-7}

Regulation of the POP content in various products can not be applied effectively, while in some countries the law does not regulate the use of certain POP, does not define resources, and their presence in nature /1/. The basic group of POP are polycyclic aromatic hydrocarbons (PAH), polychlorinated biphenyls (PCB) and organochloric pesticides (OCP).

They can enter the organism by food or through the respiratory tract. In the bloodstream, these hydrophobic compounds are transformed by enzymes into water-soluble compounds that can still go into forms capable of leading to mutations or damage of DNA cells, causing the appearance of cancer. Their accumulation takes place in adipose tissue, kidneys, liver and spleen [26, 27].

On the list of hazardous substances according to United States Environmental Protection Agency (US EPA) is 16 PAH, which are divided into lower (with 2-3 condensed benzene rings in the molecule) and higher (with 4-6 condensed benzene rings in the molecule). Since most of these compounds show mutagenic or carcinogenic effects, Table 7. shows an overview of the physical properties of most important PAH [30].

Presence of Persistent Organic Pollutants in Food

The main intake of persistent ogranic compounds in the human body is through the digestive tract, while breathing brings only a small part. Nutrition is a major source of PAH. The most of the PAH enter the body through the cereals up to 1/3 of total intake, followed by oils and fats also 1/3, while vegetables and sugar make up the majority of the remaining amount. The amount of PAH in meat and milk is significantly lower [31]. Although the highest concentration of PAH was not found in cereals, a daily intake of cereals is the largest, and therefore the highest PAH enter through cereals [32]. Different eating habits affect the daily intake of different amounts of PAH. So, the amount of PAH that enters the human body in Italy is 3 mg/day, of which 1.4 mg/day per person is carcinogenic [33]. In the Netherlands, this amount is increased slightly and is between 5-17 mg/day per person [32]. Unlike Italy and the Netherlands, where the daily amount is increased, in New Zealand is only 1.2 mg/day per person [34]. In Italy, fat intake is 75 g/day per capita, while in the Netherlands 40.2 g/day, and therefore the lower intake of PAH through the fat is in the Netherlands.

Based on the data from the literature it can be concluded that the highest intake of PAH is through cereals, vegetables, fruits, meat and meat products, milk and dairy products, which are also the most common in the diet.

The minimal risk level (MRL) established by the Organization of American Toxic Substances and Registration of Deases (ATSDR) is only an indicator of possible sources of risk to human health, and are not precise values that can be used to determine the exact level of pollution and hazards [35]. Exposure to concentrations of less than the minimum amount of risk does not mean that there will be no occurrence of some disease.

De Vos says in his paper that phenanthrene and chrysene are most present in food, and fluoranthene as non carcinogenic [32].

Regardless of the geographic area it was found that the smoked meat, meat products and meat from the grill are the most dangerous sources of PAH [34]. In nondairy product equivalent, margarine, a considerable amount of PAH is present in form of carcinogenic benzo(a)pyrene 0.2 to 5.2 μg/kg [36]. Regarding to carcinogenic properties of some PAH (benzo(a)pyrene, benzo (a)anthracene, chrysene) some countries established specific restrictions of PAH intake. Germany, Austria and Poland have limited the intake of benzo(a)pyrene over smoked meat products at 1mg/kg, while in Finland for example there is no such kind of restrictions [38].

The influence of the environment, particularly in industrial areas, as well as near major roads, on the PAH content in plants is very pronounced. Almost all 16 PAH, except acenaften and benzo(a)anthracene were found in samples [38].

The general conclusion is that the vegetables that grow near roads and in industrial regions have an increased PAH content. It is also noted that the PAH concentration is considerably higher in leafy vegetables due to the greater exposure to air pollution.

Presence of Polycyclic Aromatic Hydrocarbons in Sugar Technology Products

The presence of polycyclic aromatic hydrocarbons in sugar technology products are most examined in dried extracted pulp, because drying process may increase the amount of PAH compounds.

Group of authors from Sweden have dealt with the PAH content in sugar beet dietary fiber, depending on the drying method (direct or indirect drying) /53/. It may be noted that the dried extracted pulp samples had a relatively low PAH content. According to the mentioned literature, the dominant PAH in all samples was phenanthrene. It is observed that there was no significant difference in the total PAH content depending on the method of drying, and the content of benzo(a)pyrene and benzo(a)anthracene was in the interval from 0.3 to 0.4 μg/kg.

The results of the PAH content in dried extracted pulp samples of sugar beet originating from Sweden, directly dried by flue gases created in the process of combustion of fuel oil, coal and natural gas were analyzed, too [39]. In all the analyzed samples the high values of total PAH concentrations were determined. The dominant compound in all tested samples was phenanthrene, also, 1-metilfenantren, 2-metilfenantren, fluoranthene and pyrene were found in large quantities. The concentration of benzo(a)pyrene and benzo (a) anthracene (from 1.0 to 4.3 μg/kg) in extracted pulp is higher comparising with concentrations in dietary fiber. The authors emphasize that a significant portion of PAH content in dried samples is result of air pollution in the area for the cultivation of these crops [39].

The increase in PAH concentrations can cause drying of some agricultural crops in order to reduce the moisture content. This is especially evident in the direct process of drying by direct heating with fuel oil, heating oil or coal. Because of these results it is recommended to use the device for drying with indirect heat. Otherwise, direct way requires fuel natural gas. Modern kilns are equipped with filters for flue gases, regardless of the type of fuel, and is therefore barely noticeable difference between dried and undried products [40].

Serra, Pupin i Toledo examined the presence of PAH in samples of sugar cane and its products and concluded the presence of PAH in almost all samples. PAH were determined by High Presure Liquid Chromatography (HPLC). In the samples of burned sugar cane, commercial sugar (except refined) and the alcohol obtained by fermentation and distillation of sugar cane juice the following PAH compounds have been found: benzo(a)pyrene, benzo(a)anthracene, phenanthrene and naphthalene [41]. Table 2.25 shows that the total PAH concentration varies between 1.3 to 21.6 μg/kg, and the amount of benzo(a)pyrene and benzo(a)anthracene ranges from 0.25 to 0.9 μg/kg. The conclusion is that process of sugar refining leads to decreased amounts of PAH, and much of PAH remain in molasses.

In Serbia, the maximum allowable amount of PAH in sugar and sugar beet products is not defined, but, according to Regulations of the quantities of various toxic substances in food only the presence of benzo(a)pyrene in smoked products up to 5 ng/g is allowed. As for organochlorine pesticides, according to the same Regulations, the presence of linolan is limited to 50 ng/g [42].

The allowed quantities of organochlorine pesticide endosulfane (α-, β- and sulfate) in sugar beet is 100 ng/g. For PAH compounds, PCB (polichlorinated bipheniles) compounds and other organochlorine pesticides permitted quantity is not defined either in the final products, raw materials and by-products of technological sugar production process.

MATERIALS AND METHODS

Representative samples of beet sugar, dried beet pulp, molasses and sugar are the samples that have been taken every day and collected in a container. After ten days the samples were mixed and the average sample was made, representative for that decade. Throughout the campaign, the the average samples for each decade were made. At the end of the campaign average samples, representative for all decade were mixed and a representative sample of campaign was obtained.

Main Characteristics of Samples

Samples of sugar beet, dried beet pulp, molasses, and sugar, which were used to examine the content of metals and PAH, originating from the same sugar factory in Vojvodina. In sugar beet samples, used for testing the presence of POP, certain characteristics were determined: polarimetric sucrose content, dry matter content, pH value, invert sugar content, the content of the core and ash content. The results are shown in Table 8. The data from Table 8. indicate that sugar beet samples have common technological characteristics.

Table 8. Main characteristics of sample of sugar beet

Sample no.	P [°Z]	DM [%]	pH	Invert [%SM]	Core [% on sugar beet]	Ash [%DM]
1	14.47	22.1	6.4	1.052	4.03	2,52
2	14.52	22.2	6.5	0.662	4.06	3,00
3	14.28	21.1	7.1	0.70	4.34	2.68
4	14.09	21.3	6.6	0.652	4.36	2.80
x	14.34	21.7	6.7	0.709	4.20	2.75

P – sucrose content, DM – dry matter content, pH – value pH, Invert –invert sugar, x – average value.

In the samples of dried pulp, in which the content of PAH is further defined, dry matter content and ash content were determined by drying, and the results are shown in Table 9. Based on the results from Table 9. it is concluded that the dry pulp samples have usual technological characteristics.

Table 9. Main characteristics of sample of dry pulp

Sample no.	DM [%]	Ash [%DM]
1	87.59	3.52
2	87.37	3.14
3	87.19	3.55
4	86.05	3.52
x	87.05	3.43

DM-dry matter, x – average value.

Table 10. Main characteristics of sample of molasses

Sample no.	P [°Z]	DM [°Bx]	pH	Invert [%SM]	Color [ICUMSA]
1	47.94	87.11	7.7	0.522	11530
2	48.23	84.79	7.6	0.374	10237
3	55.63	85.07	6.8	0.846	9107
4	61.34	84.54	6.8	0.623	7773
x	53.29	85.38	7.2	0.591	9662

P – sucrose, DM – dry matter, Invert – invert sugar, B – color,
x – average value.

In the samples of molasses, used for further analysis, the following characteristics were determined: polarimetric sucrose content, refractometric dry matter content, pH value, invert sugar content and color in solution. Test results are shown in Table 10. According to the results from Table 10 it can be noticed that the technological characteristics of molasses are common.

In the samples of sugar, the following characteristics were determined: moisture, invert sugar content, ash content, sulfur dioxide content and the content of coloring matter in solution. The results are shown in Table 11. Based on the results it can be concluded that the samples of sugar, applied to examine the content of POP have usual technological characteristics.

Table 11. Main characteristics of sample of sugar

Sample no.	Humudity [%]	Invert [%]	Ash [%]	SO_2 [mg/kg]	Color [ICUMSA]
1	0.024	0.003	0.014	0.17	49.0
2	0.028	0.002	0.013	0.17	46.0
3	0.028	0.006	0.012	0.08	50.2
4	0.028	0.004	0.013	0.09	50.8

Determination of parameters of all samples within the main characteristics was performed according to Methods for laboratory control of the production process in sugar factory [44]. The representative samples of sugar beet, dried sugar beet pulp, molasses and sugar used for the determination of the content of metals were obtained from a sugar plant in Vojvodina. The examined samples were of usual technological characteristics [43], as shown in Table 1.

Metal Content Determination

The chemicals used for the determination of metals are of a satisfactory degree of cleanness for the analysis of the content of metals in traces. In this research the samples were prepared using two methods: wet burning and heating to ashes. In the case of sugar beet and dried sugar beet pulp samples, the method of wet burning involves treating the samples using nitric and perchloric acids and gradual heating to 200°C. The temperature is then maintained until a completely colourless and clear solution is obtained. After cooling, the contents are quantitatively placed into a measuring receptacle of 50 $cm^{3,}$ which is then filled up with demineralized water. Two blind tests are simultaneously prepared with the same quantity of the acids used for the preparation of the samples. Employing the method of wet burning, molasses is steamed with nitric acid for 12 hours, after which it is treated using a mixture of nitric, sulphuric and perchloric acids. The steaming is done until dry matter is obtained and, having added dissolved nitric acid, it is filtered into a measuring receptacle of 100 cm^3. Metals are determined in the obtained filtrate. Employing the method of wet burning, sugar is dissolved in demineralized water, it is then treated using nitric and sulphuric acids and carefully heated. Nitric acid is added in portions in order to prevent carbonization and continue with heating carefully to avoid excessive appearance of foam. Eventually, a colourless solution containing no suspended solid matter is obtained. Two blind tests are simultaneously prepared with the same quantity of the acids used for the oxidation of the sample. Standard solutions for the determination of metals are prepared in a 5% sulphuric acid solution. Simultaneously with the wet burning method, the content of metals was determined in the samples of sugar without any previous preparation. A sugar sample is dissolved so that the content of solid matter in the solution is 10%. Metals are directly determined in this solution. Standard solutions for gauging the apparatus are filled up using a solution of pure sucrose containing 10% of dry matter (producer "Kemika" Zagreb).

The method of heating to ashes involves treating the samples of sugar beet and dried sugar beet pulp at 600°C for 2 hours and dissolving the remains in hydrochloric acid. After dissolved nitric acid has been added, the contents are filtered into a measuring receptacle of 50 cm^3 which is then filled up with dissolved nitric acid.

Two blind tests are simultaneously prepared with the same quantity of the acids used for the preparation of the samples [45]. The measurements were carried out using PERKIN-ELMER 703 atomic absorption spectrophotometer. Potassium and sodium were determined by means of flame photometry, where potassium was determined at the wave length of 381.5 nm, and sodium at 293.5 nm. Calcium, magnesium, iron, copper and zinc were determined using atomic absorption spectrophotometer. Calcium was determined at the wave length of 211 nm, magnesium 285.2 nm, iron 248.3 nm, copper 324.7 nm and zinc 213.9 nm. The air-acetylene flame of the atomic absorption spectrophotometer is used for determination.

Polycyclic Aromatic Hydrocarbons Content Determination

The applied solvents were all with certain level of cleanliness for the analysis of organic compounds in trace. Chemicals for preparation of samples for the determination of persistent organic pollutants were:

- Methanol;
- Cyclohexane;
- N, N'-dimethylformamide, DMF;
- Silica gel, for column chromatography, neutral, particle size 63-200 μm (70-230 mesh) /12, 45/;
- *Potassium hydroxide, KOH;*

- *Anhydrous sodium sulfate, Na_2SO_4*, which is prepared by annealing at 360°C for 4 hours, then cooled and stored in a desiccator;
- *Distilled water, extracted twice by cyclohexane.*
- *Technical acetone for dishes rinsing.*

Determination of PAH was done by a modified Larsson's method [39]. In the preparation of plant tissues and food the process of saponification was used, i. e. alkaline degradation. In determination of PAH degradation was carried out in an alkaline solution of a strong base (KOH) in 24 hours, followed by extraction [46].

In order to allocate as cleaner fraction the extract was purified by liquid-liquid extraction, and/or by column chromatography. Due to the complexity of the matrix, dried pulp, molasses, sugar beets underwent to matrix destruction. After the destruction PAH were separated by column chromatography. The column filled with silica gel is an essential part of the sample preparation for the determination of POP by gas chromatography, as this leads to a separation of PAH, PCB, and OCP in order of expiration from the gel layer..

In column chromatography the cyclohexane is used as a medium of fractionation. The second fraction of 23-100 ml (ie, fraction pushed with 77 ml of cyclohexane) is captured and collected. This fraction (24 - 100 ml) contains polycyclic aromatic hydrocarbon compounds. Fraction is evaporationed until it becomes dry. Prior to the gas chromatography analysis the paired extract is dissolved in 50 μl of hexane.

Analysis of individual PAH content was performed on a gas chromatograph with hydrogen flame - ionization detector - FID [39]. Determination of the investigated compounds was performed using external standard method [40].

Table 12. The limit of detection of the method (LODmet)

Sample	m_{sample} [g]	V_{eks}PAH [□l]	LOD_{met}PAH [ng/g]
Sugar beet	161.0000	50	0.3106
Dried sugar beet pulp	80.0000	50	0.6250
Sugar	150.0000	50	0.3333
Molasses	150.0000	50	0.3333

m_{sample} – mass of the sample, V_{eks}PAH – final volume of the extract for PAH determination, LOD_{met}PAH – detection limit of the method for PAH determination.

The average detection limit of the applied gas chromatograph (GC) for analysis of PAH is about 2 ng. Volume of injected extract is 2 μl. The results of the detection limit of the method for the investigated samples are shown in Table 12.

Table 12. shows that limit of detection of the method, for extracted dry pulp samples is the highest 0.6250 ng/g, for sugar and molasses 0.3333 ng/g, while for sugar beet is the smallest 0.3106 ng/g.

RESULTS AND DISCUSSION

Metal Content

The contents of micro and macroelements in sugar beet (Table 13) are high and influenced by the conditions of sugar beet growing, i.e. agrotechnical and climatic conditions. Potassium, sodium, calcium and magnesium are determined with the aim of estimating the technological ripeness of beet [47]. The highest content in beet is that of potassium, approximately 7000 mg/kg, followed by sodium and magnesium, and then calcium with about 1000 mg/kg. Regarding the microelements, the most dominating are iron (362.29 mg/kg) and manganese (50.14 mg/kg), which is most likely the consequence of their high content in the soil in which sugar beet has been grown [48]. The values for metals obtained using the methods of wet burning and heating to ashes do not differ significantly.

Table 13. Metal content in sample of sugar beet

Metals	Wet burning		Heating to ashes	
	Average value	Standard deviation	Average value	Standard deviation
K [mg/kg]	7388.00	635.95	6884.00	986.86
Na [mg/kg]	2228.00	106.14	2464.00	191.22
Ca [mg/kg]	968.00	69.04	852.00	65.32
Mg [mg/kg]	2340.00	126.10	2096.00	93.45
Cu [mg/kg]	7.03	0.70	8.69	0.93
Zn [mg/kg]	6.71	1.30	5.61	1.07
Fe [mg/kg]	361.89	58.76	n.a.	--
Mn [mg/kg]	50.14	11.58	n.a.	--

n.a. – not analyzed.

The content of metals in the samples of dried sugar beet pulp is shown in Table 14. As it was expected, the content of alkali metals is approximately three times lower than in sugar beet. Most of these metals were extracted into juice during the technological process of producing sugar. The content of calcium increased as a result of adding calcium oxide into the water for the hydraulic transportation of beet with the aim of disinfection. The content of magnesium does not practically change. A greater amount of this alkaline-earth metal remains in sugar beet pulp. The same is with copper and zinc. This is very convenient for dried sugar beet pulp is used as fodder, and copper, iron and zinc are essential microelements. The content of copper is increased in comparison to the values (by approximately 0.01 mg/kg) obtained in the year 2002 for dried sugar beet pulp from Backa and Srem [49]. The content of iron in dried sugar beet pulp is reduced by half when compared to sugar beet. It is noticeably lower in comparison to the data from the references concerning the pulp from Northern Backa (311 mg/kg). It is, however, similar to the content of iron in dried sugar beet pulp from Southern Backa (134 mg/kg). Different methods of sample preparation bring about identical results.

Table 14. Metal content in sample of dried sugar beet pulp

Metals	Wet burning		Heating to ashes	
	Average value	Standard deviation	Average value	Standard deviation
K [mg/kg]	2532.00	433.70	2616.00	291.09
Na [mg/kg]	932.00	184.21	1096.00	238.89
Ca [mg/kg]	5144.00	270.92	4820.00	184.84
Mg [mg/kg]	2396.00	233.60	2240.00	273.86
Cu [mg/kg]	6.20	0.42	6.40	1.07
Zn [mg/kg]	10.14	0.27	7.18	0.57
Fe [mg/kg]	151.60	18.27	n.a.	-
Mn [mg/kg]	36.00	4.69	n.a.	-

n.a. – not analyzed.

Molasses remains after a three-level crystallization of sucrose and contains all the behindhand compounds and elements of the technological process of producing sugar. The content of metals in molasses is shown in Table 15. 100 kilograms of beet give 4 kilograms of molasses. According to the results, approximately 20% of potassium and sodium goes to molasses, while about 30% goes to dried sugar beet pulp. About 0.4% of the overall mineral matter in sugar beet goes to the row juice, while approximately 0.2% per beet remains in the thin juice. The content of calcium in molasses cannot be interpreted the same way since the content of calcium increases as a result of the fact that lime salts remain after the row juice has been cleaned. There is very little magnesium in molasses for the greater part remains in dried sugar beet pulp. Zinc goes to molasses in very small quantities as well. The content of iron in molasses equals 139.20 mg/kg, which is in accordance with the data found in the references [3]. Table 16. shows the data about the values of the content of metals in sugar. It is obvious that in sugar metals remain in traces, which was expected. Potassium and sodium in sugar originate from the raw material and suplements, and as dissolved compounds they go through the phase of juice refinement. In the course of the sugar production process, the ions of calcium leave sediment as carbonates, phosphates, sulfites, sulfates, etc. However, their removal is not complete and depends on the juice composition, pH value and the temperature. It should be mentioned that calcium originates from the raw material and calcium oxide which is added in the juice refinement phase. As far as the microelements are concerned, copper, zinc and iron were analysed. The values for the mentioned elements satisfy the criteria of both national and foreign regulations. The values for metals obtained using the method of wet burning and metal analysis without preparation do not differ significantly. Employing the statistical method of pair comparison for probability $\alpha=0.05$, t <1.99 is obtained for each metal, which means that the differences are not significant.

Table 15. Metal content in sample of molasses

Metals	Wet burning	
	Average value	Standard deviation
K [mg/kg]	36812	1906.64
Na [mg/kg]	8608	1270.47
Ca [mg/kg]	2971.20	406.28
Mg [mg/kg]	137.88	53.97
Cu [mg/kg]	2.24	0.44
Zn [mg/kg]	11.04	1.02
Fe [mg/kg]	138.90	26.90
Mn [mg/kg]	n.a.	-

n.a. – not analyzed.

Table 16. Metal content in sample of sugar

Metals	Wet burning		Without preparation	
	Average value	Standard deviation	Average value	Standardnddeviation
K [mg/kg]	18.52	2.37	17.26	2.90
Na [mg/kg]	6.39	0.77	6.18	0.98
Ca [mg/kg]	13,82	2.47	14.19	1.45
Mg [mg/kg]	0.12	0.09	0.13	0.10
Cu [mg/kg]	0.07	0.02	0.09	0.02
Zn [mg/kg]	0.02	0.01	0.03	0.01
Fe [mg/kg]	n.a.	-	0.37	0.08
Mn [mg/kg]	n.a.	-	n.d.	-

n.a. – not analyzed.
n.d. – not detected.

Polycyclic Aromatic Hydrocarbons Content

Representative samples, which were investigated, are presented in Table 17, that shows the weight of samples with the dry matter content. The highest mass of the sample for the determination of POP is measured in sugar beet, where it has the lowest dry matter content. Sugar has the highest dry matter content, almost 100%.

Sugar beet is a raw material for technology of sugar production process. Of 12 examined types of PAH compounds in the representative sample of sugar beet 11 compounds are present. Only acenaftilene was not detected, which may mean that the amount is below the detection limit. Test results of PAH content in the sample of sugar beet (mash), originating from Vojvodina, are shown in Table 18.

Table 17. List of analyzed samples

Cont. No.	Sample	Sample mass [g]	Dry matter content in the sample [%]	Dry matter content in the sample [g]
1	Sugar beet	161	21.70	34.94
2	Dry matter	80	87.05	69.64
3	Molasses	150	85.38	128.07
4	Sugar	150	99.97	149.96

Table 18. Results of PAH content in sample of sugar beet

PAH	[pg/g uzorka]	[pg/g SM uzorka]
acenafthilene	nd	nd
fluorene	0.8	3.7
krizen	2.6	12.0
benzo(a)anthracene	1.6	7.4
benzo(b)fluoranthene	4.2	19.3
indeno(1,2,3-cd)pyrene	0.4	1.8
fenanthrene	11.0	50.7
anthracen	0.2	0.9
pyrene	2.2	10.1
benzo(k)fluoranten	7.0	32.3
benzo(b)pyrene	31.2	143.8
dibenzo(ah)antracen	2.9	13.4
□ PAH	64.1	295.4

In a representative sugar beet sample the total PAH content is in amount of 64.1 pg/g. The total PAH content of sugar beet, calculated on a dry matter of the sample, amounts to 295.4 pg/g of d.m. That amount is about 2.5 times higher than the value of PAH content in extracted dry pulp (Table 19), respectively, for more than three times higher of the PAH content in molasses (Table 20). Based on the presented it can be concluded that raw material contains the greatest amount of PAH that enters the tissue of sugar beet from the soil.

In sugar beet the most present PAH is benzo(b)pyrene in amount of 31.2 pg/g, following by phenanthrene in the amount of 11.0 pg/g. Calculated on the dry matter content of sugar beet benzo(b)pyrene amounts to 143.8 pg/g d.m.. It is noteworthy that the benzo(b)pyrene is one of the most cancerous compounds. Interestingly, the benzo(b)pyrene accounts for 50% of the total PAH compounds in sugar beet. Other PAH compounds are present in smaller amounts.

According to current Regulations on the amount of pesticides and other toxic substances in food the maximum allowable amount of PAH in sugar beet is not defined [50].

Extracted dried pulp are used as animal feed or as an additive for human consumption. It is therefore necessary to examine the content of PAH in these types of samples. Also, it is very important to pay attention on drying way of extracted pulp, since it greatly affects the PAH content in them. Test results of examined PAH content in a representative sample of the extracted dry pulp, originating in Vojvodina, are shown in Table 19. Of 12 examined types of PAH compounds 9 is detected. The total PAH content amounts 98.4 pg/g of dried pulp, which is about 40% higher than the PAH content in sugar beet. If the PAH content, calculated to the dry matter of dried pulp, compares with the PAH content in sugar beet, also to the dry matter, total PAH content is 2.5 times higher in sugar beet.

In the examined representative sample of dried pulp the most present PAH is benzo(b)pyrene in amount of 37.0 pg/g, following by dibenzo(ah)anthacene in amount of 23.4 pg/g. These compounds are more cancerous comparing to others that are presented in the sample, and represented about 60% of the total amount of PAH. In the extracted dry pulp the presence of acenaftilene, fluorene and indeno(1,2,3-cd)pyrene was not detected. Under the current Regulations on the amount of pesticides and other toxic substances in food, the maximum allowable amount of PAH in extracted dry pulp is not defined [50].

Molasses is a by-product of the technological process of sugar production, in which all nonsaccharose compounds are collected, and is an essential starting raw material for many other technologies. For this reason, the control of molasses is very important.

Table 19. Results of PAH content in the sample of extracted dry pulp

PAH	[pg/g uzorka]	[pg/g SM uzorka]
Acenaftilene	nd	nd
fluorene	nd	nd
krizen	5.8	6.7
benzo(a)anthracen	2.9	3.3
benzo(b)fluoranthene	6.0	6.9
indeno(1,2,3-cd)pyrene	nd	nd
Fenanthren4	11.9	13.7
antracen	0.1	0.11
piren	2.8	3.2
benzo(k)fluoranten	8.5	9.8
benzo(b)piren	37.0	42.5
dibenzo(ah)antracen	23.4	26.9
□ PAH	98.4	113.11

nd – not detected.

In a representative sample of molasses 11 PAH compounds were detected of 12 examined. The total PAH content in molasses amounts to 76.4 pg/g. The total PAH content in the molasses calculated of the dry matter is 89.5 pg/g d.m.. The PAH compounds come into molasses from sugar beet, and during its treatment from used water, and other aids that are used in technological process. The largely represented PAH in molasses is also benzo(b)pyrene, in the amount of 38.1 pg/g. In this case, benzo(b)pyrene, also represents 50% of the total PAH content. Phenanthrene and benzo(k)fluoranthene are present in the sample in amount of 19.2 and 12.6 pg/g. Other compounds are present in much smaller quantities. Acenaftilene compound was not detected. Under the current Regulations on the amount of pesticides and other toxic substances in food the maximum allowable amount of PAH in sugar is not defined [50]. Test researching results of PAH content in the sample of molasses originating in Vojvodina, are shown in Table 20. Sugar is the end product of the technological process of sugar production. The results of PAH content in the sample of sugar, originating in Vojvodina are shown in Table 21. In a representative sample of sugar, as expected, cancerous PAH compounds were not detected. Only phenanthrene was found as noncancerous, which is present in the environment in large amounts. Perhaps during storage of sugar occurred the adsorption of phenanthrene on the sugar crystals from the air. Phenanthrene was detected in the amount of 21.0 ng/g.

Table 20. Results of PAH content in the sample of molasses

PAH	[pg/g samples]	[pg/g dry matter of samples]
acenaftilene	nd	nd
fluorene	1.1	1.3
krizene	2.8	3.3
benzo(a)anthracen	1.8	2.1
benzo(b)fluoranthen	5.3	6.2
indeno(1,2,3-cd)piren	0.2	0.23
Fenantrene	12.8	15.0
antracene	0.3	0.35
pyrene	2.2	2.6
benzo(k)fluoranthen	8.4	9.8
benzo(b)pyrene	38.1	44.6
dibenzo(ah)antracen	3.4	4.0
□ PAH	76.4	89.48

nd – not detected.

Table 21. Results of PAH content in the sample of sugar

PAH	[ng/g samples]	[ng/g dry matter of samples]
acenaftilene	nd	nd
fluorene	nd	nd
krizen	nd	nd
benzo(a)anthracene	nd	nd
benzo(b)fluoranthene	nd	nd
indeno(1,2,3-cd)pyrene	nd	nd
fenanthrene	21.0	21.01
antracene	nd	nd
pyrene	nd	nd
benzo(k)fluoranthene	nd	nd
benzo(b)pyrene	nd	nd
dibenzo(ah)anthracene	nd	nd
□ PAH	21.0	21.01

nd – not detected.

According to current Regulations on the amount of pesticides and other toxic substances in food the maximum allowable amount of PAH in sugar is not defined [50].

Of all examined samples, extracted dried pulp contain the highest amount of PAH (113.11 pg/g d.m.). The part of PAH compounds, which are located in dried pulp is probably caused by drying process.

The sum of the amounts of PAH compounds in molasses is 89.48 pg/g of dry matter, which is about 20% less than in extracted dried pulp. Since all nonsaccharose compounds are collected in molasses, PAH compounds behave in an identical way. It should not be neglected the assumption that water, lime and other substances, which are used in technology of sugar production, contain a certain amount of PAH compounds, which pass into molasses.

If PAH content in dried sugar beet pulp originating in the territory of Vojvodina (the total amount of PAH is 98.8 pg/g of sample), is compared with results that are obtained by Larsson and colleagues from Sweden (75 – 110 µg/kg) /45/, it can be observed that total PAH content in domestic dried pulp in lower. From the results of the PAH content in the dried sugar beet pulp it can be concluded that, in the factory, filters for flue gases are used during the process of drying. In Sweden, in all extracted pulp and fibers [11], as in Brazil in the products of sugar cane [13], the occurrence of cancerous benzo (a) pyrene is registrated. The presence of benzo(a)pyrene is probably because of flue gases that are used directly in the drying treatment of extracted fibers.

Comparing the PAH content in the samples investigated in the graduate thesis and PAH content, which was done by Serra and colleagues from Brazil [13] in sugar cane, it can be concluded that the polycyclic aromatic hydrocarbon phenanthrene is present in all products of sugar beet and sugar cane. In sugar obtained from of the sugar cane the presence of cancerous benzo(a)pyrene is detected, while it was not the case in sugar obtained from local sugar factory.

CONCLUSION

Based on the results of the determination of metals in the samples of sugar industry products, it is possible to conclude the following:

- The values of the content of metals obtained using the method of wet burning and the method of heating to ashes do not differ significantly. Both methods can be employed for metal content determination in sugar beet and dried sugar beet pulp.
- When determining metals in sugar employing the method of wet burning and the direct method, the obtained values do not differ significantly. Therefore, both methods can be equally used.
- The content of the examined metals in sugar is in compliance with the national standards and the regulations of Hungary and the EU as well.
- The regulations concerning the quantities of pesticides, metals, metaloids and other poisonous and anabolic substances in food products should include set limits determining the maximum content of metals in sugar beet, dried sugar beet pulp and molasses.
- The highest content in beet is that of potassium, approximately 7000 mg/kg, followed by sodium, magnesium and calcium.
- The content of alkali metals in dried sugar beet pulp is about three times lower than in sugar beet. The majority of these metals were extracted into juice in the course of the technological process of producing sugar. About 20% of the potassium and sodium content found in sugar beet was detected in molasses.

- As opposed to alkali metals, practically all the magnesium from sugar beet remains in dried sugar beet pulp. Only a small quantity goes to molasses.
- Of all the examined microelements in sugar beet, the highest content is that of iron, ranging from 307 to 437 mg/kg. About a half (129-179 mg/kg) remains in dried sugar beet pulp, while the rest converges in molasses (86-159 mg/kg).
- Microelements copper and zinc remain largely in dried sugar beet pulp (more than 80%).

Based on the results of examination of the presence of polycyclic aromatic hydrocarbons in representative samples of sugar beet, dried extracted pulp, molasses and sugar, using modified method by Larsson, the following can be concluded:

- 11 PAH compounds were detected in sugar beet of 12 examined. Only acenaftilene was not found, which may mean that the amount is below the detection limit.
- The total PAH content in sugar beet is in the amount of 64.1 pg/g.
- The total PAH content in sugar beet, calculated on a gram of dry weight of the sample, amounts to 295.4 pg. That amount is about 2.5 times higher than the value of PAH content in extracted dry pulp and for more than three times higher than the PAH content in molasses. Based on the above, it can be noticed that raw material contains the greatest amount of PAH that enters the tissue of sugar beet from the soil.
- Cancerous PAH compound benzo(b)pyrene is present in sugar beet in the largest quantity, in the amount of 31.2 pg/g. In gram of dry matter of the sugar beet sample the content benzo(b)pyrene amounts to 143.8 pg. Benzo(b)pyrene presents 50% of the total PAH compounds.
- The toxic compound phenanthrene is present in sugar beet in the amount of 11.0 pg/g.
- In extracted dried sugar beet pulp 9 PAH compounds were detected of 12 examined.
- The total PAH content in the extracted dried pulp is 98.4 pg/g (113.1 pg/g of dry matter of sample). PAH compounds come into dried pulp from sugar beet and produce during the drying process.

- In dried pulp, PAH compound benzo(b)pyrene is present in the largest quantity of 37.0 pg/g, followed by dibenzo(a)anthacene in the amount of 23.4 pg/g. These compounds are more cancerous then other presented in the sample, and represent about 60% of the total amount of PAH.
- Acenaftilene, fluorene and indeno(1,2,3-cd)pyrene were not detected in extracted dried sugar beet pulp.
- Low PAH content in extracted dried pulp (the total amount of PAH is 98.8 pg/100 g of sample) is caused by use of filters for flue gases, that serve as a source heat in drying process.
- In dried pulp cancerous PAH compound benzo(b)pyrene represents 50% of the total PAH compounds. These obtained results lead to the conclusion that our climate is dominated by the benzo(b)pyrene, that gets into the tissue of sugar beet from the soil. In processing of sugar beet benzo(b)pyrene distributes in the pulp and then in the fibers produced from them.
- The presence of PAH in sugar is probably due to soil contamination and/or air in the area where sugar beet is grown, and/or air pollution in the factory, where sugar is stored.

ACKNOWLEDGMENTS

These experiments are part of the investigations, supported by the Serbian Ministry of Science (Project no. TR 31014).

REFERENCES

[1] Poel, van der P. W.; Schiweck, H.; Schwartz, T. *Sugar Technology: Beet and Cane Sugar Manufacture*; Albert Bartens: Berlin, 1998; 5-78.

[2] Dronnet,V. M.; Axelos, M. A; V.; Renard, C. M.; Thibault, J. F. *Carbohyd. polym.* 1998, *35*, 239-247. 1. Improvement of the binding capacity of metal cations by sugar-beet pulp. 2. Binding of divalent metal cations by modified sugar-beet pulp.

[3] Olbrich, H. *Die Melasse*; Inst. Fur Garungsgewerbe: Berlin, 1960.

[4] Lee, H.; Dookhran,G.; Chau, A. *Analyst* 1987, *112*, 31-40. Analytic reference materials, Part VI. Development and certification of sediment reference material for selected polycyclic aromatic hydrocarbons.

[5] Šušić, S.; Petrov, S.; Kukić, G.; Sinobad, V.; Perunović, P.; Koronsovac, B.; Bašić, Đ. *Osnovi Tehnologije Šećera 1*; Univerzitet u Beogradu: Beograd, 1994; pp 10-24.

[6] Vogel, M. *Zuckerind.* 1991, *116*, 265-270. Alternative utilization sugar beet pulp.

[7] Broughton, N.; Dallon, C.; Jones, G.; Williams, E. *Int. Sugar J.* 1995, *57 – 60*, 93 – 95. Adding value to sugar beet pulp.

[8] Micard, V.; Grabler, C.; Thibault, J. F. *Enzime Microb. Tehnol.*1996, 162 – 170. Enzimic Sahharification of Sugar beet pulp.

[9] Perrson, K. *Ernahrungs – Umschau* 1986, *3*, 98 –99. Dietery fibre from sugar beet – Fibrex.

[10] Fasatiova, L. *Listy cukrovar.* 1988, *104*, 201 – 205. Vlaknina pro potravinarske učely – Sinecal 1 (Fibrous material for food purposes).

[11] Gyura, J.; Petrov, S.; Sekulić, R.; Psodorov, Đ. *Žito hleb.* 1991, 373 – 376. I deo: Dobijanje i svojstva aditiva. Primena aditiva dobijenih iz izluženih rezanaca šećerne repe u pekarskim proizvodima.

[12] Rede, R.; Gyura, J.; Petrov, S. *Teh. mesa.* 1992, *34*, 28 – 31. Celulozno pektinski aditivi iz izluženih rezanaca šećerne repe – Primena u proizvodima od oblikovanog usitnjenog mesa i u fermentovanim kobasicama.

[13] Milosavljević, Ž.; Puača, V. *Stočna hrana*; Privredni pregled: Beograd,1978.

[14] Einsminger, M.; Oddfield, J.; Heinemann, W.; *Feeds and Nutricion digest Ensminger*; Publishing Company: USA, 1990.

[15] Sólyom L., Lásztity R. *A melasz*; Mûszaki Könyvkiadó, Mezôgazdasági Könyvkiadó: Budapest, 1980.

[16] Yugoslav standards, JUS E.13.020, *Molasses.*

[17] Yugoslav standards, Official letters no. 7, 1992.

[18] Ronda, F.; Sancho, D.; del Alamo, M.; Gomez, M. *Zuckerind.* 2001, *126*, 208-212. Direct determination of arsenic, cadmium, cobalt, copper, chromium, lead, tin and zinc in white beet sugar using graphite furnace atomic absorption spectrophotometry.

[19] Leblebici, J; Volkan, M. *Journal of Agriculture and Food Chem.* 1998, *46*, 173-177.

[20] Sample Preparation for Arsenic, Copper, Iron, and Lead Determination in Sugar.

[21] Mohamed, A.E. *Food Chem.* 1998, *65*, 503-507. Environmental variations of trace element concentrations in Egyptian cane sugar and soil samples (Edfu factories).

[22] Official letters SRJ. 2000, 20. Proizvodi industrije šećera i sporedni proizvodi industrije šećera i proizvodnja askorbinske kiseline.

[23] Službeni glasnik SRJ. 1992, 5. Pravilnik o količinama pesticida, metala i metaloida i drugih otrovnih supstancija, hemioterapeutika, anabolika i drugih supstancija koje se mogu nalaziti u namirnicama.

[24] FAO/WHO, Codex Alimentarius Pesticide residue Contaminants. Codex Alimentarius Commision, FAO and WHO, Rome, 1990.

[25] Hatályos Jogszabályok Gyűjteménye, EuM rendelet az élelmiszerek vegyi szennyezettségének megengedhető mértékéről, Budapest (VI.16.) 17/1999.

[26] Locatelli, C.; Torsi, G. *Microchem. J.* 2003, *75*, 233-240. Analytical procedure for the simultaneous voltametric determination of heavy metals in meals.

[27] Škrbić, B. Cvejanov, J. *Nafta.* 1988, *39*, 433. Postupci određivanja policikličnih aromatičnih ugljovodonika u vazduhu.

[28] Gomao, G.; Grey, J.; Rabie, S.; Lopez-Bote, C.; Boren, A. *Food Addit. Contam.* 1993, *10*, 503. Polycyclic aromatic hydrocarbons in smoked food products and liquid smoke flavourings.

[29] Edlund, S. *PAH as a POP*; The International Institute for Industrial Environmental Economics: Lund, Sweden, 2001.

[30] Nisbet, C.; Lagoy, P. *Reg. Tox. Pharmacol.* 1992, *16*, 290. Toxic equivalency factors (TEF) for polycyclic aromatic hydrocarbons (PAHs).

[31] Manz, M.; Wenzel, K. – D.; Dietze, U.; Schuurmann, G. *The Sci. Total Env.* 2001, *277*, 187. Persistent organic pollutants in agricultural soils of central Germany.

[32] Dennis, M.; Massez, R.; Cripps, G.; Venn, I.; Howrth, N.; Lee, G. *Food. Addit. Contam.* 1991, *8*, 517-530. Factors affecting the polycycloc aromatic hydrocarbons content of cereals, fats and other food products.

[33] de Vos, R.; van Dokkum, W.; Schouten, A.; de Jong-Berkhout, P. *Fd. Chem. Toxic.* 1990, *28*, 263. Polycyclic aromatic hydrocarbons in Dutch total diet samples (1984 – 1986).

[34] Lodovici, M.; Dolara, P.; Casalini, C.; Ciappellano, S.; Testolin, G. *Food Addit. Cont.* 1995, no. 5, 703-713. Polycyclic aromatic hydrocarbon contamination in Italian diet.

[35] Phillips, H. D. *Mutation res.* 1999, *443*, 137 – 147. Polyciclic aromatic hydrocarbons in the diet. www.atsdr.cdc.gov/

[36] Thomson, B.; Lake, R.; Lill, R. *Polycyclic Aromatic Compd.* 1996, *11*, 177-184. The contribution of margarine to cancer risk from polycyclic aromatic hydrocarbons in New Zealand diet.

[37] Tuominen, J.; Pyysalo, H.; Sauri, M. *Food. Chem.* 1988, *36*, 118. Cereal products as a source of polycyclic aromatic hydrocarbons.

[38] Voutsa, D.; Samara, C. The Science of Total Environment 1998, 203 – 216. Dietery intake of trace elements and polyciclic aromatic hydrocarbons via vegetables grown in industrial Greek area.

[39] Larsson, B.K., Osterdahl, B.–G., Regner, *S. Swedish J. Agric.* 1990, *49*, 5. Polyciclic Aromatic Hydrocarbons and Volatile N-Nitrosamines in Some Dried Agricultural Products.

[40] Bolling, H. *Die Muhle.* 1989, *126*. Kontamination bei direkter Rausgastrockung und Möglichkaiten ihrer Reduzierung.

[41] Serra, G. E.; Pupin, A. M.; Toledo, M. C. F. *Bol. SBCTA.* 1995, *29* (2), 134 – 137. Ensaios preliminares sobre a contaminacao da cana – de – acucare e derivados por hidrocarbonetos policiclicos aromaticos.

[42] Službeni glasnik SRJ. 1992, br. 5,p. 67. Pravilnik o količinama pesticida, metala i metaloida i drugih otrovnih supstancija, hemioterapeutika, anabolika i drugih supstancija koje se mogu nalaziti u namirnicama.

[43] Reinefeld, E.; Schneider, F.: *Analytische Betriebskontrolle der Zuckerindustrie*; Teil A. Verlag Dr. Albert Bartens: Berlin, 1978.

[44] Službeni list SRJ. 2000, br. 20, 5. Proizvodi industrije šećera i sporedni proizvodi industrije šećera i proizvodnja askorbinske kiseline.

[45] Wieteska, E.; Zioek, A.; Drzewinska, A. *Analytica Chim. A.* 1996, *330*, 251-257. Extraction as a method for preparation of vegetable samples for the determination of trace metals by atomic absorption spectrometry.

[46] Škrbić, B.; Filipčev, B.*Žito-hleb.*2003, *3*, 103-112. Prisustvo policikličnih aromatičnih ugljovodonika u sirovini i hrani biljnog porekla i mogući uticaj na zdravlje.

[47] Šušić, S.; Petrov, S.; Kukić, G.; Sinobad, V.; Perunović, P.; Koroncovac, B.; Bašić, Đ. *Osnovi Tehnologije šećera*; «Jugošećer» d.d.: Beograd, 1994.

[48] Ubavić, M.; Bogdanović, D.; Hadžić, V. *Savremena poljoprivreda* 1993, 1993:1, 47 – 51 p. Osnovna hemijska svojstva zemljišta Vojvodine i mogućnosti njihovog zagađenja teškim metalima.

[49] Gyura, J.; Filipović, N.; Škrbić, B.; Šereš, Z.; Ćupić, S. *Central Eur. J. Occup. Env.l Med.* 2003, *9*(4), 304-309. Heavy metals and inorganic cations in soil and sugar beet pulp in northern Serbia.

[50] European Commission, 2002. Scientific Committee on Food, Polyciclic Aromatic Hydrocarbons – Occurence in foods, dietary exposure and health effects, Brussels, Belgium, http://europa.Eu.Int./comm/food /fs/sc/scf/out154en.Pdf.

In: Sucrose
Editor: Salvatore Magazù

ISBN: 978-1-62417-984-6

Chapter 2

BIOPROTECTIVE EFFECTS OF SUCROSE AND TREHALOSE ON PROTEINS

Salvatore Magazù,[1,*] Federica Migliardo,[1,2] Antonio Benedetto,[1] Emanuele Calabrò,[1] Roberto La Torre[3] and Maria Teresa Caccamo[1]

[1]Dipartimento di Fisica e di Scienze della Terra, Università di Messina, Messina, Italy
[2]Laboratoire de Dynamique et Structure des Matériaux Moléculaires, Unesco-L'Oreal University of Lille I, France
[3]Department of Matter Physics and Electronic Engineering, University of Messina, Messina, Italy

ABSTRACT

The aim of the present chapter is to report some experimental findings on the dynamical effects induced by the addition of homologous disaccharides, i.e. sucrose and trehalose, to hydrated proteins. On purpose Elastic Incoherent Neutron Scattering (EINS) data, collected by the IN10 ILL spectrometer in the T=20 K ÷320 K temperature range, on dry and hydrated Lysozyme, also in the presence of disaccharides, are reported and discussed. Furthermore, Fourier Transform InfraRed (FTIR)

* Corresponding author: Salvatore Magazù. Dipartimento di Fisica e di Scienze della Terra, Università di Messina, Viale F. Stagno D'Alcontres, n° 31, P.O. Box 55, S. Agata 98166 Messina, Italy. E-mail: smagazu@unime.it, tel. +39 0906765025 fax. +39 090395004.

spectroscopy data are reported in order to show the bioprotective effectiveness of trehalose connected with the application of an extremely low frequency electromagnetic field, at 180 μT.

In particular, the neutron scattering results highlight that the dynamical transition, registered at about T=220 K in hydrated Lysozyme, in the presence of disaccharides is shifted to a temperature of T=255 K; on the other hand, FTIR spectra show an increase of the CH_2 group spectral contributions at 1921 cm^{-1} and 1853 cm^{-1} after 3 hours of exposure, and that such effect is not observed after the addition of disaccharides at the same exposure conditions.

Keywords: Mean square displacement, neutron scattering, FTIR spectroscopy, magnetic field, dynamical transition, lysozyme, disaccharides, sucrose

INTRODUCTION

The purpose of this chapter is to show the bioprotective effectiveness of two homologous disaccharides, i.e. sucrose and trehalose, with respect to two environmental stress, i.e. to the temperature variation and to the extremely low frequency electromagnetic fields exposure, on a typical protein, the Lysozyme.

As reported in literature, several investigations carried out on protein thermal denaturation have put in evidence the bio-protection effectiveness of disaccharides [1, 2].

In particular, investigations carried out on Lysozyme evidenced the bioprotectant effectiveness of disaccharides [1, 3, 4], trehalose being the most efficient in preserving the native conformation of the protein against high temperatures [3].

So far different hypotheses to explain why disaccharides are particularly effective have been proposed. Crowe et al. [5] formulated the so called "water replacement hypothesis", for which a direct disaccharide-biostructure interactions occurs.

Cryptobiosis, from Greek *Kriptos*, which means both "hidden" and "coated", refers to a particular state of organisms, during which undetectable hidden levels of metabolic functions are maintained for mending prohibitive environmental conditions [6, 7]. Experimental data show that not only the structural and dynamical properties of water are strongly perturbed by disaccharides but also that these co-solvents are referentially excluded from the hydration shell of proteins [8]. Inelastic neutron spectra reveal a more marked downshift of the OH stretching mode and a narrower bandwidth for the trehalose/H_2O mixture which are indicative of a higher disaccharide-water interaction and of a higher order [9]. Further results evidenced that the structural properties of water are locally perturbed more strongly by disaccharides. The intramolecular OH stretching Raman spectra of disaccharide aqueous solutions show that, at the same concentration and temperature value, the area of the tetrahedric contribution is lower in the case of trehalose, so indicating that a more marked destructuring effect occurs. This result constitutes a crystal-clear proof which furnishes an accounting of the fact that trehalose frustrates better than the other disaccharides ice formation [10].

Other experiments on trehalose/H_2O, maltose/H_2O and sucrose/H_2O mixtures, show that the intensity profiles of the bending modes, identified by density functional simulations, are more structured, indicating that trehalose forms with water molecules entities which show a more “cryptocrystalline” behaviour: the macroscopically glassy protective shell hides a local crystalline character [11-12].

Finally the Self-Distribution-Function (SDF) procedure, applied on Elastic Incoherent Neutron Scattering (EINS) data obtained by the IN13 spectrometer on trehalose/H_2O and sucrose/H_2O, highlighted a different Q-dependence for the two disaccharides: the partial MSD behaviours of sucrose and trehalose are equivalent in the high r-domain, whereas they are different in the small-r domain; this circumstance induces a difference in the total MSDs, so suggesting that the higher structure sensitivity of sucrose in respect to trehalose is related to the small spatial observation windows [13-21].

The microscopic characterization of the protein dynamics in the presence of disaccharides plays a key role in many biotechnological fields, such as pharmaceutics, cosmetics and food science, where the use of disaccharides improves both the product quality and the shelf-life.

MATERIALS AND METHODS

Experimental neutron data were collected at the Institute Laue Langevin (Grenoble, France) by the IN10 spectrometer, employed in the elastic scan configuration. This spectrometer is characterized by a relatively high energy of the incident neutrons which allows to span a quite wide range of momentum transfer. More specifically, for the IN10 spectrometer the incident wavelength is 6.27 Å, the Q-range is 0.30÷2.00 $Å^{-1}$ and the elastic energy resolution (FWHM) is 1 μeV, which corresponds to a time resolution of about 2192 ps.

Thus scattering particles which move in a time scale much slower than this characteristic time are seen as elastic scatterers, whereas a decrease of the elastic intensity is observed for scattering particles which moves faster. For the experiments samples of partially deuterated lysozyme in dry, H_2O, trehalose/H_2O and sucrose/H_2O environments have been employed. More specifically, the hen-egg white Lysozyme protein was used. The protein was dialyzed in order to remove salts and then lyophilized. The lyophilized powder was hydrated in H_2O at a hydration value of h=0.4 (with h=water/protein weight fraction) and in trehalose/H_2O and in sucrose/H_2O environments at a hydration value of h=0.4 [with h=(water+disaccharide)/protein weight fraction].

Ample time after the mixing was taken. Lyophilized Lysozyme was directly used as dry sample. The hydration value of 0.4 has been chosen because to have a monolayer of water covering the protein surface [22-24]; in fact it is well known that the activity of proteins depends on the presence of at least a minimum amount of solvent water. Data were collected in the temperature range of 20÷320 K and for 12 hours. Empty cell contribution was subtracted and spectra were normalized to a vanadium standard. This data treatment was performed with the Lamp code relative to the employed spectrometer; other programs and specific new codes were used for data analysis.

As far as Fourier Transform InfraRed (FTIR) measurements are concerned, a couple of Helmholtz coils linked to a AC voltage regulating up to 230 volt, at the frequency of 50 Hz, was used to generate time-varying electromagnetic fields. This device was used to expose samples at a magnetic flux density whose intensity was fixed at 180 μT. Lysozyme was prepared in D_2O solution 60 mg/ml for control and exposed samples. Analogue samples were added with trehalose 150mg/ml. FTIR absorption spectra were recorded at room temperature by a spectrometer Vertex 80v of Bruker Optics. Assorbance method was chosen for spectrum collection. Lysozyme solution samples, in absence and in the presence of disaccharides, were placed between a pair of CaF_2 windows. For each spectrum 64 interferograms were collected and co-added employing a Happ-Genzel apodization function to generate a spectrum with a spectral resolution of 4 cm^{-1}. InfraRed (IR) spectra of D_2O solution were subtracted from the spectra at the corresponding temperature. Each measure was performed under vacuum to eliminate minor spectral contributions due to residual water vapor. IR spectra were baseline corrected and area normalized. In addition, second-derivative analysis of IR spectra was performed to enhance the fine spectral structure [25].

RESULTS AND DISCUSSION

Characterizing the dynamics of biological macromolecules is a key step for understanding their function since the knowledge of their structure alone is not always sufficient. One of the dynamical phenomena of great interest is the so-called "dynamic transition" which has been observed in hydrated proteins as a rapid rise of the measured MSD at a temperature value around T=220-240 K, which adds itself to others MSD kinks in dry and hydrated proteins [26-28].

It is commonly accepted that the temperature behaviour of the measured molecular MSD in H_2O and D_2O hydrated lysozyme, starting from the lowest temperatures, can be interpreted in the following way: (i) at first the measured MSD follows the typical trend of the low frequency vibrational contribution; (ii) then an enhancement of motion amplitudes at 125 K is attributed to the rotational motion of methyl groups; (iii) then, in sequence, a dynamical transition at a temperature of T=220 K is registered.

In Figure 1a a comparison between the temperature behaviour of the measured MSD of dry and D_2O hydrated lysozyme, obtained from data collected by IN10 spectrometer, is shown. The MSD of the hydrated lysozyme shows a dynamical transition at a temperature of about T=220 K. In Figure 1b the comparison between the measured MSD temperature behaviour of dry and of H_2O hydrated lysozyme in sucrose is shown. As it can be seen, the dynamical transition is shifted at a higher temperature value, i.e. T=255 K. This shift of 35 K can be connected with the presence of the disaccharides. In particular, the presence of the disaccharides slows down the dynamics of the hydrated protein; as a consequence, the measured relaxation time 'enters' in the resolution windows at higher temperature values in respect to the simple hydrated Lysozyme, as it has been shown in Reference [28].

As far as the effects of exposure of Lysozyme in D_2O solution (in absence and in presence of trehalose) to a low frequency (50 Hz) electromagnetic field are concerned, the spectral contributions of the protein linkages IR vibration bands in the mid-infrared spectroscopy region were investigated. It is well known that FTIR can be considered as a valuable tool for analyzing protein structure [25, 29, 30]. In fact, unlike UV-VIS spectroscopy which probes transitions between electronic states, IR spectroscopy detects transitions between rotational or vibration energy levels, yielding precious information on the molecular structure. One of the most representative bands of the protein secondary structure spectrum is that of the amide I around 1650 cm^{-1}; this arises mainly from the C = O stretching vibration, with minor contributions of the C – N stretching vibration and of the N – H in-plane bend.

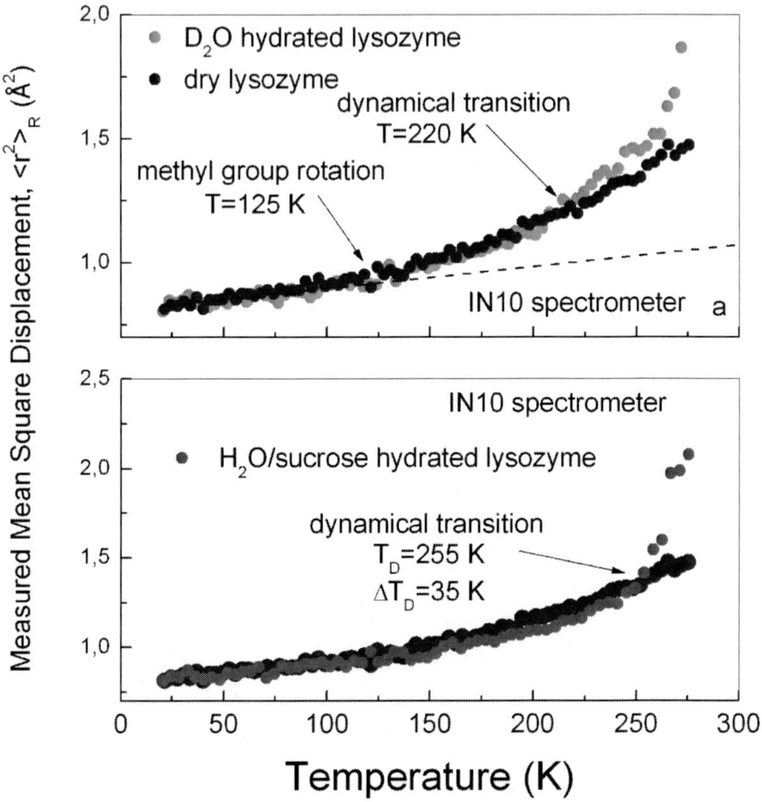

Figure 1. (a) (top) Comparison between the temperature behaviour of the measured MSD of dry (blue) and D_2O hydrated (green) Lysozyme, obtained from data collected by IN10. (b) (bottom) Comparison between the MSDs obtained for sucrose H_2O-hydrated lysozyme (red) and dry Lysozyme (blue) by the IN10 spectrometer. The hydrated sample shows a transition at a temperature of about (a) T=220 K; the presence of disaccharide shifts the transition to a temperature of about (b) T=255 K.

The shape of the amide I band can be considered as due to overlapping sub-bands representing α-helices, β-sheets, turns and random structures. The weak intense band around 1550 cm^{-1} is the amide II band. It mainly corresponds to a mixture of N – H in-plane bend and C – N stretch. The secondary structure of Lysozyme is characterized by α-helices (41%) and β-sheets (21%) [31, 32]. Lysozyme was prepared in D_2O because there is no vibrational contribution of D_2O to the spectrum of the protein in the amide I region, while FTIR spectrum of H_2O is characterized by a broad band around 1630 cm^{-1} corresponding to the bending vibration of the molecule. The FTIR spectrum was analyzed for monitoring changes of the secondary structure of Lysozyme due to ELF-EMF exposure. After three hours of exposure at the intensity value of 180 μT no appreciable alteration was detected in the amide I and II regions. In contrast, relevant changes were observed after exposure in the range from 2800 to 3000 cm^{-1}, as shown in Figure 2. In this region symmetric and asymmetric CH_2 and CH_3 stretching vibrations of protein side chains are generally observed, assigned to methylene and methyl group. In particular, the bands close to 2960 and 2870 cm^{-1} originate, respectively, from the asymmetric stretching $\nu_{as}CH_3$ and the symmetric stretching ν_sCH_3 of CH_3 methyl groups, whereas vibration bands around 2921 and 2853 cm^{-1} are assigned to symmetric and asymmetric bending ν_sCH_2 $\nu_{as}CH_2$, respectively [33, 34]. The intensity of both bands of methylene group were observed to increase after the exposure to the electromagnetic field, as it can be observed in Figure 2. In order to enhance the fine spectral structures in this spectral region, a second-derivative analysis of Lysozyme IR spectra was performed. As it is well known, in the second-derivative spectrum, the intrinsic shape of an infrared absorbance is approximated by a Lorentzian function [22]; in such a case the peak frequency is practically identical with the original peak frequency, but the half-bandwidth is reduced.

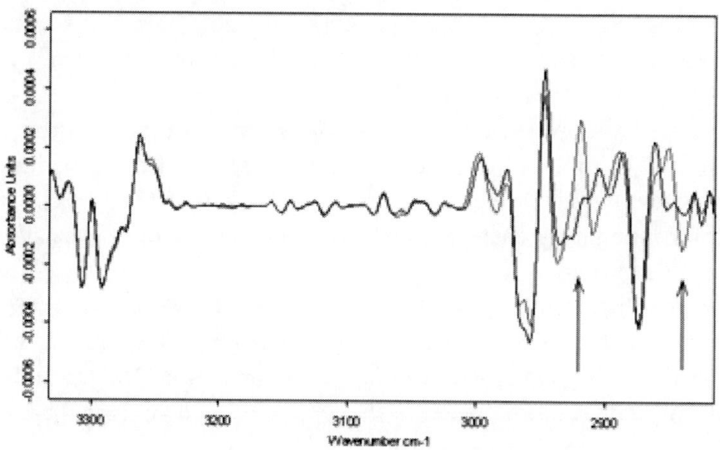

Figure 2. Acquired spectra in mid-infrared region from 3400 cm^{-1} to 2800 cm^{-1} of Lysozyme in D_2O solution. The red line represents the exposed sample spectrum, after 3 h of exposure to a magnetic field of 180 μT. The increases of the CH_2 bands at 2921 cm^{-1} and 2853 cm^{-1} for exposed sample are indicated by arrows.

The second derivative spectrum analysis confirms the increase of the intensity of $\nu_s CH_2$ and $\nu_{as} CH_2$, as it is shown in Figure 3a.

Furthermore, the addition of disaccharides reduces drastically these effects due to the exposure to electromagnetic field. Spectra of Lysozyme in disaccharides D_2O solution were acquired after analogue exposure time. Second-derivative analysis was performed to enhance the fine spectral structure in the examined spectral region; any appreciable change of methylene and methyl groups, as shown in Figure 3b was evidenced.

CONCLUSION

EINS allows to characterize the dynamical properties of dry and hydrated Lysozyme also in the presence of disaccharides. The accessible Q-range of the IN10 spectrometer extends from 0.5 $Å^{-1}$ to 2.0 $Å^{-1}$ and has allowed to evaluate the MSDs as a function of temperature for sucrose/H_2O/lysozyme and for trehalose/H_2O/ lysozyme.

From the present study it clearly emerges that, when disaccharides are added to hydrated protein, the protein dynamical transition, registered at about T=220 K in the D_2O hydrated Lysozyme, is shifted at a higher temperature value, i.e. T=255 K. This 35 K temperature shift puts into evidence that the presence of the disaccharides slows down the dynamics of the hydrated protein.

FTIR spectroscopy has allowed to show the effects of exposure of lysozyme in D_2O solution (in absence and in presence of disaccharides) to a low frequency (50 Hz) electromagnetic field. The FTIR spectrum was analyzed for monitoring changes of the secondary structure of Lysozyme due to ELF-EMF exposure.

After three hours of exposure at the intensity of 180 μT no appreciable alteration was detected in the amide I and II regions. In contrast, relevant changes were observed after the exposure in the range from 2800 to 3000 cm^{-1}. However, the addition of trehalose is shown to drastically reduce these effects due to the exposure to electromagnetic field.

The entire body of the experimental findings highlights the bioprotective effectiveness of disaccharides with respect to two environmental stress, i.e. to the temperature variation and to the extremely low frequency electromagnetic fields exposure.

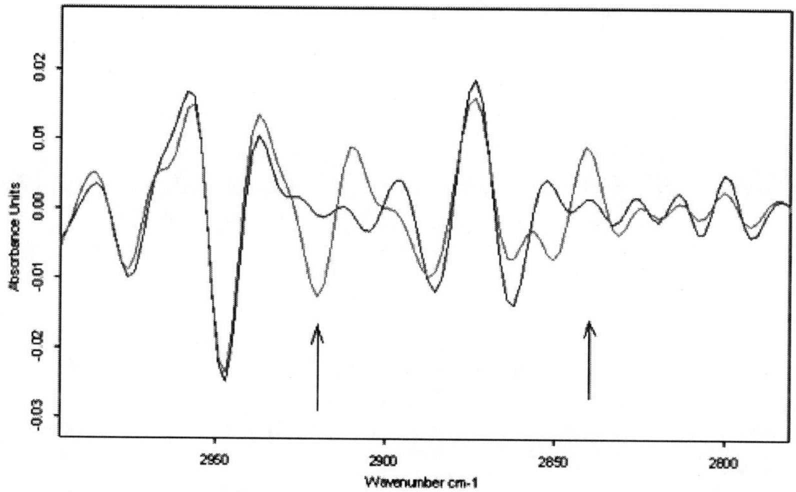

a)

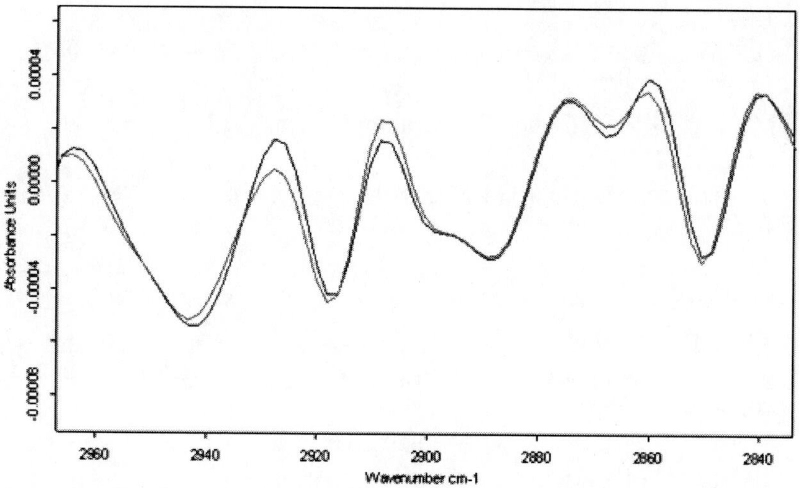

b)

Figure 3. (A) Second derivative spectra from 3000 cm^{-1} to 2800 cm^{-1} of Lysozyme in D_2O solution. The red line represents the exposed sample spectrum, after 3 h of exposure to a magnetic field of 180 μT. The increases of the CH_2 bands at 2921 cm^{-1} and 2853 cm^{-1} (indicated by arrows) is evidenced. (B) Second derivative spectra from 3000 cm^{-1} to 2800 cm^{-1} of Lysozyme in trehalose D_2O solution acquired after analogue exposure conditions (the red line represents the exposed sample spectrum). No appreciable difference can be observed with respect to control sample spectrum.

References

[1] Hédoux, A.; Ionov, R.; Willart, J. F.; Lerbret, A.; Affouard, F.; Guinet, Y.; Descamps, M.; Prevost, D.; Paccou, L.; Danède, F. *J. Chem. Phys.* 2006, 124, 14703-7.

[2] Hédoux, A.; Willart, J. F.; Paccou, L.; Guinet, Y.; Affouard, F.; Lerbret, A.; Descamps, M. *J. Phys. Chem. B* 2009, 113, 6119-6126.

[3] Hédoux, A.; Willart, J. F.; Ionov, R.; Affouard, F.; Guinet, Y.; Paccou, L.; Lerbret, A.; Descamps, M. *J. Phys. Chem. B* 2006, 110, 22886-22893.

[4] Hedoux, A.; Affouard, F.; Descamps, M.; Guinet, Y.; Paccou, L. *J. Phys.: Cond. Matt.* 2007, 19, 2051421-8.

[5] Crowe, J. H.; Carpenter, J. F.; Crowe, L. M. *Ann. Rev. Physiol.* 1998, 60, 73-103.

[6] Sussich, F.; Urbani, R.; Princivalle, F.; Cesàro, A. *J. Amer. Chem. Soc.* 1998, 120, 7893-7899.

[7] Sussich, F.; Bortoluzzi, S.; Cesaro, A. *Thermochim. Acta* 2002, 391, 137-150.

[8] Cesàro, A.; De Giacomo, O.; Sussich, F. *Food Chem.* 2008, 106, 1318-1328.

[9] Magazù, S.; Migliardo, F.; Ramirez-Cuesta, A. J. *J. Roy. Soc. Inter.* 2005, 2, 527-532.

[10] Magazù, S.; Maisano, G.; Migliardo, P.; Villari, V.; *J. Phys. Chem. B* 1999, 111, 9086-9092.

[11] Affouard, F.; Bordat, P.; Descamps, M.; Lerbret, A.; Magazù, S.; Migliardo, F.; Ramirez-Cuesta, A. J.; Telling, M. F. T. *Chem. Phys.* 2005, 317, 258-266.

[12] Magazù, S.; Migliardo, F.; Telling, M. T. F. *J. Phys. Chem. B* 2006, 110, 1020-1025.

[13] Magazù, S.; Maisano, G.; Migliardo, F.; Benedetto, A. *J. Mol. Struct.* 2008, 882, 140-145.

[14] Magazù, S.; Maisano, G.; Migliardo, F.; Benedetto, A. *J. Phys. Chem. B* 2008, 112, 8936-8942.

[15] Magazù, S.; Maisano, G.; Migliardo, F.; Benedetto, A. *Phys. Rev. E* 2008, 77, 0618021-6.

[16] Magazù, S.; Maisano, G.; Migliardo, F.; Galli, G.; Benedetto, A.; Morineau, D.; Affouard, F.; Descamps, M. *J. Chem. Phys.* 2008, 129, 155103-8.

[17] Magazù, S.; Maisano, G.; Migliardo, F.; Benedetto, A. *Phys. Rev. E* 2009, 79, 0419151-9.
[18] Magazù, S.; Maisano, G.; Migliardo, F.; Benedetto, A. *Spectroscopy* 2010, 24, 387-391.
[19] Magazù, S.; Maisano, G.; Migliardo, F.; Benedetto, A. *Biochim. Biophys. Act.* 2010, 1804, 49-55.
[20] Magazù, S.; Migliardo, F.; Benedetto, A. *J. Phys. Chem. B* 2010, 114, 9268-9274.
[21] Magazù, S.; Migliardo, F.; Benedetto, A.; Mondelli, C.; Gonzalez, M. A. *J. Non-Cryst. Sol.* 2011, 357, 664-670.
[22] Teeter, M.M. *Ann. Rev. Bioph. Biophysic. Chem.* 1991, 20, 577-600.
[23] Careri, G. *Progr. Biophys. Molec. Bio.* 70, 223-249.
[24] Gregory, R. B. *Protein-Solvent Interactions*; Dekker: New York, NY, 1995.
[25] Surewicz, W. K.; Mantsch, H. H. *Biochim. Biophys. Act.* 1988, 952, 115−130.
[26] Khodadadi, S.; Pawlus, S.; Roh, J. H.; Garcia Sakai, V.; Mamontov, E.; Sokolov, A. P. *J. Chem. Phys.* 2008, 128, 1951061-5.
[27] Doster, W. *Europ. Biophys. J.* 2007, *37*, 591-602.
[28] Magazù, S.; Migliardo, F.; Benedetto, A. *J. Phys. Chem. B* 2011, 115, 7736-7743.
[29] Byler, D. M.; Susi, H. *Biopolymer* 1986, 25, 469−487.
[30] Dong, A.; Huang, P.; Caughey, W. S. *Biochemistry* 1990, 29, 3303−3308.
[31] Anderle, G.; Mendelsohn, R. *Biophys. J.* 1987, 52, 69-74.
[32] Cai, S.; Singh, B. R. *Biophys. Chem.* 1999, 80, 7-20.
[33] Stuart, B. *Biological applications of infrared spectroscopy*; Analytical Chemistry of Open Learning; John Wiley and Sons: 1997; 115.
[34] Dumas, P.; Miller, L. *Vibr. Spectr.* 2003, 32, 3–21.

In: Sucrose
Editor: Salvatore Magazù

ISBN: 978-1-62417-984-6

Chapter 3

INFLUENCE OF SUCROSE ON SURROUNDING WATER BY EXTENDED FREQUENCY RANGE DEPOLARIZED LIGHT SCATTERING

***L. Lupi*[1], *L. Comez*[1,2], *M. Paolantoni*[3], *P. Sassi*[3], *A. Morresi*[3] and *D. Fioretto*[1,4]**

[1]Dipartimento di Fisica, Università di Perugia, Perugia, Italy
[2]IOM-CNR c/o Dipartimento di Fisica, Università di Perugia, Perugia, Italy
[3]Dipartimento di Chimica, Università di Perugia, Perugia, Italy
[4]Centro di Eccellenza sui Materiali Innovativi Nanostrutturati (CEMIN), Università of Perugia, Perugia, Italy

ABSTRACT

The role of disaccharides as bioprotectors is intimately connected with their interaction with hydration water. To investigate this issue, depolarized light scattering spectra of aqueous solutions of sucrose have been recorded in the range 0.3 GHz – 30 THz by combining the use of a double monochromator and a multipass Fabry-Perot interferometer. The spectra give us information on both the rotational diffusion of a single sucrose molecule and the effect induced by this solute on the picosecond dynamics of water. In particular, two distinct relaxation processes have been identified, and assigned to hydration and bulk water molecules.

The mobility of water localized within the sugar hydration shell is found to be lower than the mobility of water in bulk. The number of molecules involved in the slower dynamics and the extent of retardation are quantified and discussed in comparison with the results recently obtained for other mono and disaccharide solutions.

INTRODUCTION

Aqueous solutions of carbohydrates are object of an increasing scientific interest. In fact, carbohydrates constitute the main part of the organic substance on Earth and play, together with water, a fundamental role in many processes of biological relevance. Simple sugars are also considered as a useful model to study the interplay between hydrophilic solutes and water dynamics and to provide an insight into the behavior of more complex biological molecules. Moreover, the structural and dynamical characteristics of sugars-water solutions are themselves very intriguing, being strongly connected with their exceptional bioprotective properties. In this respect, the stabilizing effect of carbohydrates towards biomolecules is deeply related with the dynamical properties of the sugar molecules and with the perturbation they induce on the surrounding water. It was proven, for instance, that sucrose is responsible for an appreciable slowing down of the dynamics of the water molecules located in its first solvation shell [1]. Therefore, the experimental characterization of both solute and solvent relaxation processes is fundamental to draw an exhaustive description of the interplay between solute and solvent dynamics. Different techniques have been used to study the dynamics of water-sucrose solutions, frequently compared with that of water-trehalose solutions, ranging from Raman scattering [2-4] to dielectric spectroscopy [5], neutron scattering [6, 7, 3], and thermodynamic measurements [8, 9]. It is common experience that separating the sugar relaxation modes from the water ones is not an easy task.

Recently, extended frequency range depolarized light scattering (EDLS) has been exploited in our laboratories, operating in a frequency range that goes from $\sim$ 0.3 to $3\text{x}10^4$ GHz by the combined use of dispersive and interferometric setups. EDLS is a powerful technique to disentangle solute from solvent dynamics in aqueous solutions. Solutions with different carbohydrates [10-15] and biological molecules [16, 17] show a retardation ratio ξ -- the ratio between the relaxation time of hydration and bulk water -- typically ranging from about 4 to 10, around room temperature. Moreover, from the comparison of the relaxation strengths of bulk and hydration water, EDLS give the average hydration number N_H -- the average number of water molecules dynamically perturbed in the close vicinity of each solute molecule -- which is found to range from a single layer in carbohydrates, up to two or more layers in peptides and proteins. In this chapter, spectra of sucrose-water solutions obtained at room temperature and different concentrations are reported. A low frequency contribution due to the rotational diffusion of the solute is clearly distinguished from hydration and bulk water relaxation modes. The perturbation induced in water by a sucrose molecule is quantitatively analyzed in terms of hydration number N_H and retardation ratio ξ and discussed in comparison with results previously obtained on glucose and trehalose-water solutions.

EXPERIMENTAL SETUP

Sucrose was purchased from Panreac with purity higher than 99.1%. Doubly distilled and deionized water was prepared in our laboratory. The solutions were prepared by weight, adding the sugar to water then stirring and heating them until the solute was completely dissolved at four different sucrose molar fractions x=0.005, x=0.009, x=0.021, and x=0.031. All the solutions were freshly prepared and conditioned for more than one hour before measurements in a 10 mm path quartz cuvette. Temperature was 25°C and fluctuations were kept within 0.1 °C during the spectra recording. Vertically polarized single mode Ar+ (λ_0=514.5 nm) and solid state (λ_0=532 nm) lasers were used as light sources with typical power lower than 500 mW and the horizontally polarized scattered light (I_{VH}) was analyzed by means of two different spectrometers.

The low-frequency region from 0.01 to 7 cm^{-1} (0.3-200 GHz) was recorded in back scattering geometry, by means of a Sandercock-type (3+3)-pass tandem Fabry-Perot interferometer, characterized by a finesse of about 100 and a contrast >5 x 10^{10}. Three different mirror separations, d = 14 mm, d = 4 mm and d = 1 mm, corresponding to distinct free spectral ranges, were used. The data acquisition was performed by means of a system developed and tested in our laboratory, composed by an electronic board connected to the interferometer control unit, and by the software running inside the board and on a laboratory PC. The software running on the acquisition PC is a dialog-based application, named GHOST, working as an advanced multi-channel analyzer. [18].

Higher frequency measurements were recorded in the 1-1200 cm^{-1} (3-36000 GHz) frequency range using an ISA Jobin-Yvon model U1000 double monochromator having 1 m focal length with holographic gratings. The detection system utilized was a thermoelectrically cooled Hamamatsu model 943XX photomultiplier, computer-controlled by the ISA Jobin–Yvon SpectraMax package. The scattered light was collected adopting a 90° scattering geometry in two different frequency regions: from -10 to 40 cm^{-1} with a resolution of 0.5 cm^{-1} and from 3 to 1200 cm^{-1} with a resolution of 1 cm^{-1}.

After subtraction of the dark count contribution, low- and high-frequency spectra were spliced taking advantage of an overlap of about half a decade in frequency. Further, the susceptibility spectra were calculated as the ratio between the $I_{VH}(\nu)$ intensity and $[n(\nu)+1]$, where $n(\nu)$ is the Bose-Einstein occupation number, namely $n(\nu) = [\exp(h\nu/kT) - 1]^{-1}$.

RESULTS AND DISCUSSION

Figure 1 shows EDLS spectra for solutions at different sucrose molar fractions, at T=25°C. Due to the presence of the sugar, a new spectral feature can be recognized in the low frequency region of the spectrum (~1GHz), well separated from the region where the characteristic solvent relaxation processes occur. The intensity of this contribution increases with the sucrose content, while its position progressively shifts toward lower frequencies, very similarly to what happens in water-trehalose solutions [12]. The larger optical anisotropy of the solute compared to water and the observed concentration dependence, suggest the attribution of this low frequency component to the rotational diffusion of sucrose.

On the other hand, the high frequency region ($\nu > 1$THz) is assigned to the intermolecular bending and stretching resonant modes of water molecules while the intermediate region, extending from 10 to 10^3 GHz, to the characteristic relaxation dynamics of water [12].

The small interference between solute and solvent components allows one to disentangle the solute from the solvent dynamics. After subtraction of the sugar relaxation mode from the spectrum [10, 12, 15], two distinct relaxation processes can be evidenced. A fast process related to bulk water molecules scarcely affected by the solute and a slower one related to hydration molecules.

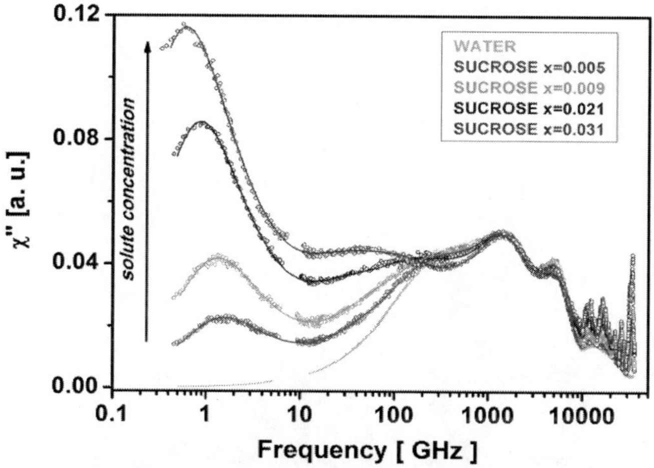

Figure 1. Imaginary part of the susceptibility of pure water and sucrose/water solutions at different sugar molar fractions. The arrow indicates the path of a concentration increase. The continuous lines refer to the fitting curves (see text for details). The lack of data around 10 GHz is due to the removal of few spurious points originated by the leakage of the Brillouin peaks.

The susceptibility spectrum can be thus modeled as the sum of five distinct contributions, as reported in Figure 2. Three Cole-Davidson functions are used to fit the relaxation components; the one located at 1 GHz ca. accounts for the dynamics of sucrose, while the components centered at about 60 and 300 GHz are associated to the relaxation process of hydration and bulk water molecules, respectively. Finally, two damped harmonic oscillator (DHO) functions are used to represent the two resonant modes of the H-bonded water network, located around 1800 and 5100 GHz (i.e. 60 and 170 cm^{-1}). As a whole, the fitting function for our spectra is:

$$\chi''(\omega) = \mathrm{Im}\left\{ -\frac{\Delta}{[1+i\omega\tau]^{\beta}} - \frac{\Delta_{slow}}{[1+i\omega\tau_{slow}]^{\beta_{slow}}} - \frac{\Delta_{fast}}{[1+i\omega\tau_{fast}]^{\beta_{fast}}} + \frac{\Delta_b\omega_b^2}{\omega^2-\omega_b^2-i\omega\Gamma_b} + \frac{\Delta_s\omega_s^2}{\omega^2-\omega_s^2-i\omega\Gamma_s} \right\} \quad (1)$$

where Δ, τ, β, Δ_{slow}, τ_{slow}, β_{slow} and Δ_{fast}, τ_{fast}, β_{fast} are the characteristic amplitude, times and stretching parameters of the sugar relaxation term and the two relaxation processes of water, respectively. ω_b, ω_s, Γ_b and Γ_s are the frequencies and the widths of the intermolecular bending and stretching modes of water, respectively.

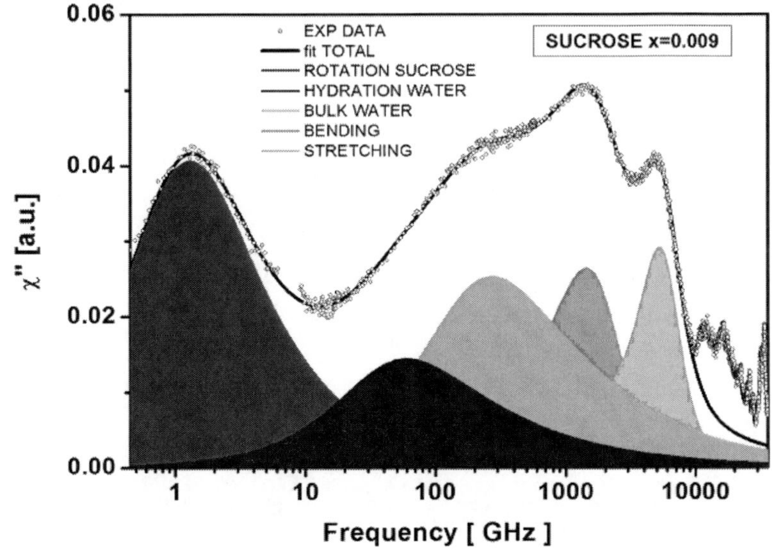

Figure 2. Susceptibility of the sucrose/water solution at 25°C and x=0.009 molar fraction. Experimental data (black O) are reported together with the total fitting curve (black line) and the single components: rotational diffusion of sucrose (violet); relaxation of hydration (blue) and bulk (cyan) water; and bending and stretching intermolecular resonant modes of water (orange and pink).

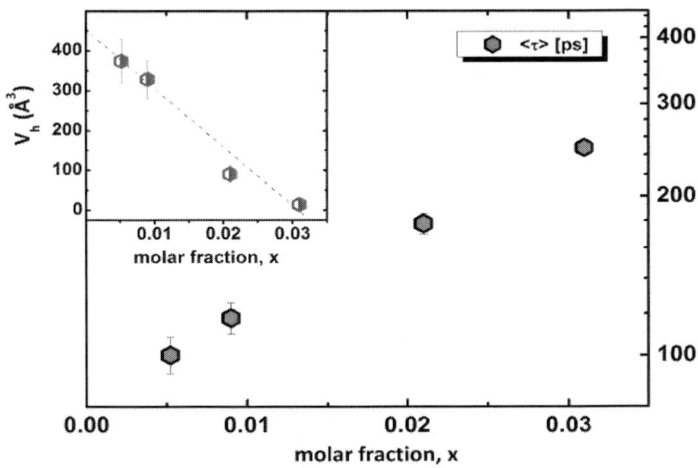

Figure 3. Average rotational relaxation time $<\tau>=\tau\beta$ of sucrose. In the inset, the hydrodynamic volume evaluated by Equation (2). The linear extrapolation to infinite dilution provides V_h = (450±40) Å^3.

Rotational Diffusion of Sucrose

Concerning the sucrose relaxation process, the stretching parameter β was found to be almost constant (around 0.8) in the whole temperature and concentration range under investigation, thus it was fixed to β=0.8 in the fitting procedure to be consistent with previous results of water-trehalose solutions [11]. The concentration dependence of the average relaxation time $<\tau>=\tau \cdot \beta$ (Figure 3) shows an exponential raise of $<\tau>$ as a function of the solute molar fraction recalling our previous findings on glucose and trehalose-water solutions [15, 11]. In analogy with those studies, this relaxation can be interpreted in terms of the rotational diffusion of the sucrose molecules in a medium of increasing viscosity. In this framework, we notice that depolarized scattering experiments detect the collective reorientation time τ, which is connected to the single particle correlation time τ_s by the relation $\tau = (g_2 / j_2)\, \tau_s$, being g_2 and j_2 the static and dynamic correlation parameter, respectively. In the high dilution limit, the ratio g_2 / j_2 tends to unit and DLS can directly probe the single particle correlation time. As a result, at least in the low concentration limit, the detected relaxation time can be described in terms of the Stokes–Einstein–Debye equation, which relates the single particle correlation time τ_s to the viscosity of the solution η:

$$\tau_s = V_h \eta / (k_B T), \qquad (2)$$

where V_h is the so-called hydrodynamic volume closely related to the molecular volume. The inset of Figure 3 depicts the values of V_h obtained with Equation 2 using the experimental values of τ and viscosity data taken from Ref. [19]. A linear extrapolation to infinite dilution, namely in the limit of negligible inter-particle interactions, provides V_h = 450±40 Å^3. This is a reasonable value for sucrose, not far from that of trehalose, V_h = 430±30 Å^3 [11]. These values for the hydrodynamic volume, very close to those of the molecular volumes of the sugars, point out an interesting difference between the dynamics of sugar and that of small charged molecules in water [20]. In fact, in case of ions, the solute rotation was found to drag the overall solvation shell. Conversely, our results suggest that the rotational diffusion of sugar is totally decoupled from that of surrounding water. In other words, water molecules rearrange at very faster rates with respect to sugar molecules so that the sugar hydration shell is destroyed and re-formed several times during the period of a single rotation of the solute. This is also consistent with the large spectral distance of about two decades between the relaxation of sucrose and that of water, as visible in Figure 1.

It is also to be noticed that carbohydrates are known to have a strong tendency to self-associate in aqueous solutions, leading to concentration-dependent clustering. [21, 22] The hydrogen bond network that sucrose forms in aqueous solutions was, for example, analyzed computationally [23] in connection with other experimental results, suggesting that the formation of sucrose clusters results in the decoupling of water and sucrose diffusion [24] and that sucrose percolation is related to the decoupling of viscosity and probe molecule diffusion [25]. The high propensity for self-association of carbohydrate molecules is not in contradiction with the experimental evidence obtained by EDLS of rotational diffusion of single sucrose, trehalose and glucose molecules up to concentrations close to the supposed percolation limit. In fact, looking at the simulations recently performed in water trehalose solutions [26], the most probable coordination number for sugar molecules remains lower than 2 in the investigated range and the average life-time of these aggregates is about 11 ps, one order of magnitude faster than the rotational correlation time we find for the sugar molecule [11]. In this condition, rotational diffusion mainly reflects the clustering as an increase of inter-trehalose interaction, i.e. a change of viscosity, and not as the development of rotating species with increased hydrodynamic radius.

Hydration and Bulk Water

The average relaxation time of the two relaxation processes of water is reported in Figure 4 as a function of sugar concentration. The fast process has a characteristic relaxation time of 0.4-0.9 ps, comparable to the relaxation time measured in pure water (~ 0.5 ps) and is assigned to the dynamics of bulk-like water molecules whose motion is only slightly affected by the sugar. The slow process, has a characteristic time of about 3-4 ps, and is assigned to those water molecules temporarily localized within the sugar hydration shell. From a physical point of view these relaxation processes should essentially relate to the local translational motion of water molecules that modulate the anisotropic polarizability of the system via intermolecular interaction-induced mechanisms. Rotational contributions are of minor importance for water molecules owing to their almost isotropic polarizabiliy. This structural rearrangement is strongly associated with the fast hydrogen bond reorganization of the system and the corresponding relaxation time is often regarded as a measure of the average hydrogen bond lifetime in water [13, 14, 27, 28]. From these relaxation times, the retardation ratio ξ has been calculated and reported in Figure 5 in comparison with the results previously obtained for trehalose aqueous solutions. As it can be seen the rearrangement dynamics of hydration water slows down of a factor between 5 and 6 when compared to bulk water.

From the relative intensity of the two water relaxation processes the average hydration number N_H can be also calculated. In our case N_H is defined as the number of water molecules contributing to the intensity of the slow relaxation term divided by the total number of sugar molecules in solution. It can be obtained from the ratio R between the amplitude of the slow process and that of the total water contribution $R = \Delta_{slow}/(\Delta_{slow} + \Delta_{fast})$, through the relationship $N_H = R / f_s$, where f_s is the sucrose/water molar ratio. Figure 6 shows R versus f_s in water-sucrose solutions together with the values obtained in water-trehalose solutions. The values obtained at low concentrations are those potentially more affected by systematic errors due either to the small relative contribution of hydrating water or to the possible interference of water-sugar cross-contributions [29] in the spectra. The values at high concentration give a hydration number ranging between 17 and 22, close to the average value 17±1 previously obtained for trehalose.

Overall these findings suggest that approximately a single layer of hydrating water molecules per sucrose experience a 5-6-fold dynamical slowing down when compared to the bulk. This picture closely recall that derived by the molecular dynamics simulations study of Lee et al.[1] In this case structural and dynamical properties of proximal and bulk water were analyzed. Sugars were found to decrease the translational and rotational mobility of proximal water and only minor differences were reported between trehalose and sucrose in their overall effects on the structural order, translational diffusion coefficient and rotational correlation time of the surrounding water.

On the whole this chapter provides an important piece of information well integrated with results obtained by previous spectroscopic investigations of water-sucrose solutions. Previous Raman scattering studies, [2 - 4] were mainly devoted to the study of the modifications induced by the sugar on the structure of water, through the analysis of the intramolecular OH stretching mode [2, 3], and on the properties of the H-bonding network through the analysis of the vibrational density of states. In this respect, the novelty of this investigation resides in the extension of the accessible frequency range towards lower frequencies by means of the Fabry-Perot interferometer, which allowed us to directly measure the diffusional dynamics of both water and sugar molecules.

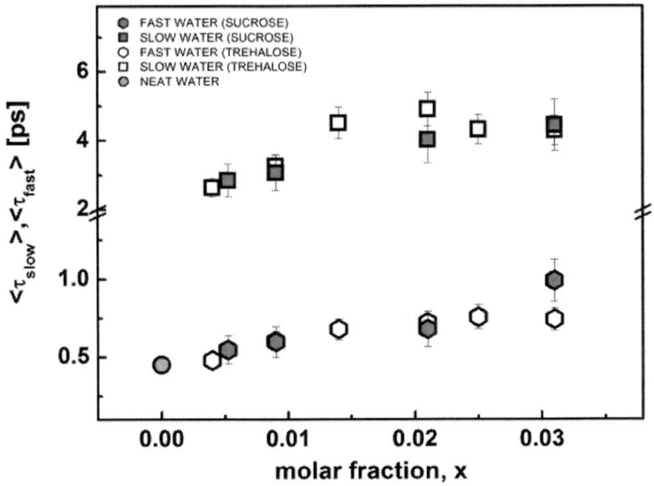

Figure 4. Average relaxation time of the hydrating $<\tau_{slow}>$ (full squares) and bulk $<\tau_{fast}>$ (full hexagons) water relaxation processes obtained by the adopted fitting procedure for the sucrose/water solution at different concentrations at ambient temperature. The relaxation time of pure water is also reported (cyan symbol) for comparison. Open symbols refer to trehalose/water solutions taken from [12].

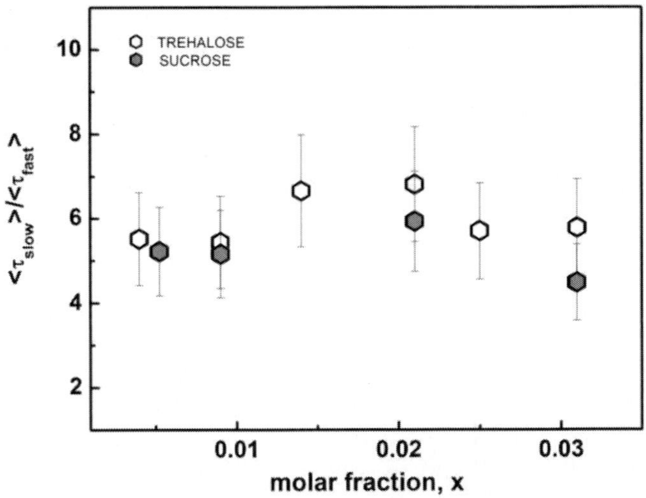

Figure 5. Retardation factor $<\tau_{slow}>/ <\tau_{fast}>$ for sucrose/water solutions (full symbols) at different concentrations compared to the results on trehalose/water solutions (open symbols) [12].

The same information could, in principle, be pursued by dielectric spectroscopy [5]. Nevertheless, the elaboration of dielectric spectra in the diluted regime here addressed is complicated by the overlapping of sugar and water relaxational bands. In fact, dielectric spectra of sugar-water solutions, show a single broad relaxation component [5]. This may be explained recalling that dielectric spectroscopy is mainly sensitive to the reorientation of OH groups (which is expected to be similar for water and sugar), rather than to the rotation of the whole sugar molecule, detected in light scattering experiments; in addition, since the dipolar relaxation of water is typically located in the ten GHz relaxation region, the slow exchange picture breaks down, thus the possibility of having two well separated spectral features for bulk and hydration water fails. In this respect, it is known that the exchange rate of water molecules solvating hydrophobic solutes is about 4 GHz, [30] very close to the relaxation rate of bulk and hydration water molecules. Dielectric spectra are thus at intermediate condition between slow exchange, where the two relaxations would be well separated, and fast exchange, where they would collapse into a single peak at intermediate frequency. In this condition, a broad non-exponential spectrum is expected, as revealed by experiments.

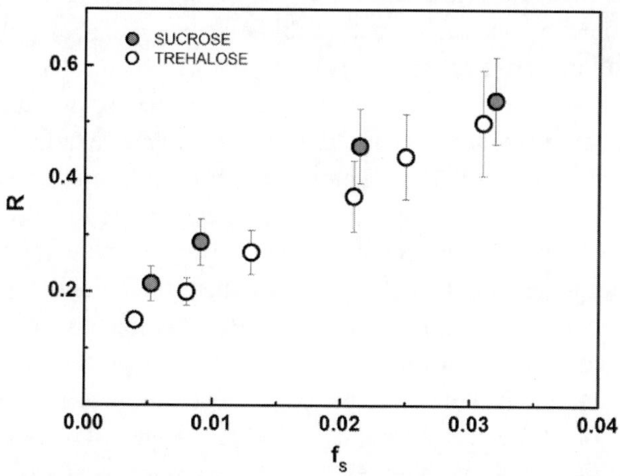

Figure 6. Relative weight $R = \Delta_{slow}/(\Delta_{slow} + \Delta_{fast})$ of the slow water relaxation process as a function of the sucrose molar ratio f_s.

Quasielastic neutron scattering was used to study the fragility of sucrose and trehalose solutions, via the temperature dependence of the mean square displacement [6, 7, 3]. It was recognized that the trehalose/water mixture at 0.05 water molar fraction is the strongest system compared to the sucrose/

water mixture at the same concentration, and this was also confirmed by time-of-flight neutron scattering results [31], supporting the hypothesis of a better attitude of trehalose to encapsulate biomolecules into more rigid and more temperature insensitive structures. This property was connected to the greater cryptobiotic effectiveness of trehalose with respect to sucrose [3, 7]. This finding, also confirmed by inelastic neutron scattering and simulation studies [6], is not in contradiction with our result of a comparable effect of sucrose and trehalose on surrounding water molecules. In fact, it should be underlined that our results are obtained in the water rich region, while the peculiar effects induced by trehalose, as revealed by neutron scattering, are obtained in the sugar-rich domain. The comparison of our findings with those obtained by neutron scattering probably suggests that the more pronounced bio-protectant effect of trehalose emerges only when the content of water is considerably reduced.

CONCLUSION

In this chapter, the influence of sucrose on surrounding water molecules has been studied by means of extended frequency range depolarized light scattering of diluted aqueous solutions.

The combined use of two different experimental setups allowed us to access a very large frequency range that includes the relaxation mode of the solute and both relaxation and resonant modes of the aqueous medium.

Depolarized light scattering experiments, depending on the anisotropic polarizability of the system, are proven to be a favorable tool to separate relaxation processes of solute and solvent in aqueous solutions.

Unambiguous evidence of a considerable slowing down of the water relaxation process has been demonstrated, isolating spectral features due to bulk and hydration water. Notably, the retardation effect induced by carbohydrates on the water dynamics may be related to the bioconservative properties of this class of compounds [32, 33]. Sucrose, similarly to trehalose, is found to strongly affect the relaxation dynamics at picosecond time scale. The rearrangement dynamics of hydrating water is found to be 5-6 times slower than that of bulk water. A future work will focus on gaining more insights on the number and spatial location of hydration water molecules, especially in connection with their possible dependence on sugar concentration, by comparing EDLS spectra with molecular dynamics simulation results [29].

REFERENCES

[1] Lee, S. L.; Debenedetti, P. G. ; Errington, J. R. *J. Chem. Phys.* 2005, 122, 204511-204520.

[2] Branca, C.; Magazù, S.; Maisano, G. and Migliardo, P. *J. Chem. Phys.* 1999, 111, 281-287.

[3] Branca, C.; Magazù, S.; Maisano, G.; Bennington, S. M. and Fåk, B. *J. Phys. Chem. B* 2003, 107, 1444-1451.

[4] Lerbret, A.; Affouard, F.; Bordat, P.; Hédoux, A.; Guinet, Y.; Descamps, M. *J. Non-Cryst. Solids* 2011, 357, 695–699.

[5] Fuchs, K. and Kaatze, U. *J. Chem. Phys.* 2002, 116, 7137-7144.

[6] Affouard, F.; Bordat, P.; Descamps, M.; Lerbret, A.; Magazù, S.; Migliardo, F.; Ramirez-Cuesta, A. J.; Telling, M. F. T. *Chem. Phys.* 2005, 317, 258–266.

[7] Magazù, S.; Maisano, G.; Migliardo, F. and Mondelli, C. J. *Phys. Chem. B* 2004, 108, 13580-13585.

[8] Gharsallaoui, A.; Rogé, B.; Génotelle, J.; Mathlouthi, M. *Food Chem.* 2008, 106, 1443–1453.

[9] Uchida, T.; Nagayama, M.; Gohara, K. *J. Crystal Growth* 2009, 311, 4747–4752.

[10] Rossi, B.; Comez, L.; Fioretto, D.; Lupi, L.; Caponi, S. and Rossi, F. *J. Raman Spectrosc.* 2011, 42, 1479-1483.

[11] Gallina, M. E.; Comez, L.; Morresi, A.; Paolantoni, M.; Perticaroli, S.; Sassi, P. and Fioretto, D. *J. Chem. Phys.* 2010, 132, 214508-214513.

[12] Paolantoni, M.; Comez, L.; Gallina, M. E.; Sassi, P.; Scarponi, F.; Fioretto, D. and Morresi, A. *J. Phys. Chem. B* 2009, 113, 7874–7878.

[13] Paolantoni, M.; Comez, L.; Fioretto, D.; Gallina, M. E.; Morresi, A.; Sassi, P.; Scarponi, F. *J. Raman Spectrosc.* 2008, 39, 238-243.

[14] Paolantoni, M.; Sassi, P.; Morresi, A.; Santini, S. *J. Chem. Phys.* 2007, 127, 024504-024512.

[15] Fioretto, D.; Comez, L.; Gallina, M.E.; Morresi, A.; Palmieri, L.; Paolantoni, M.; Sassi, P.; Scarponi, F. *Chem. Phys. Letters* 2007, 441, 232-236.

[16] Perticaroli, S.; Comez, L.; Paolantoni, M.; Sassi, P.; Morresi, A. and Fioretto, D. *J. Am. Chem. Soc.* 2011, 133, 12063–12068.

[17] Perticaroli, S.; Comez, L.; Paolantoni, M.; Sassi, P.; Lupi, L.; Fioretto, D.; Paciaroni, A. and Morresi, A. *J. Phys. Chem. B* 2010, 114, 8262-8269.

[18] Fioretto, D.; Scarponi, F. *Materials Science and Engineering A* 2009, 521–522, 243-246.

[19] Seoncheol, C.; Kim, S. H. and Kim, D. *J. Korean Phys. Soc.* 2010, 56, 1315-1318.

[20] Bakker, H. J.; Kropman, M. F. and Omta, A. W. *J. Phys.: Condens. Matter* 2005, 17, S3215-S3224.

[21] Sidebottom, D. L.; Tran, T. D. *Phys. Rev. E* 2010, 82, 051904-051910.

[22] Sonoda, M. T.; Skaf, M. S. *J. Phys. Chem. B* 2007, 111, 11948-11956.

[23] Molinero, V.; Cagin, T.; Goddard, W. A. *Chem. Phys. Lett.* 2003, 377, 469-474.

[24] Rampp, M.; Buttersack, C.; Ludemann, H. D. *Carbohydr. Res.* 2000, 328, 561-572.

[25] Champion, D.; Hervet, H.; Blond, G.; LeMeste, M.; Simatos, D. *J. Phys. Chem. B* 1997, 101, 10674-10679.

[26] Sapir, L. and Harries, D. *J. Phys. Chem. B* 2011, 115, 624-634.

[27] Torre, R.; Bartolini, P.; Righini, R. *Nature* 2004, 428, 296-299.

[28] Teixeira, J.; Luzar, A.; Longeville, S. *J. Phys.: Condens. Matter* 2006, 18, S2353-S2362.

[29] Lupi, L. Ph. D. *Thesis,* 2012, Department of Physics, University of Perugia.

[30] Fioretto, D.; Marini, A.; Massarotti, M.; Onori, G.; Palmieri, L.; Santucci, A.; Socino, G. *J. Chem. Phys.* 1993, *99*, 8115–8119.

[31] Branca, C.; Magazù, S.; Maisano, G. and Migliardo, F. *Phys. Rev. B* 2001, *64*, 224204-224211.

[32] Magazù, S.; Migliardo, F.; Telling, M. T. F. *Eur. Biophys. J.* 2007, *36*, 163-171.

[33] Heyden, M.; Bründermann, E.; Heugen, U.; Niehues, G.; Leitner, D. M.; Havenith, M. *J. Am. Chem. Soc.* 2008, *130*, 5773-5779.

In: Sucrose
Editor: Salvatore Magazù

ISBN: 978-1-62417-984-6

Chapter 4

IMPROVEMENT OF COLOR AND FUNCTIONAL STABILITY OF STRAWBERRY JAM BY IMPREGNATION WITH SUCROSE

Yoshiyuki Watanabe*
Department of Biotechnology and Chemistry, Faculty of Engineering,
Kinki University, Takaya, Higashi-Hiroshima, Japan

ABSTRACT

Strawberry impregnated with sucrose was used for the jam preparation, and the effect of various impregnating conditions on the stability of anthocyanins in the jam was examined. The amount of sucrose in impregnated strawberry depended on the concentration of sucrose solution and the operation time for the impregnation. It was kinetically indicated that the impregnation of strawberry in advance of the jam preparation stabilized anthocyanins in the jam. The rate constants by the Weibull model for the color deterioration of the jam impregnated with sucrose and the degradation of anthocyanins in the jam were estimated, and the relationship between the two rate constants was observed to be almost linear.

The antioxidative ability of the strawberry jam correlated with the amount of anthocyanin in the jam. It was shown that the impregnation of strawberry with sucrose was effective for improvement of functional stability of strawberry jam.

* E-mail address: wysyk@hiro.kindai.ac.jp.

Keywords: Antioxidative ability; color and functional stability; impregnation; strawberry jam; sucrose

INTRODUCTION

Impregnation is a technique for replacing gas and liquid through the internal pores of a material by an external liquid [1, 2]. Impregnation can be used to accelerate mass transfer and promote a more homogeneous distribution in fruits, because solutes in the solution can be introduced more efficiently into the tissue. Immersing of the material in the solution and vacuum processing are needed, and this process can enrich food products with nutrients and vitamins, and aid the incorporation of useful additives. In addition, it may improve the sensorial taste, smell, and appearance properties of food.

Although anthocyanins are the most abundant flavonoid constituents of fruits and vegetables, and are bioactive compounds, they are susceptible to heat and light during manufacturing, transportation, and preservation. They cause color deterioration of processed food containing anthocyanins, such as strawberry jam.

Thus, the improvement of the stability of anthocyanin in food is important in jam production and the food industry, and many studies on the color stability of strawberry jam have been reported [3-8]. The main anthocyanin involved in strawberry is known to be pelargonidin 3-glucoside [9, 10], but the type of cultivar, ripening degree, storage conditions, and other components in strawberry affect the anthocyanin [11]. The effects of high-pressure processing in jam manufacture [12], as well as various saccharides, not only monosaccharides but oligo- and polysaccharides [13] on the stabilization of anthocyanin have been examined. Some saccharides, such as cyclodextrins and maltodextrin, are reported to be effective for the stabilization of anthocyanin in food [14]. Sucrose is a *disaccharide* composed of *glucose* and *fructose.*

It is universal in plants and fulfills many roles: transport sugar, storage reserve, compatible solute and signal compound [15]. Sucrose with a sweet taste is generally used for the jam manufacturing. The application of the above-mentioned impregnation technique using the sucrose solution for the jam production may contribute to improvement of the product quality and the stability.

In this chapter, effect of impregnating with sucrose on the color and functional stability of strawberry jam is described. First, the effect of impregnating conditions using the sucrose solution on the stability of anthocyanins in the jam was examined. Second, the color stability of impregnated strawberry jam with sucrose was evaluated. In third section, the relationship between the antioxidative ability, which is one of the functional properties, of the impregnated jam and anthocyanins in the jam was studied. The degradation of anthocyanins and the color deterioration processes were expressed by the Weibull equation, and their stabilities were kinetically analyzed.

EFFECT OF IMPREGNATING CONDITIONS USING SUCROSE ON THE STABILITY OF ANTHOCYANINS IN STRAWBERRY JAM

Ten grams of a piece of strawberry (*Fragaria x ananassa*), the moisture on the surface of which was removed using a wiper, was added to 30 mL of sucrose solution at the concentrations from 0.29 to 2.34 mol/L [8]. Impregnation from 5 to 60 min was carried out under reduced pressure (4 kPa). The impregnated strawberry was ground down in a mortar with 0.1 g of sea sand. After filtration, the distilled water was added to the filtrate to obtain 20 mL of the extract. Fifteen milliliters of distilled water, 25 g of sucrose, and 0.5 g of pectin were added to 50 g of the impregnated strawberry. The mixture was heated at 102°C for 2 min. One gram of the jam was weighed in flat-bottomed glass cups (1.5 cm i.d. and 3.0 cm height). The cups were placed in a plastic container with a Petri dish containing the distilled water to regulate the relative humidity at 100%. The container was stored in the dark at 65°C for 50 to 100 h. The cups were removed at appropriate intervals for observation of the transient changes in the total amount of anthocyanins, and 1 mL of the hydrochloric acid/methanol mixture (5/95(v/v)) was added to the cup to fully dissolve anthocyanins in the strawberry jam. Then, the mixture was centrifuged using a centrifugal separator. The extraction and centrifugation were repeated 5 times.

The total concentration of anthocyanins in the extract was measured at 510 nm using a Ultra violet-visible spectrophotometer [16]. The total amount of anthocyanins in the jam was measured 2 to 3 times. The concentration of sucrose in the extract was measured using HPLC with a YMC-Pack NH_2 column (4.6 mmϕ x 150 mm) and a refractive index detector. After dilution 2 to 10 times with an eluent, acetonitrile/water mixture (75/25(v/v)), for HPLC analysis, the diluted extract was passed through a disposable membrane filter cartridge, which held the hydrophilic polytetrafluoroethylene membrane with a pore diameter of 0.20 μm. Twenty microliters of the filtrate was applied to the column and eluted at 1.0 mL/min. Each measurement of the concentration was carried out in triplicate and the mean value was calculated.

Figure 1 shows the relationship between the concentration of sucrose in impregnating solution and the amount of sucrose in strawberry extract was examined with impregnation carried out for 30 min. For the concentrations from 0 to 1.75 mol/L, the amount of sucrose extracted from the strawberry was proportional to the sucrose concentration in the impregnating solution. At concentrations over 1.75 mol/L, the amount of sucrose in the used strawberry reached the maximum under these processing conditions. It may be impossible to transfer the sucrose from the solution to the strawberry owing to the high viscosity of the impregnating solution.

Figure 2 shows the dependence of the amount of sucrose impregnated into the strawberry on the processing time was measured at the concentration of 1.17 mol/L. The impregnation rapidly proceeded for 10 min, whereas the amount of sucrose in the strawberry extract was almost constant from 10 to 30 min.

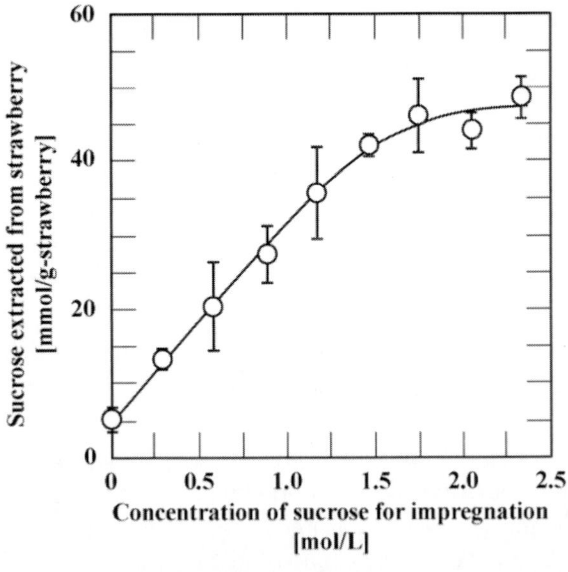

Figure 1. Relationship between the concentration of sucrose in impregnating solution and the concentration of sucrose in strawberry extract. The sucrose solution was impregnated for 30 min. Statistical significance was determined at $p < 0.05$.

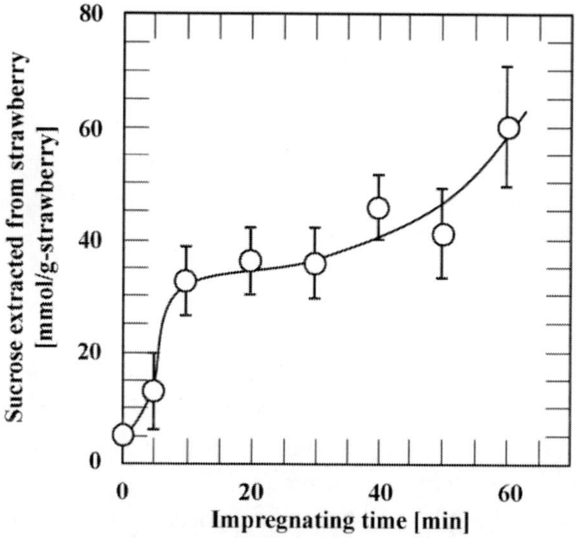

Figure 2. Relationship between impregnating time and the concentration of sucrose in strawberry extract. The sucrose solution was impregnated at 1.17 mol/L. Statistical significance was determined at $p < 0.05$.

In operating for more than 40 min, the amount markedly increased again. During the initial period of the impregnation, the sucrose in the solution was promptly transferred from the outer pericarp to unoccupied positions, to which it could easily move, in the strawberry. Afterwards, the rate of transfer slowed as the empty spaces were filled with the sucrose from the solution. Further impregnating process under reduced pressure for a long time might break the internal structure of the strawberry, resulting in the large increment of sucrose in it. Thereafter, the processing at 30 min was adopted for evaluation of the effects of the impregnation on the stability of anthocyanins in the strawberry jam and the color stability of the jam. Strawberry jam mixed with or produced from strawberry impregnated with sucrose from 0.29 to 1.46 mol/L was prepared. Figure 3 shows the transient changes in the fractions of remaining anthocyanin in the strawberry jam mixed with or produced from strawberry impregnated with 0.29, 0.88, and 1.46 mol/L sucrose at 65°C and 100% relative humidity. The degradation kinetics of the anthocyanins were empirically expressed by the Weibull equation (Eq. 1), which is flexible and can be used to describe many deterioration kinetics [17, 18]:

$$\frac{A}{A_0} = \exp[-(k_{\mathrm{Ant}}t)^n] \tag{1}$$

where A_0 and A are the initial amount of anthocyanins and that at time t, respectively, k_{Ant} is the rate constant, and n is the shape constant. The kinetic parameters, k and n, were estimated by fitting the experimental results by nonlinear regression using Solver of Microsoft® Excel 2007. The curves in Figure 3 were drawn on the basis of the Weibull equation using the estimated parameter. Figure 4 shows the relationship between the rate constant, k_{Ant}, or the shape constant, n, of the Weibull model for the degradation of anthocyanin and the concentration of sucrose in the solution.

The k_{Ant} values both with and without impregnation decreased with the increasing concentration of sucrose, but the decrement with the impregnation was larger than that without it. These suggested that the impregnation of sucrose in advance of the jam preparation stabilized the anthocyanin in the jam more strongly than the mere addition of sucrose during the preparation. Firthermore, a high concentration of sucrose in the impregnation was effective for the stabilization of anthocyanins in jam preservation. The intensity of color of anthocyanin is known to increase by the addition of saccharides, such as glucose, maltose, and sucrose [13].

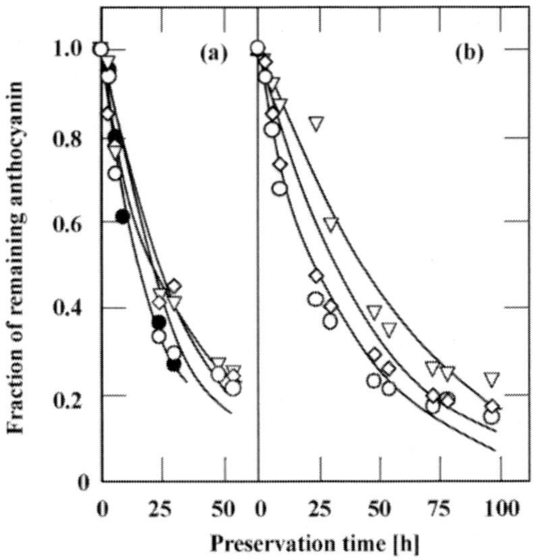

Figure 3. Degradation of anthocyanins in strawberry jam at 65°C and 100% relative humidity. The sucrose solutions at the concentrations of (○) 0.29, (◇) 0.88, and (▽) 1.46 mol/L were (a) mixed with the jam or (b) impregnated into strawberry for 30 min before the preparation of the jam. The control (●) represents neither addition nor impregnation of sucrose into the jam. The solid curves were calculated using the estimated kinetic parameters of the Weibull model.

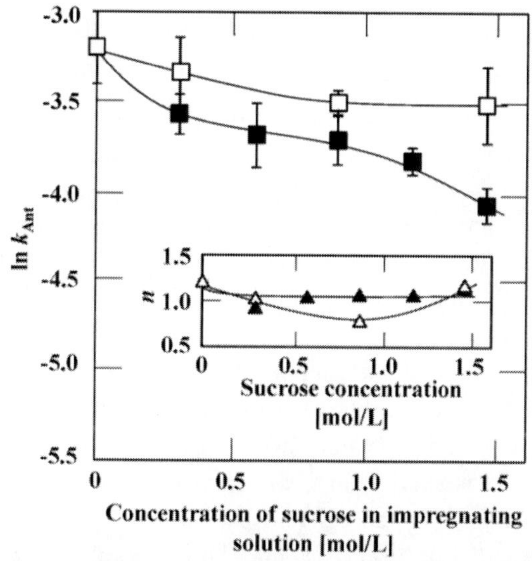

Figure 4. Effect of the concentration of sucrose in impregnating solution on the rate constant, k [h^{-1}], of the Weibull model for the degradation of anthocyanins in strawberry jam. The inset shows the relationship between the sucrose concentration and the shape constant, n. The closed (■, ▲) and open (□, Δ) symbols represent the parameters with and without the impregnation using sucrose solution, respectively. Statistical significance was determine at $p < 0.05$.

The removal of water by saccharides causes this increase through the displacement of the hydration/dehydration equilibrium towards the colored species. The cause of the protective effect of sucrose was also suggested: inhibition of pigment degradative enzymes, namely, polyphenol oxidase and β-glucosidase, steric interference with condensation, namely, anthocyanin-phenolic polymerization; anthocyanin-ascorbate, or provision of a partial oxygen barrier [19]. These would support on the effectiveness of the impregnation for the stability of anthocyanin in the jam. Regardless of the impregnation processing, the n value for each concentration of the sucrose was about 1.

The Color Stability of Impregnated Strawberry Jam with Sucrose

Color analysis of the jam was conducted with a colorimeter. The instrument was calibrated with a standard white and black reflective plate. The instrumental values, L^*, a^*, and b^*, were recorded and the color difference, ΔE (= $\sqrt{\Delta L^{*2} + \Delta a^{*2} + \Delta b^{*2}}$), the chroma, C^*(= $\sqrt{a^{*2} + b^{*2}}$), and the hue angle, θ (= arctan b^*/a^*), were calculated from these values. All color measurements were carried out in triplicate, and the mean value was reported.

Figure 5 shows the transient changes in color parameters for strawberry jam impregnated using the sucrose solution at several concentrations. The preservation of the jam were carried out at 65°C and 100% relative humidity. The L^* values for the jam without impregnation also decreased from 33.1 to 15.8 (Figure 5(a)).

However, there was no difference among the values with and without impregnation, and the value did not depend on the sucrose concentration in the impregnating solution. The a^* value for each jam rapidly decreased during the early stage of the preservation and was almost constant after 50 h (Figure 5(b)). The b^* value for the impregnated jam slowly decreased, while that for the non-impregnated one did not change markedly (Figure 5(c)). The difference for the color difference, ΔE, for the jam was not found (Figure 5(d)).

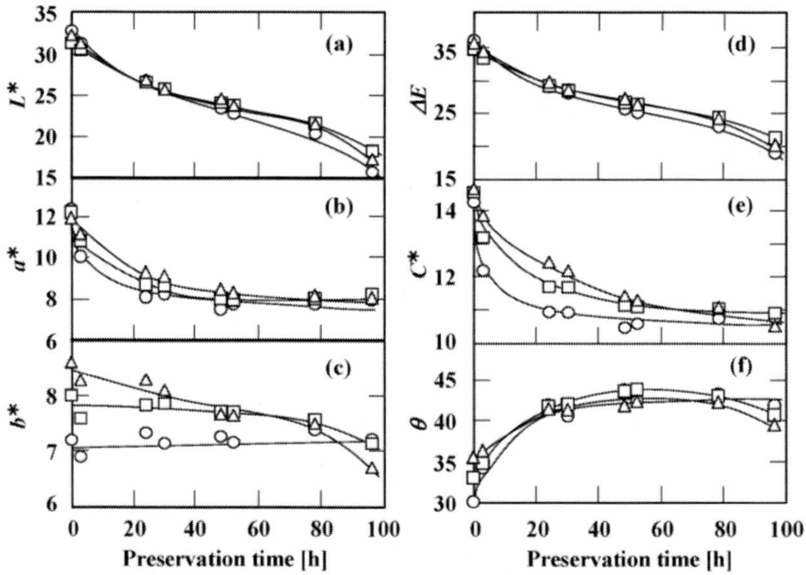

Figure 5. The transient changes in color parameters, (a) L^*, (b) a^*, (c) b^*, (d) ΔE, (e) C^* and (f) θ, for strawberry jam impregnated using (□) 0.88 and (Δ) 1.46 mol/L sucrose solution at 65°C and 100% relative humidity. The control (○) represents no impregnation into strawberry.

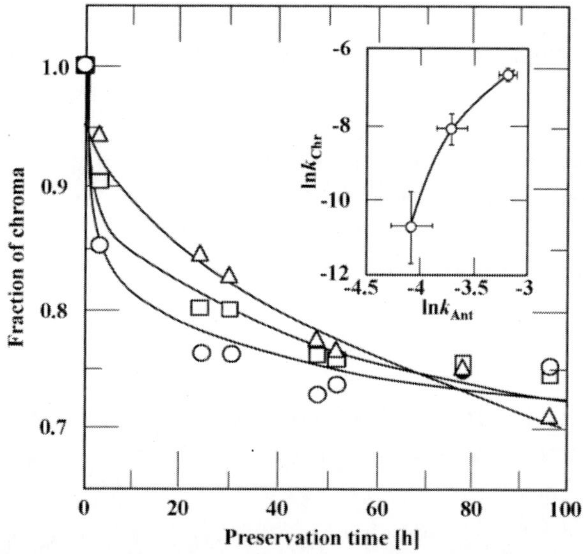

Figure 6. The transient changes in the fraction of chroma, C^*/C_0^*, for strawberry jam impregnated using the sucrose solution at 65°C and 100% relative humidity. The symbols are the same as in Figure 5. The solid curves were calculated using the estimated kinetic parameters of the Weibull model for the fraction. The inset shows the relationship between the rate constants, k_{Ant} and k_C [h^{-1}], of the model for the degradation of anthocyanins in strawberry jam and the chromatic deterioration of the jam, respectively. Statistical significance was determined at $p < 0.05$.

The ΔE value did not differ by the larger contribution of L^* value, compared with those of the a^* and b^* values, to the ΔE value. For the chroma, C^*, derived from the a^* and b^* values, a similar tendency was shown to that of the a^* value, though the difference between the C^* values for the jams with the different concentrations of sucrose solution was larger than that for the a^* values (Figure 5(e)). The difference for the hue angle, θ, for the jam was hardly observed (Figure 5(f)). For the a^*, b^* and C^* values, a higher value was observed at a higher concentration of the sucrose solution in the impregnation at almost all time points.

Thus, the C^* value was used as an index for the color stability of the impregnated jam. Figure 6 shows the chromatic deterioration of strawberry jam impregnated using 0.88 and 1.46 mol/L sucrose solution at 65°C and 100% relative humidity. The above-mentioned Weibull model was applied for the fraction of chroma, and the rate constant, k_{Chr}, for the chromatic deterioration of the jam was estimated. The relationship between the two rate constants, k_{Ant} and k_{Chr}, was almost linear, as shown in the inset in Figure 6. It has been reported that the decrease in the pigments in strawberry jam at temperatures from 20 to 37°C is not always correlated with a decrease in the a^* value [5].

Since the jam was preserved at higher temperature in this study, the thermal degradation of anthocyanins rather than enzymatic reaction in the strawberry might have resulted in the different influence on the color property of the jam. It was shown that the stabilization of anthocyanin by the impregnation of sucrose into strawberry prior to the production of the jam also contributed to the color stability, especially the chroma.

RELATIONSHIP BETWEEN IMPREGNATION WITH SUCROSE AND ANTIOXIDATIVE ABILITY OF STRAWBERRY JAM

In accordance with reported methods [20], the radical scavenging activities of the jam extract were evaluated. Fifteen milliliters of 0.4 mmol/L DPPH (1,1-diphenyl-2-picrylhydrazyl) free radical solution was mixed with 15 mL of 0.2 mol/L MES buffer (pH 6.0) and the same volume of 3.4 mol/L ethanol solution.

The sample solution was prepared at six concentrations by diluting the jam extract sampled at appropriate intervals with 13.7 mol/L ethanol solution. Then, 0.6 mL of the sample solution and 1.8 mL of the mixture containing DPPH radicals were added to an amber vial. The headspace of the vial was filled with nitrogen gas, and it was tightly sealed. The vial was shaken and incubated for 20 min at 25°C. The sample was removed and the absorption at 520 nm was measured using the spectrophotometer, yielding A. Instead of the anthocyanin solution from the jam, 13.7 mol/L ethanol was used as blank B. The DPPH radical scavenging activity was determined using the following formula:

$$\text{DPPH radical scavenging activity} = \left(\frac{\mathrm{B}-\mathrm{A}}{\mathrm{B}}\right)\times 100 \qquad (2)$$

Each measurement of the DPPH radical scavenging activity of the jam extracts was carried out in duplicate and the mean value was calculated.

Figure 7 shows the transient changes in the 50% scavenging concentration, SC_{50}, for DPPH radicals of the extract from strawberry jam impregnated using 0.88 and 1.46 mol/L sucrose solution and preserved at 65°C and 100% relative humidity. For each jam, the SC_{50} value increased with preservation time, indicating that the antioxidative ability of the jam decreased during the preservation.

The increment of the SC_{50} value was suppressed by the impregnation with sucrose. Furthermore, the suppressive effect was stronger at higher concentration of sucrose-impregnating solution. Figure 8 shows the relationship between the fraction of remaining anthocyanins in the jam impregnated using the sucrose solution and the SC_{50} values for DPPH radicals of the jam extract.

The plots lie on a straight line ($R^2 = 0.90$). That is, the SC_{50} value was in inversely proportional to the fraction of remaining anthocyanins in the impregnated jam. Thermal degradation of anthocyanins results in the formation of polyphenolic degradation products, though it is not clear if the formation of these components results in an overall reduction in antioxidant activity [21]. In this case, the antioxidative activity of the strawberry jam would be due to the remaining anthocyanin in it. The sucrose impregnation into strawberry prior to the production of jam is effective for not only the color stability but also the maintenance of its function.

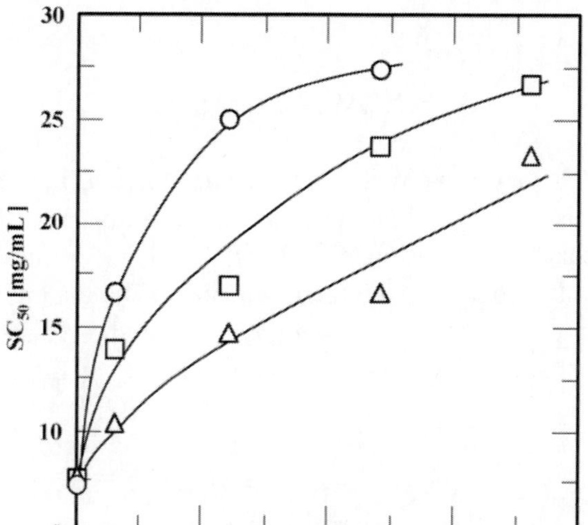

Figure 7. The transient changes in the 50% scavenging concentration, SC_{50}, for DPPH radicals of the extract from strawberry jam impregnated using (□) 0.88 and (Δ) 1.46 mol/L sucrose solution and preserved at 65°C and 100% relative humidity. The control (○) represents no impregnation into strawberry.

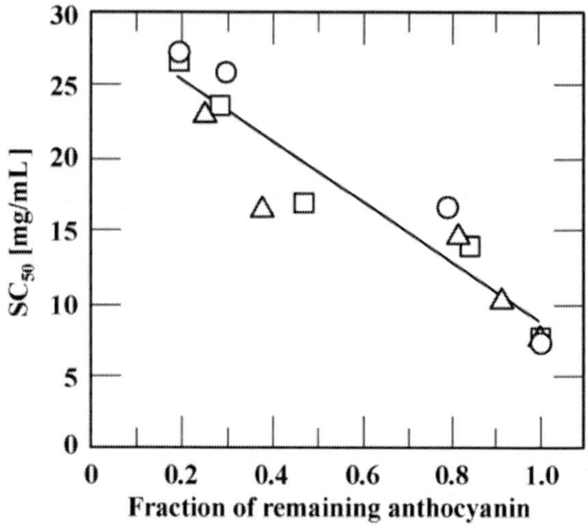

Figure 8. Relationship between the fractions of remaining anthocyanin in strawberry jam impregnated using the sucrose solution and the SC_{50} values for DPPH radicals of the corresponding jam extract preserved at 65°C and 100% relative humidity. The symbols are the same as in Figure 7. The solid curve represents the correlation between the two values ($R^2 = 0.90$).

ACKNOWLEDGMENTS

The author is very grateful to Dr. Masato Nomura, Professor of Kinki University, for his valuable discussions and advises throughout this study, and sincerely appreciate Dr. Yoshiharu Okada, Associate Professor of Kinki University, for his patient and accurate guidance. The author would like to thank all the members of the Laboratory of Biomolecular Engineering, Department of Biotechnology and Chemistry, Faculty of Engineering, Kinki University.

REFERENCES

[1] Hújica-Paz, H.; Vaidez-Fragoso, A.; López-Malo, A.; Palou, E.; Welti-Chanes, J. *J. Food Eng.* 2003, *57*, 305-314.

[2] Castelló, M. L.; Fito, P. J.; Chiralt, A. *J. Food Eng.* 2010, *97*, 64-71.

[3] Abers, J. E.; Wrolstad, R. E. *J. Food Sci.* 1979, *44*, 75-78, 81.

[4] O'Beirne, D.; Kelly, G. *Lebensm. Wissen. Technol.* 1985, *18*, 47-51.

[5] García-Viguera, C.; Zafrilla, P.; Romero, F.; Abellán, P.; Artés, F.; Tomás-Barberán, F. A. *J. Food Sci.* 1999, *64*, 243-247.
[6] Wicklund, T.; Rosenfeld, H. J.; Martinsen, B. K.; Sundfør, M. W.; Lea, P.; Bruun, T.; Blomhoff, R.; Haffner, K. *Lebensm. Wissen. Technol.* 2005, *38*, 387-391.
[7] Watanabe, Y.; Kurata, A.; Yamanaka, K.; Suginaka, T. *New Food Ind.* 2007, *49*, 31-35.
[8] Watanabe, Y.; Yoshimoto, K.; Okada, Y.; Nomura M. *LWT Food Sci. Technol.* 2011, *44*, 891-895.
[9] Sondheimer, E.; Kertesz, Z. I. *J. Am. Chem. Soc.* 1948, *70*, 3476-3479.
[10] Viguera, C. G.; Zafrilla, P.; Barberan, F. T. *J. Sci. Food Agric.* 1997, *73*, 207-213.
[11] Olsson, M. E.; Ekvall, J.; Gustavsson, K. E.; Nilsson, J.; Pillai, D.; Sjöholm, I.; Svensson, U.; Åkesson, B.; Nyman, M. G. L. *J. Agric. Food Chem.* 2004, *52*, 2490-2498.
[12] Dervisi, P.; Lamb, J.; Zabetakis, I. *Food Chem.* 2001, *73*, 85-91.
[13] Lewis, C. E.; Walker, J. R. L.; Lancaster, J. E. *Food Chem.* 1995, *54*, 315-319.
[14] Chandra, A.; Nair, M. G.; Iezzoni, A. F. *J. Agric. Food Chem.* 1993, *41*, 1062-1065.
[15] Lunn, J. E.; MacRae, E. *Curr. Opin. Plant Biol.* 2003, *6*, 208-214.
[16] Dangles, O.; Wigand, M. C.; Brouillard, R. *Phytochem.* 1992, *31*, 3811-3812.
[17] Cunha, L. M.; Oliveira, F. A. R.; Oliveira, J. C. *J. Food Eng.* 1998, *37*, 175-191.
[18] Watanabe, Y.; Nakanishi, H.; Goto, N.; Otsuka, K.; Kimura, T.; Adachi, S. *J. Am. Oil Chem. Soc.* 2010, *87*, 1475-1480.
[19] Wrolstad, R. E.; Skrede, G.; Lea, P.; Enersen, G. *J. Food Sci.* 1990, *55*, 1064-1065.
[20] Fujita, A.; Masumoto, K.; Kawakami, K.; Mikami, T.; Nomura, M. *J. Oleo Sci.* 2006, *55*, 585-591.
[21] Patras, A.; Brunton, N. P.; O'Donnell, C.; Tiwari, B. K. *Trends Food Sci. Technol.* 2010, *21*, 3-11.

In: Sucrose
Editor: Salvatore Magazù

ISBN: 978-1-62417-984-6

Chapter 5

THE EFFECTS OF SUCROSE ON NEURONAL ACTIVITY

Elena Timofeeva and Arojit Mitra
Faculté de Médecine, Département Psychiatrie et Neurosciences,
Centre de recherche de l'Institut universitaire de cardiologie
et de pneumologie de Québec, Université Laval,
Québec (QC), Canada

ABSTRACT

During the past few centuries humans have transformed from rear to voracious consumers of sugar. The present chapter sheds light on the questions of why we did increased our sugar consumption and what effects sucrose intake can produce on our mood and mind. Once consumed, sucrose sends signals to the brain via specialized taste receptors and glucosensing mechanisms. Sucrose intake activates in the brain the primary gustatory pathway and the brain reward system, which recognizes sweet taste of sucrose as rewarding. The role of the sweet taste system is to detect potentially high-energy sweet food that normally is relatively rare in the nature. The glucosensing mechanisms stimulate or inhibit food intake according to the energy needs. Because of the scarcity of sweet food in the nature, seeking this type of food requires some effort. Therefore, once such a food is found and consumed, this effort would be awarded by the brain reward system. These sophisticated systems work properly when their functions are not compromised by the unlimited availability of sweet palatable food, which may counteract the precise mechanisms controlling food intake. The experimental results obtained in animal models have shown that seeking and consumption of the regular non-sweet foods activate the medial hypothalamus which is directly related to the control of energy homeostasis and stress response. In contrast, seeking and consumption of sucrose inhibit the activity of the medial hypothalamus, but strongly activate the brain reward areas. This sucrose-induced shift in neuronal activity results in consumption of more and more palatable sweet foods at the expense of regular low-energy foods. Repeated overeating of sucrose can alter the neurochemical state of the brain reward regions, promoting sucrose craving and triggering sucrose binge-eating episodes. On the other hand, a sucrose-induced decrease in the activity of the medial hypothalamus directly affects the response of neuroendocrine system to stress. The stress-induced neuronal expression of stress neuropeptides as well as the release of plasma stress hormones is blunted by sucrose consumption. This 'anti-stress' effect of sucrose may explain overconsumption of sweets during stress even in the absence of hunger or needs for calories. This chapter reviews the neuronal effects of sucrose that from one side is beneficial by giving us energy and helping to relieve stress, or, from the other side, it may be detrimental by leading to uncontrolled craving for sucrose, eating disorders and obesity.

ABBREVIATIONS

ACTH	adrenocorticotropic hormone;
CRF	corticotropin-releasing factor;
CRF1	CRF type 1 receptor;
CRF2	CRF type 2 receptor;
DMH	dorsomedial hypothalamic nucleus;
DMHc	compact part of the dorsomedial hypothalamic nucleus;
DMHv	ventral part of the dorsomedial hypothalamic nucleus;
GE	glucose-excited glucosensing neurons;
GI	glucose-inhibited glucosensing neurons;
GK	glucokinase;
HPA	hypothalamic-pituitary-adrenal axis;
LH	lateral hypothalamic area;
LS	lateral septum;
NTS	nucleus of the solitary tract;
PB	parabrachial nucleus;
PVH	paraventricular hypothalamic nucleus;

PVHm	magnocellular part of the paraventricular hypothalamic nucleus;
PVHp	parvocellular part of the paraventricular hypothalamic nucleus;
PVT	paraventricular thalamic nucleus;
SON	supraoptic nucleus;
T1R	sweet taste receptor;
VMH	ventromedial hypothalamic nucleus;
VPM	ventral posterior thalamic nucleus;
VTA	ventral tegmental area.

1. Introduction. Statistics Show that We Have Dramatically Increased Our Sugar Production and Intake over the Last Several Centuries

Sucrose is the organic compound commonly known as table sugar. The sucrose molecule is a disaccharide composed of glucose and fructose. Responsiveness to the sweetness of sugar has very ancient evolutionary beginnings, being manifested as chemotaxis even in motile bacteria such as *E. coli* [1]. Attractiveness to sweets is evolutionarily justified because sweetness intensity generally indicates energy density in contrast to bitterness, which tends to indicate toxicity [2].

The people of New Guinea were probably the first to domesticate sugarcane, sometime around 8000 BC. Originally, people chewed sugarcane raw to extract its sweetness. Crystallization of sugar began in India during the Gupta dynasty, around AD 350 [3]. Early refining methods involved grinding the cane to extract the juice, and then boiling down the juice or drying it in the sun to yield sugary solids that looked like gravel. The English word "sugar" (which is phonetically similar to the French "*sucre*", the German "*Zucker*" and the words assigned to sugar in many other languages) originates from the Sanskrit word "*sharkara*" that means "gravel" or "sand". Similarly, Chinese use the term "gravel sugar" and Russians "sugar sand" for what is also known as "table sugar".

Sugar production in ancient times was so limited that sugar was highly prized and its use subjected to strict rules. Among the ancient Greeks and Romans, sugar was known as an imported medicine, not as a food. For example, Dioscorides in Greece in the 1st century (AD) wrote: "There is a kind of coalescent honey called sugar found in reeds in India and Arabia, similar in consistency to salt and brittle enough to be broken between the teeth like salt. It is good dissolved in water, and taken as a drink to help a painful bladder or the kidneys" [4]. At that time, the primary sweetener was honey, but because it was relatively rare and not mass produced, the majority of people, especially the poorer classes, had no sweeteners at all in their normal diet [5].

During the Middle Ages, the cultivation of sugarcane and production of sugar spread from India to Europe via trading ports. However, sugar production during the medieval period remained extremely low, and sugar was considered mostly a "fine spice" with a high price [3]. The value of sugar and its rarity at that time are reflected by the historical fact that King Emmanuel I of Portugal, "the Fortunate" (1469 –1521), sent life-sized sugar statues of cardinals and the Pope to the Vatican in 1513 as a gift [6].

The situation with sugar production radically changed after the New World was discovered and sugarcane was planted in the Caribbean islands, Brazil and the southern United States. Producing and trading sugar in the 17th and 18th centuries in the Caribbean British colonies was so lucrative that it was known as white gold [7]. After the British blocked sugar exports to Europe in the 18th century, Germany, France, and Austria developed a thriving industry by producing sugar from the beetroot. The combined manufacture of sugar from sugarcane and beets led to a marked increase in global sugar production, from 250,000 tons in 1800 to 8 million tons in 1900 [8]. At the end of the 20th century, the global production of sugar increased to more than 110 million tons per year [9].

Therefore, during only the past few centuries have humans transformed themselves from rear to voracious consumers of sugar. The present chapter sheds light on the questions of why we increased our consumption of sugar and what effects sucrose intake may produce on our mood and mind.

2. The Neuronal Network Activated by Sucrose

Sushruta Samhita, the classic book of Ayurvedic medicine, describes an herbal extract from the plant *Gymnema sylvestre*. This extract was called 'gur-mar' ('sugar-destroying') due to its ability to block specifically the sensation of sweet taste [10]. This particular effect suggests that the sweet-taste receptors on the surface of the taste bud cells are different from the receptors for other taste stimuli. A proteolytic enzyme applied to the dorsal tongue almost completely suppressed sweet taste [11], indicating that the sweet-taste receptors are the proteins. Recent progress in molecular biology and genetics has finally revealed candidates for sweet perception, the members of T1R family of receptors [12]. More precisely, these studies showed that perception of sweetness in mammals depends on the expression of the receptor T1R3 that, at the apical membrane of the taste receptor cells, forms a complex with a related protein, T1R2. This T1R2-T1R3 heterodimer is a G-protein coupled receptor that binds with sugar and artificial sweeteners [13-16].

Binding of sweet molecules to the T1R2-T1R3 receptor complex triggers a conformational change in the molecules of the complex. This change activates the G-protein, alpha-gustducin, which in turn activates adenylate cyclase and phospholipase C. Activation of these signalling molecules results in an increase in intracellular free calcium [17, 18]. The increase in calcium activates the transient receptor potential channel M5 (TRPM5) [17], which causes release of the neurotransmitter and activation of the primary afferent neurons. Taste information ascends to the brain by the sensory fibers of the facial nerve (cranial nerve VII), which innervates the anterior tongue, and the glossopharyngeal nerve (cranial nerve IX) and the vagus nerve (cranial nerve X), which innervate the posterior tongue. Because the sweet taste buds are more concentrated at the anterior part of the tongue, the information about sweet taste enters the brain mostly by the facial nerve. According to the labelled line theory [19], sweet-related information is encoded and transmitted by the specific subgroup of fibers, the sucrose-best fibers, that is more responsive to sucrose than to the four other basic taste stimuli (salty, sour, bitter, and umami). Alternatively, sweet-related information may be transferred by an "across-fiber pattern" to the brain where this information is encoded by specific neuronal populations [20].

The first relay for the ascending gustatory information in the brain is the nucleus of the solitary tract (NTS) (Figure 1), whose neurons demonstrate topographic responses to the taste stimuli according to the receptive field in the oral cavity [21].

In addition to the afferent fibers originating in the oral cavity, the NTS receives the vagal afferents coming from the gastrointestinal tract (Figure 1). Recent investigations suggest that the gastrointestinal tract may transfer to the brain information related to sweet molecules. The expression of all types of T1Rs was found in the gastrointestinal tract, including the stomach, duodenum, jejunum, ileum, and colon [22]. These taste receptors signal via the enteric nervous system to the brain. The enteric nervous system is now considered the third, in addition to the sympathetic and the parasympathetic, branch of the autonomic nervous system, which transfers gut sensory signals to the brain and can participate in forming long-term representations of gut sensations [23]. These gut feelings, called 'homeostatic emotions' [24] or even 'extended consciousness'[25], may affect our emotional state and underlie intuitive decision making [23].

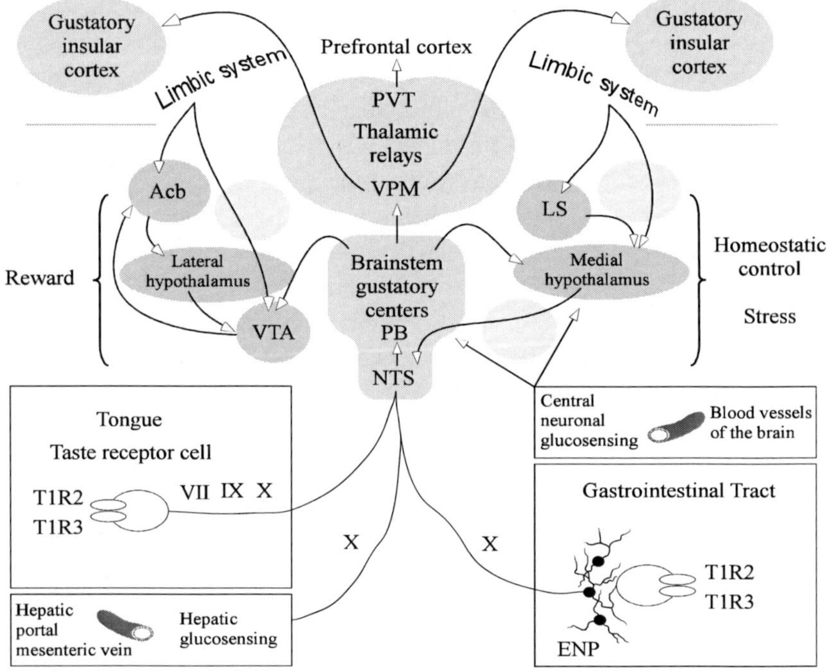

Figure 1. The neuronal network activated by sucrose intake. VII – facial nerve; IX – glossopharyngeal nerve; X – vagus nerve; Acb – nucleus accumbens; Amy – amygdala; ENP – enteric nervous plexus; LS – lateral septum; NTS – nucleus of the solitary tract; PB – parabrachial nucleus; PVT – paraventricular thalamic nucleus; T1R2/3 – sweet taste receptor subunits; VPM – ventral posteromedial nucleus of the thalamus; VTA – ventral tegmental area.

From the medullar NTS, the sensory information is directed to the parabrachial nucleus (PB; Figure 1) located in the pons [26, 27]. In addition to the main stream from the NTS to the PB, some NTS fibers run directly to the central amygdala, paraventricular thalamic (PVT), and paraventricular hypothalamic (PVH) nuclei [28]. The brainstem gustatory centers may generate the mimetic response to the taste of sucrose in rats. The brainstem's ability to generate a behavioral response to the application of sucrose to the tongue was first revealed by Norgen and Grill [29, 30]. In their experiments, the decerebrated rats, with the brainstem separated from the upper forebrain, demonstrated similar mimetic responses to sucrose in taste reactivity tests compared to the intact rats [29].

In the PB, the sweet signals generated by sucrose or saccharin are coded by the central lateral subnucleus [31]. The lesion of the PB impairs the increase in sucrose licking as a function of sucrose concentration seen in intact rats [32]. Conversely, stimulation of the cannabinoid receptors CB1 in the PB selectively stimulates feeding of palatable foods in rats [33]. From the PB, the gustatory pathway branches to densely innervate the medial hypothalamus, ventral tegmental area (VTA), and midline thalamic nuclei [34-36]. From the parvocellular part of the ventral posterior thalamic nucleus (VPM), the gustatory information is directed to the primary gustatory insular cortex (Figure 1). In the gustatory insular cortex, the neurons responsive to taste are located in the anterior, dysgranular region [37]. Another thalamic gustatory-related pathway travels from the PB to the PVT, and, after synapsing in the PVT, reaches the prefrontal cortex (Figure 1). The interconnecting loop formed by the prefrontal cortex, nucleus accumbens, lateral hypothalamus, and VTA is intimately related to the rewarding effects of sucrose. The taste of sucrose activates the dopaminergic neurons of the VTA [38] and elevates dopamine levels in the nucleus accumbens [39]. The dopamine levels increase in the accumbens in proportion to the sucrose concentration [40], and the neurons of the nucleus accumbens explicitly encode for the hedonic value of sucrose [41, 42].

Although the orosensory system is important for the sucrose-triggered dopamine release in the nucleus accumbens, as has been shown in real and sham sucrose feeding [40], the lack of sweet taste perception does not prevent the development of a preference for sweets! Indeed, mice genetically lacking the TRPM5 channel mediating the effects of sweet receptors and required for sweet taste perception, can develop a robust preference for sucrose solutions based solely on caloric content [43]. Sucrose, but not the non-caloric sweetener sucralose, induces dopamine release in the accumbens of mice lacking functional sweet taste transduction [43]. Therefore, the physiological events starting in the gastro-intestinal tract and providing information on the metabolic value of nutrients may along with the taste signals affect the brain reward system. But how does the brain receive information about consumed sweets? Accumulating evidence suggests that ingested sweets may signal to the brain via peripheral and central glucosensing.

Once consumed, sucrose is digested in the small intestine by hydrolysis to monosaccharides, glucose, and fructose [44, 45]. In the intestines, monosaccharides cross the mucosal cell membranes by simple diffusion or by mechanisms involving a specific transport system [46-49]. The monosaccharides pass via the portal circulation to the liver, where part of the glucose and virtually all the fructose are metabolized to glycogen or enter the tricarboxylic acid cycle [50]. The remainder of the glucose passing into the peripheral circulation enters the peripheral tissues normally under the influence of insulin. Into the brain glucose is transported across the blood-brain barrier by specific insulin-independent transporter mechanisms [51]. The brain almost exclusively depends on glucose as an energy supply, because fatty acids or proteins cannot traverse the blood-brain barrier. Only in special situations, such as hyponutrition or the ketogenic diet, does the organism produces a significant amount of alternative substrates such as ketones or lactate that can traverse the blood-brain barrier and assume a role in supplying energy to the brain [52]. Astrocyte-derived lactate is not an important metabolic substrate for neurons compared to glucose use [53-55]. Therefore, the brain metabolism almost exclusively depends on glucose as an ATP-substrate. The brain cannot store glucose in energetic reserves, but it requires much more energy compared to other organs. Indeed, the mass of the human brain constitutes only 2% of the entire body weight, but consumes 50% of the carbohydrates ingested over a 24-h period [52]. Not surprisingly, during an energy shortage the "selfish" brain may stimulate the intake of sweet carbohydrates and allocate more glucose for energy needs through an increase in glucose transport across the blood-brain barrier, a decrease in energy metabolism, and an adjustment of the energy supply to the peripheral organs [56].

According to the "glucostatic theory" proposed by Jean Mayer in 1953, the brain can monitor plasma and cerebrospinal fluid glucose [57, 58]. To maintain glucose within narrow limits, which are 3.0-5.6 mM in the plasma and 0.5-2.5 mM in the cerebrospinal fluid, the brain may adjust the glucose levels with a counter-regulatory response that includes autonomic (activation of the sympathetic or parasympathetic nervous system), endocrine (secretion of hormones), and behavioral (intake of nutrients) adjustments [59]. In the periphery, the important glucosensing elements were found in the hepatic portal mesenteric vein. The hepatic glucosensing mechanism was revealed in experiments showing the ability of the local glucose infusion in the portal hepatic vein to suppress hypoglycemia-induced hunger and sympathoadrenal response [60-62]. Hepatic glucosensing elements monitor plasma glucose just before it enters the liver from the gut. This information is conveyed to the brainstem by the vagal and spinal afferents [63-66].

Glucose concentration in the cerebrospinal fluid is monitored in the brain by the glucosensing neurons detected in the brainstem, including the NTS, area postrema, and dorsal motor nucleus of the vagus nerve [67-69], and in the hypothalamus, including the lateral hypothalamic area and the ventromedial hypothalamic nucleus [70, 71]. Similar to peripheral glucosensing elements that trigger a counter-regulatory response, the neuronal glucosensing mechanisms regulate plasma glucose concentration and feeding behavior. Thus, the intracerebroventricular infusion of non-metabolic glucose analogue 5-thioglucose at microdoses (as low as 0.5 μM) potentially increases the plasma glucose concentration by hormonal and autonomic counter-regulation and eliciting feeding [72].

Glucosensing neurons are generally classified as "glucose-excited" (GE) or "glucose-inhibited" (GI), according to whether their mean firing rate increases or decreases, respectively, in response to local changes in extracellular glucose [73-75]. Two alternative mechanisms of neuronal glucose sensing have been proposed. The first glucosensing mechanism involves intracellular glucose oxidation, and the second mechanism is based on oxidation-independent membrane-bound glucosensing. When the oxidative mechanism of glucosensing is involved, glucose is transported into the cytoplasmic pool by specific glucose transporter proteins [73]. Cytoplasmic metabolism of glucose is controlled by glucokinase (GK), the rate-limiting factor in glycolysis [76, 77]. GK action on glucose results in a series of intracellular events eventually leading to increases in the cytosolic ATP:ADP ratio and subsequent closure of ATP-sensitive potassium (K_{ATP}) channels, which in turn causes cell depolarization of the GE neurons [73, 74]. Alternative mechanisms of inhibiting GI neurons by glucose may involve activation of the tandem-pore K_{2p} ion channels [78]. The mechanism of oxidation-independent membrane-bound glucosensing involves activation of transmembrane G-protein coupled dimers of the taste receptors T1R1/T1R2 and T1R2/T1R3 expressed by neurons in different forebrain regions, such as the hypothalamus, thalamus, hippocampus, and cortex [79]. The brain expression of T1Rs is increased by the metabolic states promoting energy intake. Thus, food deprivation increases levels of T1R1 and T1R2 in the mice hypothalamus [79]. Likewise, hypothalamic expression of T1R1 and T1R2 is increased in hyperphagic genetically obese ob/ob mice in a non-food-deprived state [79]. Cultured mouse embryonic hypothalamic cells upregulate the expression of T1R2 in a low-glucose medium. This effect was reversed by increased glucose concentration [79].

Therefore, sucrose signals to the brain via specialized taste receptors located in the tongue and expressed along the gastrointestinal tract. Once sucrose is digested to glucose and fructose in the small intestine, glucose is detected by peripheral and central glucosensing mechanisms. In the brain, sucrose intake activates the primary gustatory pathway that includes the brainstem, thalamic relays, and the primary gustatory cortex. In addition, sucrose-related signals are conveyed to the reward system that includes the dopaminergic VTA neurons, nucleus accumbens, lateral hypothalamus, and prefrontal cortex. Finally, the sweet taste signals and glucosensing affect the activity of the medial hypothalamus regulating energy metabolism and stress response (Figure 1).

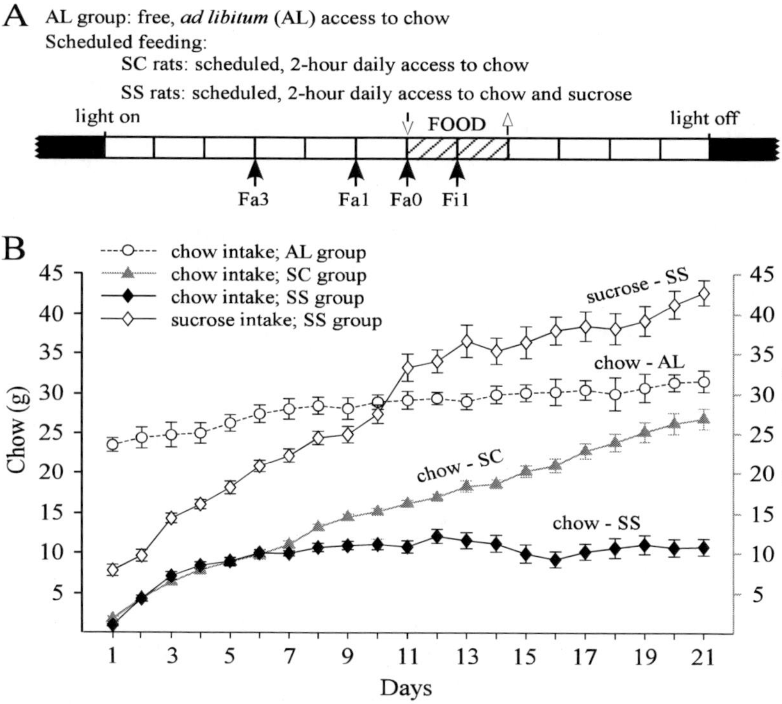

Figure 2. The rats submitting to scheduled 2-h daily access to chow (SC group, as shown in A) gradually increased daily intake of chow while the rats maintained on 2-h daily access to chow and 10% sucrose solution (SS group, as shown in A) significantly increased intake of sucrose but not chow (as shown in B). To detect neuronal activation in the brain, at the end of the 3-week feeding schedules, the animals were sacrificed (shown in A with the arrows) during food anticipation [3 (Fa3) and 1 (Fa1) h before and at the moment (Fa0) of expected food] as well as 1 h after feeding (Fi1). Modified from [100].

3. Why Do We Consume more Sugar than We Should, According to our Metabolic Needs?

The role of the sweet taste system is to detect the potentially high-energy sweet foods that normally are relatively rare in the nature. The glucosensing stimulates or inhibits food intake according to the energy needs estimated by this mechanism as the levels of plasma and brain glucose. Because of the scarcity of sweet foods in the nature, seeking these foods requires some effort. Therefore, once these foods are found and consumed, this effort would be awarded by the brain reward system. These sophisticated systems work properly when their function is not compromised by the unlimited availability of sweet palatable foods. This availability of palatable foods may counteract the precise mechanisms controlling food intake and instigate the development of eating disorders. The misbalance in eating underlines the development of obesity, diabetes, metabolic syndrome, and related disorders. In the following parts, we will take a close look on how sucrose may be responsible for these misbalances.

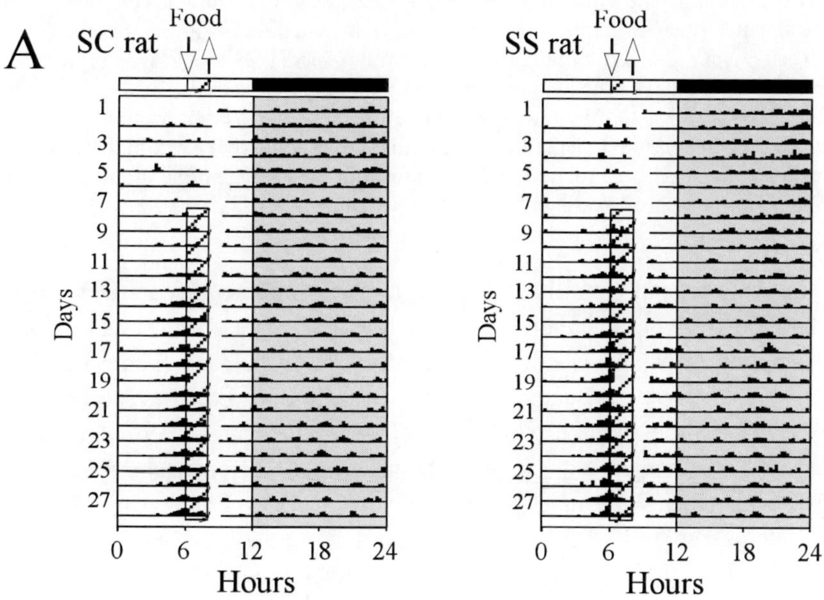

Figure 3. (Continued).

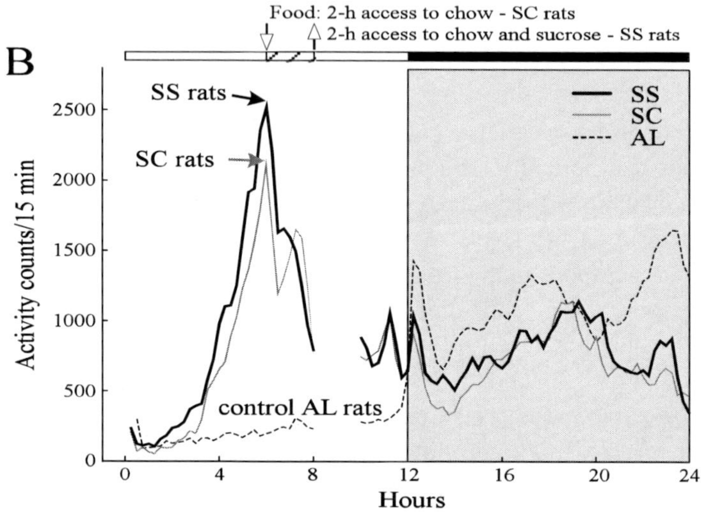

Figure 3. The rats anticipating sucrose demonstrated higher locomotor food-anticipating activity. The rats were maintained on a 12:12-h light-dark cycle (shown by the light and dark horizontal bars). The rats were fed regular chow *ad libitum* for the first 7 days, and for the following days (8-28), access to food (chow for the SC rats and chow and 10% sucrose solution for the SS rats) was scheduled as 2-h daily access (between 6 and 8 Zeitgeber time). On the actograms (panel A), the horizontal lines correspond to the days of the experiment, and the locomotor activity was plotted by the vertical bars for each 15 min as a percentage of the absolute maximal activity recorded over the entire experiment. Note the increase in locomotor activity within the few hours preceding access to food. B, The waveform of the average of locomotor activity during *ad libitum* chow feeding (1-7 days) or scheduled (11-28 days) chow (SC rats) or chow and sucrose (SS rats) feeding. Modified from [100].

In experimental conditions, when rats have unlimited access to mundane rat chow and highly palatable foods, such as pork spread and sweet cookies, consumption of palatable foods may rise to 90% of the daily food ration [80]. Similarly, when a 10% sucrose solution was introduced to chow-fed rats, the rats decreased their intake of chow and took a high amount of the sucrose solution. For example, the control, chow-fed rats daily consumed 32.2 g of chow, while their littermates maintained on *ad libitum* access to chow and 10% sucrose consumed 20.3 g chow and 175.4 ml of the sucrose solution every day [81]. In the same experiment, another group of rats had an intermittent (4 days per week) access to sucrose. The rats with intermittent access to sucrose consumed 29.3 g of chow per day during the days on regular chow, but when the rats regained access to sucrose, they decreased their daily intake of chow to 21.8 g and, in addition to this chow, consumed 167.4 ml of the 10%

sucrose solution [81]. The results obtained in Mary Dallman's laboratory also demonstrated that adding sucrose to diets significantly decreased regular chow intake [82, 83]. Relative hypophagia of less-preferred food may depend on a compensatory response attempting to re-balance the increased caloric intake due to consumption of calorie-rich palatable food [84, 85]. A recent investigation of feeding behavior suggested additional mechanisms that may regulate food intake according to its palatability by a decrease in the reinforcing efficacy of less preferred foods [86]. Access to the preferred diet rich in chocolate-flavored sucrose significantly decreased motivation to work to obtain chow, as revealed by the decreased breakpoint, the last completed ratio of non-reinforced versus reinforced lever pressing for chow, as well as the total lever pressing for chow on the progressive ratio schedules [86]. Analogously, rats withdrawn from access to the substances of abuse, such as amphetamine, methamphetamine, morphine, or nicotine, show decreased motivation to work for a natural reward such as sucrose [87-90].

The increase in sucrose intake at the expense of regular chow may suggest that sucrose intake may strongly activate the reward brain areas. To investigate this possibility and characterize the neuronal network activated during the motivational state for sucrose intake, we performed a series of experiments with rats trained to eat at a fixed time of the day (as shown in Figure 2, A). These restricted feeding schedules trigger development of food anticipation activity, a specific increase in locomotion and food seeking within a few hours preceding scheduled access to food (Figure 3). When rats had scheduled 2-h daily access to chow (SC groups), they gradually increased their chow intake so that at the end of the 3-week scheduled feeding their 2-h chow intake was comparable to the 24-h chow consumption of the *ad libitum* chow-fed rats (AL groups) (Figure 2, B). This adaptation to consuming the daily ration of food within a few hours of scheduled feeding is not surprising and has been shown repeatedly [91, 92]. Surprisingly, the rats maintained on 2-h daily scheduled access to chow and the 10% sucrose solution (SS group) dramatically increased their intake of sucrose but not chow (Figure 2, B). The sucrose-consuming rats also demonstrated higher locomotor activity within 2-3 h preceding scheduled access to food (Figure 3). Similar development of anticipation of palatable food was shown in Carolina Escobar's work, in which non-food-restricted, *ad libitum* chow-fed rats receiving 5 g of palatable chocolate at a fixed time of the day developed chocolate anticipation revealed by an increase in locomotor activity just before the expected access to chocolate [93, 94]. Interestingly, sweet glucose, but not vegetable or mineral oil, was able to shift the time of the food anticipating activity in the rats [95].

The nutritive value of palatable food is an important factor for entraining food anticipation. Several studies have demonstrated that restricted daily access to palatable, nutrient-rich (such as sugar, chocolate, glucose), but not to palatable non-nutritive (such as saccharin) food can engender food anticipation [95, 96]. It seems that the amount of palatable nutritive food has to be high enough to create the nutrient 'pulses' at the metabolic level. The minimum threshold to shift circadian activity was achieved with 4 g of palatable mash [96], 6 g of glucose [95], 6 g of standard chow [97], or 30% of the daily intake [98]. Another study demonstrated that brief (~5 min) daily access to sucrose increased anticipatory wheel-running activity, body temperature, and plasma corticosterone in food-restricted (to 85% of the body weight of the control rats) but not in *ad-libitum*-fed rats [99]. It has been suggested that the combination of a deprivation regimen and scheduled access to sucrose may give rise to a more global anticipatory mechanism because the temporal cycles of energy balance may be strongly modulated by the incentive properties of sucrose [99]. Anticipation of food in food-restricted rats strongly activated the medial hypothalamic regions regulating energy balance and stress response. Within 3 h before access to chow, neuronal activation, detected by the induction of expression of mRNA of immediate early gene c-*fos*, was seen in the dorsomedial (DMH) and paraventricular (PVH) hypothalamic nuclei (Figures 4, 5) [92, 100]. Similar results have been shown with the increase in the expression of the Fos protein in the DMH and PVH of chow-anticipating rats [101]. Conversely, chocolate-anticipating rats did not demonstrate neuronal activation in the medial hypothalamus, but showed a positive signal for the Fos protein in the limbic forebrain, the nucleus accumbens, and the prefrontal cortex [93]. In our experiments, adding sucrose to the feeding schedules completely abolished induction of the expression of c-*fos* mRNA in the DMH and PVH during food anticipation (Figures 4, 5). Conversely, sucrose-anticipating rats demonstrated strong neuronal activation in the prefrontal cortex, the nucleus accumbens, and the anterior perifornical part of the lateral hypothalamus (Figures 5, 6) [100]. In contrast, the medial hypothalamic regions demonstrated lower activation in the sucrose-eating rats compared to their chow-eating littermates (Figures 4, 5). Thus, the sucrose-eating rats demonstrated a striking absence of neuronal activation in the magnocellular PVH and the supraoptic nucleus (SON) (Figure 5) [100]. These hypothalamic regions express oxytocin [28], a nonapeptide strongly linked to feeding termination mechanisms. Intracerebroventricular [102, 103] or peripheral [102, 104] administration of oxytocin decreases food intake, while administration of oxytocin receptor antagonists prevents this inhibition [102,

104] [105, 106]. Mice lacking the oxytocin gene overconsume the palatable sucrose solution [107]. The avidity for sucrose was evident in these mice from the first exposure, when the oxytocin-lacking mice's consumption of sucrose was 20-fold greater compared to the wild-type controls [108]. Conversely, chronic sugar intake decreased the activity of the neurons expressing oxytocin [109]. This sugar-induced downregulation of oxytocin neurons may contribute to a decrease in satiety signals and overeating of sucrose.

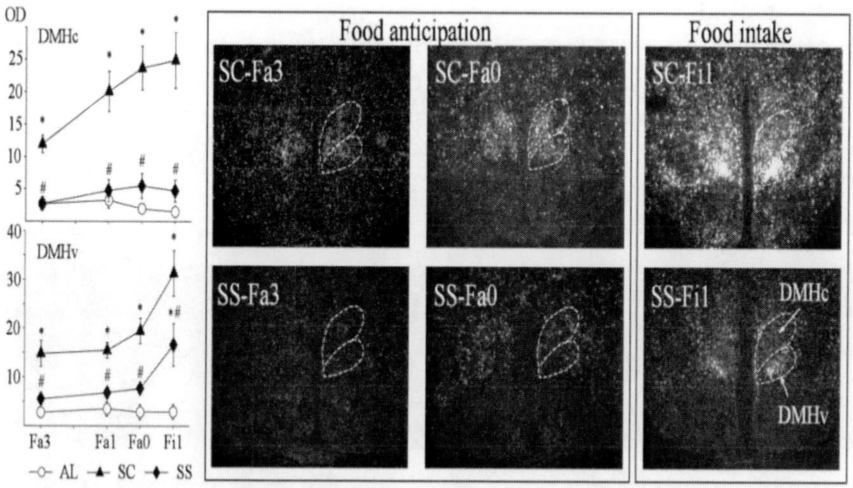

Figure 4. Chow-anticipating (SC) but not sucrose-anticipating (SS) rats strongly activated the inductionof expression of c-*fos* mRNA in the dorsomedial hypothalamic nucleus (DMH). Chow feeding (SC-Fi1) also strongly affected the compact (DMHc) and ventral (DMHv) parts of the DMH. Sucrose feeding triggered activation in the ventral but not compact DMH, but the levels of c-*fos* mRNA expression in the DMHv of the sucrose-fed rats were significantly lower compared to those in the chow-fed rats. The photomicrographs depict the positive hybridization signal of c-*fos* mRNA in the DMH. The histograms demonstrate the analyses of optical density (OD) of the hybridization signal of c-*fos* mRNA in the DMHc and DMHv. The rats were fed chow *ad libitum* [AL (○) rats], or maintained during 3 weeks on 2-h daily access to chow [SC (▲) rats] or chow and 10% sucrose solution [SS (♦) rats] and were sacrificed during food anticipation [3 (Fa3) and 1 (Fa1) h before and at the moment (Fa0) of expected food] as well as 1 h after feeding (Fi1). *Significantly different from AL. #Significant difference between SC and SS. Modified from [100].

In addition to the limbic structures, sucrose-consuming rats showed higher activation of the NTS (Figure 7). This result is in agreement with the reported increase in postprandial Fos immunoreactivity in the NTS of rats maintained on repeated scheduled access to palatable food compared to rats maintained on chow-restricted schedules [110]. As was described above, the NTS is an important relay for the gustatory signals informing the brain about the availability and consumption of palatable sweet foods. The visceral afferents synapse in the NTS in a precise topographic distribution with the taste tongue afferents occupying the most rostral portion and gastrointestinal afferents synapsing in the intermediate portion of the nucleus [21, 111]. However, because the sweet food-related signals enter the NTS not only from the oral cavity, but also from the sweet taste receptors expressed along the gastrointestinal tract and from the hepatic glucosensing elements, all portions of the NTS, the rostral, medial, and caudal, demonstrate higher neuronal activation during sucrose feeding in sucrose-consuming rats compared to chow-fed rats [100].

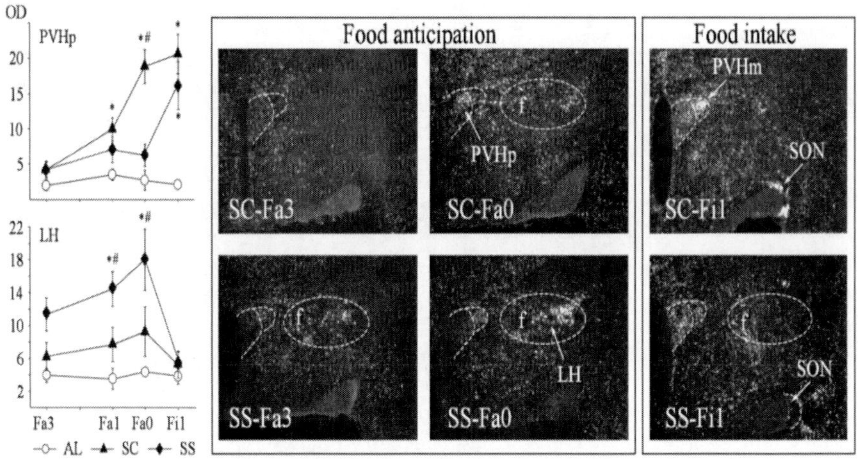

Figure 5. Chow anticipation (SC rats) activated the parvocellular part of the paraventricular hypothalamic nucleus (PVHp) while sucrose anticipation (SS rats) triggered anterior perifornical lateral hypothalamus (LH) activity. The photomicrographs depict the positive hybridization signal of c-*fos* mRNA. The histograms demonstrate the analyses of optical density (OD) of the hybridization signal of c-*fos* mRNA in the PVHp and LH. The rats were fed chow *ad libitum* [AL (○) rats], or maintained during 3 weeks on 2-h daily access to chow [SC (▲) rats] or chow and 10% sucrose solution [SS (♦) rats] and were sacrificed during food anticipation [3 (Fa3) and 1 (Fa1) h before and at the moment (Fa0) of expected food] as well as 1 h after feeding (Fi1). f – fornix; PVHm – magnocellular part of the paraventricular hypothalamic nucleus. SON – supraoptic nucleus. *Significantly different from AL. #Significant difference between SC and SS. Modified from [100].

Therefore, experimental rats maintained on restricted feeding of chow demonstrate high neuronal activation of the medial hypothalamic structures during food-anticipating time. The activity of these medial hypothalamic structures directly relates to the control of energy homeostasis and stress response. Adding sucrose to feeding schedules displaces the neuronal activity from the medial tuberal hypothalamus to the limbic prefrontal cortex and the regions intimately interconnected with the prefrontal cortex, the nucleus accumbens, and the lateral anterior hypothalamus (Figure 8). These limbic-related structures are known as the brain regions responsible for generating the reward. In these circumstances, the consumption of sucrose is not balanced according to metabolic needs, but is instigated by activation of the reward system. This shift in neuronal activity results in consumption of more and more palatable sweet foods at the expense of regular low-energy foods.

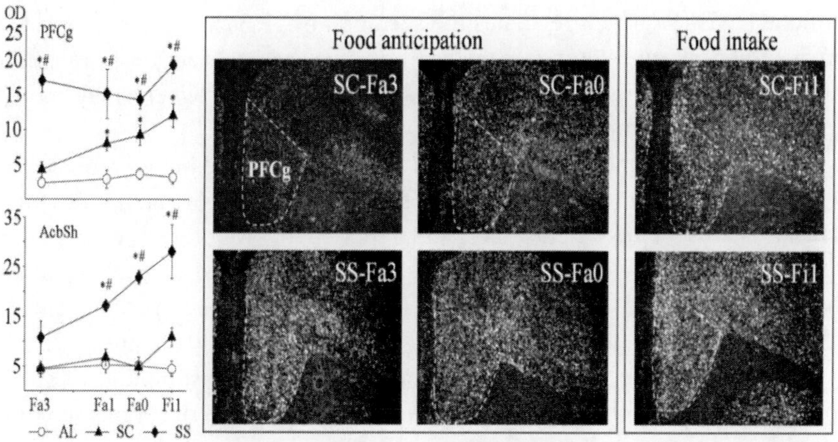

Figure 6. Sucrose but not chow anticipation and feeding activated the nucleus accumbens shell (AcbSh; bottom histogram). Sucrose anticipation and feeding higher and earlier activated the prefrontal cingulate cortex compared to chow anticipation and feeding (PFCg; top histograms and photomicrographs). The rats were fed chow *ad libitum* [AL (○) rats], or maintained during 3 weeks on 2-h daily access to chow [SC (▲) rats] or chow and 10% sucrose solution [SS (♦) rats] and were sacrificed during food anticipation [3 (Fa3) and 1 (Fa1) h before and at the moment (Fa0) of expected food] as well as 1 h after feeding (Fi1). OD - optical density of the hybridization signal of c-*fos* mRNA. *Significantly different from AL. #Significant difference between SC and SS. Modified from [100].

4. Why Sugar is Comforting during Stress?

The results obtained in our laboratory [92, 100] and reported by others [93, 101] suggest that sucrose and sweet palatable food may decrease the activity of the medial hypothalamic regions. The medial hypothalamus contains the regions regulating the neuroendocrine and behavioral response to stress. The principal neuroendocrine response to stress is the activation of the hypothalamic-pituitary-adrenal (HPA) axis. The key hypothalamic player of this axis is the parvocellular PVH. Stress activates the neurons of the parvocellular PVH that produce 41-amino acid neuropeptide corticotropin-releasing factor (CRF) [112, 113]. Axons of the parvocellular PVH neurons descend to the medial eminence, where CRF is secreted and, by embarking to the pituitary portal system, reaches the anterior pituitary. In the anterior pituitary, CRF stimulates release into the bloodstream of adrenocorticotropic hormone (ACTH), which regulates the secretion of glucocorticoids, cortisol in humans, and corticosterone in rats, from the adrenal cortex. Lipophilic glucocorticoids readily reach the central nervous system, where they inhibit expression of CRF (for reviews, see Refs. [114-116]).

Stress exposure increases in minutes the levels of blood glucocorticoids by hundred folds [81, 117]. The high, stress-like levels of glucocorticoids may increase sucrose intake. This fact was reported by Mary Dallman. In her experiments, low-to-high levels of plasma corticosterone were clamped by adrenalectomia and corticosterone replacement. The results clearly demonstrated an increase in sucrose and saccharine intake by the high levels of plasma corticosterone [118, 119]. This increase in the consumption of sweet foods by glucocorticoids may explain the increased intake of sweets in some stressful conditions.

Although glucocorticoids increase saccharin and sucrose intake [118, 119], in the three-bottle choice tests of saccharin, sucrose, and water, adrenalectomized rats showed a consistent preference for sucrose compared to saccharin, suggesting that drinking sucrose made them feel better than drinking saccharin [120, 121]. Indeed, sucrose but not saccharin normalized the levels of CRF mRNA in the PVH of adrenalectomized rats [120]. Similarly, continuous intake of sucrose decreased CRF mRNA expression in the PVH of stressed rats (Figure 9) [81]. In addition to decreasing the hypothalamic expression of CRF, voluntary consumption of sucrose decreases the ACTH level in adrenalectomized rats [118] as well as the levels of corticosterone in stressed rats (Figure 9) [81]. The remarkable effects of sucrose in adrenalectomized rats are not limited to “normalization” of the activity of the HPA axis. Caloric intake, body weight gain, insulin, fat depot weights, and an uncoupling protein in the brown adipose tissue were restored in the adrenalectomized rats drinking sucrose to the levels observed in the sham-adrenalectomized rats not given sucrose to drink [118].

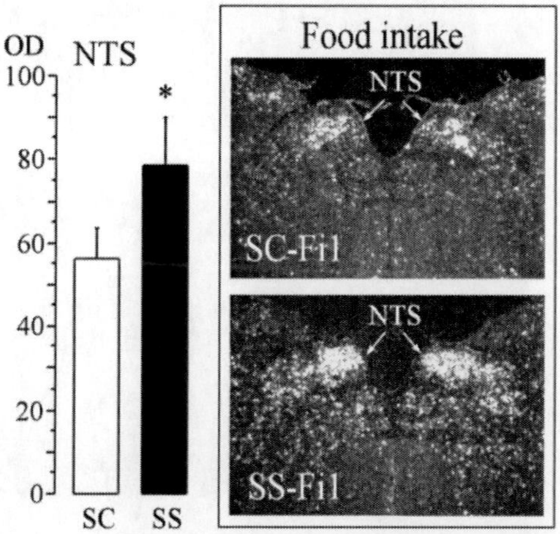

Figure 7. The c-*fos* mRNA expression levels were significantly higher after 1 h of feeding (Fi1) in the nucleus of the solitary tract (NTS) of rats maintained on scheduled 2-h daily feeding of 10% sucrose solution and chow (SS rats) compared to those seen in the rats maintained on 2-h daily access to chow (SC rats). The photomicrographs depict the positive hybridization signal of c-*fos* mRNA in the NTS. The histogram demonstrates the optical density (OD) of the positive hybridization signal of c-*fos* mRNA in the NTS. *Significantly different from SC. Modified from [100].

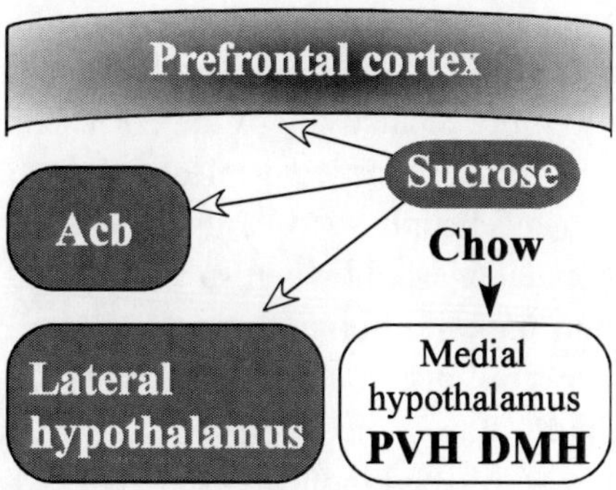

Figure 8. Chow anticipation activates the regions of the medial hypothalamus such as the paraventricular (PVH) and the dorsomedial (DMH) hypothalamic nuclei. Adding of sucrose to the feeding schedules displaced neuronal activity during food anticipation to the prefrontal cortex, nucleus accumbens (Acb), and anterior lateral hypothalamus.

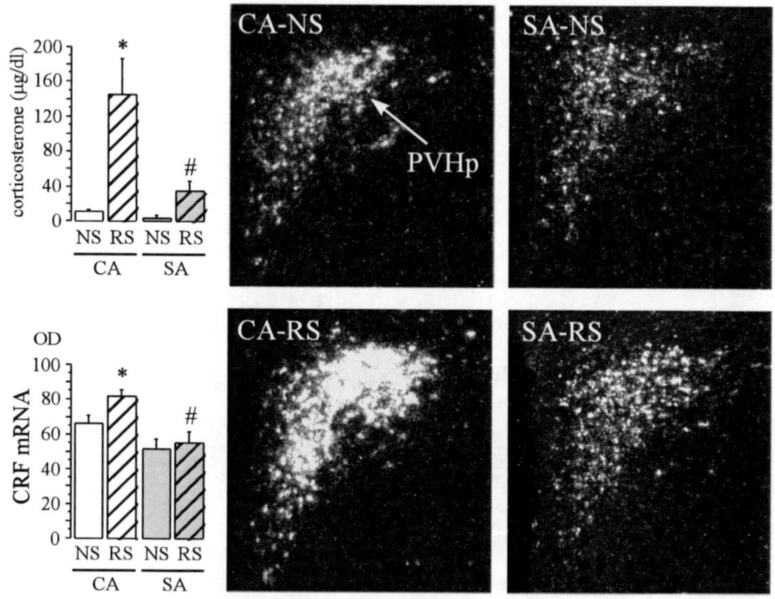

Figure 9. Continuous 6-week *ad libitum* access to sucrose (SA rats) significantly blunted the restraint stress-induced increase in plasma corticosterone (top histogram) and corticotropin-releasing factor (CRF) mRNA levels in the parvocellular part of the paraventricular hypothalamic nucleus (PVHp). The photomicrographs depict the positive hybridization signal of CRF mRNA. The bottom histogram demonstrates the optical density (OD) analyses of the hybridization signal of CRF mRNA. The rats were fed for 6 weeks *ad libitum* chow (CA) or chow and 10% sucrose solution (SA) and were sacrificed in the non-stressed condition (NS) or after 1 h of restraint stress (RS). *Significantly different from NS in the same feeding condition. #Significantly different from CA in the same stressful condition.

Activation of the HPA axis is a key neurohormonal response to stress. Sucrose eating is able to blunt the activity of the HPA axis at the level of CRF expression, and ACTH and glucocorticoid release. This ‘anti-stress’ effect of sucrose may explain why people and animals are more predisposed to consuming pleasurable palatable food when stressed [83, 122-128] even when they are not hungry and have no homeostatic needs for calories [129, 130]. Therefore, sugar and sweets may be taken as ‘anti-stress’ self-medication [131]. Stressor-associated non-homeostatic feeding may promote obesity [132]. Conversely, removal of food induces strong stress-like activation of the HPA axis in obese animals. Indeed, the genetically obese Zucker rats show significant induction of expression of c-*fos* in the CRF PVH neurons at 3-6 h and a strong increase in plasma corticosterone at 6-12 h after food removal, whereas their lean littermates do not show any signs of hunger and HPA axis activity at this time [133, 134]. This result suggests that the obese phenotype may promote feeding to 'self-medicate' the hyperactivity of the HPA axis.

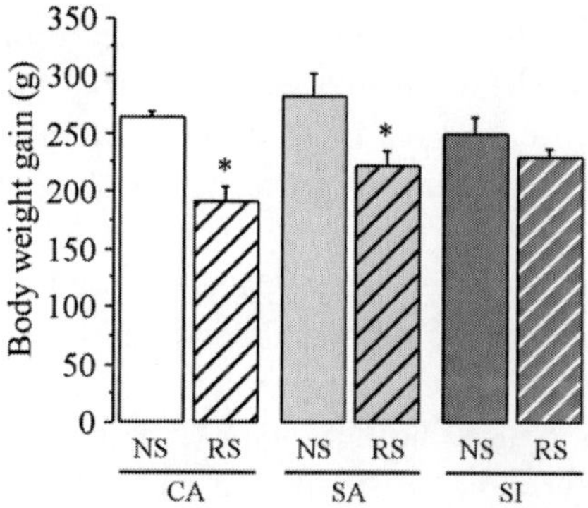

Figure 10. The rats maintained on intermittent access to sucrose (SI rats; 4-day-per-week access to 10% sucrose) were resistant to the anorectic effect of chronic restraint stress and did not show a stress-induced decrease in body weight gain compared to rats with continuous *ad libitum* access to chow (CA rats) or chow and 10% sucrose solution (SA rats). All rats were maintained on their respective feeding regimen during 6 weeks and were non-stressed (NS rats) or stressed (RS rats) by 1-h restraint stress applied once per week. *Significantly different from NS rats in the same feeding condition. Modified from [81].

When access to food is not under control, people show a wide variety of feeding responses to stress. Approximately 20% of people do not change their feeding behavior during stressful periods, 40% or more increase their caloric intake, and 40% or less decrease their caloric intake when stressed [122, 132, 135-137]. In experimental conditions when animals have access only to mundane chow, repeated or acute stress generally promotes anorectic response [138-140]. The anorectic effects of CRF are at the core of the stress-induced decrease in food intake. Depending on the stress paradigm and the dose used, the nonspecific CRF antagonist alpha-helical CRF partially or completely reverses emotional and physical stress-induced anorexia [140-142]. Continuous access to sucrose decreases stress-induced activation of the expression of CRF and c-*fos* mRNAs in the parvocellular PVH (Figure 9) [81]. This sucrose-mediated decrease in stress-induced activation of the PVH underlies the lower HPA axis activation in response to stress in sucrose-fed rats [81, 82, 121, 129]. However, the anorectic response to stress was strongly inhibited in rats with intermittent but not continuous access to sucrose (Figure

10) [81]. In our experiment, the intermittent consumption of sucrose without food restriction (4 days per week, given *ad libitum*) or in combination with food restriction (4 days per week, limited to 2-h daily access) effectively dampened the decrease in the body weight gain induced by weekly sessions of 1-h restraint stress in the control groups maintained on *ad libitum* chow or chow and sucrose [81]. The results reported by Kinzig et al. showed that post-stress intake of sucrose and lard was decreased in rats maintained on continuous but not intermittent access to palatable food [143]. Therefore, continuous access to palatable food dampens stress-induced activation of the HPA axis, while intermittent feeding of palatable food more potently affects the behavioral anorectic effects of stress. These particular diet effects on the stress-related CRF system depend on the differential role of the CRF receptors mediating the CRF signals. The CRF type 1 receptor (CRF1) is strongly expressed in the parvocellular PVH in response to stress and mediates the CRF-induced activation of the HPA axis during stress [144, 145]. Mice lacking CRF1 failed to exhibit the characteristic activation of the HPA axis to stress due to insufficient ACTH production [146]. The CRF type 2 receptor (CRF2) is expressed in the brain in the ventromedial hypothalamic nucleus (VMH) and in the lateral septum (LS). Central blockade of CRF2 with specific antagonists or antisense oligonucleotides counteracts the CRF anorectic effects [147, 148]. Likewise, mice deficient in CRF2 consume substantially more food when maintained on a palatable high-fat diet [149, 150]. Intermittent access to sucrose significantly decreased CRF2 mRNA levels and stress-induced c-*fos* mRNA expression in the LS (Figure 11) [81]. The rats maintained on intermittent access to sucrose and demonstrating lower LS activity also showed “impulsive”-like licking of sucrose. Indeed, the rats maintained on intermittent sucrose (SI rats) showed high and persistent overnight sucrose- but not water-licking activity (Figure 12) [81]. Interestingly, the LS lesion led to a dramatic increase in sucrose-licking activity but not water-licking activity [151]. This increase in sucrose-licking activity in the LS-lesioned rats was independent of thirsting or fasting and was not eliminated by sucrose preloading [151]. In contrast, direct stimulation of CRF2 in the LS by specific CRF2 agonist inhibits feeding [152]. Therefore, a decrease in LS activation and the expression of CRF2 in the LS may contribute to increased sucrose intake in rats maintained on intermittent sucrose access [81]. But why might intermittent access to sucrose trigger the development of certain impulsivity of sucrose consumption? On the next pages, we will discuss what is special in intermittent sucrose intake and why this regimen may change feeding behavior in experimental animals.

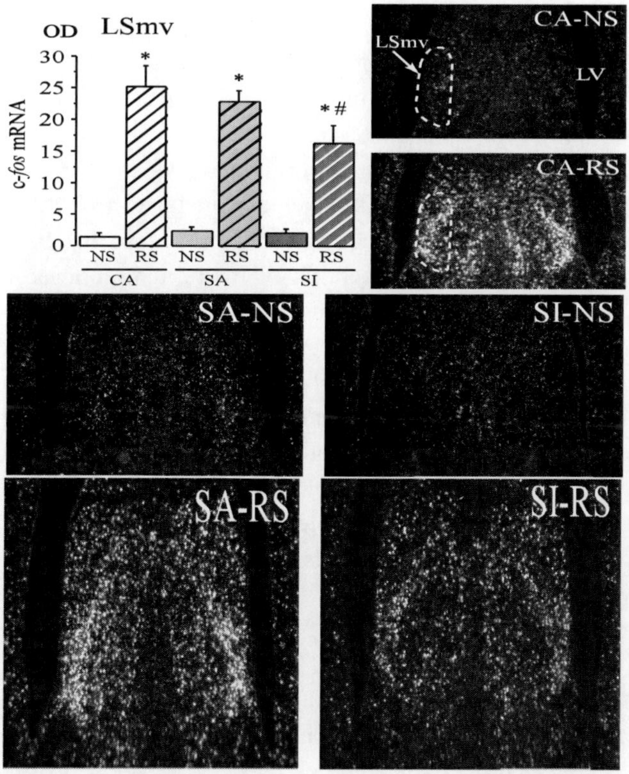

Figure 11. The rats maintained on intermittent access to sucrose (SI rats; 4-day-per-week access to 10% sucrose) showed blunted stress-induced induction of expression of c-*fos* mRNA in the lateral septum (LS) compared to the rats with continuous *ad libitum* access to chow (CA rats) or chow and 10% sucrose solution (SA rats). All rats were maintained on their respective feeding regimen for 6 weeks and were non-stressed (NS rats) or stressed (RS rats) by 1-h restraint stress applied once per week. The rats were sacrificed immediately after the last, sixth session of restraint stress. The histogram demonstrates the optical density (OD) of the positive hybridization signal of c-*fos* mRNA in the medioventral LS (LSmv). *Significantly different from NS rats in the same feeding condition. #Significantly different from CA rats in the same stressful condition. Modified from [81].

5. Could Sucrose Be Addictive?

The concept of "sugar addiction" has been discussed in scientific and popular literature for many years, but consensus on this topic is far from unanimous. Clinical accounts of "sugar addiction" have been reviewed by a number of books and were the focus of popular diet programs [153-156]. In these accounts, people describe food cravings, particularly for sugar and sweets that can trigger irresistible impulsive eating. Attempts to control intake of sugar-rich foods or imposing self-restriction for sweets may trigger withdrawal and dysphoria symptoms. In this negative state of the mood, any stressful situation or even slight disturbance can trigger irresistible impulsive episode of binge eating [127]. Although addiction to food has been discussed with interest in the popular and scientific literature and proposed to be based on brain neurochemistry [157, 158], this phenomenon only recently has been seen as clinically relevant. The binge-eating disorder is defined in the DSM-5 (Diagnostic and Statistical Manual of Mental Disorders) Development as follows: (1) eating in a discrete period of time an amount of food that is definitely larger than most people would eat in a similar period of time under similar circumstances; and (2) a sense of lack of control over eating during the episode. To study the neuronal and molecular mechanisms of food addiction, resorting to experimental animal models is inevitable. Given some subjective definition for food addiction, such as a sense of a lack of the control or a feeling of guilt, developing a convincing animal model of food addiction is not easy. However, certain criteria that can be assessed with high precision have been proposed. These criteria include (1) the escalation of food intake with a high proportion of intake at one time, and (2) behavioral sensitization [159, 160]. Several animal models of binge eating were developed by intermittent access to highly palatable food such as sucrose. Thus, rats maintained on intermittent access to sugar binge-eat sugar in the first hour of daily access and show progressive escalation of their daily intake of sugar [160, 161]. What is special in intermittent excessive intake of sucrose? Consumption of palatable food, such as sucrose, by naïve rats produces release of dopamine in the accumbens shell [162]. However, this response can wane during a long meal and does not reappear during following tests [162, 163]. This decrease in dopamine release upon habituation to familiar taste [164] is dissimilar from repeated dopamine release to the nucleus accumbens each time the drugs of abuse are consumed [165, 166]. However, when sucrose is given to rats intermittently, in 12-h daily access following 12 h of food deprivation, the animals gradually escalate their sucrose intake from 37 ml to 112 ml per day, and the release of dopamine to the accumbens shell is produced repeatedly and is significant even on the 21st day of the access to sucrose [162]. Control groups, eating sucrose *ad libitum* or chow intermittently, failed to repeatedly increase dopamine in the nucleus accumbens during sucrose-eating tests and showed signs of habituation to the taste of sucrose [162]. In addition to increased dopamine, the sucrose-sensitized rats maintained on intermittent sucrose demonstrated delayed release in accumbens acetylcholine [162]. Repeated increase in dopamine secretion to the nucleus accumbens may reinforce the eating of sucrose [165, 167, 168] while delaying acetylcholine may hinder satiation [169, 170]. Complete inhibition of acetylcholine satiety response by sucrose sham feeding in sucrose-sensitized rats additionally increased their intake of sucrose [171]. This result is relevant to the stronger binge episodes accompanied by purging in the cases of bulimia nervosa.

Sucrose-sensitized rats not only change the dopamine/acetylcholine secretion to the ventral striatum. The intermittent sucrose regimen results in long-lasting alterations at the levels of expression of the neurotransmitters and their receptors. Thus, sugar-dependent rats show alterations in the mRNA levels of the dopamine receptors and opioids similar to that seen in morphine-dependent rats, but compared to morphine, the effects of sugar on the mRNA levels were of a greater magnitude in the nucleus accumbens than in the caudate-putamen [172]. Specifically, after the chronic schedule of intermittent bingeing on sucrose solution, the mRNA levels of the D2 dopamine receptor, and the preproenkephalin and preprotachykinin genes were decreased, while D3 dopamine receptor mRNA was increased in the dopamine-receptive regions of the forebrain [172]. The sucrose-bingeing rats also demonstrated long-term alterations at the level of receptor binding. The intermittent sucrose regimen increased dopamine D1 receptor binding in the accumbens core and shell. In contrast, D2 receptor binding was decreased in the striatum, while the binding to the dopamine transporter increased in the midbrain [161]. In addition, sucrose-dependent rats demonstrated increases in μ-1 opioid receptor binding in the cingulate cortex, hippocampus, locus coeruleus and accumbens shell [161].

Long-term modifications in brain neurotransmission in the sucrose-dependent rats were reflected in their behavior. As mentioned above, the sucrose-sensitized rats maintained on intermittent access to sucrose dramatically escalated their sucrose intake within the first hour of access to sucrose. Moreover, these rats showed extremely higher, significantly more than ever before, motivation to lever press for sugar on the fixed ratio schedules after 2 weeks of sugar deprivation [173]. This result provides evidence that the altered neurochemical state of sucrose-sensitized rats lasts at least for 2 weeks of sugar abstinence and leads to enhanced sugar intake.

Sugar-dependent rats showed cross-sensitization to drugs of abuse. Cross-sensitization is increased sensitivity, usually manifested as an increased locomotor response, to a new drug or substance in an animal addicted to another drug [160]. Animals sensitized to one drug may increase consumption of a different drug. Figuratively saying, one drug acts as a "gateway" to another. For example, animals sensitized to amphetamine show accelerated escalation of their cocaine intake [174], and animals sensitized to nicotine consume more alcohol compared with non-sensitized animals [175].

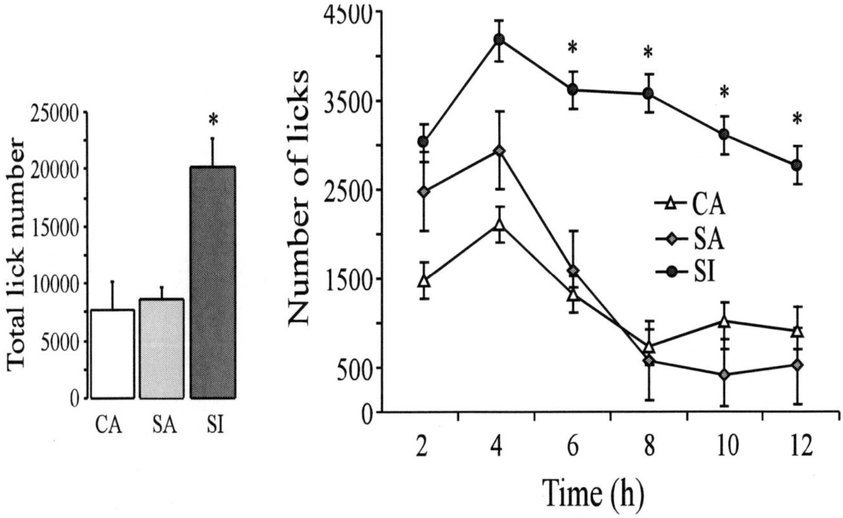

Figure 12. The rats maintained for 6 weeks on intermittent access to sucrose (SI rats; 4-day-per-week access to 10% sucrose) demonstrated a higher total overnight number of licks of sucrose (left histogram) as well as overnight persistence of high levels of sucrose licking (right waveforms) compared to the rats maintained for 6 weeks on continuous *ad libitum* access to chow (CA rats) or chow and 10% sucrose solution (SA rats). *Significantly different from other groups. Modified from [81].

This behavior is thought to occur when different drugs activate the same neural circuitry [176]. Interestingly, sugar-dependent rats show enhanced intake of unsweetened ethanol [177]. The rats sensitized to amphetamine by repeated injection of this drug show sugar-induced hyperactivity and sugar hyperphagia [178].

Conversely, the rats maintained on intermittent access to sucrose demonstrated a hyperactive response to amphetamine [179]. These results suggest that the drug of abuse may invade the neuronal mechanisms designed for the natural reward such as sucrose. But on the other hand, these data warn that sugar may be addictive, similar to drugs of abuse [160]. There is evidence that sensitization to sugar due to long-term intermittent consumption causes endogenous opioid dependence.

Administration of naloxone, an opioid antagonist with a high affinity for μ-opioid receptors, in sucrose-dependent rats causes spontaneous somatic withdrawal signs, such as teeth chattering, forepaw tremor, and head shaking [159].

In addition, naloxone increased the anxiety of these rats, revealed by reduced time spent on the exposed arm of an elevated plus maze. In the nucleus accumbens of sucrose-sensitized rats, naloxone decreased extracellular dopamine, while dose-dependently increased acetylcholine.

The indices of anxiety and dopamine/acetylcholine imbalance in the naloxone-treated sugar-sensitized rats were quantitatively similar to that seen in withdrawal from morphine or nicotine, suggesting development of sugar dependence [159].

Similar to naloxone, food deprivation of sucrose-sensitized rats increases anxiety and causes somatic withdrawal signs, such as teeth chattering [159]. Food deprivation affects the dopaminergic neurotransmission in the nucleus accumbens. Specifically, food deprivation decreases extracellular dopamine in the ventral striatum while accumulating dopamine in the presynaptic terminals that ensure higher dopamine release in response to refeeding or intra-accumbens administration of amphetamine [180].

In addition to a decrease in dopamine, food deprivation strongly increases acetylcholine in the nucleus accumbens of sucrose-dependent rats [181]. Although these effects of food deprivation may potentiate feeding of palatable food, a binge-eating model can be developed without referring to food deprivation.

Thus, a rat model bingeing on palatable hydrogenated vegetable shortening was developed in Rebecca Corwin's laboratory [182]. This model was developed by intermittent access to palatable food, a treatment that triggered progressive increase in intake of palatable food by shortening the access to this food. Long-term neuronal plasticity is suspected for this model, as its development takes about 4 weeks, but, once established, the bingeing behavior is manifested persistently [183-185].

Binge-eating models demonstrate increased anxiety and are vulnerable to stress [186]. Foot shock stress specifically increased the intake of palatable food but not regular chow in rats with a history of repeated food restriction and refeeding with highly palatable food ingredients, such as sweet cookies [187-189].

In our experiments, the regimens of food restriction and intermittent access to sucrose considerably escalated the intake of palatable sucrose but not chow [100]. Intermittent access to sucrose decreased the anorectic effects of stress with the concomitant decrease of neuronal activation in the lateral septum [81].

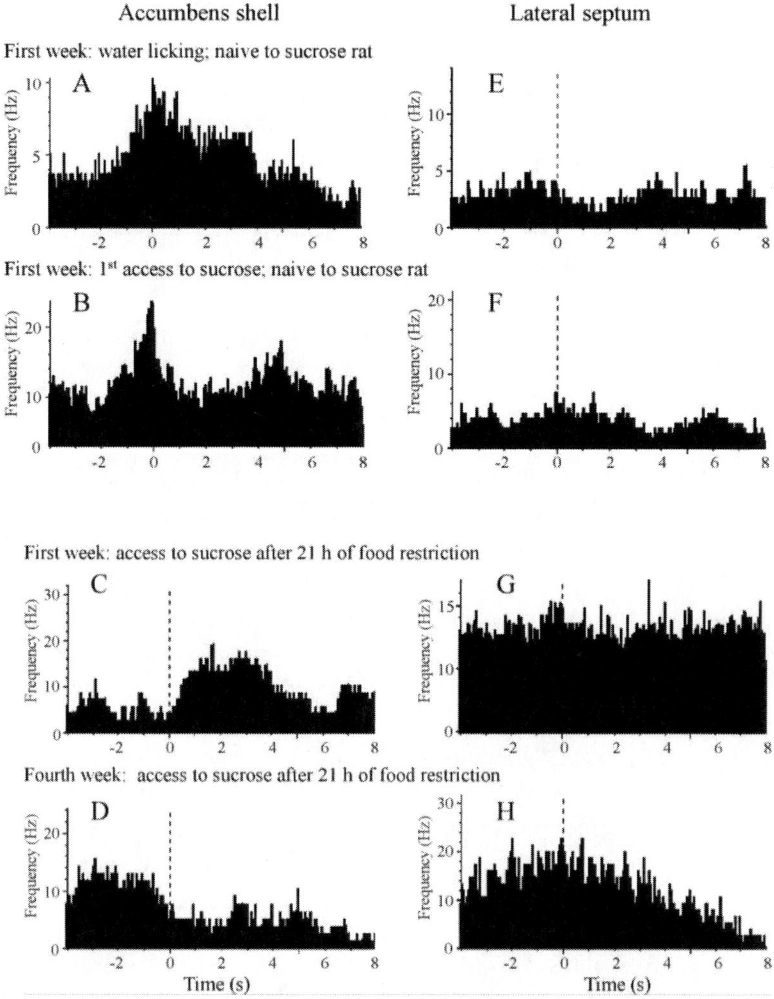

Figure 13. The regimen triggering development of bingeing on sucrose produced alterations in neuronal activity in the nucleus accumbens shell (AcbSh; A-D) and the lateral septum (LS; E-H). Specifically, sucrose-bingeing rats developed a strong sucrose-anticipatory response in the AcbSh (D *versus* C), while consumption of sucrose inhibited neuronal activity in the LS (G *versus* H). The rats (n=6) were submitted to weekly cycles of food restriction (4 days per week the access to food was limited to 3 h daily), intermittent access to sucrose (3-h daily; 4 days per week), and chronic foot shock (0.6 mA for 60 s; 1 time per week). The rats were implanted with

chronic platinum-iridium electrodes aimed at the AcbSh and the LS. The extracellular neuronal firing was recorded using the TDT multichannel acquisition system. Water- and sucrose-liking events were recorded simultaneously with neuronal activity using a Med Associates behavioral test chamber equipped with two photobeam lickometers. The peri-event histograms, with a bin width of 1 ms, represent the firing frequency of the majority of the neurons in the recorded structures 4 s before and 8 s after the onset (time 0) of licking clusters defined as persistent licking activity with inter-licking intervals of less than 1 s. Water-licking in the naïve-to-sucrose rats produced an increase in the firing frequency immediately (~500 ms) before and during licking in the AcbSh (A) but not in the LS (E). At their first access to sucrose, these rats showed an increase in firing frequency immediately (~500 ms) before sucrose licking in the AcbSh (B) but not in the LS (F). Access to sucrose after food restriction in the first week of cyclic treatments showed a delayed (by 500 ms) increase in the firing rate in the Acb (C), while at these conditions the LS demonstrated a significant increase in the basal activity but no response to sucrose licking (G). Escalation of sucrose intake at the end of the fourth week was accompanied by the development of a strong sucrose-anticipatory (from -4 s to -200 ms) firing in the AcbSh (D) and sucrose-induced decrease (from +4 s) in neuronal firing in the LS (H) [Mitra and Timofeeva, unpublished].

In addition, intermittent sucrose intake displaced neuronal activity during food-anticipatory periods from the medial hypothalamus to the ventral striatum [100]. To monitor the neuronal activity in the lateral septum and the nucleus accumbens shell in the rats submitted to feeding conditions triggering sucrose bingeing, we extracellularly recorded the neuronal firing in these structures using chronically implanted bunches of platinum-iridium electrodes. The preliminary test of sucrose-naïve rats to water and sucrose intake showed no response in the lateral septum (Figure 13, E, F). In contrast, the majority of the neurons in the accumbens shell increased their firing rate 500 ms before and 4 s during the clusters of water licking (Figure 13, A).

In the accumbens shell, the first access to sucrose showed an increase in the firing rate 500 ms before the initiation of sucrose licking, following by a decrease in neuronal firing during sucrose licking (Figure 13, B). Food restriction increased significantly the firing rate of the neurons in the lateral septum (Figure 13, G) but not in the accumbens shell (Figure 13, C). Access to sucrose after the first food restriction increased the firing rate of the majority of the neurons in the accumbens shell but not in the lateral septum (Figure 13, C, G). Four weekly cycles of food restriction, intermittent access to sucrose, and 1-h weekly foot shock stress led to the development of an anticipatory, 4 s before the clusters of sucrose licking, increase in the firing rate in the accumbens shell (Figure 13, D), and a significant decrease in the firing rate upon sucrose licking in the lateral septum (Figure 13, H). These results show that the regimen triggering development of bingeing on sucrose is accompanied by dynamic alterations in the neuronal activity of the brain regions involved in sucrose reward and stress-related effects.

Therefore, sucrose intake affects the activity of the neuronal circuitries that mediate the rewarding effects of sucrose. Through evolution, these mechanisms were developed to ensure the seeking and consumption of energy-rich foods. However, as the animal models suggest, excessive intermittent intake of sucrose especially combined with chronic stress and food restriction may trigger long-term plasticity in the brain reward- and stress-related pathways that may promote craving for sucrose and trigger sucrose binge-eating episodes.

CONCLUSION

The statistics shows that during the past few centuries humans increased their intake of sucrose by hundreds of times. Are we aware of this dramatic alteration in our diet? How might sucrose change our neuronal activity and our mood and mind? Is sucrose our friend or enemy? This review attempted to find answers to these questions. Generally, our brain recognizes sucrose as rewarding. This effect of sucrose is hardwired in the brain to assure seeking and consumption of high-energy food, assuring therefore survival of an individual and a species. However, clinical records and experimental results suggest that sucrose may be addictive and its consumption may in some conditions become uncontrollable. Between the conditions triggering uncontrollable binge-eating of palatable food, food restriction, chronic stress, and repeated overeating of sweets seem to be the most dangerous. Some mechanisms underlying the sucrose feeding behavior remain obscure. Not every person who consumes alcohol becomes alcohol-dependent. The same is true for consumption of palatable food: only some people develop uncontrollable bingeing on sweet foods. The mechanisms of individual resistance or vulnerability to sucrose remain to be investigated. The physiological and morphological research of the several last decades characterized in detail the neuronal pathways activated by sucrose. These studies have revealed the ascending gustatory pathways as well as the neuronal glucosensitivity informing the brain about sucrose consumption and glucose availability. Recent studies have demonstrated that consuming sucrose may decrease the activity of the stress-related brain structures while increasing the anticipatory activation of the brain reward system. These mechanisms may increase the craving for sucrose but also may help in managing the stress reaction. Allegorically, sucrose can be compared to Janus, a Roman gate-keeping god who had two faces - one was friendly and was turned to his friends, and the other was scary and turned to his enemies. We have to use sucrose as our friend that gives us energy and helps us to ease stress, while avoiding overeating sucrose, which may lead to uncontrolled craving for sucrose, eating disorders and obesity.

REFERENCES

[1] Blass, E. M. In *Sweetness*; Springer-Verlag: London, 1987; pp 115-124.

[2] Logue, A. W. *The psychology of eating and drinking*; Brunner-Routledge: New York, 2004.

[3] Bernstein, W. J. *A Splendid Exchange: How Trade Shaped the World*; Atlantic Books: London, 2008.

[4] Riddle, J. M. In *Catalogus translationum et commentariorum: Mediaeval and Renaissance Latin translations and commentaries: annoted lists and guides.*; Catholic Univ. of America Press: Washington, DC, 1984.

[5] Revel, J. F. *Culture and cuisine*; Doubleday: New York, 1982.

[6] Galloway, J. H. *The sugar cane industry*; Cambridge University Press: Cambridge, UK, 1989.

[7] Parker, M. *The Sugar Barons: Family, Corruption, Empire and War*; Hutchinson: London, 2011.

[8] Mintz, S. W. *Sweetness and power: the place of sugar in modern history*; Penguin Books: New York, 1986.

[9] Johnson, R. J.; Segal, M. S.; Sautin, Y.; Nakagawa, T.; Feig, D. I.; Kang, D. H.; Gersch, M. S.; Benner, S.; Sanchez-Lozada, L. G. *Am J Clin Nutr*. 2007, 86, 899-906.

[10] Kanetkar, P.; Singhal, R.; Kamat, M. *J Clin Biochem Nutr*. 2007, 41, 77-81.

[11] Hiji, T. *Nature*. 1975, 256, 427-429.

[12] Montmayeur, J. P.; Liberles, S. D.; Matsunami, H.; Buck, L. B. *Nat Neurosci*. 2001, 4, 492-498.

[13] Nelson, G.; Hoon, M. A.; Chandrashekar, J.; Zhang, Y.; Ryba, N. J.; Zuker, C. S. *Cell*. 2001, 106, 381-390.

[14] Li, X.; Staszewski, L.; Xu, H.; Durick, K.; Zoller, M.; Adler, E. *Proc Natl Acad Sci U S A*. 2002, 99, 4692-4696.

[15] Nakagawa, Y.; Nagasawa, M.; Yamada, S.; Hara, A.; Mogami, H.; Nikolaev, V. O.; Lohse, M. J.; Shigemura, N.; Ninomiya, Y.; Kojima, I. *PLoS One*. 2009, 4, e5106.
[16] Xu, H.; Staszewski, L.; Tang, H.; Adler, E.; Zoller, M.; Li, X. *Proc Natl Acad Sci U S A*. 2004, 101, 14258-14263.
[17] Ishimaru, Y.; Matsunami, H. *J Dent Res*. 2009, 88, 212-218.
[18] Hisatsune, C.; Yasumatsu, K.; Takahashi-Iwanaga, H.; Ogawa, N.; Kuroda, Y.; Yoshida, R.; Ninomiya, Y.; Mikoshiba, K. *J Biol Chem*. 2007, 282, 37225-37231.
[19] Frank, M. *J Gen Physiol*. 1973, 61, 588-618.
[20] Erickson, R. P. *Behav Brain Sci*. 2008, 31, 59-75.
[21] Travers, S. P.; Norgren, R. *J Neurophysiol*. 1995, 73, 2144-2162.
[22] Treesukosol, Y.; Smith, K. R.; Spector, A. C. *Physiol Behav*. 2011, 105, 14-26.
[23] Mayer, E. A. *Nat Rev Neurosci*. 2011, 12, 453-466.
[24] Craig, A. D. *Nat Rev Neurosci*. 2002, 3, 655-666.
[25] Damasio, A. R. *The feeling of what happens: body and emotion in the making of consciousness*; Harcourt Brace: New York, 1999.
[26] Norgren, R.; Leonard, C. M. *Science*. 1971, 173, 1136-1139.
[27] Norgren, R.; Leonard, C. M. *J Comp Neurol*. 1973, 150, 217-237.
[28] Timofeeva, E.; Baraboi, E. D.; Richard, D. *Eur J Neurosci*. 2005, 22, 1489-1501.
[29] Grill, H. J.; Norgren, R. *Brain Res*. 1978, 143, 281-297.
[30] Grill, H. J.; Norgren, R. *Brain Res*. 1978, 143, 263-279.
[31] Yamamoto, T.; Shimura, T.; Sakai, N.; Ozaki, N. *Physiol Behav*. 1994, 56, 1197-1202.
[32] Spector, A. C.; Grill, H. J.; Norgren, R. *Physiol Behav*. 1993, 53, 277-283.
[33] DiPatrizio, N. V.; Simansky, K. J. *J Neurosci*. 2008, 28, 9702-9709.Phillipson, O. T. *J Comp Neurol*. 1979, 187, 117-143.
[34] Alden, M.; Besson, J. M.; Bernard, J. F. *J Comp Neurol*. 1994, 341, 289-314.
[35] Krout, K. E.; Loewy, A. D. *J Comp Neurol*. 2000, 428, 475-494.
[36] Cechetto, D. F.; Saper, C. B. *J Comp Neurol*. 1987, 262, 27-45.
[37] Wise, R. A. *Philos Trans R Soc Lond B Biol Sci*. 2006, 361, 1149-1158.
[38] Hernandez, L.; Hoebel, B. G. *Life Sci*. 1988, 42, 1705-1712.
[39] Hajnal, A.; Smith, G. P.; Norgren, R. *Am J Physiol*. 2004, 286, R31-R37.
[40] Taha, S. A.; Fields, H. L. *J Neurosci*. 2005, 25, 1193-1202.

[41] Krause, M.; German, P. W.; Taha, S. A.; Fields, H. L. *J Neurosci.* 2010, 30, 4746-4756.
[42] de Araujo, I. E.; Oliveira-Maia, A. J.; Sotnikova, T. D.; Gainetdinov, R. R.; Caron, M. G.; Nicolelis, M. A.; Simon, S. A. *Neuron.* 2008, 57, 930-941.
[43] Robayo-Torres, C. C.; Quezada-Calvillo, R.; Nichols, B. L. *Clin Gastroenterol Hepatol.* 2006, 4, 276-287.
[44] Gudmand-Hoyer, E.; Skovbjerg, H. *Scand J Gastroenterol Suppl.* 1996, 216, 111-121.
[45] Riby, J. E.; Fujisawa, T.; Kretchmer, N. *Am J Clin Nutr.* 1993, 58, 748S-753S.
[46] Crane, R. K. In *Symposia of the International Society for Cell Biology*; Academic Press: New York, 1966; 71-102.
[47] Caspary, W. F. In *Na-linked transport of organic solutes*; Springer: Berlin, 1972; 99-108.
[48] Wright, E. M. *Annu Rev Physiol.* 1993, 55, 575-589.
[49] Southgate, D. A. T. *Am J Clin Nutr.* 1995, 62, 203S-211S.
[50] Gjedde, A. In *Physiology and pharmacology of the blood-brain barrier*; Springler: Berlin, 1992; 65-115.
[51] Peters, A.; Schweiger, U.; Pellerin, L.; Hubold, C.; Oltmanns, K. M.; Conrad, M.; Schultes, B.; Born, J.; Fehm, H. L. *Neurosci Biobehav Rev.* 2004, 28, 143-180.
[52] Mangia, S.; Simpson, I. A.; Vannucci, S. J.; Carruthers, A. *J Neurochem.* 2009, 109 Suppl 1, 55-62.
[53] DiNuzzo, M.; Mangia, S.; Maraviglia, B.; Giove, F. *J Cereb Blood Flow Metab.* 2010, 30, 586-602.
[54] Mangia, S.; DiNuzzo, M.; Giove, F.; Carruthers, A.; Simpson, I. A.; Vannucci, S. J. *J Cereb Blood Flow Metab.* 2011, 31, 1346-1353.
[55] Peters, A.; Pellerin, L.; Dallman, M. F.; Oltmanns, K. M.; Schweiger, U.; Born, J.; Fehm, H. L. *Prog Neurobiol.* 2007, 81, 61-88.
[56] Mayer, J. *N Engl J Med.* 1953, 249, 13-16.
[57] Mayer, J. *Ann N Y Acad Sci.* 1955, 63, 15-43.
[58] Watts, A. G.; Donovan, C. M. *Front Neuroendocrinol.* 2010, 31, 32-43.
[59] Russek, M. *Nature.* 1963, 197, 79-80.
[60] Donovan, C. M.; Hamilton-Wessler, M.; Halter, J. B.; Bergman, R. N. *Proc Natl Acad Sci U S A.* 1994, 91, 2863-2867.
[61] Hevener, A. L.; Bergman, R. N.; Donovan, C. M. *Diabetes.* 1997, 46, 1521-1525.
[62] Niijima, A. *Ann N Y Acad Sci.* 1969, 157, 690-700.

[63] Niijima, A. *Prog Neurobiol.* 1989, 33, 135-147.
[64] Thorens, B.; Larsen, P. J. *Curr Opin Clin Nutr Metab Care.* 2004, 7, 471-478.
[65] Fujita, S.; Donovan, C. M. *Diabetes.* 2005, 54, 3258-3264.
[66] Funahashi, M.; Adachi, A. *Brain Res Bull.* 1993, 32, 531-535.
[67] Balfour, R. H.; Hansen, A. M.; Trapp, S. *J Physiol.* 2006, 570, 469-484.
[68] Mizuno, Y.; Oomura, Y. *Brain Res.* 1984, 307, 109-116.
[69] Oomura, Y.; Ono, T.; Ooyama, H.; Wayner, M. J. *Nature.* 1969, 222, 282-284.
[70] Ono, T.; Nishino, H.; Fukuda, M.; Sasaki, K.; Muramoto, K.; Oomura, Y. *Brain Res.* 1982, 232, 494-499.
[71] Slusser, P. G.; Ritter, R. C. *Brain Res.* 1980, 202, 474-478.
[72] McCrimmon, R. *Diabet Med.* 2008, 25, 513-522.
[73] Gonzalez, J. A.; Jensen, L. T.; Fugger, L.; Burdakov, D. *Diabetes.* 2008, 57, 2569-2576.
[74] Oomura, Y. In *Advances in Metabolic Disorders. CNS Regulation of Carbohydrate*; Academic Press: New York, 1983; 10, 31-65.
[75] Matschinsky, F. M. *Diabetes.* 1996, 45, 223-241.
[76] Schuit, F. C.; Huypens, P.; Heimberg, H.; Pipeleers, D. G. *Diabetes.* 2001, 50, 1-11.
[77] Burdakov, D.; Jensen, L. T.; Alexopoulos, H.; Williams, R. H.; Fearon, I. M.; O'Kelly, I.; Gerasimenko, O.; Fugger, L.; Verkhratsky, A. *Neuron.* 2006, 50, 711-722.
[78] Ren, X.; Zhou, L.; Terwilliger, R.; Newton, S. S.; de Araujo, I. E. *Front Integr Neurosci.* 2009, 3, 12.
[79] Timofeeva, E.; Baraboi, E. D.; Poulin, A. M.; Richard, D. *J Neuroendocrinol.* 2009, 21, 982-992.
[80] Martin, J.; Timofeeva, E. *Am J Physiol.* 2010, 298, R1383-R1398.
[81] Bell, M. E.; Bhargava, A.; Soriano, L.; Laugero, K.; Akana, S. F.; Dallman, M. F. *J Neuroendocrinol.* 2002, 14, 330-342.
[82] Pecoraro, N.; Reyes, F.; Gomez, F.; Bhargava, A.; Dallman, M. F. *Endocrinology.* 2004, 145, 3754-3762.
[83] Treit, D.; Spetch, M. L. *Physiol Behav.* 1986, 36, 311-317.
[84] Snowdon, C. T. *J Comp Physiol Psychol.* 1969, 69, 91-100.
[85] Cottone, P.; Sabino, V.; Steardo, L.; Zorrilla, E. P. *Am J Physiol.* 2008, 295, R1066-R1076.
[86] Hoefer, M. E.; Voskanian, S. J.; Koob, G. F.; Pulvirenti, L. *Pharmacol Biochem Behav.* 2006, 83, 403-409.

[87] LeSage, M. G.; Burroughs, D.; Pentel, P. R. *Pharmacol Biochem Behav*. 2006, 83, 585-591.

[88] Orsini, C.; Koob, G. F.; Pulvirenti, L. *Neuropsychopharmacology*. 2001, 25, 789-792.

[89] Zhang, D.; Zhou, X.; Wang, X.; Xiang, X.; Chen, H.; Hao, W. *Addict Biol*. 2007, 12, 152-157.

[90] Landry, G. J.; Simon, M. M.; Webb, I. C.; Mistlberger, R. E. *Am J Physiol*. 2006, 290, R1527-1534.

[91] Poulin, A. M.; Timofeeva, E. *Brain Res*. 2008, 1227, 128-141.

[92] Mendoza, J.; Angeles-Castellanos, M.; Escobar, C. *Neuroscience*. 2005, 133, 293-303.

[93] Angeles-Castellanos, M.; Salgado-Delgado, R.; Rodriguez, K.; Buijs, R. M.; Escobar, C. *Neuroscience*. 2008, 155, 297-307.

[94] Stephan, F. K.; Davidson, A. J. *Physiol Behav*. 1998, 65, 277-288.

[95] Mistlberger, R.; Rusak, B. *Physiol Behav*. 1987, 41, 219-226.

[96] Stephan, F. K. *Physiol Behav*. 1997, 62, 995-1002.

[97] Mistlberger, R. E. *Neurosci Biobehav Rev*. 1994, 18, 171-195.

[98] Pecoraro, N.; Gomez, F.; Laugero, K.; Dallman, M. F. *Behav Neurosci*. 2002, 116, 757-776.

[99] Mitra, A.; Lenglos, C.; Martin, J.; Mbende, N.; Gagne, A.; Timofeeva, E. *Neuroscience*. 2011, 192, 459-474.

[100] Angeles-Castellanos, M.; Aguilar-Roblero, R.; Escobar, C. *Am J Physiol*. 2004, 286, R158-165.

[101] Arletti, R.; Benelli, A.; Bertolini, A. *Peptides*. 1989, 10, 89-93.

[102] Olson, B. R.; Drutarosky, M. D.; Chow, M. S.; Hruby, V. J.; Stricker, E. M.; Verbalis, J. G. *Peptides*. 1991, 12, 113-118.

[103] Arletti, R.; Benelli, A.; Bertolini, A. *Physiol Behav*. 1990, 48, 825-830.

[104] Blevins, J. E.; Schwartz, M. W.; Baskin, D. G. *Am J Physiol*. 2004, 287, R87-R96.

[105] Olson, B. R.; Drutarosky, M. D.; Stricker, E. M.; Verbalis, J. G. *Endocrinology*. 1991, 129, 785-791.

[106] Miedlar, J. A.; Rinaman, L.; Vollmer, R. R.; Amico, J. A. *Am J Physiol*. 2007, 293, R1063-R1068.

[107] Amico, J. A.; Vollmer, R. R.; Cai, H. M.; Miedlar, J. A.; Rinaman, L. *Am J Physiol*. 2005, 289, R1798-R1806.

[108] Mitra, A.; Gosnell, B. A.; Schioth, H. B.; Grace, M. K.; Klockars, A.; Olszewski, P. K.; Levine, A. S. *Peptides*. 2010, 31, 1346-1352.

[109] Bello, N. T.; Guarda, A. S.; Terrillion, C. E.; Redgrave, G. W.; Coughlin, J. W.; Moran, T. H. *Am J Physiol*. 2009, 297, R622-R631.

[110] Travers, J. B.; Travers, S. P.; Norgren, R. *Annu Rev Neurosci*. 1987, 10, 595-632.

[111] Timofeeva, E.; Huang, Q.; Richard, D. *Neuroendocrinology*. 2003, 77, 388-405.

[112] Turnbull, A. V.; Rivier, C. *Proc Soc Exp Biol Med*. 1997, 215, 1-10.

[113] Dallman, M. F.; Akana, S. F.; Levin, N.; Walker, C. D.; Bradbury, M. J.; Suemaru, S.; Scribner, K. S. *Ann N Y Acad Sci*. 1994, 746, 22-31.

[114] Herman, J. P.; Prewitt, C. M.; Cullinan, W. E. *Crit Rev Neurobiol*. 1996, 10, 371-394.

[115] Sawchenko, P. E.; Li, H. Y.; Ericsson, A. *Prog Brain Res*. 2000, 122, 61-78.

[116] Ling, S.; Jamali, F. *J Pharm Pharm Sci*. 2003, 6, 246-251.

[117] Bell, M. E.; Bhatnagar, S.; Liang, J.; Soriano, L.; Nagy, T. R.; Dallman, M. F. *J Neuroendocrinol*. 2000, 12, 461-470.

[118] Bhatnagar, S.; Bell, M. E.; Liang, J.; Soriano, L.; Nagy, T. R.; Dallman, M. F. *J Neuroendocrinol*. 2000, 12, 453-460.

[119] Laugero, K. D.; Bell, M. E.; Bhatnagar, S.; Soriano, L.; Dallman, M. F. *Endocrinology*. 2001, 142, 2796-2804.

[120] Dallman, M. F.; Akana, S. F.; Laugero, K. D.; Gomez, F.; Manalo, S.; Bell, M. E.; Bhatnagar, S. *Physiol Behav*. 2003, 79, 3-12.

[121] Gibson, E. L. *Physiol Behav*. 2006, 89, 53-61.

[122] O'Connor, D. B.; Jones, F.; Conner, M.; McMillan, B.; Ferguson, E. *Health Psychol*. 2008, 27, S20-31.

[123] Kandiah, J.; Yake, M.; Jones, J.; Meyer, M. *Nutrition Research*. 2006, 26, 118-123.

[124] Zellner, D. A.; Loaiza, S.; Gonzalez, Z.; Pita, J.; Morales, J.; Pecora, D.; Wolf, A. *Physiol Behav*. 2006, 87, 789-793.

[125] Epel, E.; Lapidus, R.; McEwen, B.; Brownell, K. *Psychoneuroendocrinology*. 2001, 26, 37-49.

[126] Gluck, M. E.; Geliebter, A.; Hung, J.; Yahav, E. *Psychosom Med*. 2004, 66, 876-881.

[127] Oliver, G.; Wardle, J.; Gibson, E. L. *Psychosom Med*. 2000, 62, 853-865.

[128] Foster, M. T.; Warne, J. P.; Ginsberg, A. B.; Horneman, H. F.; Pecoraro, N. C.; Akana, S. F.; Dallman, M. F. *Endocrinology*. 2009, 150, 2325-2333.

[129] Rutters, F.; Nieuwenhuizen, A. G.; Lemmens, S. G.; Born, J. M.; Westerterp-Plantenga, M. S. *Obesity*. 2009, 17, 72-77.

[130] Dallman, M. F.; Pecoraro, N. C.; la Fleur, S. E. *Brain Behav Immun.* 2005, 19, 275-280.
[131] Dallman, M. F. *Trends Endocrinol Metab.* 2010, 21, 159-165.
[132] Timofeeva, E.; Richard, D. *J Comp Neurol.* 2001, 441, 71-89.
[133] Timofeeva, E.; Richard, D. *Neuroendocrinology.* 1997, 66, 327-340.
[134] Torres, S. J.; Nowson, C. A. *Nutrition.* 2007, 23, 887-894.
[135] Block, J. P.; He, Y.; Zaslavsky, A. M.; Ding, L.; Ayanian, J. Z. *Am J Epidemiol.* 2009, 170, 181-192.
[136] Serlachius, A.; Hamer, M.; Wardle, J. *Physiol Behav.* 2007, 92, 548-553.
[137] Dallman, M.; Bhatnagar, S. In *Handbook of physiology, sextion 7: the endocrine system*; Oxford University Press: New York, 2001; 179-210.
[138] Rybkin, II; Zhou, Y.; Volaufova, J.; Smagin, G. N.; Ryan, D. H.; Harris, R. B. *Am J Physiol.* 1997, 273, R1612-R1622.
[139] Shibasaki, T.; Yamauchi, N.; Kato, Y.; Masuda, A.; Imaki, T.; Hotta, M.; Demura, H.; Oono, H.; Ling, N.; Shizume, K. *Life Sci.* 1988, 43, 1103-1110.
[140] Hotta, M.; Shibasaki, T.; Arai, K.; Demura, H. *Brain Res.* 1999, 823, 221-225.
[141] Krahn, D. D.; Gosnell, B. A.; Grace, M.; Levine, A. S. *Brain Res Bull.* 1986, 17, 285-289.
[142] Kinzig, K. P.; Hargrave, S. L.; Honors, M. A. *Physiol Behav.* 2008, 95, 108-113.
[143] Timofeeva, E. *Can J Addiction Med.* 2010, 1, 4-11.
[144] Pelleymounter, M. A.; Joppa, M.; Ling, N.; Foster, A. C. *J Pharmacol Exp Ther.* 2002, 302, 145-152.
[145] Smith, G. W.; Aubry, J. M.; Dellu, F.; Contarino, A.; Bilezikjian, L. M.; Gold, L. H.; Chen, R.; Marchuk, Y.; Hauser, C.; Bentley, C. A.; Sawchenko, P. E.; Koob, G. F.; Vale, W.; Lee, K. F. *Neuron.* 1998, 20, 1093-1102.
[146] Smagin, G. N.; Howell, L. A.; Ryan, D. H.; De Souza, E. B.; Harris, R. B. *Neuroreport.* 1998, 9, 1601-1606.
[147] Pelleymounter, M. A.; Joppa, M.; Carmouche, M.; Cullen, M. J.; Brown, B.; Murphy, B.; Grigoriadis, D. E.; Ling, N.; Foster, A. C. *J Pharmacol Exp Ther.* 2000, 293, 799-806.
[148] Bale, T. L.; Anderson, K. R.; Roberts, A. J.; Lee, K. F.; Nagy, T. R.; Vale, W. W. *Endocrinology.* 2003, 144, 2580-2587.
[149] Bale, T. L.; Contarino, A.; Smith, G. W.; Chan, R.; Gold, L. H.; Sawchenko, P. E.; Koob, G. F.; Vale, W. W.; Lee, K. F. *Nat Genet.* 2000, 24, 410-414.

[150] Beatty, W. W.; Schwartzbaum, J. S. *J Comp Physiol Psychol*. 1968, 65, 93-102.
[151] Bakshi, V. P.; Newman, S. M.; Smith-Roe, S.; Jochman, K. A.; Kalin, N. H. *J Neurosci*. 2007, 27, 10568-10577.
[152] Appleton, N. *Lick the Sugar Habit*; Nancy Appleton: Santa Monica, 1996.
[153] DesMaisons, K. *Your Last Diet! The Sugar Addict's Weight-loss Plan*; Random House: Toronto, 2001.
[154] Katherine, A. *Anatomy of a Food Addiction: An Efective Program to Overcome Compulsive Eating*; Gurze Books: Carlsbad, 1996.
[155] Rufus, E. *Sugar addiction: a step-by-step guide to overcoming sugar addiction*; Elizabeth Brown Rufus: Bloomington, 2004.
[156] Hoebel, B. G.; Hernandez, L.; Schwartz, D. H.; Mark, G. P.; Hunter, G. A. In *The psychobiology of Human Eating Disorders: Preclinical and Clinical Perspewctives*; Annals NY Acad Scienc: New York, 1989; 575, 171-193.
[157] Le Magnen, J. In *Taste, experience, and feeding*; American Psychological Association: Washington, 1990; 241-252.
[158] Colantuoni, C.; Rada, P.; McCarthy, J.; Patten, C.; Avena, N. M.; Chadeayne, A.; Hoebel, B. G. *Obes Res*. 2002, 10, 478-488.
[159] Avena, N. M.; Rada, P.; Hoebel, B. G. *Neurosci Biobehav Rev*. 2008, 32, 20-39.
[160] Colantuoni, C.; Schwenker, J.; McCarthy, J.; Rada, P.; Ladenheim, B.; Cadet, J. L.; Schwartz, G. J.; Moran, T. H.; Hoebel, B. G. *Neuroreport*. 2001, 12, 3549-3552.
[161] Rada, P.; Avena, N. M.; Hoebel, B. G. *Neuroscience*. 2005, 134, 737-744.
[162] Di Chiara, G.; Tanda, G. *Psychopharmacology*. 1997, 134, 351-353.
[163] Bassareo, V.; Di Chiara, G. *Eur J Neurosci*. 1999, 11, 4389-4397.
[164] Pothos, E.; Rada, P.; Mark, G. P.; Hoebel, B. G. *Brain Res*. 1991, 566, 348-350.
[165] Wise, R. A.; Newton, P.; Leeb, K.; Burnette, B.; Pocock, D.; Justice, J. B., Jr. *Psychopharmacology*. 1995, 120, 10-20.
[166] Di Chiara, G.; Imperato, A. *Proc Natl Acad Sci U S A*. 1988, 85, 5274-5278.
[167] Wise, R. A.; Rompre, P. P. *Annu Rev Psychol*. 1989, 40, 191-225.
[168] Hoebel, B. G.; Avena, N. M.; Rada, P. *Curr Opin Pharmacol*. 2007, 7, 617-627.

[169] Mark, G. P.; Weinberg, J. B.; Rada, P.; Pothos, E.; Hoebel, B. G. *Appetite*. 1992, 19, 201.
[170] Avena, N. M.; Rada, P.; Moise, N.; Hoebel, B. G. *Neuroscience*. 2006, 139, 813-820.
[171] Spangler, R.; Wittkowski, K. M.; Goddard, N. L.; Avena, N. M.; Hoebel, B. G.; Leibowitz, S. F. *Brain Res Mol Brain Res*. 2004, 124, 134-142.
[172] Avena, N. M.; Long, K. A.; Hoebel, B. G. *Physiol Behav*. 2005, 84, 359-362.
[173] Ferrario, C. R.; Robinson, T. E. *Eur Neuropsychopharmacol*. 2007, 17, 352-357.
[174] Blomqvist, O.; Ericson, M.; Johnson, D. H.; Engel, J. A.; Soderpalm, B. *Eur J Pharmacol*. 1996, 314, 257-267.
[175] Wise, R. A. *J Abnorm Psychol*. 1988, 97, 118-132.
[176] Avena, N. M.; Carrillo, C. A.; Needham, L.; Leibowitz, S. F.; Hoebel, B. G. *Alcohol*. 2004, 34, 203-209.
[177] Avena, N. M.; Hoebel, B. G. *Pharmacol Biochem Behav*. 2003, 74, 635-639.
[178] Avena, N. M.; Hoebel, B. G. *Neuroscience*. 2003, 122, 17-20.
[179] Pothos, E. N.; Creese, I.; Hoebel, B. G. *J Neurosci*. 1995, 15, 6640-6650.
[180] Avena, N. M.; Bocarsly, M. E.; Rada, P.; Kim, A.; Hoebel, B. G. *Physiol Behav*. 2008, 94, 309-315.
[181] Corwin, R. L. *Appetite*. 2006, 46, 11-15.
[182] Corwin, R. L. *Appetite*. 2004, 42, 139-142.
[183] Corwin, R. L.; Wojnicki, F. H. *Curr Protoc Neurosci*. 2006, 9, 23B.
[184] Corwin, R. L.; Wojnicki, F. H.; Fisher, J. O.; Dimitriou, S. G.; Rice, H. B.; Young, M. A. *Physiol Behav*. 1998, 65, 545-553.
[185] Corwin, R. L.; Avena, N. M.; Boggiano, M. M. *Physiol Behav*. 2011, 104, 87-97.
[186] Hagan, M. M.; Wauford, P. K.; Chandler, P. C.; Jarrett, L. A.; Rybak, R. J.; Blackburn, K. *Physiol Behav*. 2002, 77, 45-54.
[187] Hagan, M. M.; Chandler, P. C.; Wauford, P. K.; Rybak, R. J.; Oswald, K. D. *Int J Eat Disord*. 2003, 34, 183-197.
[188] Hagan, M. M.; Moss, D. E. *Int J Eat Disord*. 1997, 22, 411-420.

In: Sucrose
Editor: Salvatore Magazù
ISBN: 978-1-62417-984-6

Chapter 6

EFFECT OF THE ADDITION OF SUCROSE IN RHEOLOGICAL PROPERTIES

Priscila Anadão*
University of São Paulo –School of Engineering, Metallurgical and Material Science Department, Avenida Professor Mello Moraes, São Paulo- SP, Brazil

ABSTRACT

Sucrose is an important macronutrient that provides humans with a source of energy. Sucrose most important advantages include low cost and easy availability. Aiming to modify the rheological properties of a system, sucrose addition has been investigated and has shown to be successful in several areas. In the food area, sucrose is very important, as it can be used as an ingredient or a preserving agent and its effect in rheological properties is investigated in order to obtain, for example, information about differences in food texture. Sucrose has also been employed as an emulsifier in oil-water emulsions that reduces the interfacial tension, denoted by viscosity changes. The ceramic area has also used sucrose to adjust the forces between the particles that compose the dispersions since sucrose provides steric hindrance, hydration repulsion or electrosteric stabilization. Ergo, the objective of this chapter is to present literature examples regarding sucrose addition and its effect on the rheological properties of the mentioned areas.

* E-mail: priscila.anadao@gmail.com.

INTRODUCTION

Sucrose, generally known as table sugar and sometimes called saccharose, is an organic compound characterized by its white color, being odorless and a crystalline powder with a sweet taste. This important macronutrient which provides humans with a source of energy occurs naturally in every fruit and vegetable. This carbohydrate is the major product of photosynthesis which is the process that occurs in plants when the sun energy is transformed into food. Its occurrence exists in high amounts in sugar cane (20% by weight) and sugar beets (15% by weight) from which it is obtained for commercial purposes in quantities of 150,000,000 tons annually.

Sucrose (Figure 1) is a disaccharide made from the combinations of the two monosaccharides in 1:1 proportion, α-D-glucose (1 equiv) and β-D-fructose (1 equiv). Its molecular formula is $C_{12}H_{22}O_{11}$.

In this disaccharide, the linkage between glucose and fructose is performed via an ether bond between the C1 of the glucosyl subunit and the C2 of the fructosyl unit. This bond is called a glycosidic bond and is sometimes mentioned as an α- β-1-2 bond, since the linkage is between an α-OH from the glucose bonding and an β-OH from the fructose, which means that the glycosidic bond is formed between the reducing ends of both glucose and fructose which inhibits the possibility of further bonds to other saccharide units. As hydrogen atoms are removed from the OH groups in the dehydration reaction, which causes ring closure, sucrose does not contain anomeric hydroxyl groups and neither of the rings is able to open; therefore, sucrose is considered a nonreducing sugar [1-3].

The use of sucrose in order to modify the viscosity of a system has been widely explored and has shown to be a powerful tool in a wide range of areas. In the food area, this sugar plays an important role as an ingredient or preserving agent in many formulations and technological processes and the knowledge of rheological properties is important for food processing operations since the flow characteristics of a food product are dependent on the fluid viscosity and density.

The properties of sucrose molecules include their equatorial hydroxyl groups which inhibit the chain organization. This behavior is important when sucrose is added to several types of starches and other macromolecules and, as a reflection of this influence, viscosity is altered.

In the literature, it is also possible to observe the use of sucrose as an emulsifier in oil-water emulsions that reduces the interfacial tension, denoted by viscosity changes.

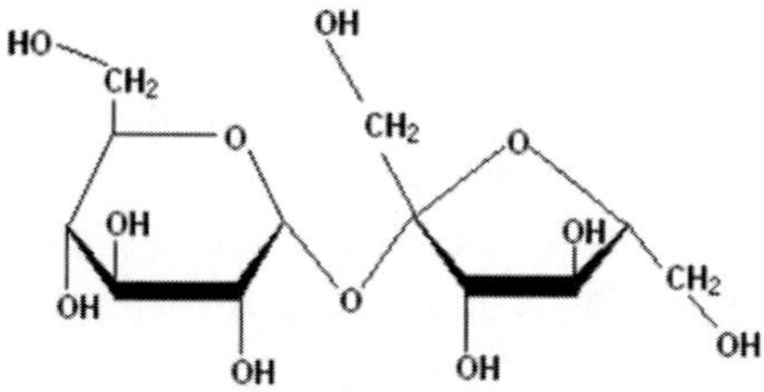

Figure 1. Schematic representation of the sucrose molecule.

The addition of sucrose is also performed in ceramic slurries and pastes aiming to adjust the forces between the particles since sucrose provides steric hindrance, hydration repulsion or electrosteric stabilization, and it presents low cost and easy availability to be largely used in ceramic field.

Therefore, this chapter presents examples of the effect of sucrose in the viscosity of the systems of the mentioned areas, besides the author's results concerning this effect.

USE OF SUCROSE IN THE FOOD AREA

As commented before, the benefit of adding sucrose to food solutions is the possibility to modulate the flow characteristics of a food product. Sucrose solutions in several concentrations and temperatures can be found in a number of food transformation processes and are used for formulating a large number of products and food ingredients, in areas such as candies formulation or the pastry industry [4]. Moreover, by mixing different simple and complex sugars, the optimal mixture mainly in terms of freezing point and sweetness capability can be obtained [5].

As an example of this importance, an investigation into the effect of sucrose on the viscosity in aqueous solutions of carboxymethylcellulose (CMC), which is a hydrocolloid largely applied in foodstuff formulation, product development and processing, was performed at different temperatures. By using the power-low model, it was found that the flow behavior index decreased polynomially with the sucrose concentration and increased linearly with the temperature and the consistency coefficient increased linearly with concentration and decreased linearly with the increase in temperature. It was concluded that the CMC viscosity was increased with the sucrose concentration and was decreased by the increase of temperature [6].

The effect of molecular weight and concentration of ethylcellulose combined with lecithin in the fluidization of sucrose–fat suspension was investigated to be applied in chocolate manufacturing, aiming to maintain or enhance the flowability of molten chocolate. Only ethylcellulose was not sufficiently functional to fluidify the sucrose suspension. A combination with a low content of lecithin ethylcellulose (0.05 wt.%) had an overwhelming effect on the fluidization and dispersibility properties of sucrose particles, improving the preparation of fat-based food confections with reduced-fat content. The conformation and adsorption phenomenon of ethylcellulose molecules at the sucrose-vegetable oil interface, especially in the presence of lecithin, was complex and not yet understood [7].

The use of sucrose in rheology was also studied in cross-linked waxy maize starch dispersions since starch dispersion viscosities are dependent on the type of starch, on the sucrose concentration and on the heating temperature. The sucrose content was not responsible for significant changes in the granule size distribution and an increase in temperature promoted antithixotropic behavior in the dispersions, that is, the apparent viscosities of the dispersion increased over time due to shearing. It was also observed that by increasing temperature, changes in granule morphology were detected and these changes increased the binding energy of the network of the water–sucrose–starch granule microstructures [8].

The effect of sucrose was also investigated in rheological properties of rice starch pastes studied by steady and dynamic shear. The addition of sucrose promoted a decrease in consistency index, apparent viscosity and yield stress. Storage and loss moduli decreased with the increase in sucrose concentration [9]. Sucrose and fructose were also added to heated amioca starch dispersions and the rheological behavior was studied by small and large deformations. All rheological parameters - elastic and viscous moduli, apparent viscosity, thixotropy, yield stress and shear modulus, except for the dynamic yield stress, increased by adding these sugars, maybe because fructose and sucrose increased the strength of the internal bonds or cohesiveness of the dispersions [10].

Studies were also performed to investigate the effect of sucrose on the rheological properties of wheat starch–milk pastes. According to the H-B model, the yield stress has shown to increase with sucrose concentration (ex.: an increase by 200% with 16 wt.% sucrose in comparison with sugar free paste). The effect on the consistency coefficient was less pronounced than on the yield stress. The flow behavior index increased at high sucrose concentrations, that is, the pastes became less shear thinning [11].

A comparison between different sugars (fructose, glucose, maltose and sucrose) in rheological properties of aqueous sago starch was made. Although sugars increased gelatinization enthalpy, the effect with sucrose was the least pronounced [12]. Sugar addition was also investigated in the gelation of oxidized starch. The loss modulus was observed to be higher than the storage modulus by adding sucrose, which meant the intermolecular interactions at that stage were largely topological. The use of glucose and fructose decreased the rate of conformational ordering during cooling [13]. The effect of these sugars was also studied in corn and potato starch rheological properties and starches were more readily gelatinized in sucrose solutions [14].

Chang, Lim and Yoo investigated the effect of different sugars (sucrose, glucose and xylose) on the dynamic rheological properties of corn starch pastes. A decrease in storage modulus and in the pseudoplateau values were observed with the increase of sugar concentration [15].

A study regarding the influence of sucrose on the gelatinization of acorn starch was carried out. Sucrose was found to retard the retrodegradation of this starch and the regelatinization enthalpy of this starch was dependent on the sucrose concentration, more than on storage days, maybe due to the higher importance of the interaction between sucrose and amylopectin than between sucrose and amylase [16].

Another food dispersion to which sucrose was added was the low-methoxyl pectin gels. Pectins, which are complex mixtures of polysaccharides present in the cell walls of fruits and vegetables, are generally used as gelling agents, stabilizers, thickeners and emulsifiers in many food products. In this study, a non-isothermal kinetic model described dynamic moduli values during gelation induced by the cooling dispersion of low-methoxyl pectin gels with two different sucrose contents (10 and 30 wt.%). The increase of both pectin and sucrose contents increased storage modulus during aging process. The number average molecular weight of chains between cross-links was higher in the dispersion without sucrose which showed that the hydroxyl groups of the sucrose played an important role in the gel formation by stabilizing the structure of junction zones [17].

Dispersions of pectin from pomelo fruit peels with sucrose and calcium ions were also studied. An increase of sucrose concentration as well as of the other components resulted in an increase of both storage and loss moduli, although the loss modulus was always greater than the storage modulus. The formation of a gel network was a slow process [18].

In the protein area, the effect of sucrose addition to the final properties has been already described. Baier and Mc Clements studied the influence of sucrose on the heat-induced gelation of bovine serum albumin (BSA) since the knowledge of the interactions between protein and additive can allow food scientists to design protein gels. Sucrose had an important role in altering the thermal stability of globular proteins, by increasing the gelation temperature, by increasing the attraction through a preferential interaction mechanism and by modifying the result into a higher viscosity. As a final result, by adding sucrose, the final gel strength and appearance of the gels were changed [19].

The influence of sucrose, besides glycerol and different salts, on rheological properties of unfrozen and frozen egg yolk at -24°C was also studied. All additives prevented egg yolk gelation at concentrations higher than 2 wt.%; therefore, they can be considered good cryoprotectant [20].

A study of the influence of sucrose on cold gelation of heat-denatured whey protein isolate was also performed aiming to preview final properties when applied to dessert products. Sucrose molecules were found to reduce the gelation rate because viscosity was increased by their addition at low concentrations. At higher concentrations, it facilitated gelation because they promoted protein-protein interactions [21, 22].

The thermal denaturation and functionality of whey protein isolate was also investigated in terms of adding sucrose. Sugar increased the gelation temperature at which maximum flocculation was observed and augmented the extent of droplet flocculation [23].

SUCROSE AS AN EMULSIFIER IN OIL-WATER EMULSIONS

Sugar-based emulsifiers, also frequently called alkyl glycosides, have received attention as they present good surface activity and functional properties. This type of emulsifier is produced through the functionalization of the sugar head group and the advantages of using it are related to its biodegradability, biocompatibility and non-toxic nature. Another important advantage is that it is much less sensitive to temperature variation as compared to other typical types of commercially available emulsifiers. The areas that usually use emulsifiers and are favored by sugar-based emulsifiers are cosmetic and pharmaceutical industry.

Niraula, King and Misran investigated the rheology properties of the sucrose dodecanoate stabilized paraffin oil-water emulsions and compared to those of similar oil-water emulsions stabilized with non-ionic surfactant Brij 35p and ionic surfactant sodium dodecyl sulfate. Sucrose-based emulsifier produced significantly smaller-sized droplets in comparison to the others emulsifiers, suggesting that the droplet size distribution is highly affected by the surfactant type. Moreover, this type of emulsifier presented a greater degree of shear thinning and higher yield stress. Sugar-emulsifier also exhibited higher values of storage and loss moduli which implied possessing better viscoelastic properties and therefore, in performing better as an emulsifying agent as compared to the Brij 35p and SDS stabilized emulsions [24].

The rheology of sucrose palmitate stabilized oil/ water emulsions was investigated and peculiar responses related to the steady state flow curves were observed with two different regions - below a shear rate of 10^{-5} s^{-1}, a Newtonian type behavior and above this value, an exponentially decaying shear-thinning behavior [25].

The influence of sucrose on the flocculation stability of n-hexadecane oil-in-water emulsions stabilized by β-lactoglobulin, a globular protein, was investigated before and after isothermal heat treatment. Sucrose addition promoted an increase of the thermal denaturation temperature and droplet flocculation was formed when sucrose was added before the heat treatment and an opposite effect was observed when sucrose was added after the heat treatment [26]. Sucrose palmitate was used in oil-in-water emulsions composed of sunflower oil and the influence of this composition and the temperature on the linear viscoelasticity properties. Higher sucrose palmitate concentration yielded higher values of the linear viscoelasticity functions and a broader plateau region in the relaxation time spectrum, probably due to an improvement in the elastic network. An increase of sucrose palmitate concentration also produced a transition from an isotropic micellar solution to a dispersion of lamellar liquid-crystalline portions in the micellar matrix, increasing the initial continuous-phase viscosity. Hence, a specific interfacial area, smaller than expected, was produced [27].

A rheology study of sunflower oil-water emulsions was carried out by varying sucrose concentration and temperature. Emulsion properties were improved by sucrose addition and presented a pseudoplastic behavior. The consistency index was influenced by sugar concentration, as well as the activation energy values, which varied from 31077 to 10716 kJ/ kg mol [28].

Oil-in-water emulsions stabilized by sucrose palmitate were studied according to sucrose ester concentration. Both sucrose ester and oil concentrations were found to increase emulsion viscosity due to the production of a more structured system with a lower droplet size and polydispersity. Moreover, although a strong structural breakdown occurred due to steady shear, master flow curves could be obtained by superposition methods [29].

SUCROSE ADDITION IN CERAMIC SLURRIES

Organic additives are widely employed in ceramic colloidal processing in order to adjust the forces between the particles and therefore, to control viscosity. By adding sucrose or other type of carbohydrate, the properties of slurries and pastes are usually defined by steric hindrance provided by the sugar molecules adsorbed on the oxide particle surface. As sucrose is low-cost and easily available, it is largely used in order to modify the system viscosity.

One example of this addition was to alumina slurries, dispersed with a polyacrylate dispersant, Darvan 821 A. This addition was observed to correspond to a decrease in apparent yield stress, viscosity, thixotropy and to an increase in non-Newtonian index in comparison with the dispersion with polyacrylate. The association of sucrose molecules with the polyacrylate molecules, which were adsorbed on alumina particle surfaces, was established through intermolecular hydrogen bond between free hydroxyl groups of sucrose and carboxylate ions of polyacrylate molecules. This hindrance led to a weakening of the interparticle network and to a decrease in viscosity. An increase in loss tangent and a decrease in thixotropy were also attributed to this weakening [30].

The effect of different sugars in the rheology of aqueous suspensions of ultrafine (40 nm diameter) g-alumina powder, including sucrose, was investigated by Schilling et al. In relation to sucrose, the rheological behavior was improved maybe due to involvement of the fructosyl moiety in sorption to the surfaces of alumina nanoparticles. This fructosyl moiety is bound to the glucosyl moiety by the glycosidic bond (axially oriented with respect to the fructofuranose ring) and this conformation could be changed and sorption to alumina facilitated [31].

The rheology properties of aqueous zirconia with ammonium polyacrylate ($PANH_4$) and sucrose were evaluated by Wang and Guo. In relation to the order of addition of both additives in the aqueous zirconia, the system was found to be sensitive to this order. By adding sucrose in the second step, sucrose interacts through free hydroxyl groups of itself and of the carboxylate ions of adsorbed $PANH_4$ molecules. When sucrose was added in the first step, sucrose occupied the active sites of zirconia and the adsorption of the $PANH_4$ was blocked, only few groups of this polymer could establish a bond to the zirconia and the stability of the system originated from the mutual repulsion of carboxylate groups between electrosteric adlayers; therefore, a more fluid system was produced. The sucrose addition also promoted a reduction in the yield stress besides improving flowability [32].

Sucrose addition was also performed in aqueous suspensions containing cetyl trimethyl ammonium bromide in order to investigate its influence on ceramic foam production. The system viscosity was decreased, stabilizing the foams by reducing the suspensions drainage. A minimization of the coalescence of the bubbles was another advantage obtained by adding sucrose which led to lower cell sizes in the sintered foams. Furthermore, ceramic foams were strengthened due to the capability of sucrose to hold the water molecules through hydrogen bonding. It was possible to conclude that sucrose allows the fabrication of ultra light ceramics that can be easily handled and also machined [33].

Different types of sugar were added to dense alumina slurries and the rheological properties were studied. The main aim of this investigation was to decrease drying shrinkage and to increase solid volume content without harming plasticity.

Rheology properties were determined by creep rheology testing methods, which are non-destructive methods to determine the viscous and elastic components of a viscoelastic substance. Slurries with sucrose showed much more deformation at a constant pressure in comparison to the other slurries. A higher rate loss modulus/ storage modulus was observed for the slurries with sucrose and this means that these slurries were more viscous than elastic in comparison to the other slurries. The described behaviors were due to the stronger charges that sucrose possesses which can prevent particle agglomeration by providing steric hindrance effect [34].

Anadão et al. prepared carbon/ sodium montmorillonite clay nano-composites from dispersions that contained sodium montmorillonite, sucrose and water, through direct carbonization of sucrose intercalated between montmorillonite platelets under mild conditions at a low reaction temperature to be applied in catalytic applications. Since clay-mineral based catalysts have shown to present good catalytic activity in several types of applications, such as oil refineries, the petrochemical industry and organic synthesis and as sucrose is known to be adsorbed in the interlamelar regions of the clay mineral, with the exclusion of water, because it forms a well defined chemical group when complexed with montmorillonite and also for being cheap and easily available in nature; sodium montmorillonite clay and sucrose were chosen to produce the carbon-clay nanocomposites.

As each dispersion had to be extruded, before undergoing at direct carbonization, the viscosity of each dispersion should be investigated, including the modifications related to the sucrose addition in clay/ water dispersions.

Two different types of dispersion were studied. The first group was related to the use of different clay contents and a half part of sucrose and in the second one, sucrose content varied while clay content remained the same for all dispersions. In the first group, dispersions composed of 2.0 (sample 1), 3.0 (sample 2) and 4.0 (sample 3) mass% montmorillonite in water were prepared under mechanical stirring for 10 minutes. A resting time of 24 hours was respected and dispersions were again stirred for 5 minutes. Hence, viscosities were measured at different rotational speeds.

Sucrose was added to the dispersion at half the proportion of the clay mass in the dispersion (ex.: 1.0 mass% sucrose was added in the dispersion with 2.0 mass% MMT). Again, the dispersion was stirred for 10 minutes and rested for a minimum of 2 hours. After that, dispersions were stirred for 5 minutes and again, viscosity was determined.

The other group was composed of dispersions with 4.0 mass% clay/ water that were prepared as above. Then, 0.4 (sample 4), 1.0 (sample 5) and 10.0 (sample 6) mass% sucrose were added, the proportion of which corresponded to the extremes between partial and total coverage of the matrix (clay) by the carbonous material (substrate) resulting from the burning of the intercalated sucrose, and the same procedure was performed. Again, viscosities were measured before and after sucrose addition. Rheological measurements were conducted with a Brookfield Model DV-II viscometer.

At higher rotational speeds, the viscosities of the dispersions with varying MMT content were observed to decrease. All dispersions could be considered non-Newtonian-fluids and the sucrose addition did not change the type of fluid. One possibility for decreasing viscosity is that agglomerates of stacked clay mineral platelets, filled by sucrose molecules, were formed and these agglomerates were aligned in the shear direction, resulting in lower values of viscosity. Sucrose addition increased the viscosity values, which meant that sucrose was adsorbed and bigger structures were formed, probably by a hydrogen bond between the hydroxyl groups of the sucrose and the oxygen atoms, linked to the silicon atom in the clay mineral layer. However, the extension of this increase was not considerably great, which allowed easy handling of these dispersions [35].

CONCLUSION

As already mentioned, sucrose is a good additive to be used in several types of solutions and dispersion provided it presents low cost and easy availability. Moreover, it does not pose human risks, which allows it to be applied in a large range of applications, including the food and cosmetic area. Therefore, it can be successfully used to modify the rheology properties of these solutions and dispersions.

It was observed from the scientific papers that the largest number of investigations about the influence of sucrose addition in rheological properties comes from food applications. However, great attention could also be observed in the ceramic area and promising results were obtained.

Finally, as sucrose presents the advantages pointed out above and a particular structure that can establish several types of bonds with different types of materials, it would be interesting that, in the future, sucrose addition, in order to modify rheology properties, is explored in a larger number of areas as a replacement for other toxic materials.

References

[1] Nelson, D. L.; Cox, M. M. *Lehninger Princípios de Bioquímica*; Sarvier: São Paulo, SP, 2002; pp 225-232.

[2] Voet, D.; Voet, J. G.; Pratt, C. W. *Fundamentos de Bioquímica*; Artmed: Porto Alegre, RS, 2000; pp 273-275.

[3] Berg J. M.; Tymoczko, J. L.; Stryer, L. *Biochemistry*; Sarvier: São Paulo, SP, 2002; pp 462-465.

[4] Quintas, M. A. C.; Fundo, J. F.; Silva, C. L. M. *Food. Eng. Rev.* 2010, *2*, 204-215.

[5] Migliori, M.; Gabriele, D.; Di Sanzo, R.; De Cindio, B.; Correra, S. *J. Chem. Eng. Data* 2007, *52*, 1347-1353.

[6] Cancela, M. A.; Álvarez, E.; Maceiras, R. *J. Food Eng.*2005,*71*,419-424.

[7] Do, T. –A. L.; Mitchell, J. R.; Wolf, B.; Vieira, *J. React. Funct. Polym.* 2010, *70*, 856-862.

[8] Acquarone, V. M.; Rao, M. A. *Carbohyd. Polym.* 2003, *51*, 451-458.

[9] Yoo, D.; Yoo, B. *Starch* 2005, *57*, 254-261.

[10] Genovese, D. B.; Acquarone, V. M.; Youn, K. –S.; Rao, M. A. *Food Sci. Tech. Int.* 2004, *10*, 51-57.

[11] Abu-Jdayil, B.; Mohameed, H. A.; Eassa, A. *J. Food Eng.* 2004, *64*, 207-212.

[12] Ahmad, F. B.; Williams, P. A. *Biopolymers* 1999, *50*, 401-412.

[13] Evageliou, V.; Richardson, R. K.; Morris, E. R. *Carbohyd. Polym.* 2000, *42*, 261-272.

[14] Sikora, M.; Mazurkiewicz, J.; Tomasik, P.; Pielichowski, K. *Int. J. Food Sci. Tech.* 1999, *34*, 371-383.
[15] Chang, Y. H.; Lim, S. T.; Yoo, B. *J. Food Eng.* 2004, *64*, 521-527.
[16] Aee, L. H.; Hyang, K. N. H.; Nishimari, K. *Thermochim. Acta* 1998, *322*, 39-46.
[17] Fu, J. –T.; Rao, M. A. *Food Hydrocolloid.* 2001, *15*, 93-100.
[18] Norziah, M. H.; Kong, S. S.; Karim, A. A.; Seow, C. C. *Food Hydrocolloid.* 2001, *15*, 491-498.
[19] Baierand, S. K.; Mc Clements, D. J. *J. Agric. Food Chem.* 2003, *51*, 8107-8112.
[20] Telis, V. R. N.; Kieckbusch, T. G. *J. Food Sci.* 1998, *63*, 20-24.
[21] Kulmyrzaev, A.; Cancelliere, C.; Mc Clements, D. J. *J. Sci. Food Agric.* 2000, *80*, 1341-1318.
[22] Mc Clements, J.; Bryant, C. M. *Food Res. Int.* 2000, *33*, 649-653.
[23] Kulmyrzaev, A.; Bryant, C. M.; Mc Clements, D. J. *J. Agric. Food Chem.* 2000, *48*, 1593-1597.
[24] Niraula, B.; King, T. C.; Misran, M. *Colloid. Surface A* 2004, *251*, 59-74.
[25] Bower, C.; Gallegos, M. R.; Mackley, J. M. *Rheol. Acta* 1999, *38*, 145-149.
[26] Kim, H. –J.; Decker, E. A.; Mc Clements, D. J. *J. Agric. Food Chem.* 2003, *51*, 766-772.
[27] Guerrero, A.; Partal, P.; Gallegos, C. *J. Rheol.* 1998, *42*, 1375-1388.
[28] Maskan, M.; Göğüş, F. *J. Food Eng.* 2000, *43*, 173-177.
[29] Partal, P.; Guerrero, AZ.; Berjanos, M.; Gallegos, C. *JAOCS* 1997, *74*, 1203-1212.
[30] Pradhan, M.; Bhargava, P. *J. Am. Ceram. Soc.* 2005, *88*, 833-838.
[31] Schilling, C. H.; Sikora, M.; Tomasik, P.; Li, C.; Garcia, V. *J. Eur. Ceram. Soc.* 2002, *22*, 917-921.
[32] Wang, X.; Guo, L. *Powder Technol.* 2008, *186*, 107-112.
[33] Pradhan, M.; Bhargava, P. *J. Am. Ceram. Soc.* 2005, *88*, 216-218.
[34] Kim, J. C.; Sdchilling, C. H.; Tomasik, P.; Auh, K. H. *Mater. Lett.* 2000, *42*, 221-224.
[35] Anadão, P.; Hildebrando, E. A.; Pajolli, I. L. R.; Pereira, K. R. O.; Wiebeck, H.; Diaz, F. R. V. *Appl. Clay Sci.* 2011, *53*, 288-296.

Reviewed by Prof. Dr. Genaro Z. Clericuzi, Professor at Federal University of Paraíba.

In: Sucrose
Editor: Salvatore Magazù

ISBN: 978-1-62417-984-6

Chapter 7

REACTIONS OF SUCROSE IN THE PRESENCE OF SOLID CATALYSTS

D. S. Pito and J. E. Castanheiro*
Centro de Química de Évora, Departamento de Química,
Universidade de Évora, Évora, Portugal

ABSTRACT

Carbohydrates are the most abundant organic compounds on the world. Consequently, sucrose is a molecule abundant and inexpensive. The products of sucrose hydrolysis are glucose and fructose, which are used in the food industry. The sucrose derivatives, such as esters and ethers, have interesting properties due to the presence of lipophilic and hydrophilic moieties, provided by sucrose and alkyl chain. Traditionally, these reactions are carried out over homogenous catalysts, which are widely used in chemical processes to synthesize fine and bulk chemicals. However, they have serious drawbacks of hazards in handling, difficult separation and production of toxic waste. Solid catalysts can replace the homogeneous ones for simpler and environmentally more benign processes. Heterogeneous catalysts have been used in hydrolysis, esterification and etherification reactions of sucrose. In this work, the use of different solid catalysts for the conversion of sucrose (by hydrolysis, esterification and etherification) will be reviewed.

* Corresponding author. Tel.+351 266745311; Fax.: +351 266744971; E-mail address: jefc@uevora.pt.

1. Introduction

Biomass is an abundant renewable resource and it can be transformed in fuel, chemical products and others materials [1-6]. The utilization of biomass could also lead to a cleaner and safer environment via reduction of greenhouse gases (CO_2, N_2O) and other toxic gases (NOx, SO_2) which are produced by the use of fossil fuels [7].

Carbohydrates, which constitute the higher portion of biomass, are the most abundant organic compounds on earth. The utilization of sugars for the production of chemical and intermediates are importance for relieving the reliance of the chemical industry on pollutants petrochemical. In the future, it will be expected that the access to fossil raw material becomes more expensive and difficult. In contrast, different types of molecules can be synthesized from biomass become the process cheaper and environmental friendly [8-10].

Sucrose is a dimmer composed of two sugar monomers, d-fructose and a-d-glucose, and it is non-reducing. Sucrose constitutes a significant part of the human diet and therefore, it is widely used in the food industry (ice cream, baked goods, desserts, confections, intermediate-moisture foods, and soft drinks) [11]. Sucrose can be functionalized and converted into different additives. However, the chemical transformation of sucrose is limited because of the poor selectivity of the reactions and the low choice of solvents, both of which result in high purification costs. Other uses in the non-food industry, such as the use of sucrose as a starting material for the formation of high added value furanic derivatives (5-hydroxymethylfurfural) are also appealing [12].

Traditionally, homogeneous catalysts are used in the chemical processes, but they have serious drawbacks of hazards in handling, corrosiveness, difficult separation, and production of toxic waste. Solid catalyst can replace the homogeneous ones for simpler and environmentally more benign processes [1]. The hydrolysis of sucrose has been carried out over different heterogeneous catalysts. However, only few works have applied heterogeneous catalysts in esterification and etherification of sucrose.

This present review focuses on solid catalysts as potential heterogeneous catalysts for reactions of sucrose, replacing homogenous ones. The first topic is related with the hydrolysis of sucrose. The second topic relates to the esterification of sucrose and the third topic deals with the conversion of sucrose by etherification over solid catalysts.

2. Hydrolysis of Sucrose

The hydrolysis of sucrose produces inverted sugars, i.e., glucose and fructose (Figure 1). Enzymes are the main industrial catalysts used for the hydrolysis of sucrose, but they present different drawbacks, such as the production of waste, low thermal stability, and problems with separation and recovery of the enzyme from the product. In order to improve the process, supported enzymes have been carried out [13]. However, long reaction time is required.

Different solid acids have been used as catalysts in hydrolysis of sucrose.

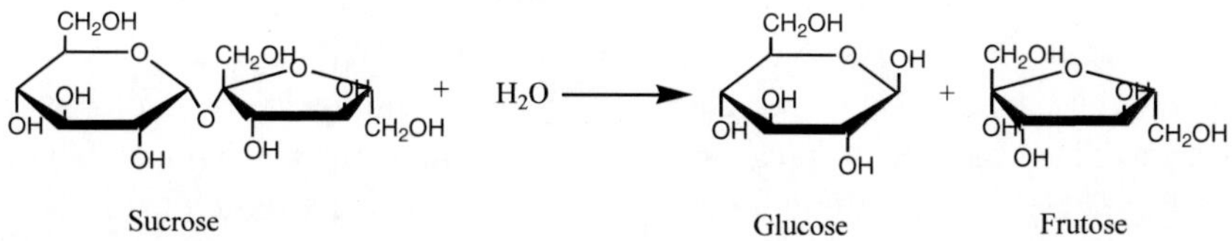

Figure 1. Schematic representation of the hydrolysis of sucrose to glucose and fructose.

Catalysts with Sulfonic Acid Groups

Hydrolysis of sucrose has been carried out over strong acidic cation-exchange resins with sulfonic groups, at relatively low temperatures. However, it is generally produced high levels of impurities and 5-hydroxymethylfurfural (HMF) [14, 15]. Strongly acidic cation exchangers were also used for the hydrolysis of sucrose at 298-343 K. It was observed that the selectivity to fructose and glucose is 48.5%, at 97% of sucrose conversion [16].

Kim et al. [17] studied the hydrolysis of sucrose over sulfonated polystyrene latex as catalyst. It was observed that this catalyst is more effective than H_2SO_4 or Dowex 50.

The hydrolysis of sucrose was carried out fixed bed reactor with acid form ion exchange resin, as catalyst. Reaction temperature was varied from 50 to 75 ^{o}C. The reaction was first-order over this range. The data indicated that the observed rate of reaction is strongly influenced by diffusion within the resin particles and that external (film) mass transfer is not significant for the range of conditions explored [18].

Mizota et al. [19] studied the hydrolysis of sucrose over sulfonic acid ($S0_3H$) group attached to polyethylene microporous hollow fiber by radiation-induced graft polymerization of sodium p-styrenesulfonate. The catalytic activity of this material was compared with the $S0_3H$ group introduced into the polystyrene chain cross-linked with divinylbenzene. The authors observed that the graft-type acid catalyst had about 10 times the hydrolytic activity for sucrose as the cross-linked acid catalyst. This behavior was explained due to a larger reactant (sucrose) have more difficult access to the $S0_3H$ group of the cross-linked catalyst. On the other hand, the catalyst attached to the grafted polymer chain provides access to sucrose due to its flexible polymer structure.

Nasef et al. [20] have reported the hydrolysis of sucrose to glucose and fructose by poly(tetrafluoroethylene-co-perfluorovinyl ether)-graft-polystyrene sulfonic acid (PFA-g-PSSA) membranes. These catalytic materials were prepared by radiation-induced grafting of styrene followed by sulfonation reaction. The reaction was carried out in a batch reactor, with different membranes and in a temperature range of 40–70 ºC. The catalytic activity of the membranes increased with the reaction temperature. The increase in the degree of grafting i.e. concentration of fixed sulfonic groups was found to enhance the catalytic activity of these membranes. The catalytic activity of the sulfonic acid membranes is found to be higher than that of commercial catalytic crosslinked ion exchange resins.

Pito et al. [21] studied the hydrolysis of sucrose over heterogeneous catalysts with sulfonic groups, at 80ºC. The catalyst consisted in poly(vinyl alcohol) (PVA) with sulfonic acid groups. A series of PVA with different crosslinking degree were prepared. It was observed that the catalytic activity of PVA matrix increases with the crosslinking degree, due to the increases of the amount of sulfonic acid groups on PVA. In order to optimise the conditions, the influence of various reaction parameters, such as, initial concentration of sucrose, catalyst loading, temperature and catalytic stability, of the most efficient catalyst, PVA_40, were carried out. It was found that at $80^{\circ}C$, with 0.511 g of catalyst loading and with an initial concentration of sucrose of 0.6 $mol.dm^{-3}$, a sucrose conversion of about 90%, after 3 hours, could be obtained. PVA_40 catalyst was recycled and reused with negligible loss in the activity. A simple kinetic model was developed assuming that the sucrose hydrolysis is an irreversible reaction and the first order with respect to the sucrose concentration. It was observed that the kinetic model fits experimental concentration data quite well.

The hydrolysis of sucrose to glucose and fructose was studied over radiation-induced graft-copolymers with sulfonic groups by Abd El-Rehim et al. [22]. In order to prepare this catalyst, acrylic acid monomer (AA) was copolymerized with sulfonated starch (SS), at different compositions, using ionizing radiation. The kinetics of the reaction was determined for various (SS/AA) graft copolymers compositions and at a temperature range of 40–60 C. The catalytic activity of the copolymers was found to be dependent on the reaction temperature and (SS/AA) graft copolymers compositions. Hydrolysis of sucrose catalyzed by SS-g-AA copolymers showed that the catalytic activity increases with the reaction temperature, because of higher reaction rate constants. Also, the increase in the SS content (amount of sulfonic groups) led to enhance the catalytic activity of copolymers.

A. El-Mohdy et al. [23] have also studied the hydrolysis of sucrose over kappa carrageenan/acrylic acid graft-copolymers (kC-g-AAc) with sulfonic acid groups. The graft-copolymers (kC-g-AAc) were prepared by using γ-radiation. This materials was acidified to convert the sulfate group ($-OSO_3-$) in kappa carrageenan into sulfuric group ($-OSO_3H$). The catalytic activity of the copolymers was found to be dependent on the reaction temperature and kC/AAc compositions, it increased with high reaction temperature and enhanced kC content in the feed solution.

Dhepe et al. [24] studied the hydrolysis of sucrose over mesoporous silicas with sulfonic acid groups. These acid groups were introduced on silica by one-pot or by grafting method. The sulfonated mesoporous silica showed higher conversion and turnover frequency than conventional Amberlyst-15, Nafion-silica and HZSM-5 catalysts. The mesoporous catalysts are recyclable and the reproducible activity is achieved.

Zeolites

Zeolites are aluminosilicates with a microporous network of channels and cavities. These materials can be synthesized with different crystal structure, framework Si/A1 ratio and proton exchange level, which allow design of catalytic properties such as pore size, hydrophobicity, strength of acid sites, and their distribution. Zeolites can be used as catalysts in oil refining, petrochemistry and in production of fine chemicals [25, 26].

Buttersack et al. [27] studied the hydrolysis of sucrose over dealuminated Y zeolites. It was observed that the sucrose molecule adopts a conformation that allows its diffusion into the pores of Y zeolite due to hydro-phobic

/hydrophilic balance and adsorption over the zeolite surface. It was also observed a 90% of sucrose conversion into inverted sugars, with a selectivity close to 90%, in the presence of dealuminated Y zeolite (Si/Al =110), at 343 K.

Hydrolysis of sucrose was also carried out over H-form dealuminated zeolites (H-BEA, H-MFI, H-MOR, H-Y-FAU) by Moreau et al. [28]. For all catalysts, hydrolysis takes place with a high selectivity, regardless of the level of conversion. The catalysts acted as specific adsorbents of colored by-products formed during the course of the reaction, 5-hydroxymethylfurfural (HMF) in particular. The amount of this by-product was reduced to less than 100 ppm. The H-Y FAU (Si/Al=15) catalyst was found to have the better balance between activity, selectivity and by-product amount.

Moreau et al. [29] studied the hydrolysis of sucrose over a commercial dealuminated H-Y zeolite (Si/Al =15). Higher reaction temperatures can be used with the former catalysts, and improvement of both activity and selectivity was obtained from their adsorbent and shape selective properties. It was reported that the low amount of by-products may result from the better adsorbent capacity of faujasites compared to resins. The formation of by-products was less important in microporous zeolites than in macroporous resins.

Heteropolyacids

Heteropoly acids (HPAs) are known active catalysts for both homogeneous and heterogeneous acid-catalyzed reactions. Heteropolyacids (HPAs) has some advantages, such as the ease of handling and removal, reusability, fewer side reactions, strong Brønsted acidity approaching the superacid region, high proton mobility, stability and catalytic activity. The major disadvantages of HPAs are their low thermal stability, low surface area (1-10 m^2/g), separation problem from reaction mixtures and solubility. In order to increase the specific area of the heteropolyacids, a variety of supports have been used as support to immobilize HPAs [30, 31].

Hydrolysis of sucrose was studied over heteropolyacid included in silica [32]. The catalyst was prepared according to Izumi et al. [33] by sol-gel method. The introduction of HPA on silica by this method created a microporous material. A first-order dependence on sucrose was observed. At the optimizing conditions, the activation parameters have been evaluated using the Arrhenius and Eyring plots. The activation parameters for hydrolysis of sucrose by silica included 12-tungstophosphoric acid was 77.29 kJ/mol, -0.127 kJ/mol.K, 80.18 kJ/mol and 4.72x10^6 for $\Delta H^{\neq}$, $\Delta S^{\neq}$, Ea and frequency factor (A), respectively.

Others Catalysts

The hydrolysis of sucrose was carried out using $V_2O_5/\gamma-Al_2O_3$ as catalyst. At the optimum conditions the activation parameters have been evaluated using the Arrhenius and Eyring plots. The activation parameters for hydrolysis of sucrose by silica included 12-tungstophosphoric acid was 51.63 kJ/mol, -0.195 kJ/mol.K, 54.39 kJ/mol and 1216 for $\Delta H^{\neq}$, $\Delta S^{\neq}$, Ea and frequency factor (A), respectively. A conversion close to 50-60% at 353 K, after 3 h, was obtained [34].

S. Sumiya et al. [35] studied the hydrolysis of sucrose over hydrated niobium oxide (niobic acid) supported on mesoporous silica SBA-15 (Nb/SBA-15). The results showed that the sucrose conversion increases linearly with Nb_2O_5 content, while the turnover number (TON, moles of sucrose converted/moles of Nb) was almost constant. This behavior was explained due to the niobic acid to be uniformly supported on surfaces of mesopores of SBA-15. The catalytic activity of these catalysts was also compared with activity obtained with bulk niobic acid and Nb/SBA-15-Oxa (prepared by impregnation of niobium oxalate). TONs for bulk niobic acid and Nb/SBA-15-Oxa were 0.28 and 2.80, respectively, which were considerably smaller than similar values for Nb/SBA-15 (about 4.8). Differences in activity for sucrose hydrolysis between Nb/SBA-15 and Nb/SBA-15-Oxa were attributable to differences in the strength and in the number of Brönsted acid sites. It was also observed that the choice of acid (HNO_3, H_2SO_4, H_3PO_4 or HCl) to be used in the preparation process influences catalytic activity. Nb/SBA-15 prepared by H_3PO_4 treatment yielded the highest sucrose conversion.

The hydrolysis of sucrose has been studied in mild conditions (50-80°C), in water, over several solid acid catalysts. Strong acidic resins (Amberlite A120 and A200), mixed oxides (silica-alumina and silica-zirconia), and niobium-containing solids (niobic acid, silica-niobia, and niobium phosphate) have been chosen as acid catalysts. The hydrolysis activity was studied in a continuous reactor with fixed catalytic bed working in total recirculation mode. The sulfonic acidic resins, as expected, gave complete sucrose conversion at 80°C. Among the other catalysts, niobium phosphate provided the most interesting results towards the sucrose hydrolysis, while acid oxide catalysts did not show interesting activity [36].

Layered and nanosheet aggregates of $HTaMoO_6$ were examined as solid acid catalysts for the sucrose hydrolysis, by Tagusagawa et al. [37]. The catalytic activity and acid properties of the $HTaMoO_6$ compounds were compared with those of layered $HNbMoO_6$ and a range of conventional solid acids. HTaMoO6 aggregated-nanosheet catalyst was found to function as a strong solid acid catalyst, exceeding the activity of layered $HTaMoO_6$ and $HNbMoO_6$, niobic acid, zeolites and ion-exchange resins for hydrolysis of sucrose. $HTaMoO_6$ nanosheets possess additional strong acid sites on the oxide formed by exposure of a single layer, along with strong acid sites within the interlayer of the layered aggregate structure, resulting in higher acid catalytic activity than that of the original layered oxide. The HTaMoO6 catalyst was recoverable by filtration and washing with water to remove residue, and the material was confirmed to be reusable with no change in activity (within 5%) after three reuse cycles at hydrolysis of sucrose.

3. Esterification of Sucrose

Sucrose esters are compounds that due to their physicochemical properties have been used in foods, cosmetics and pharmaceuticals. Sucrose esters have the presence of lipophilic and hydrophilic moieties, provided by sucrose and alkyl chain (ester). The hydrophilic/lipophilic balance (HLB) of sucrose esters can be changed by varying the number of ester groups per molecule, or the degree of unsaturation of the acyl chains or the alkyl chain length of the acyl groups. Consequently, sucrose ester can range from those of a water soluble surfactant (high HLB) to an oil-soluble emulsifier (low HLB) [38, 12]. They are completely biodegradable, harmless to the environment, nontoxic, skin-compatible, odorless and tasteless, and are digested as a blend of sucrose and fatty acids in the stomach. Because of their properties as antimicrobials, they are of interest for the storage of food, and their antitumoral [39] and insecticidal [40]. Although for many applications these mixtures of mono-, di-, and triesters are convenient, chemical reactions that preferentially produce sucrose monoesters in a single and economical procedure may represent an attractive approach to new uses [12].

Sucrose esters can be obtained by esterification and transesterification in the presence of chemical or biological catalysts. The chemical processes are frequently carried out in presence of basic catalyst at high temperatures, being obtained poor selectivity [41]. The use of enzyme, as catalysts, becomes the sucrose esters processes most selective and can be carried out lower temperatures. Lipases and proteases were found to selectively esterify sugars, in non-aqueous solvent [42-44].

A series of sucrose monoesters and homogeneous or mixed diesters, which have various chain lengths and saturation levels, were prepared under Mitsunobu conditions with good regioselectivity. Among the anhydro derivatives arising from competitive intramolecular etherification, 3',6'-anhydrosucrose 6-O-monoesters, which have never been reported, were identified. Monoesters and diesters were prepared in high purity [45].

The base-catalyzed synthesis of four sucrose fatty acid esters (caprylate, laurate, myristate, and palmitate) was performed in dimethylsulfoxide by transesterification of sucrose with the corresponding vinyl esters using Na_2HPO_4 as catalyst, at 313 K. In using a molar ratio sucrose/vinyl ester 4:1 and mild reaction conditions (40°C and atmospheric pressure), yields were higher than 85%. The isolated sucroesters had a higher percentage of monoesters (≥90%) and a lower content of diesters in comparison with commercial derivatives [46].

Different studies were carried out in homogeneous phases and in biocatalysis. However, few examples of sucrose esters preparation over heterogeneous catalysis were found.

Coent et al. [47] studied a kinetic model for the synthesis of sucrose esters without solvent. This synthesis is a heterogeneous reaction between the sucrose (solid) and the methyl palmitate (liquid) in the presence of a solid catalyst. The reaction was carried out at 403 K, and after 5 h, they achieved yields to mono- and diesters close to 11 and 76%, respectively, with a sucrose/methyl ester molar ratio of 2.4. It has established the kinetic model by steps. The model showed a good agreement with the experimental data.

Fitremann et al. [48] studied the synthesis of sucrose fatty acid esters, with good yields in a solvent-free medium. High contents of monoesters and low saponification rate were observed. The co-melting of sucrose and a multivalent cation soap such as magnesium or zinc soaps, under basic conditions, allowed the formation of a homogeneous reaction mixture, where solid sucrose was fully dissolved. The kinetic monitoring profiles are similar to reactions in homogeneous solutions, with fast initial formation of monoesters. As a consequence, conversion of sucrose in sucrose esters occurred in good yields. The specificity of multivalent cation soaps compared to monovalent cation soaps, for example, potassium stearate, was pointed out.

The esterification of sucrose with octanoyl chloride was carried out in basic aqueous medium [49]. It was observed that the acylation of sucrose can be directed towards the formation of variously substituted esters by choosing the sucrose content of the starting aqueous solution. It was also observed that when the sugar concentration increased, more substituted esters were obtained. Monoesters can be obtained from a more dilute solution.

The transesterification of sucrose with aliphatic esters to produce sucrose fatty acid esters was carried out under ultrasound irradiation. It was observed good yield (>73%). The optimum reaction conditions for the transesterification reaction included a molar ratio of sucrose to fatty acid ethyl ester of 2:1 and the use of a 13% mol anhydrous K2CO3 catalyst. The optimum reaction temperature was set at 70 °C, the optimum reaction time was 2 h, and the optimum reaction pressure was 11 kPa. The reaction had excellent monoester selectivity [50].

4. Etherification of Sucrose

Due to the hydrophilic/lipophilic balance, sucrose ethers show different properties. These compounds can be used as nonionic surfactants in food and cosmetics, or in plastics and polymers, depending of the alkyl chain and the degree of substitution or etherification. They are biodegradable and nontoxic. The synthesis of sucrose ethers can be carried out by two methods. Method 1 involves the ring opening of epoxide in the presence of a tertiary amine under tedious experimental conditions. However, this method has got some problems with the homogeneity of the reaction media because there are differences in polarity of the reactants. The method 2 is the telomerization of butadiene with sucrose in the presence of a palladium complex and a phosphine as catalyst. This method is used to prepare long-chain substituted ethers [12].

Gagnaire et al. [51] described the preparation of amphiphilic hydroxyalkyl sucrose ethers by ring-opening of 1,2-epoxydodecane from unprotected sucrose in water. It was showed that among the monosubstituted products, the 2- and 1'- regioisomers account for 60% of the mixture. The high reactivity of these positions was confirmed in water as it is in dipolar aprotic solvents. After 4 h and at 383 K, in the presence of N-methylmorpholine, with cetyltrimethyl-ammonium bromide as surfactant, with a sucrose/epoxide molar ratio of 4, the authors observed that the yields of mono-ether and di-ester are 36 and 19%, respectively. In the presence of Me4NBu, similar results were obtained. A careful analysis also showed evidence of the formation of oligomerisation products as by-products.

Danel et al [52] studied the synthesis of amphiphilic sucrose ethers from two fatty epoxides (1,2-epoxydodecane and 1,2-epoxydodecan-3-ol) in water and DMSO. The study of the reaction kinetics showed that the 1,2-epoxydodecan-3-ol is more reactive for both interfacial and electronic reasons.

Gagnaire et al. [53] also studied the heterogeneous reaction of sucrose with 1,2-epoxydodecane in water. It was showed that with a good emulsification, a high interfacial area, obtained by both a good stirring and the addition of a surfactant, change the distribution of the products, namely sucrose monoethers, sucrose diethers, polysubstituted and oligomerisation products. The yield of sucrose ethers was increased to the detriment of hydrolysis and oligomerisation reactions. From the results of the kinetic monitoring, it was suggested a model explaining the competition between the different reactions depending on their location in the micro-heterogeneous medium.

Sucrose etherification with the 1,2-epoxydodecane was carried out using various tertiary amines as catalysts [54]. The reversible addition of the tertiary amine on the epoxide led to the formation of a strongly basic quaternary ammonium salt, responsible for the catalytic activity observed. A strongly basic anion-exchange resin (OH– form) A26 catalyzed the sucrose etherification at low temperature. This heterogeneous catalyst exhibited the same catalytic activity than the homogeneous catalyst. A26 resin was more selective than the tetramethylammonium hydroxide and it can be easily separated from the reaction products become the process cleaner. However, the resin was not stable and its reuse gave only a 25% yield of sucroethers.

Villandier et al. [55] studied the etherification of sucrose with 1,2-epoxydodecane over anion exchange resins (PS–NMe2 and PS–NOH), SiO2–NMe2 (silica functionalized with dimethylamine), SiO2–Im (silica functionalized with 2-methylimidazole) and PS–Im catalyst (polystyrene functionalized with methylimidazole goups). It was observed that the silica catalysts were too hydrophilic and prevents the rapid adsorption of the fatty epoxide to the catalytic sites. Consequently, thc thermal epoxide degradation occurred more rapidly than the catalytic process and disaccharide ethers were consequently produced with poor yields. Polystyrene functionalized with dimethylamino groups showed high yields. Best catalytic activity was obtained with the PS–Im catalyst. Disaccharide hydroxyalkylethers yields greater than 90% were obtained in a DMSO–water mixture in the presence of the recoverable PS–NOH solid catalyst.

The sucroethers were synthesized by telomerization of butadiene with sucrose, catalyzed by $Pd(acac)_2$ and phosphine ligand, at 343 K, in a mixture of isopropanol/water. Sucroethers (octadienyl) with a high degree of substitution of 4.7-5.3 were obtained. High turnover numbers of 40000 was obtained [56].

Pennequin et al. [57] studied the sucrose-butadiene telomerization in water or water/isopropanol medium, using as catalytic system a hydrosoluble palladium salt and trisodium tris(m-sulfonatophenyl)phosphine (TPPTS). Telomerization was carried out in water or water-organic medium in the presence of a palladium salt and TPPTS as catalyst. Mono- and dioctadienylether compounds were selectively obtained using a NaOH 1 M/isopropanol mixture. With NaOH (1 M), it was found a good compromise between sucrose conversion (85%) and selectivity and it was obtained mono- and dioctadienyl ethers with yields of 43 and 45%, respectively, with a degree of substitution of 1.6. When the reaction was carried out in isopropanol/NaOH (1 M) system, the authors observed a sucrose conversion (73%) with yield of 66 and 32%, with only 2% of side products.

The etherification of sucrose was carried out by telomerization with butadiene, over palladium complexes [58]. Experimental conditions (temperature, butadiene/sucrose ratio and the nature of catalyst) affected the degrees of substitution, which ranging from 1 to 6. The authors observed that the palladium precursor salt ($Pd(OAc)_2$ and $PdCl_2$) were the most efficient catalysts.

Conclusion

Biomass is a renewable class of materials has been attracted much attention on the last years. Sugars, which are intermediates from biomass to chemicals, are the most abundant organic compounds. The hydrolysis of sucrose allows its conversion into glucose and fructose, which are used in the food industry. The sucrose esters and ethers have numerous interesting properties due to the presence of lipophilic and hydrophilic moieties. Traditionally, homogeneous catalysts have been used in the synthesis of esters and ethers. However, solid catalysts have many advantages over liquid ones. They do less harm to the environment and have not corrosion or disposal of effluent problems. They are reusable and easy to be separated from liquid products. In order to become this process as “green processes”, the hydrolysis of sucrose has been carried out over different heterogeneous catalysts.

However, only few heterogeneous catalysts have been used in esterification and etherification of sucrose.

References

[1] Snell, K. D.; Peoples, O. P. *Biofuels Bioprod. Bioref.* 2009, 3, 456-467.

[2] Zheng, Y.; Chen, X.; Shen, Y. *Chem. Rev.* 2008, 108, 5253-5277.

[3] Clark, J. H.; Budarin, V.; Deswarte, F. E. I.; Hardy, J. J. E.; Kerton, F. M.; Hunt, A. J.; Luque, R., Macquarrie, D. J.; Milkowski, K.; Rodriguez, A.; Samuel, O.; Tavener, S. J.; White, R. J.; Wilson, A. J. *Green Chem.* 2006, 8, 853-860.

[4] Huber, G. W.; Iborra, S.; Corma, A. *Chem. Rev.* 2006, 106, 4044- 4098.

[5] Perego, C.; Bianchi, D. *Chem. Eng. J.* 2010, 161, 314-322.

[6] Perego, C.; Bosetti, A. *Microporous Mesoporous Mater.* 2011, 144, 28-39.

[7] Iliopoulou, E. F.; Antonakou, E. V.; Karakoulia, S. A.; Vasalos, I. A.; Lappas, A. A.; Triantafyllidis, K. S. *Chem. Eng. J.* 2007, 134, 51-57.

[8] Gallezot, P. *ChemSusChem* 2008, 1, 734-737.

[9] Tong, X.; Ma Y.; Li Y. *Appl. Catal. A: Gen.* 2010, 385, 1-13.

[10] Cabiac, A.; Guillon, E.; Chambon, F.; Pinel, C.; Rataboul, F.; Essayem, N. *Appl. Catal. A: Gen.* 2011, 402, 1-10.

[11] Lichtenthaler, F. W.; Peters, S. *C. R. Chim.* 2004, 7, 65-90.

[12] Corma, A.; Iborra, S.; Velty, A. *Chem. Rev.* 2007, 107, 2411-2502.

[13] Khobragade, C. N.; Chandel, S. G. *Indian J. Chem. Technol.* 2002, 9, 535-539.

[14] Masroua A.; Revillon, A.; Martin, J. C.; Guyot, A.; Descotes, G. *Bull. Soc. Chim. Fr.* 1988, 561-566.

[15] Satyanar, B.; Varma, Y. B. G., *Indian J. Technol.* 1970, 8, 58-62.

[16] Zhang, H.; Yang, J.; C., Zhang CN Patent 1048233, 1991.

[17] Kim, J. H.; El-Aasser, M. S.; Klein A.; Vanderhoff, J. W. *Polym. Mater. Sci. Eng.* 1987, 27, 819-823.

[18] Reed, E. W.; Dranoff, J. S. *Ind. Eng. Chem. Fund.* 1964, 3, 304-307.

[19] Mizota, T.; Tsuneda, S.; Saito, K.; Sugo, T. *Ind. Eng. Chem. Res.* 1994, 33, 2215-2219.

[20] Nasef, M. M.; Saidi, H.; Senna, M. M. *Chem. Eng. J.* 2005, 108, 13-17.

[21] Pito, D. S.; Fonseca, I. M.; Ramos, A. M.; Vital, J.; Castanheiro, J. E. *Bioresour. Technology* 2009, 100, 4546-4550.

[22] Abd El-Rehim, H. A.; Diaa, D. A. *Carb. Poly.* 2011, doi:10.1016/j.carbpol.2011.09.072.

[23] Abd El-Mohdy, H. L.; Abd El-Rehim, H. A. *Chem. Eng. J.* 2008, 145, 154-159.

[24] Dhepe, P. L.; Ohashi, M.; Inagaki, S.; Ichikawa, M.; Fukuoka, A. *Catal. Lett.* 2005, 102, 163-169.

[25] Venuto, P. B. *Micropor. Mater.* 1994, 2, 297-411.

[26] Corma, A. *Chem. Rev.* 1997, 97, 2373- 2420.

[27] Buttersack, C.; Martin, J. C. *J. Mol. Catal.* 1994, 94, 283L-L290.

[28] Moreau C.; Durand, R.; Alies, F. R.; Cotillon, M.; Frutz, T.; Theoleyre, M.A. *Ind. Crops Prod.* 2000, 11, 237-242.

[29] Moreau, C.; Durand, R.; Duhamet, J.; Rivalier, P. *J. Carbohydr. Chem.* 1997, 16, 709-714.

[30] Kozhevnikov, I. V. *Chem. Rev.* 1998, 98, 171-198.

[31] Misono, M.; Nojiri, N. *Appl. Catal.* 1990, 64, 1-30.

[32] Iloukhani, H.; Azizian, S.; Samadani, N. *Phys. Chem. Liq.* 2002, 40, 159-165.

[33] Izumi, Y.; Hisano, K.; Hida, T. *App. Catal. A: Gen.* 1999, 181, 277-282.

[34] Iloukhani, H.; Azizian, S.; Samadani, N. *React. Kinet. Catal. Lett.* 2001, 72, 239-244.

[35] Sumiya, S.; Oumi, Y.; Sadakane M.; Sano, T. *Appl. Catal. A: Gen.* 2009, 365, 261-267.

[36] Marzo, M.; Gervasini, A.; Carniti, P. *Carb. Res* 2011, doi:10.1016/j.carres.2011.10.018.

[37] Tagusagawa, C.; Takagaki, A.; Takanabe, K.; Ebitani, K.; Hayashi, S.; Domen, K. *J. Catal.* 2010, 270, 206-212.

[38] Foley, P.; Kermanshahi, A.; Beach, E.S.; Zimmerman, J.B. *Chem. Soc. Rev.* 2011, DOI: 10.1039/c1cs15217c.

[39] Okabe, S.; Suganuma, M.; Tada, Y.; Ochiai, Y.; Sueoka, E.; Kohya, H.; Shibata, A.; Takahashi, M.; Mizutani, M.; Matsuzaki, T.; Fujiki, H. *Jpn. J. Cancer Res.* 1999, 90, 669-676.

[40] Puterka, G.J.; Farone, W.; Palmer, T.; Barrington, A. *J. Econ. Entomol.* 2003, 96, 636-644.

[41] Nakamura, S. *Oleochemicals* 1997, 8, 866-874.

[42] Potier, P.; Bouchu, A.; Descotes, G.; Queneau, Y. *Tetrahedron Lett.* 2000, 41, 3597-3600.

[43] Potier, P.; Bouchu, A.; Gagnaire, J.; Queneau, Y. *Tetrahedron: Asymmetry* 2001, 12, 2409-2419.

[44] Riva, S.; Chopineau, J.; Kieboom, A. P. G.; Klibanov, A. M. *J. Am. Chem. Soc.* 1988, 110, 584-589.

[45] Molinier, V.; Fitremann, J.; Bouchu, A.; Queneau, Y. *Tetrahedron: Asymmetry* 2004, 15, 1753-1762.

[46] Cruces, M. A.; Plou, F. J.; Ferrer, M.; Bernabe, M.; Ballesteros, A. *J. Am. Oil Chem. Soc.* 2001, 78, 541-546.

[47] le Coent, A. L.; Tayakout-Fayolle, M.; Couenne, F.; Briancon, S.; Lieto, J.; Fitremann-Gagnaire, J.; Queneau, Y.; Bouchu, A. *Chem. Eng. Sci.* 2003, 58, 367-376.

[48] Fitremann, J.; Queneau, Y.; Maître, J.-P.; Bouchu, A. *Tetrahedron Lett.* 2007, 48, 4111-4114.

[49] Thevenet, S.; Descotes, G.; Bouchu, A.; Queneau, Y. *J. Carbohydr. Chem.* 1997, 16, 691-696.

[50] Huang, D.; Jiang, X.; Zhu, H.; Fu, X.; Zhong, K.; Gao, W. *Ultrason. Sonochem.* 2010, 17, 352-355.

[51] Gagnaire, J.; Toraman, G.; Descotes, G.; Bouchu, A.; Queneau, Y. *Tetrahedron Lett.* 1999, 40, 2757-2760.

[52] Danel, M.; Gagnaire, J.; Queneau, Y. *J. Mol. Catal. A:Chem.* 2002, 184, 131-138.

[53] Gagnaire, J.; Cornet, A.; Bouchu, A.; Descotes, C.; Queneau, Y. *Colloids Surf. A:Physicochem. Eng. Aspects* 2000, 172, 125-138.

[54] Pierre, R.; Adam, I.; Fitremann, J.; Jerome, F.; Bouchu, A.; Courtois, G.; Barrault, J.; Queneau, Y. *Comp. Rend. Chim.* 2004, 7, 151-160.

[55] Villandier, N.; Adam, I.; Jerome, F.; Barrault, J.; Pierre, R.; Bouchu, A.; Fitremann, J.; Queneau, Y. *J. Mol. Catal. A:Chem.* 2006, 259, 67-77.

[56] Hill, K.; Gruber, B.; Weese, K. J. *Tetrahedron Lett.* 1994, 35, 4541-4542.

[57] Pennequin, I.; Meyer, J.; Suisse, I.; Mortreux, A. *J. Mol. Catal. A:Chem.* 1997, 120, 139-142.

[58] Desvergnes-Breuil, V.; Pinel, C.; Gallezot, P. *Green Chem.* 2001, 3, 175-177.

In: Sucrose
Editor: Salvatore Magazù

ISBN: 978-1-62417-984-6

Chapter 8

CYTOTOXIC POTENTIAL OF SUCROSE OCTAACETATE FROM THE ETHANOL EXTRACT OF THE SEEDS OF *ANNONA CORNIFOLIA* A. ST.-HIL. (ANNONACEAE)

Luciana A. R. S. Lima[1,*], Tânia M. A. Alves[2], Carlos L. Zani[2], Lúcia P. S. Pimenta[3] and Maria Amélia D. Boaventura[3]

[1]Campus Centro-Oeste Dona Lindu, Universidade Federal de São João Del-Rei, Divinópolis, MG, Brazil
[2]Laboratório de Química de Produtos Naturais, Centro de Pesquisas René Rachou/Fiocruz, Belo Horizonte, MG, Brazil
[3]Departamento de Química, Instituto de Ciências Exatas, Universidade Federal de Minas Gerais, Belo Horizonte, MG, Brazil

ABSTRACT

Annona cornifolia A. St.-Hil. is a small annual perennial tree found in the Brazilian savannah and is popularly known as "araticum-mirim".

[*] Correspondence: Prof. Dr. Luciana Alves Rodrigues dos Santos Lima - Campus Centro-Oeste Dona Lindu, Universidade Federal de São João Del-Rei, Rua Sebastião Gonçalves Coelho 400, Chanadour, Divinópolis, 35501-296, MG, Brazil. Tel.: +55 (37) 3221-1392. Fax.: +55 (37) 3221-1614. E-mail: luarsantos@ufsj.edu.br.

The ripe orange fruit pulp is sweet and aromatic. The green fruit is popularly used in the treatment of ulcers. Sucrose octaacetate was obtained from the ethanol extract of *Annona cornifolia* seeds by acetylation with pyridine and acetic anhydride, and purified using column chromatography (silica gel and Sephadex LH-20). In a previous study, the antifungal activity of sucrose octaacetate was detected against the pathogenic fungus *Paracoccidioides brasiliensis*. *P. brasiliensis* isolates (Pb-18, Pb-11, Pb-01, Pb-B339, Pb-8 and virulent Pb-18) were susceptible to sucrose octaacetate. In the present work, the possible cytotoxic activity of sucrose octaacetate was evaluated by studying its effects against human tumor cell lines, including melanoma (UACC-62), renal carcinoma (TK-10) and breast cancer (MCF-7), using the sulforhodamine B assay. Sucrose octaacetate showed a cytostatic effect at 59.32, 63.98 and 32.51 μg/mL against the UACC-62, TK-10 and MCF-7 cell lines, respectively. In summary, this study provides evidence of the cytotoxic effect of sucrose octaacetate from the ethanol extract of *Annona cornifolia* seeds and also reports on the bioactivity of this compound for the first time. These results represent a step toward the use of this product as a drug candidate.

Keywords: *Annona cornifolia*, sucrose octaacetate, tumor cell lines

1. Introduction

Cancer is a generic term used for a large number of diseases that can affect any part of the body. Other synonyms used are malignant tumor and neoplasm. Cancer arises from one single cell. The transformation from a normal cell into a tumor cell occurs as a multistage process, typically a progression from a pre-cancerous lesion to a malignant tumor. One defining feature of cancer is the rapid multiplication of abnormal cells that grow beyond their usual boundaries, which can invade and spread to other organs of the body. This process is called metastasis. Metastasis is the major cause of death from cancer [1]. Cancer can result from the interaction between a person's genetic factors and three categories of external agents, including physical carcinogens (ultraviolet and ionizing radiation), chemical carcinogens (asbestos, components of tobacco smoke, aflatoxin and arsenic) and biological carcinogens (infections from certain viruses, bacteria or parasites). Ageing is another significant factor in the development of cancer. The incidence of cancer rises dramatically with age, probably due to a buildup of risk factors for specific cancers that increase with age. The overall risk accumulation is combined with a tendency for less effective cellular repair mechanisms as a person grows older [1].

Cancer is among the leading causes of death worldwide, accounting for 7.6 million deaths (around 13% of all deaths) in 2008. The main types of cancer are lung, stomach, liver, colorectal and breast. More than 70% of all cancer deaths occur in low- and middle-income countries. Projections show that deaths from cancer worldwide should reach to over 11 million in 2030 [1].

The present generation of antineoplastic agents offers limited therapeutic benefits for most human malignancies, and the problem of resistance compromises the effectiveness of these drugs. Thus, there is a continuing need for the identification and development of new agents with novel mechanisms of action and improved therapeutic potential [2].

Among the many different strategies for drug discovery, screening the local biodiversity for bioactive natural products using appropriate bioassays is an interesting alternative for researchers, especially in countries with rich biodiversity. There is a vast literature describing natural products produced by plants, fungi and other organisms as a direct source of or inspiration for many of the currently available medicines [3].

Several *Annona* species of the Annonaceae family furnish edible fruits, some of them very much appreciated in Brazil, such as *Annona crassiflora* ("araticum"), *A. cherimola* ("cherimoya"), *A. squamosa* ("fruta do conde") and *A. muricata* ("graviola"). The fruits are usually consumed "in natura" or used in juices, desserts or ice cream preparations [4]. *Annona* species have wide use in traditional medicine against diabetes, malaria and infections [5]. These activities, from the phytochemical viewpoint, are associated with the isolation natural compounds such as alkaloids and acetogenins [6].

Annona cornifolia A. St.-Hil. is a small annual perennial tree found in the Brazilian savannah, more specifically in the states of Minas Gerais, São Paulo and Goiás, and is popularly known as "araticum-mirim". The ripe orange fruit pulp is sweet and aromatic. The green fruit is popularly used in the treatment of ulcers [4]. To our knowledge, the only phytochemical study on this species has been performed by our group, and the isolation and characterization of fatty acids, sucrose octaacetate and thirteen acetogenins have been described [7-13]. The fruits of several *Annona* species are an important source of proteins, carbohydrates and amino acids [4]. *Annona cornifolia* can also provide these metabolites, and the annonaceous acetogenins have shown antioxidant activities [10]. Further research may shed light on the use of the fruit of *A. cornifolia* in future dietary supplementation. Sucrose is a natural disaccharide widely spread throughout the plant kingdom. Sucrose octaacetate is a synthetic derivative of sucrose with the hydroxyl (OH) groups replaced by acetyl ($OCOCH_3$) groups [12].

In our previous study, the antifungal activity of sucrose octaacetate was evaluated against 16 fungal strains of clinical interest; as well, the interaction of this compound with commercial antifungal drugs was tested. The results of this study showed that the *C. albicans*, *C. tropicalis, C. parapsilosis* and *C. gattii* strains were not affected by sucrose octaacetate. However, *P. brasiliensis* isolates (Pb-18, Pb-11, Pb-01, Pb-B339, Pb-8 and virulent Pb-18) were susceptible to sucrose octaacetate, with MIC values that varied from 55.5 to 333 μg/mL. Sucrose octaacetate showed a synergistic effect with itraconazole [12]. In the present work, sucrose octaacetate was evaluated for its possible cytotoxic activity by studying its effect against several human tumor cell lines, including melanoma (UACC-62), renal carcinoma (TK-10) and breast cancer (MCF-7), by employing the sulforhodamine B assay.

2. MATERIALS AND METHODS

2.1. General

The 1D and 2D NMR spectra were obtained using a Brucker Avance DRX 400 spectrometer (Ettlingen, Germany) in $CDCl_3$, containing 0.1% tetramethylsilane as the internal chemical shift standard.

2.2. Chemicals

Roswell Park Memorial Institute (RPMI) medium, fetal bovine serum (FBS), sulforhodamine B (SRB), gentamicin, trypsin-EDTA, tris [hydroxyl-methyl]aminomethane (Tris buffer), trichloroacetic acid (TCA), etoposide, silica gel and Sephadex LH-20 were obtained from Sigma (St. Louis, MO, USA). All other reagents were from Vetec (Brazil).

2.3. Plant Material

The fruits of *Annona cornifolia* A. St.-Hil. were collected in the Curvelo city region of Minas Gerais State, Brazil, from January to March 1998. The species was identified by Dr. R. Mello-Silva, and a voucher specimen (BHCB 68114) was deposited at the Instituto de Ciências Biológicas Herbarium, Universidade Federal de Minas Gerais, Belo Horizonte, MG, Brazil.

2.4. Extraction and Isolation

The extract and fractions were evaporated to dryness before column chromatography (CC). Extraction of dried and powdered seeds (850.0 g) by percolation (EtOH, 7 L, 50 h) gave a brown residue (120 g, F01) that was dissolved in MeOH/H_2O (3:7) and successively extracted with C_6H_{14} and $CHCl_3$, resulting in 79.5, 7.3 and 21.1 g of the hexanic (F02), chloroformic (F03) and hydroalcoholic (F04) fractions, respectively.

Next, 10.56 g of F04 was refluxed with 35 mL of pyridine and 105 mL of acetic anhydride for 24 hours. After extraction and solvent elimination, 13.47 g of the material (F04Ac) were obtained. F04Ac was chromatographed (6.4 x 57.0 cm column, 326 g of SiO_2 230-400 mesh with C_6H_{14}/EtOAc/MeOH as the eluents, either neat or in mixtures of increasing polarity) to yield 56 fractions of 250 mL each, subsequently combined into 14 fractions on the basis of TLC. Fraction 10 (617 mg) was purified using column chromatography (Sephadex LH-20, C_6H_{14}/EtOAc 8:2) and provided 137.4 mg of sucrose octaacetate.

2.5. Cytotoxic Assay

The cytotoxic potential of sucrose octaacetate against the human melanoma (UACC-62), renal carcinoma (TK-10) and breast cancer (MCF-7) cell lines was evaluated using the sulforhodamine B (SRB) assay adopted by the National Cancer Institute, USA [14]. All cells were cultured in RPMI medium supplemented with 5% FBS and gentamicin, at 37°C with 5% CO_2. Shortly before reaching confluence, the cells were detached with trypsin-EDTA and seeded into 96-well plates so that 100 μL in each well contained 10,000 UACC-62 and MCF-7 cells or 15,000 TK-10 cells. Sucrose octaacetate was dissolved in 1% DMSO and tested at different concentrations (100-0.19 μg/mL). After 48 hours in the presence of the compound, the cells were fixed by adding 50 μL of cold 50% (w/v) trichloracetic acid (TCA) to each well and incubating the plate at 4°C for 1 h. The supernatant was then discarded and the cells were washed five times with water.

After drying at room temperature, 50 μL of SRB solution (0.4% w/v in 1% acetic acid) was added to each well, and the plate incubated for 30 min at 4°C. Unbound SRB was removed by washing five times with 1% acetic acid and the plates were dried at room temperature overnight. The plates were read at 515 nm (Molecular Devices SpectraMax M5) after dissolution of the dye with Tris buffer (tris[hydroxymethyl] aminomethane). Etoposide was used as the positive control and 0.2% DMSO as the negative control. Each experiment was performed in triplicate. The compound concentration that produced 50% of growth inhibition (GI_{50}, cytostatic effect) and the compound concentration that killed 50% of cells (LC_{50}, cytocidal effect) were obtained from data of three independent experiments by non-linear regression using SOFTmax pro 5.3.

3. Results and Discussion

Sucrose octaacetate (Figure 1) was isolated as a yellow wax. The ^{1}H-NMR spectrum of sucrose octaacetate showed multiples signals in the δ 4.18-5.7 region. The doublet at δ 5.69 was attributed to the anomeric hydrogen (Table 1).

The ^{13}C-NMR spectrum showed twelve signals that suggested a disaccharide. Two signals at δ 103.88 and 89.33 were attributed to the anomeric carbons. The ^{1}H- and ^{13}C-NMR spectra were consistent with those previously published in the literature [15].

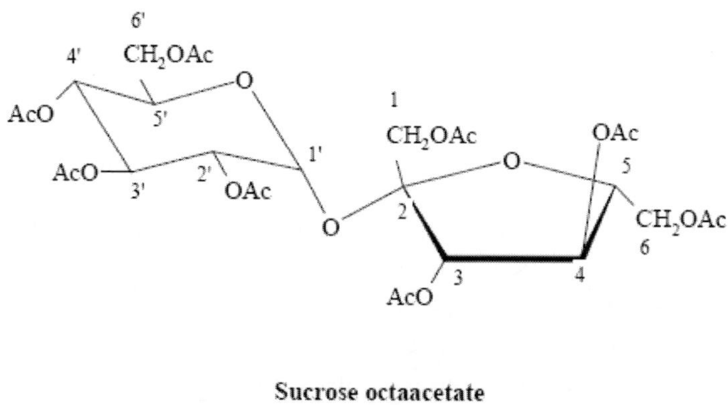

Figure 1. Structure of sucrose octaacetate isolated from the ethanol extract of *A. cornifolia* seeds.

Table 1. ^{1}H NMR [400 MHz, $CDCl_3$, δ, J(Hz)] and ^{13}C NMR [100 MHz, $CDCl_3$, δ] data for sucrose octaacetate

^{1}H NMR		^{13}C NMR	
H_1	4.18-4.37 m	C_1	62.73
H_2	-	C_2	103.88
H_3	5.34-5.49 m	C_3	75.63
H_4	5.34-5.49 m	C_4	74.93
H_5	4.18-4.37 m	C_5	79.00
H_6	4.18-4.37 m	C_6	63.47
H_1’	5.69 d (3.46)	C_1’	89.83
H_2’	4.87 dd (10.31; 3.46)	C_2’	70.13
H_3’	5.34-5.49 m	C_3’	69.48
H_4’	5.07 t (9.71)	C_4’	68.11
H_5’	4.18-4.37 m	C_5’	68.37
H_6’	4.18-4.37 m	C_6’	61.66
CH_3	1.97-2.13	CO	169.32-170.43
		CH_3	20.39

Table 2. *In vitro* cytotoxic activity of sucrose octaacetate isolated from the ethanol extract of *A. cornifolia* seeds

Cell lines	Sucrose octaacetate		Etoposide	
	$GI_{50} \pm$ SD µg/mL (µM) *	LC_{50} µg/mL (µM) *	$GI_{50} \pm$ SD µg/mL (µM) *	LC_{50} µg/mL (µM) *
MCF-7	32.51 ± 7.77 (61.24 ± 14.55)	> 100.00 (> 187.26)	0.017 ± 0.006 (0.03 ± 0.01)	57.32 (97.4)
TK-10	63.98 ± 13.15 (119.81 ± 24.62)	> 100.00 (> 187.26)	12.00 ± 1.35 (20.4 ± 2.30)	> 100.00 (>169.9)
UACC-62	59.32 ± 11.10 (111.08 ± 20.78)	> 100.00 (> 187.26)	1.82 ± 0.23 (3.1 ± 0.40)	> 100.00 (>169.9)

Etoposide: positive control. GI_{50}: the concentration of the compound that produces 50% of growth inhibition (cytostatic effect), LC_{50}: the concentration of the compound that kills 50% of cells (cytocidal effect). Human tumor cell lines: breast cancer (MCF-7), renal carcinoma (TK-10) and melanoma (UACC-62). * Concentration of the compound in µg/mL (concentration of the compound in µM).

The possible cytotoxic activity of sucrose octaacetate against human melanoma (UACC-62), renal carcinoma (TK-10) and breast cancer (MCF-7) cell lines was evaluated using the sulforhodamine B (SRB) assay adopted by the National Cancer Institute, USA (Table 2). The results showed that compound exhibited growth inhibition against human tumor cell lines. Sucrose octaacetate possessed cytotoxic potency against all cell lines (Table 2) and exhibited selective growth inhibition against the MCF-7 tumor cell line. The GI_{50} values (cytostatic effect) of the compound against UACC-62, TK-10 and MCF-7 cell lines were 59.32, 63.98 and 32.51 μg/mL, respectively. Sucrose octaacetate did not show a cytocidal effect, with LC_{50} values > 100 μg/mL against the three human tumor cell lines tested. Sucrose octaacetate showed lower cytotoxic potential than etoposide (positive control) against all human tumor cell lines tested.

There are no reports in the literature of the cytotoxic activity of sucrose octaacetate against these human tumor cell lines. Several classes of compounds have been evaluated in the search for new antitumor agents. In the treatment of cancer, most chemotherapeutic agents exhibit severe toxicity and cause many undesirable side effects; moreover, they are highly expensive, mutagenic, carcinogenic and teratogenic. Therefore, it is necessary to find other drugs. Natural products are a good source, since from 1983 to 1994 more than 60% of the approved anticancer drugs were from natural products [16].

Nine annonaceous acetogenins isolated from *A. cornifolia* were evaluated against the same human tumor cell lines (MCF-7, TK-10 and UACC-62). Annofolin was more active than the positive control, etoposide, in all cell lines tested with LC_{50} values of 48.64, 86.97 and 71.39 μg/mL in MCF-7, TK-10 and UACC-62, respectively; this compound had an GI_{50} of 3.99 μg/mL against TK-10 (study ongoing).

The antitumoral activity of a series of acetylated *bis*-tetrahydrofuranic acetogenins with a *threo/trans/threo/trans/erythro* relative configuration isolated from seeds of *Annona aff. spraguei* (Annonaceae) was evaluated using an MTT cytotoxicity assay. The acetogenins showed a cytostatic effect against the MCF-7 cell line, with ED_{50} values (effective dose observed for a 50% inhibition of cell growth) of 107, 68, 33 and 77 μg/mL for guanaconetin-1, guanaconetin-2, guanaconetin-3 and guanaconetin-4, respectively [17]. Sucrose octaacetate presented greater cytotoxicity than the acetogenins against the breast cancer cell line tested (GI_{50} 32.51 μg/mL).

Annonaceous acetogenins are natural products isolated exclusively from the Annonaceae family prior to 2008 [18] and exhibit a broad range of biological properties, such as cytotoxic, immunosuppressive, pesticidal, antiparasitic and antimicrobial activities [19]. The potential of acetogenins to inhibit cells exhibiting multiple-drug resistance has attracted increasing interest [19]. Acetogenins can reduce ATP levels via the inhibition of complex I (NADH: ubiquinone oxidoreductase) in the mitochondrial transport system and by inhibiting the NADH oxidase of plasma membranes of tumor cells, explaining their potential cytotoxic activities [20-25].

Palladium (II) complexes of 2-benzoylpyridine thiosemicarbazone (H2Bz4DH) and its N(4)-methyl (H2Bz4M) and N(4)-phenyl (H2Bz4Ph) derivatives were evaluated *in vitro* against the MCF-7, TK-10 and UACC-62 human tumor cell lines. The complex [Pd(2Bz4DH)Cl] showed activity in the three studied cell lines, with GI_{50} values of 75.5, 120.3 and 99.5 μM against MCF-7, TK-10 and UACC-62, respectively [26]. Sucrose octaacetate showed higher cytostatic effects against MCF-7 (GI_{50} 61.24 μM) and similar effect against TK-10 (GI_{50} 119.81 μM).

These results are important because palladium (II) and platinum (II) complexes of some thiosemicarbazones have shown cytotoxic activity against cisplatinum-resistant tumor cells transformed by the *ras* oncogene [27], a gene that stimulates cell growth when it is hyperactive. It is found in normal cells, where it helps to relay signals by acting as a switch. When receptors on the cell surface are stimulated, *ras* is activated and transduces signals that tell the cell to grow. If the cell-surface receptor is not stimulated, *ras* is not activated and cell growth is not stimulated. However, in about 30% of human cancers, *ras* is mutated so that it is permanently switched on, stimulating the cell to grow regardless of whether receptors on the cell surface are activated or not [28]. The biochemical mechanism by which *ras* oncogenes stimulate cisplatinum resistance is not totally understood. They might function by affecting intracellular drug concentrations or by increasing the levels of glutathione. However, there is increasing evidence that *ras* oncogenes mainly affect the expression of genes involved in DNA repair [27].

Only one report was found in the literature in which sucrose was used in the evaluation of antitumor activity. Platinum complexes of sucrose have been synthesized, characterized and evaluated for anticancer activity. Complexes containing one, two and three platinum centers bound to sucrose-derived ligands were prepared and evaluated for their biological activities, and exhibited the following characteristics: greater water solubility and less general systemic toxicity than cisplatinum, the ability to transport more than one platinum complex per molecule of sucrose to the tumor cell and binding to both strands of DNA, so that replication of tumor cells resistant to cisplatinum and carboplatin can be effectively arrested [29].

Biological studies of complexes containing one platinum center bound to sucrose-derived ligands have shown that these are non-cytotoxic and have no anticancer activity. On the other hand, the bis(platinum)complex is water soluble and comparable to cisplatinum in terms of the cytotoxicity to human KB cells in culture and anticancer activity against Lewis lung carcinoma and P388 leukemia implanted in mice. However, unlike cisplatinum, this compound in mice showed no severe toxic side effects beyond recoverable weight loss over the 50-day observation period. The tris(platinum)complex was sparingly soluble in water and showed marked *in vitro* cytotoxicity against human KB cells in culture and *in vivo* anticancer activity against implanted Lewis lung carcinoma [29]. The bis(platinum)complex presented higher solubility and activity when compared with mono(platinum) and tris(platinum) complexes.

CONCLUSION

The search for new drugs and natural products as lead compounds has been pursued in anticancer drug research. Sucrose octaacetate may be a good candidate for this purpose. Sucrose octaacetate obtained from the ethanol extract of *Annona cornifolia* seeds showed a cytostatic effect with values of 59.32, 63.98 and 32.51 μg/mL against the UACC-62, TK-10 and MCF-7 cell lines, respectively. Sucrose octaacetate presented greater cytotoxicity than acetogenins and complex [Pd(2Bz4Ph)Cl] against the MCF-7 cell line and similar effect to the complex [Pd(2Bz4Ph)Cl] against TK-10 (GI_{50} 119.81 μM). These results are important considering the search for new antineoplastic agents from natural products with novel mechanisms of action and improved therapeutic potential.

ACKNOWLEDGMENTS

Thanks go to FAPEMIG for financial support to LPSP and to CNPq for grants to LARSL and MADB. The authors are grateful to Dr. R. Mello-Silva for his assistance with plant identification.

CONFLICT OF INTEREST

The authors declare that there are no conflicts of interest.

References

[1] World Health Organization (2011). Cancer. http://www.who.int/mediacentre/factsheets/fs297/en/index.html.

[2] Ma, G.; Khan, S. I.; Mustafa, J.; Walker, L. A.; Khan, I. A. *Lipids* 2005, *40*, 303-308.

[3] Newman, D. J.; Cragg, G. M. *J. Nat. Prod.* 2007, *70*, 461-477.

[4] Correa, M. P. *Dicionário de plantas úteis do Brasil e de plantas exóticas cultivadas*; Imprensa Nacional: Rio de Janeiro, RJ, 1987; pp 151-162.

[5] Sousa, M. P.; Matos, M. E. O.; Matos, F. J. A. *Constituintes químicos de plantas medicinais brasileiras;* Imprensa Universitária: Fortaleza, CE; 1991.

[6] Alali, F. Q.; Liu X.-X.; McLaughlin, J. L. *J. Nat. Prod.* 1999, *62*, 504-540.

[7] Santos, L. A. R.; Boaventura, M. A. D.; Pimenta, L. P. S. *Biochem. Syst. Ecol.* 2006, *34*, 78-82.

[8] Santos, L. A. R.; Boaventura, M. A. D.; Pimenta, L. P. S. *Braz. J. Med. Plants* 2007, *9*, 48-51.

[9] Lima, L. A. R. S.; Pimenta, L. P. S.; Boaventura, M. A. D. *Planta Med.* 2009, *75*, 80-83.

[10] Lima, L. A. R. S.; Pimenta, L. P. S.; Boaventura, M. A. D. *Food Chem.* 2010, *122*, 1129-1138.

[11] Lima, L. A. R. S.; Boaventura, M. A. D.; Takahashi, J. A.; Pimenta, L. P. S. *In Efficacy, Safety and Clinical Evaluation;* Gupta, V. K.; Ed.; Comprehensive Bioactive Natural Products; Studium Press LLC: Houston, TX, 2010; Vol. 2, pp 231-237.

[12] Lima, L. A. R. S.; Johann, S.; Cisalpino, P. S.; Pimenta, L. P. S.; Boaventura, M.A.D. *Food Res. Int.* 2011, *44*, 2283-2288.

[13] Lima, L. A. R. S.; Johann, S.; Cisalpino, P. S.; Pimenta, L. P. S.; Boaventura, M.A.D. *J. Braz. Soc. Trop. Med.* 2011 (in press).

[14] Monks, A.; Scudiero, D.; Skehan, P.; Shoemaker, R.; Paull, K.; Vistica, D.; Hose, C.; Langley, J.; Cronise, P.; Vaigro-Wolff, A.; Gray-Goodrich, M.; Campbell, H.; Mayo, J.; Boyd, M. *Journal Natl. Cancer I* 1991, *83*, 757-766.

[15] Nishida, T.; Enzell, C. R.; Morris, G. A. *Magn. Reson. Chem.* 1986, *24*, 179-182.

[16] Newman, D. J.; Cragg, G. M.; Snader, K. M. *J. Nat. Prod.* 2003, *66*, 1022-1037.

[17] Chahboune, N.; Barrachina, I.; Royo, I.; Romero, V.; Saez, J.; Tormo, J. R.; De Pedro, N.; Estornell, E.; Zafra-Polo, M. C.; Peláez, F.; Cortes, D. *Bioorgan. Med. Chem.* 2006, *14*, 1089-1094.

[18] Pettit, G. R; Venugopal, J. R. V.; Mukku, G. C.; Herald, D. L; Knight, J. C.; Herald, C. L.; Chapuis, J. C. *J. Nat. Prod.* 2008, *71*, 130-133.

[19] Bermejo, A.; Figadère, B.; Zafra-Polo, M. C.; Barrachina, I.; Estornell, E.; Cortes, D. *Nat. Prod. Rep.* 2005, *22*, 269-303.

[20] Gallardo, T.; Zafra-Polo, M. C.; Tormo, J. R.; González, M. C.; Franck, X.; Estornell, E.; Cortes, D. J. *J. Med. Chem.* 2000, *43*, 4793-4800.

[21] Royo, I.; De Pedro, N.; Estornell, E.; Cortes, D.; Peláez, F.; Tormo, J. R. *Oncol. Res.* 2003, *13*, 521-528.

[22] Tormo, J. R.; Royo, I.; Gallardo, T.; Zafra-Polo, M. C.; Hernández, P.; Cortes, D.; Peláez, F. *Oncol. Res.* 2003, *14*, 147-154.

[23] Tormo, J. R.; De Pedro, N.; Royo, I.; Barrachina, I.; Zafra-Polo, M. C.; Cuadrillero, C.; Hernández, P.; Cortes, D.; Peláez, F. *Oncol. Res.* 2005, *15*, 129-138.

[24] Londershausen, M.; Leicht, W.; Lieb, F.; Moeschler, H.; Weiss, H. *Pestic. Sci.* 1991, *33*, 427-438.

[25] Degli Esposti, M.; Ghelli, A.; Ratta, M.; Cortes, D.; Estornell, E. *Biochem. J.* 1994, *301*, 161-167.

[26] Rebolledo, A. P.; Vieites, M.; Gambino, D.; Piro, O. E.; Castellano, E. E.; Zani, C. L.; Souza-Fagundes, E. M.; Teixeira, L. R.; Batista, A. A.; Beraldo, H. *J. Inorg. Biochem.* 2005, *99*, 698-706.

[27] Quiroga, A. G.; Pérez, J. M.; Montero, E. I.; West, D. X.; Alonso, C.; Navarro-Ranninger, C. *J. Inorg. Biochem.* 1999, *75*, 293-301.

[28] National Center for Biotechnology Information Genes and Disease (2011). Harvey Ras oncogene. http://www.ncbi.nlm.nih.gov/books/NBK22261.

[29] Sachinvala, N. D.; Chen, H.; Niemczura, W. P.; Furusawa, E.; Cramer, R. E.; Rupp, J. J.; Ganjiant, J. I. *J. Med. Chem.* 1993, *36*, 1791-1796.

In: Sucrose
Editor: Salvatore Magazù

ISBN: 978-1-62417-984-6

Chapter 9

MYTHS AND FACTS ON CYTOSOLIC SUCROSE HYDROLYSIS

Walter A. Vargas[1,2,*,≠]***, Mariana L. Martin***[1,†,≠]
and Graciela L. Salerno[1]
[1]Instituto de Investigaciones en Biodiversidad y Biotecnología (INBIOTEC-CONICET) and Centro de Investigaciones Biológicas (FIBA), Argentina
[2]Centro Hispano-Luso de Investigaciones Agrarias (CIALE), Departamento de Microbiología y Genética, Universidad de Salamanca, Campus de Villamayor-Parque Científico, Spain

ABSTRACT

Sucrose plays an essential role in Nature as part of the CO_2 assimilation pathway in the biosphere. In plants, sucrose is important for the allocation of carbon resources, and participates in a regulatory network that coordinates metabolism and development. Its metabolism is coordinated with the expression of photosynthesis-related genes by a feed-back regulation, and a sugar signaling pathway. Also, sucrose is

* Corresponding author: Walter A. Vargas. E-mail: wvargas@usal.es.
≠ These authors contributed equally to this work.
† E-mails: marimartin@fiba.org.ar, gsalerno@fiba.org.ar.

accumulated in response to environmental stresses and its degradation has been associated with a high demand of carbon and energy in sink tissues.

In the last decades, several studies on sucrose degradation in plants brought to light novel trails on carbon trafficking and the metabolic paths leading to the regulation of gene expression. However, recent findings point to an intricate relationship between sucrose metabolism and the whole plant physiology. This review is focused on the elusive Alkaline/Neutral-Invertase (A/N-Inv) isoforms. These enzymes have been long believed as cytosol-exclusive proteins that hydrolyze the disaccharide for general or maintenance functions in plant cells. Nevertheless, the story has changed in the last few years when novel subcellular localizations and essential functions have been demonstrated for A/N-Invs. From being neglected as unimportant proteins, these enzymes became leading actors in sucrose catabolism with significant roles in root morphogenesis, photosynthetic apparatus biosynthesis, and abiotic stress adaptation.

The aim of this review article is to present a detailed and updated discussion of the most significant findings on the physiological properties of A/N-Invs. Also, we incorporate this group of invertases into the metabolic paths leading sucrose into the different circuits that govern carbon partitioning, storage and regulation of whole plant metabolism.

1. Introduction

Sucrose is one of the most important metabolites in plants and plays pivotal roles in cell biology, development and metabolic regulation. The physicochemical properties of this non-reductant disaccharide are crucial for its integration into plant cell biology. In addition to its high free-energy of hydrolysis, sucrose can act as a donor of glucosyl or fructosyl residues, a crucial step for the synthesis of other important carbohydrates, such as polysaccharides and sugar nucleotides.

In most plants, sucrose is synthesized in the cytosol of photosynthetic cells and is the major form of carbohydrate transported from source leaves to support cell metabolism in heterotrophic tissues [1]. In this way, plant metabolism is integrated in a regulatory network controlling photosynthesis and primary metabolism in source leaves together with the energy and carbon requirements of the heterotrophic tissues.

Sucrose hydrolysis and its regulation is a central issue in plant carbon metabolism. Three different sucrose-degrading enzymes, ubiquitous in plants, are responsible of the disaccharide breakdown and further metabolism through different metabolic pathways: i) sucrose synthase (SuS, EC 2.4.1.13, a glucosyltransferase that catalyzes a ready reversible reaction), ii) acid invertase (Ac-Inv, a β-fructofuranosidase, EC 3.2.1.26), and iii) alkaline/neutral invertase (A/N-Inv, an α-glucosidase, no EC number assigned yet).

SuS is a key component for carbon partitioning and sucrose utilization [2, 3]. Although the enzyme is able to synthesize sucrose under *in vitro* conditions, some lines of evidence suggest that (*in vivo*) SuS is primarily involved in sucrose cleavage to supply hexoses and sugar-nucleotides into more complex metabolic pathways (such as the biosynthesis of cell-wall-associated glucans and cellulose) [4-7]. The importance of SuS in carbohydrate metabolism and cell biology has been also evidenced during abiotic stresses, organ and sink tissue development [4-8].

On the other hand, invertases offer a different outcome for sucrose breakdown. These enzymes split the disaccharide into glucose and fructose, which enter the general glycolytic pathway as phosphorylated sugars, or generate glucose-mediated signals to coordinate cell metabolism [4-9]. In general, Ac-Invs have been widely studied in many plant species [10]. They can be found inside the vacuoles or associated with the plant cell-wall, where they integrate carbohydrate metabolism into sugar signaling, cell expansion, cell differentiation, interactions with microorganisms, and osmotic regulation [4-10].

Despite sucrose hydrolysis by Ac-Inv and A/N-Inv may be seen as a metabolic redundancy, these enzymes belong to different protein families and display different catalytic mechanisms [9-11]. The co-existence of both types of enzymes inside the plant cell confers a broader array of physiological fates for sucrose.

A/N-Invs have long been disregarded and considered as maintenance enzymes associated mostly with the delivery of hexoses into respiration. However, recent studies disclosed novel roles for A/N-Invs uncovering unforeseen aspects of sucrose degradation in carbon partitioning and general plant physiology. Recent reports have demonstrated the presence of intraorganellar sucrose metabolism by proving the presence of A/N-Inv isoforms in chloroplasts, mitochondria and nucleus [12-15]. For a long time, it has been debated whether sucrose entered into organelles [16-21]. However, due to the low concentrations detected in those compartments, or objections to the methodological approaches used for organelle separations, the occurrence of intraorganellar sucrose has been long questioned. In consequence, the identification of sucrose-degrading enzymes inside mitochondria, nucleus and chloroplasts shed some light on one of the most elusive issues of plant cell metabolism.

In this chapter we describe the sucrose-hydrolyzing enzymes in plant cells with emphasis on the most recent findings about A/N-Invs and introduce all those findings into the context of the plant cell metabolism. Finally, we present a summary of the most recent advances on the study of sucrose hydrolysis and its physiological relevance in organelle metabolism, cell homeostasis and the whole plant physiology.

2. Occurrence and Biochemical Properties of Sucrose-degrading Enzymes

SuS, Ac-Inv, and A/N-Invs are ubiquitous enzymes in plants and responsible of sucrose breakdown. Sucrose hydrolysis by invertases is initially differentiated by the optimum pHs of the reactions: i) Ac-Invs, β-fructofuranosidases, show a characteristic optimum pH between 4.5 and 5.0, and ii) A/N-Inv activity is maximum at pHs in the range of 6.5 to 8.0 (Table 1). This difference in optimum pH is likely necessary to cope with *in vivo* pH variations, such as the acidic conditions inside the vacuoles or in the surroundings of cell walls, and the neutral to slightly alkaline environments in other cell locations.

A contrasting feature between invertases and SuSs is that all invertases catalyse the net hydrolysis of sucrose, while SuS cleaves the dissacharide into fructose and UDP-glucose/ADP-glucose (in plants or cyanobacteria, respectively), conserving the high energy of the glycosidic linkage of sucrose in the sugar nucleotide. These are key metabolites that act as glucose donor in the synthesis of polysaccharides such as cellulose and callose in plant species [4-7]. The difference in the reaction products of invertases and SuS has a direct impact on sugar sensing and transduction mechanisms mediated by glucose, since its phosphorylation is pivotal for sugar perception [22], but it is only produced by the enzymatic action of invertases.

With the exception of Ac-Invs, sucrose-degrading enzymes have also been reported in prokaryotic cyanobacterial strains [11, 23]. The presence of SuS and A/N-Invs in cyanobacteria suggested an evolutive relationship between the origin of sucrose metabolism and the radiation of the cyanobacterial lineage [11, 24]. In fact, A/N-Invs are the only sucrose-hydrolyzing enzymes demonstrated in cyanobacteria that emerged at early stages of the phylogenetic radiation of photosynthetic organisms [11]. This observation suggests that A/N-Inv originated early in the evolution of sucrose biosynthetic pathway [24] and might represent the most ancient mecanisms for sucrose hydrolysis in photosynthetic organisms.

A remarkable aspect of plant and cyanobacterial A/N-Invs is their high sequence identity. They define a large protein family with no significant similarity with other proteins [11]. In fact, this phenomenon is not observed even among the other sucrose metabolizing enzymes characterized in both cyanobacteria and plants [24, 25]. In agreement with that sequence similarity, both plant and cyanobacterial A/N-Inv present similar biochemical properties such as the action of inhibitors and affinity for sucrose (Table 1). The only difference is that plant A/N-Invs assembles into homotetrameric forms and the two cyanobacterial enzymes, characterized so far, do not display quaternary structures.

Table 1. Biochemical properties of enzymes involved in sucrose brakedown

	Plant enzymes			**Cyanobacterium enzymes**	
	SuS	**AcInv**	**A/N-Inv**	**SusA**	**A/N-Inv**
K_mSuc (Mm)	30-300	1.0-3.5	10.0-20.0	290	10.0-27.0
Optimal pH	5.8-7.0	4.5-5.0	6.5-8.0	5.9-6.5	6.5-7.8
Native M_r (kDa)	Tetramer/ Higher olgomers	200-240	220-280	Tetramer	51-54
Monomeric M_r (kDa)	80-92	55.0-70.0	54.0-70.0	92	53-54
Inhibition by Products	Yes	Yes	Yes	No	Yes
Inhibition by Heavy Metals	Yes	Yes	Yes	*Nd*	Yes
Inhibition by Tris	Nd	No	Yes	No	Yes
Inhibitions by Divalent Ions	Inhibition	Inhibition	Inhibition	Inhibition	Yes
Posttranlational Modifications	Phosphorylation	Glycosylation	No	Nd	Nd

Nd, no determined.

[1] Data are referred to SuS activity measurements in the sucrose cleavage direction using UDP (in the case of plant SuS) or ADP (in the case of Anabaena sp. PCC 7119 which are similar to those obtained for the strain PCC 7120).

Besides the differences in optimum pH, another remarkable distinction between both groups of invertases is the affinity for substrate: while Ac-Inv display K_m for sucrose is in the range of low millimolar values, A/N-Inv K_m are between 10 and 20 mM. The importance of this differential biochemical property relies on the fact that they act in different subcellular scenarios with varying sucrose concentrations. For instance, sucrose concentration in the cytosol of spinach and barley mature leaves was reported to be in the 50-80 mM range and about 10 mM inside the vacuoles [21, 26]. These differential sucrose concentrations are consistent with the lower affinity for sucrose found in cytosolic A/N-Inv and the requirement of higher substrate concentration for optimal activity of the enzymes (Table 1). In addition, it is worth to mention that affinity for sucrose is close to 200 mM for SuS, suggesting that at least in the cytosol sucrose is mostly metabolized through A/N-Inv hydrolysis.

As mentioned above, Ac-Invs and A/N-Inv belong to different protein families; and therefore, a completely different protein folding and architecture of the catalytic sites is expected. So far, three-dimensional structure analyses were assed only for Ac-Inv [27, 28] and tridimensional structure for A/N-Inv remains to be determined. To improve our knowledge on structural features and catalytic properties of A/N-Invs, we conducted structural analysis and surveyed for the identification of common domains between both A/N-Invs (Inv-A and Inv-B) from the cyanobacterial strain *Nostoc* sp. PCC 7120 [11] and other well-known glycosyl hydrolase enzymes. We compared the protein sequences of *Nostoc* Inv-A and Inv-B with the information available in the public database ProDom and pfam [29, 30]. At a first glance, using both enzymes as query, similar results were retrieved suggesting no major differences in structures or catalytic sites. In consequence, in the rest of the paragraph we will make general conclusions as to *Nostoc*-Invertases (*Nos*-Invs).

Nos-Invs define the minimum catalytic unit for A/N-Invs, which is highly conserved in the enzymes of plant origin (pfam04853.3 domain) (Figure 1). This protein domain is exclusive of A/N-Invs and no similarity was found in any of the proteins annotated in public databases. In general, *Nos*-Invs contain structural features common to several groups of glycosyl hydrolases (Figure 1). The prokaryotic enzymes share structural similarity with the domains pfam02324, pfam01204, PD329475 and PD000650 (conserved in dextranases, trehalases, debranching enzymes and α-glycosidases, respectively). This comparative analysis suggests that the C-terminus of *Nos*-Invs conserves structural features from dextranases (sucrose-6-glycosyl transferases) and trehalases. Dextranases consecutively transfer one glucosyl moiety from sucrose to an acceptor molecule (generally a monosaccharide or another sucrose molecule) generating a growing glucan molecule composed of α-1,6 bonded glucose residues [31]. The finding of common features between dextranases and A/N-Invs is in agreement with the possibility of common catalytic mechanisms. Both groups of enzymes bind sucrose and catalyze its hydrolysis followed by the transference of one glucosyl residue to an acceptor molecule, either to a receptor carbohydrate molecule or to a water molecule, respectively. Adding more importance to the mechanisms of action of A/N-Invs, in the same region there are structural features conserved with trehalases. These α-glucosidases hydrolyze the disaccharide trehalose (glucose-α1,1-glucose) releasing two glucose molecules. Due to the similarity between sucrose and trehalose, together with the structural similarity between the hydrolytic enzymes, it is likely that A/N-Invs share a similar catalytic mechanism with other α-glucosidases [32].

To further explore structural aspects of *Nos*-Invs, secondary and tertiary structures were predicted using the protein modeling service Swiss-Model (Gen-THREDER and Psipred). Consistently, all the algorithms calculated a high percentage of secondary structure (at least 14 α-helixes, β-sheets and 22 coiled coils). The disposition of the secondary structure predicted for *Nos*-Inv presents a strong similarity with the α-domain of glucoamylases from bacteria (PDB P1lf6) and fungi (PDB 1ayx, PDB 1gai), bacterial chitobiose phosphorylase (PDB 1lf9) and bacterial maltose phosphorylase (PDB 1h54). The tridimensional folding predicted for *Nostoc* Inv-A resembles the structure of yeast glucoamylase (PDB1ayx) determined by X-ray diffraction after crystallization (Vargas and Salerno, unpublished results). This observation suggested that *Nos*-Invs are very likely to adopt a barrel-$(\alpha/\alpha)_6$ conformation organized into 5-7 hairpin-loops structures. Due to this possibly structure, *Nos*-Inv may be catalogued into the family 15 of glycosyl hydrolases and this classification might be extrapolated to all A/N-Invs from plants.

3. A/N-INVERTASES: MULTIPLE SURPRISING LOCATIONS

Until recently, A/N-Invs were thought to be localized exclusively in the cytosol [33, 34]. However, nowadays the presence of these enzymes in organelles is out of discussion. The existence of organellar A/N-Invs was first predicted by Ji et al. (2005) after computational analysis revealing the presence of signal for mitochondrial and chloroplastic targeting in some enzymes from plant origin.

Later, the knowledge of complete genome sequences expanded our knowledge on A/N-Invs, disclosing putative multigene families encoding these proteins in *A. thaliana* (nine genes), *Oryza sativa* (eight genes), *Populus trichocharpa* (sixteen genes), *Vitis vinifera* (nine genes) and *Lotus japonicus* (seven genes) [12, 14, 35, 36]. Phylogenetic analysis based on protein sequence revealed that plant A/N-Invs can be categorized into two major clades (protein families). The sequences carrying subcellular targeting peptides (either to mitochondria or to chloroplasts) define a single clade (clade α) apart from the sequences lacking subcellular targeting signals (clade β) [12, 35-39] These results strongly support the idea that the presence of A/N-Invs in organelles is common to distantly related plants, including the moss *Physcomitrella patens* (Vargas WA, unpublished results). In consequence, the prediction of A/N-Inv forms as subcellular proteins opened the possibility to discover novel physiological functions for these enzymes and highlighted the participation of sucrose in subcellular metabolism.

3.1. Cytosolic A/N-Inv in the Crosstalk of Signaling Pathways

Several lines of evidence indicate that cytosolic sucrose hydrolysis, by A/N-Inv activity, is critical to regulate many processes such as carbon distribution, cellular differentiation, tissue development and responses to environmental challenges [13, 36, 37, 39-44]. Cytosolic A/N-Invs are induced in response to environmental stresses simultaneously with and increase in sucrose accumulation [37, 41]. It was suggested that sucrose cycling probably occurs to have a higher sensitivity to environmental changes, which quickly and efficiently modulates sucrose synthesis and degradation, to control hexose delivery into respiration, to maintain osmotic potential and aid in sugar signaling [45, 46].

In *Arabidopsis thaliana* it was demonstrated that cytosolic A/N-Invs are indispensable for normal root growth [39, 40]. The loss of two closely related cytosolic isoforms (CINV1 and CINV2) dramatically decreased root growth in *Arabidopsis* plants. These A/N-Inv isoforms are likely to be critical in supplying carbon from sucrose to non-photosynthetic cells and also to control cell development. In rice (*O. sativa*), the loss of function of a cytosolic A/N-Inv had more dramatic effects on development than in Arabidopsis [42, 43].

Likewise, in lotus (*Lotus japonicus*) was demonstrated that a cytosolic A/N-Inv is crucial for development [36].

In Arabidopsis, an important role for a cytosolic A/N-Inv isoform (CINV1) has recently been reported. This isoform acts as a link between the phosphatidylinositol- (PI) and the sucrose-mediated signaling pathways that control plant growth and development [4, 22, 47-49]. CINV1 was shown to interact with the isoform 9 of phosphatidylinositol 4-phosphate 5-kinase (PIP5K9), a component of PI pathways necessary for normal root growth [13]. The *in vivo* association of both proteins was demonstrated by coimmunoprecipitation assays using protein extracts from Arabidopsis transgenic plants over-expressing both proteins. The conclusion that CINV1 can also participate in signal transductions is supported by its sequestration inside the nucleus and its activity inhibition after association with PIP5K9. Although CINV1 was found mainly in the cytosol, the subcellular co-localization of PIP5K9 and CINV1 in membranes and nucleus was demonstrated by confocal microscopy in *Nicotiana benthamiana* leaf and onion epidermal cells. Since CINV1 sequence do not include subcellular localization signals, its fate is likely to be determined by its interaction with PIP5K9.

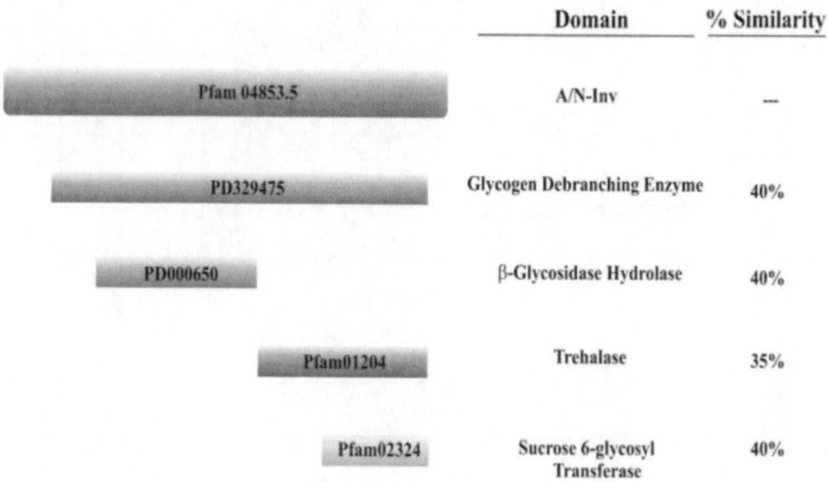

Figure 1. Schematic representation of A/N-Inv from *Nostoc* sp. PCC 7120. The representation depicts the conserved structural domains found in pfam and prodom databases. The percentage of similarity with the different conserved domains is indicated to the right.

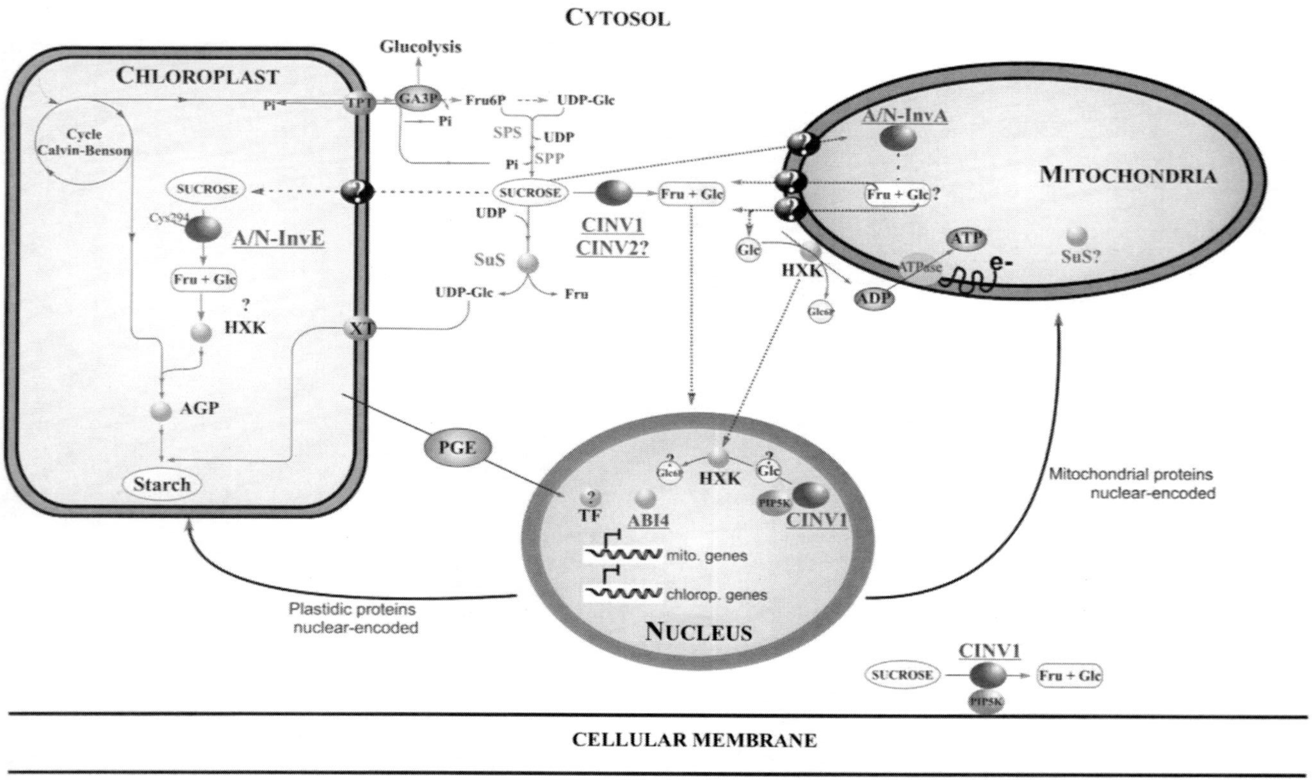

CYTOSOL
CHLOROPLAST
Cycle
Calvin-Benson
Pi
TPT
GA3P
Glucolysis
Fru6P
UDP-Glc
Pi
SPS
UDP
Pi
SPP
SUCROSE
UDP
SuS
UDP-Glc
Fru
SUCROSE
Cys294
A/N-InvE
Fru + Glc
?
HXK
XT
AGP
Starch
CINV1
CINV2?
Fru + Glc
MITOCHONDRIA
A/N-InvA
Fru + Glc ?
Glc
HXK
ATP
ATPase
ADP
e-
SuS?
PGE
HXK
Glc
?
TF
ABI4
PIP5K
CINV1
mito. genes
chlorop. genes
NUCLEUS
Plastidic proteins
nuclear-encoded
Mitochondrial proteins
nuclear-encoded
CINV1
SUCROSE
Fru + Glc
PIP5K
CELLULAR MEMBRANE

Figure 2. Model of subcellular localization of A/N-Inv isoforms in an Arabidopsis photosynthetic cell, based on the results reviewed in this report. A/N-Invs are localized in cytosol (CINV1 and CINV2), membrane (CINV1), inside the chloroplast (A/N-InvE), mitochondria (A/N-InvA) and nucleus (CINV1). Sucrose and/or the hexose produced by its hydrolysis may enter into different metabolic pathways in chloroplast, mitochondria and nucleus. A/N-Invs could regulate sucrose level en each compartment, molecule that could act in signaling. But also A/N-Inv isoforms localized in organelles may continuously and efficiently supply glucose to HXK. In chloroplast, this signaling pathway may contribute to the regulation of starch accumulation; in mitochondria, to the production of ADP that in turn could be used to regenerate ATP for supporting oxidative phosphorylation and prevent oxidative stress; and finally, in nucleus, to regulate the expression of nuclear genes that encode mitochondrial and chloroplastic proteins through ABI4 or others transcription factors. PIP5K9-CINV1 interaction probably may determine the localization of CINV1 in the nucleus and/or membrane. SPS and SPP, enzymes responsible of sucrose synthesis in the cytosol are also indicated. ABI4, ABscicic acid Insensitive factor 4; ADP, adenosine diphosphate; AGP, ADP-Glc pyrophosphorylase; A/N-InvA, At-A/N-InvA; A/N-InvE, At-A/N-InvE; AT, ADP-Glc translocator; ATP, adenosine triphosphate; ATPase, ATP synthase; CINV1/2, cytosolic A/N-Inv1/2; e^-, mitochondrial chain electron transport respiratory; e^-, mitochondrial chain electron transport respiratory; Fru, fructose; Fru6P, fructose-6-phosphate; Glc, glucose; Glc6P, glucose-6-phosphate; GA3P, glyceraldehyde-3-phosphate; HXK, hexokinase; mito- and chloro- genes, nuclear genes that encoded for mitochondrial and chloroplastic proteins; Pi, inorganic phosphate; PGE, plastid gene expression; PIP5K9, isoform 9 of phosphatidylinositol 4-phosphate 5-kinase; TPT, triose-phosphate translocator; UDP-Glc, uridine diphosphate-glucose; XT, XDP-Glc translocator. Sugars and sugar transporters (black oval) with question marks indicate that their presence in organelle was not demonstrated (nucleus) or only demonstrated in non-photosynthetic cells in *H. tuberosus* (mitochondria). Full lines, indicate signals that have been demonstrated; dotted lines indicate signals that have not already been reported.

PI metabolism contributes to the synthesis of both structural lipids and signaling molecules for multiple processes, including root growth, pollen and vascular development, and cell response to environmental stimuli [47]. Although the regulation of these pathways is largely unknown, the emerging functional link between plant phospholipids signaling and sugar metabolism suggests a more sophisticated and flexible mechanism to integrate whole-plant metabolic networks. Arabidopsis plants impaired in the expression of the gene encoding CINV1 resulted to be less sensitive to glucose, had developmental defects and transcriptional alterations in wide variety of genes [13]. Similar phenoptypes were also described in Arabidopsis glucose insensitive mutants, which are impaired in the expression of a specific hexokinase (AtHXK1) that coordinates intrinsic sugar-signals with extrinsic light intensity [50]. Even though AtHXK1 is involved in a nuclear protein complex that modulates specific gene transcription, it is predominantly associated with mitochondria [51]. Consistently, rice OsHXK isoforms (AtHXK1 orthologs) retains a dual targeting ability to mitochondria and nucleus [51], and it is possible that plant HXKs shuttle between mitochondria and nucleus.

On the other hand, in the PIP5K9-CINV1 interaction it is difficult to establish if it is sucrose or its hydrolysis products that act as signal molecules. In fact, it is well documented that the disaccharide regulates specific responses, but also many effects on growth and metabolism can be attributed to the action of glucose and fructose, or their downstream metabolic intermediates [22, 52].

In summary, CINV1 plays a relevant role in sugar signaling by regulating sucrose concentration and/or to the production of hexoses for HXK-mediated transcriptional regulation. However, to date the presence of glucose or sucrose inside the nucleus has not been reported and the molecular mechanisms underlying this sugar-signaling pathway still need to be revealed [9]. Further research is needed to identify how a carbohydrate signal is transferred from the cytosol to the nucleus and whether CINV1 activity and the HXK1-related protein complex works synergistically in Arabidopsis to control sugar-dependent gene expression.

3.2. A/N-Inv Isoforms and Plastid Metabolism

For more than two decades, the question whether sucrose could enter into plastids, and particularly into chloroplasts, was a subject of debate. Stitt and Held [19] reported that preparations of spinach chloroplasts, whether isolated from protoplasts or from whole leaves, contained sucrose or related oligosaccharides, which were hydrolyzed into glucose and fructose during incubation in the dark. However, neither sucrose metabolizing enzymes nor sucrose transporters were found in these organelles and the very low levels of sucrose detected were argued to be artifacts of the isolation procedures. Ten years ago, the presence of sucrose in plastids was indirectly inferred from transgenic tobacco plants expressing a plastid-targeted levansucrase gene from *Bacillus subtilis* [53]. Fructan accumulation in chloroplasts of the transformed tobacco plants (*Nicotiana tabacum*) could only be ascribed to the presence of sucrose, the fructosyl donor used as substrate of the levansucrase [54]. Also targeting of this enzyme to the plastids of potato plants (*Solanum tuberosum*), led to high-level fructan accumulation in amyloplasts. However, this experimental approach was questioned by Cairns (2003) [55] after a thoroughly analysis of the dataset, concluding that the subcellular targeting in bacterial levan transformed plants had not been fully demonstrated. Although to date, the origin and fate of plastidic sucrose is still waiting to be unraveled, recent evidence unequivocally indicate that sucrose may be hydrolyzed inside plastids. Firstly, Murayama and Handa [12] showed that an A/N-Inv isoform could be directed into rice (*Oryza sativa*) plastids and later Vargas et al. [14] identified a chloroplast-specific A/N-Inv (named At-A/N-InvE) in *A. thaliana*, and also demonstrated A/N-Inv activity in isolated chloroplasts from spinach (*Spinacia oleracea*). In addition, studies on Arabidopsis plants impaired in the expression of *At-A/N-InvE* suggested that this activity is linked to starch accumulation (Figure 2). These findings brought to light a novel checkpoint in the regulation of carbon partitioning between the cytosol and the plastids, and also added a new proof on a more general phenomenon in plants regarding the possible fate of sucrose inside the organelles.

Recently, it was isolated an Arabidopsis mutant (*sicy-192*) where cotyledon greening was inhibited by treatment with sucrose, glucose or fructose. In this mutant, the gene encoding At-A/N-InvE has a point-mutation in codon 294 (C294Y) [56]. This mutation confers an increased stability to the enzyme, suggesting that Cys 294 residue is necessary to regulate its *in vivo* stability during greening and may be involved in At-A/N-InvE interaction with other proteins to regulate activity and/or stability. The interaction of A/N-Invs with other proteins that regulate its activity had been already reported [13, 57]. In addition, after treatment with sucrose the mutant plants displayed modified expression of photosynthesis-related genes and nitrate reductase activity. These phenotypes suggested that At-A/N-InvE activity is involved in the coordination between carbohydrate metabolism, nitrogen assimilation and the development of the photosynthetic apparatus. Thus, Cys-294 is likely to be essential to regulate the activity of At-A/N-InvE under conditions where the balance of carbon and nitrogen sources is disrupted.

Although direct evidence of the presence of sucrose and hexose transporters in chloroplasts is still lacking, a growing body of evidence indicate that sucrose is being metabolized inside chloroplasts. The hexoses produced after sucrose hydrolysis by A/N-Inv activity may be phosphorylated by plastidic hexokinases (HXK) [4, 58] before entering into carbon metabolism [59]. Accordingly, chloroplastic A/N-Inv not only affect carbon metabolism in the organelle [14] but also produce inhibition of the development of the photosynthetic apparatus in sugar-treated seedlings [56].

Further understanding of the function of sucrose hydrolysis inside plastids may help to comprehend how sucrose mediates carbon partitioning between the organelles and the effects exerted on the photosynthetic process.

3.3. Mitochondrial A/N-Inv and the Respiration Process

Mitochondrial respiration is an important fate for hexoses in plant cell. However, neither sucrose nor glucose/fructose are usually accumulated in the mitochondrial matrix. Even though cytosolic sugars could cross the mitochondrial outer membrane [60], the entrance to the matrix is likely to occur via sugar transporters located in the mitochondrial inner membrane [15].

The occurrence of mitochondrial A/N-Invs was suggested by Ji et al. [38] and recently demonstrated using different experimental systems: a) transient expression of a chimerical construction (the fusion of the N-terminal region of rice OsNIN1 with GFP) demonstrated the mitochondrial fate of OsNIN1 [12]; b) *in vivo* experiments using GFP translational fusions also revealed the mitochondrial subcellular localization of A/N-InvA from Arabidopsis [39]; and c) by using a mitochondrial preparations, the presence of active A/N-Inv in the mitochondrial matrix of *H. tuberosus* tubers was confirmed [15]. Further studies suggested that sucrose is transported into the mitochondria through a sucrose transporter, may be hydrolyzed by an A/N-Inv activity and the hexoses could be subsequently transported back to the cytosol [15]. However, it still remains to be determined what the physiological role of this mitochondrial invertase system in plants would be [15].

Arabidopsis mutant plants were used as tools to further study the physiological function of mitochondrial A/N-Invs. *At-A/N-InvA* knockout plants (called *atinva*) showed a severe growth phenotype, affecting both leaf growth and root development [36, 40]. In addition, root length of these plants was more affected under sugar starvation conditions, excess of sugar or osmotic stress [39]. Considering that either biotic or abiotic stresses usually generate reactive oxygen species in plants [61], this phenotype could be related to a deficient protection against oxidative stress [62]. In fact, additional evidence suggests that *At-A/N-InvA* is part of the antioxidant system involved in cellular ROS homeostasis: a) the expression of *At-A/N-InvA* and oxidative-stress responsive genes increased upon application of H_2O_2; b) *atinva* mutant plants showed increased expression of genes involved in antioxidant defense; and c) transient overexpression of *At-A/N-InvA* in leaf mesophyll protoplasts down-regulated the ascorbate peroxidase 2 (APX2) promoter [39]. Further studies of the phenotypes of *atinva* mutant plants to identify additional developmental defects led us to find a delayed flowering time (Martin ML et al., unpublished). This additional phenotype emphasizes the role of mitochondrial sucrose hydrolysis in varying development processes and the importance of A/N-Inv in plant physiology.

Glycolytic enzymes, including HXK, are associated with the outer mitochondrial membrane in a respiration-dependent manner [63]. It was hypothesized that A/N-Inv isoforms localized in mitochondria can continuously and efficiently supply glucose to HXK to produce ADP, which may be used to regenerate ATP and support oxidative phosphorylation [39]. This mechanism would be important to avoid a limitation in respiration due to low ATP synthesis, and subsequent H_2O_2 accumulation in the plant cells [64]. A second control mechanism could also be provided by end product inhibition of A/N-Invs. This hypothesis is supported by the mitochondrial invertase system [64]. In that sense, it was demonstrated that sugars are transported independently of mitochondrial respiration and membrane potential, as neither KCN (an inhibitor of the mitochondrial respiratory chain) nor the uncoupler 2,4-dinitrophenol produced any effect on the uptake of sugars by mitochondria [15]. It is likely that the A/N-Inv activity, rather than the sugar uptake process, controls the respiration rate and ATP generation.

The way mitochondrial invertase system is integrated into intermediary metabolism and the role of these isoforms inside the organelle, is still not understood. Further experimental evidence is needed to prove the connection between carbon assimilation (sucrose synthesis) and respiration-related pathways.

It should be mentioned that SuS, the other sucrose degrading enzyme, was also reported as targeted to mitochondria in maize and to play an important role in the inter-compartmental signaling [65]. However, no evidence of a role beyond sucrose degradation has been reported to date.

4. A/N-INVS AND ORGANELLAR COMMUNICATION

Protein complexes inside organelles are usually composed of both organellar and nuclear encoded subunits. To guarantee energy-saving assembly and efficient functioning of such protein complexes, a proper regulatory network is required. This implies the existence of regulatory mechanisms that coordinate gene expression in several compartments. To achieve such coordination, a retrograde (organelles-to-nucleus) control mechanism has evolved. This regulatory mechanism tightly coordinates the expression of nuclear genes with the metabolic and developmental state of plastids and mitochondria by detecting signals generated inside the organelles [66-69].

The study of Arabidopsis *sicy-192* mutants reveals more interesting aspects of the function of At-A/N-InvE in chloroplasts, highlighting the role of At-A/N-InvE in plastidic retrograde regulation [48, 62]. The phenotype of *sicy-192* mutant is similar to that of *sig6* and *sco1* Arabidopsis mutants [70-73]. These plants contain a mutation in the genes *AtSIG6* (coding for a sigma factor 6) and *SCO* (coding for the elongation factor G), respectively, that alter gene expression in plastids. It is likely, that the expression of these regulatory proteins is altered in *sicy-192* mutant plants treated with sucrose. The plastidic dysfunction produced by the point mutation in the *At-A/N-InvE* gene neglected the expression of nuclear genes related to photosynthesis [56]. These results suggest that sucrose hydrolysis by At-A/N-InvE is associated with plastidic signaling and nuclear gene expression, likely mediated by plastidic retrograde regulation.

A functional association between A/N-Invs and HXK was suggested to occur in plant subcellular compartments. Organellar A/N-Invs may produce sucrose-derived glucose, which could be further sensed by HXK as part of the sugar sensing and signal transduction mechanisms. This functional link between A/N-Invs and HXK may contribute to control mitochondrial ROS production [39], modulate sugar-dependent nuclear gene expression [13, 51], and contribute to starch accumulation [14].

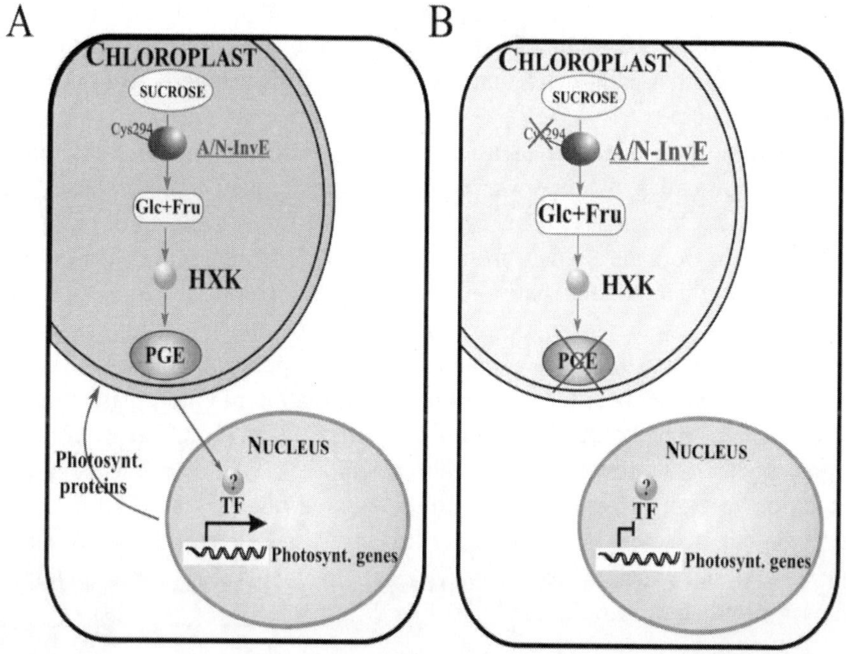

Figure 3. Role of plastidic A/N-InvE in plastid-to-nucleus retrograde signaling. a) In wild type plants, plastidic A/N-InvE could produce sucrose-derived glucose, which may be further sensed by HXK and initiate a signal transduction pathway to the nucleus (retrograde signaling), transmitting information of the developmental or functional state of the organelle. Photosynthetic protein subunits encoded in the nucleus are transported to the chloroplast where are properly assembled in functional complex. The nuclear transcription factor involved this/these process/es is unknown. b) In *sicy-192* mutant plants containing a point mutation in *A/N-InvE* the link between A/N-InvE and plastidic HXK may be altered, the plastid gene expression would be impaired and the retrograde signal would not be sent to the nucleus. As a consequence, the expression of enzymes related to photosynthesis encoded by the nuclear genome may be suppressed, which could explain the damage in the photosynthetic apparatus and the inhibition of cotyledon greening.

Sugar signals generated in mitochondra and chloroplasts by A/N-Invs, after being sensed by HXKs, may activate a signal transduction pathway to the nucleus, transmitting information of the metabolic or functional status of the organelles [66, 69]. Taking together all the results described above, we believe that when the link between At-A/N-InvE and plastidic HXK is altered the retrograde signal that keeps the chloroplast functional is not sent back to the nucleus and consequently, the photosynthetic apparatus is damaged and cotyledon greening is inhibited (Figure 3). In consequence, it is likely that the interruption of A/N-Invs and HXKs association inside the chloroplast is self-destructive for the plant cells, and a similar mechanism might also operate in the mitochondria.

The first molecular link identified between mitochondrial and chloroplast retrograde signaling pathway was a nuclear transcription factor named ABI4 (Abscicic acid Insensitive). This protein regulates the expression of genes that respond to retrograde signals from chloroplast [74] and mitochondria [75]. ABI signaling components have also been found to be closely associated with sugar signalling since, for instance, *abi4* mutants are allelic to multiple glucose -insensitive mutants [76, 77]. As photosynthesis supplies plants with sugars, it would be convenient for plant cells that the regulation of chloroplast function, carbohydrate metabolism, and mitochondrial respiration share common regulatory factors. However, the phenotypes of *sicy-192* mutants, leading to an alteration in expression of photosynthesis-related nuclear genes seems to be independent of *ABI4* [56], which led us to suggest that multiple forms of retrograde signaling pathways may exist in plants [67] and additional transcription factors would also be involved.

REFERENCES

[1] Turgeon, R. *BioScience*. 2006, *56*, 15-24.
[2] Sun, J.; Loboda, T.; Sung, S. J.; Black, C. C. *Plant Physiol*. 1992, *98*, 1163-1169.
[3] Zrenner, R.; Salanoubat, M.; Willmitzer, L.; Sonnewald, U. *Plant J*. 1995, *7*, 97-107.
[4] Koch, K. *Curr Opin Plant Biol*. 200, *47*, 235-246.
[5] Amor, Y.; Haigler, C. H.; Johnson, S.; Wainscott, M.; Delmer, D. P. *Proc Natl Acad Sci USA*. 1995, *92*, 9353-9357.
[6] Winter, H.; Huber, S. C. *Crit Rev Biochem Mol Biol*. 2000, *35*, 253-289.
[7] Coleman, H. D.; Yan, J.; Mansfield, S. D. *Proc Natl Acad Sci USA*. 2009, *106*, 13118-13123.
[8] Sturm, A; Tang, Q. *Trends Plant Sci*. 1999, *4*, 401-407.
[9] Vargas, W. A.; Salerno, G. L. *Plant Sci*. 2010, *178*, 1-8.
[10] Sturm, A. *Plant Physiol*. 1999, *121*, 1-8.
[11] Vargas, W.; Cumino, A.; Salerno, G. L. *Planta*. 2003, *216*, 951-960.
[12] Murayama, S.; Handa H. *Planta*. 2007, *225*, 1193-1203.

[13] Lou, Y.; Gou, J-Y.; Xue H-W. *Plant Cell*. 2007, *19*, 163-181.
[14] Vargas, W. A.; Pontis, H. G.; Salerno, G. L. *Planta*. 2008, *227*, 795-807.
[15] Szarka, A.; Horemans, N.; Passarella, S.; Tarcsay, A.; Orsi, F.; Salgo, A.; Banhegyi, G. *Planta*. 2008, *228*, 765-775.
[16] Heldt, H. W.; Sauer, F. *Biochim Biophys Acta*. 1971, *234*, 83-91.
[17] Wang, C. T.; Nobel P. S. *Biochim Biophys Acta*. 1971, *241*, 200-212.
[18] Santarius, K. A.; Milde H. *Planta*. 1977, *136*, 163-166.
[19] Stitt, M.; Heldt, H. W. *Plant Physiol*. 1981, *68*, 755-761.
[20] Heineke, D.; Wildenberger, K.; Sonnewald, U.; Willmitzer, L.; Heldt H. *Planta*. 1994, *194*, 29-33.
[21] Winter, H.; Robinson, D. G.; Heldt, H. W. *Planta*. 1994, *193*, 530-535.
[22] Rolland, F.; Baena-Gonzalez, E.; Sheen, J. *Annu Rev Plant Biol*. 2006, *57*, 675-709.
[23] Porchia, A. C.; Curatti, L.; Salerno G. L. *Planta*. 19992, *10*, 34-40.
[24] Salerno, G. L.; Curatti, L. *Trends Plant Sci*. 2003, *8*, 63-69.
[25] Cumino, A.; Curatti, L.; Giarrocco, L.; Salerno G. L. *FEBS Lett*. 2002, *517*, 19-23.
[26] Winter, H.; Robinson, D.; Heldt, H. *Planta*. 1993, *191*, 180-190.
[27] Alberto, F.; Bignon, C.; Sulzenbacher, G.; Henrissat, B.; Czjzek, M. *J Biol Chem*. 2004, *279*, 18903-18910.
[28] Verhaest, M.; Le Roy, K.; Sansen, S.; De Coninck, B.; Lammens, W.; De Ranter, C. J.; Van Laere, A; Van den Ende, W.; Rabijns, A. *Acta Crystallogr*. 2005, *61*, 766-768.
[29] Servant, F.; Bru, C.; Carrère, S.; Courcelle, E.; Gouzy, J.; Peyruc, D.; Kahn, D. *Brief Bioinformatics*. 2002, *3*, 246-251.
[30] Marchler-Bauer, A.; Lu, S.; Anderson, J. B.; Chitsaz, F.; Derbyshire, M. K.; DeWeese-Scott, C.; Fong, J. H.; Geer, L. Y.; Geer, R. C.; Gonzales, N. R.; Gwadz, M.; Hurwitz, D. I.; jackson, J. D.; Ke, Z.; Lanczycki, C.; Lu, F.; Marchler, G. H.; Mullokandov, M.; Omelchenko, M. V.; Robertson, C. L.; Song, J. S.; Thanki, N.; Yamashita, R. A.; Zhang, D.; Zhang, N.; Zheng, C.; Bryant, S. H. *Nucleic Acids Res. 2011, 39*, 225-229.
[31] Monchois, V.; Willemot, R. M.; Monsan P. *FEMS Microbiol Rev*. 1999, *23*, 131-151.
[32] Voit, E.O. *J Theor Biol*. 2003, *223,* 55-78.
[33] Chen, J. Q.; Black, C. C. *Arch Biochem Biophys*. 1992, *295*, 61-69.

[34] 34. Van den Ende, W.; Van Laere, A. *Physiol Plantarum. 1995, 93*, 241-248.

[35] Nonis, A.; Ruperti, B.; Pierasco, A.; Canaguier, A.; Adam-Blondon, A. F.; Di Gaspero, G.; Vizzoto, G. *Planta.* 2008, *229*, 129-142.

[36] Welham, T.; Pike, J.; Horst, I.; Flemetakis, E.; Katinakis, P.; Kaneko, T.; Sato, S.; Tabata, S.; Perry, J.; Parniske, M; Wang, T. L. *J Exp Bot.* 2009, *60*, 3353-3365.

[37] Vargas, W. A.; Pontis, H. G.; Salerno, G. L. *Planta.* 2007, *226*, 1535-1545.

[38] Ji, X.; Van den Ende, W.; Van Laere, A.; Cheng, S.; Bennett, J. *J Mol Evol.* 2005, *60*, 615-634.

[39] Xiang, L.; Le Roy, K.; Bolouri-Mghaddam, M. R.; Vanhaecke, M.; Lammens, W.; Rolland, F.; Van den Ende, W. *J Exp Bot.* 2011, *62*, 3849-3862.

[40] Barratt D. H. P.; Derbyshire, P.; Findlay, K.; Pike, M.; Wellner, N.; Lunn, J.; Feil, R.; Simpson, C.; Maule, A. J.; Smith, A. M. *Proc Natl Acad Sci USA*. 2009, *106*, 13124-13129.

[41] Qi, X; Wu, Z.; Li, J.; Mo, X.; Wu, S.; CHU, J.; WU, P. *Plant Mol Biol.* 2007, *64*, 575-587.

[42] Jia, L.; Zhang, B.; Mao, C.; Li, J.; Wu, Y.; Wu, P.; Wu, Z. *Planta.* 2008, *228*, 51-59.

[43] Yao, S-G.; Kodama, R.; Wang, H.; Ichii, M.; Taketa, S.; Yoshida, H. *Plant Sci*. 2009, *176,* 627-634.

[44] Flemetakis, E.; Efrose, R. C.; Ott, T.; Stedel, C.; Aivalakis, G.; Udvardi, M. K.; Katinakis, P. *Plant Mol Biol.* 2006, *62*, 53-69.

[45] Rohwer, J. M.; Botha, F. C. *Biochem J. 2001, 358*, 437-445.

[46] Roby, C.; Cortès, S.; Gromova, M.; Le Bail, J-L.; Roberts, J. K. M. *Mol Biol Rep.* 2002, *29*, 145-149.

[47] Xue, H-W.; Chen, X.; Mei, Y. *Biochem J.* 2009, *421*, 145-156.

[48] Smeekens, S.; Ma, J.; Hanson, J.; Rolland, F. *Curr Opin Plant Biol.* 2010, *13*, 274-279.

[49] Valluru, R.; Van den Ende, W. *Plant Sci.* 2010, *181,* 387-400.

[50] Moore, B.; Zhou, L.; Rolland, F.; Hall, Q.; Cheng, W. H.; Liu, Y. X.; Hwang, I.; Jones, T.; Sheen, J. *Science*. 2003, *300*, 332-336.

[51] Cho, Y-H;, Yoo, S-D.; Sheen, J. *Cell.* 2006, *127*, 579-589.

[52] Hummel, M.; Rahmani, F.; Smeekens, S.; Hanson, J. *Ann Bot.* 2009, *104*, 1-7.

[53] Gerrits, N; Turk, S. C.; Van Dun, K. P.; Hulleman, S. H.; Visser, R. G.; Weisbeek, P. J.; Smeekens, S. C. *Plant Physiol.* 2001, *125*, 926-934.
[54] Delobbe, A.; Dedonder, R. *C R Acad Sci Hebd Seances Acad Sci D.* 1996, *262*, 2187-2190.
[55] Cairns, A. J. *J Exp Bot.* 2003, *54*, 549 -567.
[56] Tamoi, M.; Tabuchi, T.; Demuratani, M.; Otori, K.; Tanabe, N.; Maruta, T., Shigeoka, S. *J Biol Chem.* 2010, *285*, 15399-15407.
[57] Hothorn, M.; D'Angelo, I.; Márquez, J. A.; Greiner, S.; Scheffzek, K. *J Mol Biol.* 2004, *335*, 987-995.
[58] Giese, J-O.; Herbers, K.; Hoffmann, M.; Klösgen, R. B. ; Sonnewald, U. *FEBS Lett.* 2005, *579*, 827-831.
[59] Claeyssen, E.; Rivoal, J. *Phytochemistry.* 2007, *68*, 709-731.
[60] Colombini, M. *Nature.* 1979, *279*, 643-645.
[61] Mittler, R.; Vanderauwera, S.; Gollery, M.; Van Breusegem, F. *Trends Plant Sci.* 2004, *9*, 490-498.
[62] Bolouri-Moghaddam, M. R.; Le Roy, K.; Xiang, L.; Rolland, F.; Van den Ende, W. *FEBS J.* 2010, *277*, 2022-2037.
[63] Graham, J. W.; Williams, T. C.; Morgan, M.; Fernie, A. R.; Ratcliffe, R. G.; Sweetlove L. J. *Plant Cell.* 2007, *19*, 3723-3738.
[64] Camacho-Pereira, J.; Meyer, L. E.; Machado, L. B.; Oliveira, M. F.; Galina, A. *Plant Physiol.* 2009, *149*, 1099-1110.
[65] Subbaiah, C. C.; Palaniappan, A.; Duncan, K.; Rhoads, D. M.; Huber, S. C.; Sachs, M. M. *J Biol Chem.* 2006, *281*, 15625-15635.
[66] Pesaresi, P.; Schneider, A.; Kleine, T.; Leister, D. *Curr Opin Plant Biol.* 2007, *10*, 600-606.
[67] Rhoads, D. M.; Subbaiah, C. C. *Mitochondrion.* 2007, *7*, 177-194.
[68] Pogson, B. J.; Woo, N. S.; Förster, B.; Small, I. D. *Trends Plant Sci.* 2008, *13*, 602-609.
[69] Leister, D. *Gene.* 2005, *354*, 110-116.
[70] Ruppel, N. J.; Hangarter, R. P. *BMC Plant Biol.* 2007, *7*, 37.
[71] Ishizaki, Y.; Tsunoyama, Y.; Hatano, K.; Ando, K.; Kato, K.; Shinmyo, A.; Kobori, M.; Takeba, G.; Nakahira, Y.; Shiina, T. *Plant J.* 2005, *42*, 133-144.
[72] Loschelder, H.; Schweer, J.; Link, B.; Link, G. *Plant Physiol.* 2006, *142*, 642-650.
[73] Albrecht, V.; Ingenfeld, A.; Apel, K. *Plant Mol Biol.* 2006, *60*, 507-518.

[74] Koussevitzky, S.; Nott, A.; Mockler, T. C.; Hong, F.; Sachetto-Martins, G.; Surpin, M.; Lim, J.; Mittler, R.; Chory, J. *Science*. 2007, *316*, 715-719.
[75] Giraud, E.; Van Aken, O.; Ho, L. H. M.; Whelan, J. *Plant Physiol*. 2009, *150*, 1286-1296.
[76] Rook, F.; Hadingham, S. A.; Li, Y.; Bevan, M. W. *Plant Cell Environ.* 2006, *29*, 426-434.
[77] Bossi, F.; Cordoba, E.; Dupre, P.; Mendoza, M. S.; Roman, C. S.; Leon, P. *Plant J.* 2009, *59*, 359-374.

INDEX

D

E

F

G

H

I

J

K

L

M

N

O

P

Q

R

S

T